Lumbar

accessory process	
inferior articular process	inferior apophyseal process
mammillary process	
superior articular process	superior apoph-yseal process

Sacrum and Coccyx

base	body
coccygeal horn	coccygeal cornu
lumbosacral junction	sacrovertebral junction
median sacral crest	medial sacral crest
pelvic sacral foramina	anterior sacral foramina
sacral horn	sacral cornu
superior articular process	articular process
vertebral canal	spinal canal

Chapter 9 Bony Thorax

body of sternum	gladiolus
jugular notch	manubrial notch
xiphoid process	ensiform cartilage

Chapter 10 Thoracic Viscera

cardiac impression	cardiac fossa
costodiaphragmatic recess	costophrenic, or phrenicostal sinus
hilum	hilus
impression	fossa
inferior lobe	lower lobe
jugular notch	manubrial notch
main bronchus	primary bronchus
pulmonary pleura	visceral
superior lobe	upper lobe
superior thoracic aperture	thoracic inlet

Chapter 11 Long Bone Measurement

limb	extremity

Chapter 12 Contrast Arthrography

limb	extremity

Chapter 13 Foreign Body Localization and Trauma Radiography Guidelines

limb	extremity

Chapter 14 Mouth and Salivary Glands

Mouth

frenulum of tongue	frenulum linguae
soft palate	velum
sublingual fold	plica sublingualis

Salivary Glands

parotid duct	Stensen's duct
sublingual caruncle	
sublingual ducts	ducts of Rivinus, or Bartholin's duct
submandibular duct	submaxillary, or Wharton's duct
submandibular gland	submaxillary gland

Chapter 15 Anterior Part of Neck

auditory tubes	eustachian tubes
choanae	
cricothyroid ligament	cricothyroid interval
inferior constrictor muscle	cricopharyngeus muscle
laryngeal inlet	laryngeal orifice
laryngeal pharynx	hypopharynx
lymphoid	lymphadenoid
piriformis recess	piriformis sinus
rima vestibuli	vestibular slit
valleculae epiglot-tica	epiglottic valleculae
vestibula folds	false vocal cords

Chapter 16 Digestive System
Abdomen, Liver, Spleen, Biliary Tract

Liver

hilum	hilus
porta	porta hepatis
visceral surface of liver	posterior surface of liver

Pancreas and Spleen

accessory pancre-atic duct	duct of Santorini
pancreatic duct	duct of Wirsung
pancreatic islets	islets of Langerhans

Biliary Tract

gall bladder	gallbladder
hepatopancreatic ampulla	ampulla of Vater
sphincter of the hepatopancreatic ampulla	sphincter of Oddi

Chapter 17 Digestive System
Alimentary Tract

Stomach

angular notch	incisura angularis
cardia	
cardiac notch	cardiac incisura
esophagogastric junction	esophageal orifice
gastric folds	rugae
pyloric antrum	pyloric vestibule
pyloric canal	
pyloric orifice	

Small Intestine

first portion	superior portion
second portion	descending portion
third portion	horizontal portion
fourth portion	ascending portion
common hepatic duct	hepatic duct
duodenojejunal flexure	angle of Treitz

Large Intestine

left colic flexure	splenic flexure
right colic flexure	hepatic flexure

Chapter 18 Urinary System

glomerular capsule	capsule of Bowman
hilum	hilus
major calyces	infundibula
renal papilla	apex
spongy portion [of male urethra]	cavernous portion
straight tubule	descending and as-cending limbs of the loop of Henle
suprarenal glands	adrenal glands
uriniferous tubules	

Chapter 19 Reproductive System

Male Reproductive System

ductus deferens	vas deferens
spongy portion [of male urethra]	cavernous portion

Female Reproductive System

cervix	neck
intestinal surface	posterior surface [of uterus]
isthmus	superior cervix, in-ternal os
lateral angles	cornua
ovarian vesicular follicles	ovisac
perineal body	
uterine ostium	external os, or ex-ternal orifice of cervix
uterine tube	fallopian tube [oviduct deleted]
vesical surface	anterior surface of uterus

Continued on inside back cover.

MERRILL'S ATLAS OF

RADIOGRAPHIC
POSITIONS
and
RADIOLOGIC
PROCEDURES

VOLUME THREE

MERRILL'S ATLAS OF

RADIOGRAPHIC POSITIONS and RADIOLOGIC PROCEDURES

Philip W. Ballinger, M.S., R.T.(R)

Director and Assistant Professor, Radiologic Technology Division
School of Allied Medical Professions
The Ohio State University
Columbus, Ohio

EIGHTH EDITION

with **2863** illustrations, including **9** in full color

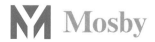

St. Louis   Baltimore   Boston   Carlsbad   Chicago   Naples   New York   Philadelphia   Portland
London   Madrid   Mexico City   Singapore   Sydney   Tokyo   Toronto   Wiesbaden

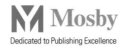

Mosby

Dedicated to Publishing Excellence

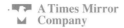

A Times Mirror
Company

Editor: Jeanne Rowland
Developmental Editor: Linda Wendling
Project Manager: Gayle May Morris
Production Editors: Deborah Vogel, Karen Allman
Manufacturing Manager: Theresa Fuchs
Design Manager: Susan Lane

EIGHTH EDITION

Printed in the United States of America
Composition by The Clarinda Company
Printing/binding by R.R. Donnelley

Mosby-Year Book, Inc.
11830 Westline Industrial Drive
St. Louis, Missouri 63146

International Standard Book Number 0-8016-7938-9

95 96 97 98 99 / 9 8 7 6 5 4 3 2

CONTRIBUTORS

Mel Allen, M.B.A., R.T.(R)(N)
Administrator
Department of Diagnostic Radiology
University of Kansas Medical Center
Kansas City, Kansas

Steven J. Bollin, Sr., B.S., R.T.(R)
Special Procedures Technologist
Radiology Department
The Ohio State University Hospitals
Columbus, Ohio

Jeffrey A. Books, R.T.(R)
Assistant Director
Medical Imaging
St. Thomas Hospital
Nashville, Tennessee

James H. Ellis, M.D.
Associate Professor
Radiology Department
University of Michigan Medical Center
Ann Arbor, Michigan

William F. Finney, III, M.A., R.T.(R)
Assistant Professor
Radiologic Technology Division
The Ohio State University
Columbus, Ohio

Sandra L. Hagen-Ansert, B.A., RDMS, RDCS
Program Director
Diagnostic Ultrasound
University of California
San Diego Medical Center
San Diego, California

Marcus W. Hedgcock, Jr., M.D.
Chief of Computed Imaging
San Francisco VA Medical Center
San Francisco, California

Richard D. Hichwa, Ph.D.
Associate Professor and Director
PET Imaging Center
The University of Iowa Medical School
Iowa City, Iowa

Kenneth C. Johnson, M.S.
Kenneth Johnson and Associates, Inc.
Columbus, Ohio

Jack C. Malott, A.S., R.T.(R), FASRT, FAHRA
Director
Radiologic Administration
University of Cincinnati Hospital
Professor, Department of Radiology
University of Cincinnati, College of
    Medicine
Cincinnati, Ohio

Charles H. Marschke, B.A., R.T.(R)(T)
Program Director, Radiation Therapy
University of Vermont
Burlington, Vermont

Deirdre A. Milne, MRT(R), ACR
Clinical Chief Technologist
Diagnostic Imaging
Hospital for Sick Children
Toronto, Ontario, Canada

Stephen T. Montelli, M.B.A., R.T.(R)
Radiographic Imaging Specialties
Murrieta, California

Richard C. Paskiet, Jr., B.A., R.T.(R)
Regional Sales Manager
Fuji Medical Systems
Stamford, Connecticut

Walter W. Peppler, Ph.D.
Clinical Associate Professor
Department of Radiology
University Hospital and Clinics
University of Wisconsin
Madison, Wisconsin

Jane A. Van Valkenburg, Ph.D., R.T.(R)
Professor
Radiological Sciences
Weber State University
Ogden, Utah

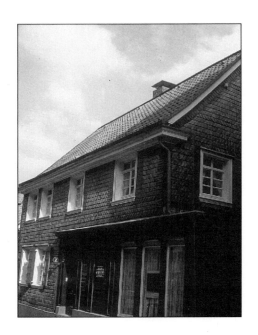

The birthplace of
Dr. Wilhelm Conrad Roentgen
in Lennep, Germany.

PREFACE

With the 1995 centennial of the discovery of x-radiation, radiography students and practitioners throughout the world are reflecting on our history, celebrating our profession's contributions, and speculating about our future in the changing health care environment. *Merrill's Atlas of Radiographic Positions and Radiologic Procedures* has quite a history of its own. It has been recognized as a classic text in the field for almost half a century. In the eighth edition we believe we have successfully built on the pioneering work begun forty-six years ago by Vinita Merrill in the first edition of the atlas. Readers familiar with the atlas will find many improvements. For those using the atlas for the first time, our hope is that you will find it a highly reliable, comprehensive resource that will serve you well for many years to come.

The planning process for the new edition included soliciting input from *Merrill's Atlas* users and from many educators, who were teaching anatomy and positioning. In response to their insightful suggestions, we have made some significant improvements.

Standardization of terminology

The use of the important radiography terms, projection and position, has been standardized throughout the atlas. In particular, the comments of Eugene D. Frank, Radiography Program Director at Mayo Clinic/Foundation, provided the catalyst for these terminology changes. After many hours of discussion with Gene, who served as a special consultant on the revision, as well as Curt Serbus, who contributed greatly to our efforts, we worked out terminology we believe will be easier for students, radiographers and physicians to understand and use. The terminology continues to be in agreement with the American Registry of Radiologic Technologists and the Canadian Association of Medical Radiation Technologists. Chapter 3 provides a complete explanation of the modified terminology, and headers throughout the text reflect the improvements.

Essential projections

As a result of surveying all radiography programs in the United States and Canada, we identified 181 essential competency projections. These projections are the ones most frequently performed and are deemed necessary for competency of entry-level practitioners.

We have designated these with a special icon to alert students and instructors that these positioning skills are essential knowledge for the beginning radiographer. Instructors may, of course, modify the list of essential competency projections as appropriate to their specific geographic locations.

Bulleted positioning descriptions

Descriptions of positioning of patient and body part have been reformatted in bulleted lists for ease of reading and understanding.

Second color

Readers will notice that headings are set in color for emphasis. The second color has been incorporated in anatomic illustrations and is also used for demonstration of central ray angle and cassette positioning.

New and modified illustrations

The new edition has hundreds of new illustrations. Of particular note are the new photographs for cranium positioning. Also important is the inclusion of degree angulation information on most illustrations involving angulation of the x-ray tube to assist the reader in quickly identifying the degree of central ray angulation or the degree of body rotation.

Historical photographs

In recognition of the 1995 centennial of the discovery of x-radiation, we have included historical photographs on the opening page of each chapter. Many are from the first edition of the atlas published in 1949, some were taken during a visit to the Röntgen Museum and birthplace of Dr. Röntgen in Lennep, Germany, and a few are from other credited sources. These photographs provide a historical perspective on the evolution of radiography and help us appreciate its significance.

Ancillaries

For the first time, the atlas has a comprehensive set of ancillaries. In addition to the third edition of *Pocket Guide to Radiography*, also available are an anatomy and positioning instructional program in slide/audiotape or CD-ROM format, student workbooks, instructor's manuals, and a 1000-question test bank on floppy disk and in bound form.

Anatomic terminology

With each new edition, anatomic terminology is updated to reflect the latest information from the International Congress of Anatomists. As in previous editions, this information is printed on the inside covers of the atlas for easy reference.

We hope you find this new edition the very best ever. Your comments and suggestions are always welcome. We are constantly striving to improve the atlas and are dependent on your input to help us in that process.

Philip W. Ballinger

ACKNOWLEDGMENTS

Sincere appreciation to the following individuals for having reviewed three or more chapters for the new edition:

Lana Andrews-Havron, B.S.R.T., R.T.(R)(T)
Baylor University Medical Center, Dallas, Texas

Michael Fugate, M.Ed., R.T.(R)
Santa Fe Community College, Gainesville, Florida

Linda Cox, M.S., R.T.(R)
Indiana University, Indianapolis, Indiana

Diane M. Kawamura, Ph.D., R.T.(R), RDMS
Weber State University, Ogden, Utah

Debra S. McMahan, B.S., PA-C, R.T.(R)
Daniel Freeman Memorial Hospital, Inglewood, California

Betty L. Palmer, A.A.S., R.T.(R)
Portland Community College, Portland, Oregon

Helen Marie Peters, ACR
Northern Alberta Institute of Technology, Edmonton, Alberta, Canada

Janet K. Scherer, DCR, RT(R), ACR
McMaster University Medical Centre, Hamilton, Ontario, Canada

Curt Serbus, M.Ed., R.T.(R)
University of Southern Indiana, Evansville, Indiana

Donald C. Shoaf, M.Ed., R.T.(R)
Forsyth Technical Community College, Winston-Salem, North Carolina

O. Scott Staley, M.S., R.T.(R)
Boise State University, Boise, Idaho

James Temme M.P.A., R.T.(R)
University of Nebraska Medical Center, Omaha, Nebraska

I am grateful to the following professionals for their constructive comments on selected chapters:

Allan C. Beebe, M.D.
Scott A. Berg, B.S., R.T.(R)
Donald R. Bernier, CNMT
Janice M. Blanchard, R.T.(R)
Steven J. Bollin Sr., B.S., R.T.(R)
Dianna Childs, R.T.(R)
Joan Clark, M.S., R.T.(R)
Kathryn S. Durand, A.S., R.T.(R)
Kevin D. Evans, B.S., R.T.(R), RDMS
Sharyn Gibson, M.H.S., RT(R)
Ruth M. Hackworth, B.S., R.T.(R)(T)
Steven G. Hayes, B.S.R.T., R.T.(R)
Keith R. Johnson, R.T.(R)(CV)
John Raphael Kenney, R.T.(R)
Michael E. Madden, Ph.D., R.T.(R)
Elaine M. Markon, M.S., R.T.(N), CNMT
Darrell E. McKay, Ph.D., R.T.(R), FASRT
Rita M. Oswald, B.S., R.T.(R)(CV)
Robert Reid, M.S., R.T.(N)
Ken Roszel, M.S., R.T.(R)
Cheryl K. Sanders, M.P.A., R.T.(R)(T), FAERS
Nancy S. Sawyer, B.S., CNMT, R.T.(N)
Rees Stuteville, M.Ed., R.T.(R)
Tom F. Torres, B.S., R.T.(R)
Beverly J. Tupper, B.S., R.T.(R)(CV)
Melinda S. Vasila, B.S., R.T.(R)(N)

Users of the atlas will notice hundreds of new illustrations. Perhaps the most noticeable additions are the new photographic illustrations for the positioning involving the cranium. **James Temme MPA, R.T.(R)**, Radiography Program Director at the University of Nebraska served as patient model and demonstrated his dedication to the profession by devoting several long, grueling, and uncomfortable days and nights of being positioned. Thank you, Jim. Thanks are also extended to the photographer, **Mr. Brent Turner** of BLT Productions, Inc. for his dedication and concern for producing high quality photographic images. Numerous photographic illustrations have also had degree angulation symbols placed on the illustration along with the degrees of angulation to assist the reader in quickly identifying the degree of central ray angulation or the degree of body part rotation.

Special thanks go to **Eugene D. Frank, M.A., R.T.(R), FASRT,** who provided invaluable help standardizing the projection and position terminology and for reviewing galleys and pages for this edition. Thanks, Gene, for devoting generous amounts of time, effort and talent during the production process and for helping to bring consistency to the atlas.

To the professional staff of the medical illustrators, medical photographers and staff of the Biomedical Communications Division in the School of Allied Medical Professions at The Ohio State University. Thanks to you the quality of the illustrations in the atlas remains high. To **Harry Condry** and **Janet Nelms** who kept track of my many orders, thank you. Thanks also to medical illustrators **Dave Schumick** and **Robert Hummel** for their competent work. To **Theron Ellinger,** thank you for printing the illustrations to demonstrate the anatomy and positioning, and to **Jenny Torbett,** senior medical photographer, thanks for your photography of numerous atlas illustrations.

To **Eileen Buckholz,** I admire your ability to manage the Radiologic Technology Division at The Ohio State University. Your skills in keeping track of student schedules, clinical and academic records, faculty, due dates and my schedule continue to amaze me. You were always there when something was needed and you always pleasantly responded to my many requests like "Eileen I can't find my copy of . . ." You would retrieve the missing item and keep all of us on schedule in your own special, caring and gentle way. A sincere thank you is not enough, but thank you again.

For more than a decade I have had the pleasure of working with **Don Ladig** of the Mosby–Year Book family. Thanks, Don. Your support and encouragement have been a constant positive driving force. During the last few years I have had the rewarding experience of working with **Jeanne Rowland,** Editor at Mosby–Year Book. Jeanne, I enjoy your honest and straight-forward manner of communicating, have found you to be readily available, and always striving to improve the atlas. Thank you, Jeanne, I have enjoyed working with you. Thanks to **Linda Wendling** for superb copyediting. You have really learned to talk like a radiographer in the last eighteen months. To **Debbie Vogel,** Project Manager, we have all appreciated your patience and calm demeanor in dealing with looming deadlines and revisions that just kept coming.

To **Terri Bruckner, M.A., R.T.(R),** where do I begin to say thank you. To keep current with the advancing profession of radiology, literally thousands of recent journal articles have been reviewed. Terri, while competently serving as my production assistant, you did an outstanding job in searching, screening, organizing and compiling the updated bibliographies for all three volumes. During the revision process, your ability to write, compile and critically evaluate new material was truly appreciated. During the production stages, your eye for consistency and detail was evident. It has indeed been a pleasure working with you, Terri.

The love and support provided by my family permitted my total involvement in this revision project. To my in-laws, **L. Neil and Ruth Hathaway,** thank you for accepting my absence too many times. I plan to improve upon the time available to spend with you as I accept early retirement from The Ohio State University. To my parents, **Dwight W. and Mildred Ballinger,** this work would not have been possible had you not supported me after I initially made the decision to enter radiology. You were always there whenever I needed something, and your love and affection truly made the project easier.

To my son and daughter, **Eric and Monica Ballinger,** now that you are in college I hope you find professions that you will enjoy as much as I do radiology. There were many times I was not available to spend time with you because "I was working on the book." I hope you understand that in spite of my sometimes absence, I do love you.

To my wife of twenty-five years, **Nancy Ballinger,** thanks for always being there when I wasn't. And thanks for saying yes when I called "Hey Nanc, got a minute?" For all the times you dropped what you were doing to proofread, check, and double check a revised manuscript, thank you. For over half of our married life you have juggled the family schedule to accommodate my involvement with the atlas. Thank you, Nancy, for your tolerance, support and love. I do love you and appreciate your active involvement in my publishing efforts.

P.W.B.

CONTENTS

VOLUME ONE

VOLUME TWO

*For a complete description of the anatomy of the facial bones, see Chapter 20 of this volume.

MERRILL'S ATLAS OF

RADIOGRAPHIC POSITIONS and RADIOLOGIC PROCEDURES

PEDIATRIC IMAGING

DEIRDRE A. MILNE

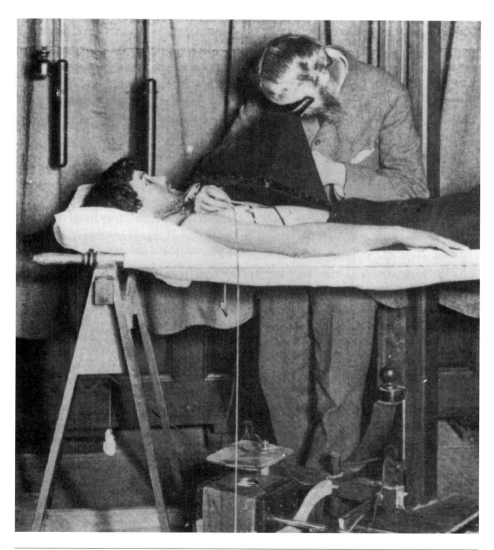

A fluoroscopist drawing outlines of the lungs on a patient's skin while looking through a hand-held fluoroscope; 1901. "The fluoroscope is held farther
away from the patient than is necessary in practice in order that the pencil
which is under it may be shown in the picture."

Reprinted from Eisenberg, RL. Radiology: An Illustrated History, Ed 2, Mosby, 1995. Original from
Pusey WA and Caldwell EW: The practical application of roentgen rays in therapeutics and diagnosis. Philadelphia, WB Saunders, 1904.

Respecting the fact that *children are not just small adults* and appreciating that they need to be approached on their level is the recipe for successful encounters with children in the imaging department. Many good cooks will agree that simply being able to read does not make one a great chef. As with any challenging recipe, the basic steps can be explained, but they must also be practiced. In pediatric radiography, radiographers often lack confidence in two main areas—communication skills and immobilization techniques.

While there are many similarities to adult radiography—such as basic positioning and film critique or assessment skills—there are some significant differences. *Approaching* the child tops the list of differences. It may help novice pediatric radiographers to think about children of various ages whom they know, and to imagine for a moment how they would explain to those children what is involved in a particular radiographic examination. This strategy, along with the descriptions that follow, will prove quite effective. An open mind, patience, creativity, and the willingness to learn and to look at the world through the eyes of a child are all that is needed to work successfully with children.

Atmosphere

The environment in which patients recover plays a significant role in the recovery process. Studies have compared the recovery course of patients whose hospital rooms looked out over parks with the recovery course of those whose view was that of a brick wall. Those patients who faced the park had a much shorter hospital stay than the other patients, and they required considerably fewer pain killers. With these differences in mind, the patient care center at the Hospital for Sick Children (Toronto) was designed and built as an atrium (Fig. 28-1). Each patient room receives natural light, from either the rooms facing outside or the rooms overlooking the atrium, where natural light comes from the glass roof. While it is easy to see how children can be amused by Miss Piggy and the barnyard animals that fly across the atrium, the environment does not have to be this elaborate to be appreciated by children. Small things can be done at relatively little cost to make a child's stay more comfortable.

ACKNOWLEDGMENT
The author wishes to thank Rob Teteruck and Ian M. Milne and illustrator Kevin Edgell for their patience, understanding, and expertise. Appreciation is also extended to Heather, Eddy, Pat, Andrea, and Debbie for their interest and assistance.
DEDICATION
To Alexander, Andrew, Erik, Richard, and the many other children who depend on us. They are our best teachers—and our future.

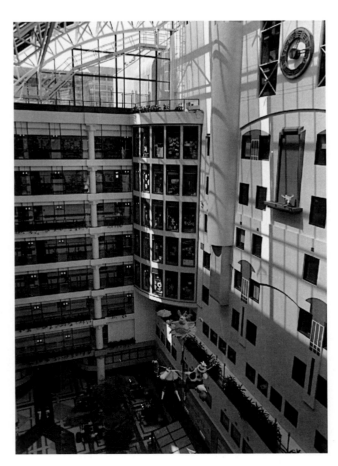

Fig. 28-1. The Atrium of the Hospital for Sick Children (Toronto), which provides inpatient care and directly related support services.

WAITING ROOM

Parents of the pediatric patient often arrive at the reception desk feeling anxious. They may be worried about what is involved in the procedure because they have not had the specifics explained to them or because they *didn't hear* all that was explained to them. They may also be worried about how much time the care of their child will take, not to mention the outcome.

Feelings of anxiousness or tension are often transferred between parent and child—the child senses a parent's tension through the parent's tone of voice or actions. A well-equipped waiting room (this does not have to be expensive) can reduce the tension. Children are attracted to and amused by the toys, while parents are free to check in or register and ask any pertinent questions.

Gender-neutral toys or activities are most appropriate, such as a small table and chairs with crayons and coloring pages. (Children should be supervised to prevent them from putting the crayons in their mouths.) Books or magazines for older children are good investments also. Any hospital's child life department could provide advice or recommendations.

IMAGING ROOM

Time can pass quickly for lengthy procedures if age-appropriate music or videos are available. A child who is absorbed in a video often requires little or no immobilization (other than the usual safety precautions designed to prevent him or her from rolling off the table). Upon request, charitable or fund-raising organizations are often happy to donate TVs and VCRs for this purpose.

Experience has shown that children are less likely to become upset or agitated if they are brought into a room which has been prepared before they enter. This preparation should include placement of the film, approximate centering of the tube to the film, and placement of all immobilization tools likely to be needed at one end of the table.

Young children are often afraid of the dark; they dislike having the lights turned out but are often comfortable with low levels of illumination. Dimming the lights enough to easily see the collimator light before the child enters can prevent the need to explain why the lights have to be dimmed. Busy radiographers often turn the lights down without explanation, causing unnecessary anxiety.

Once the procedure is completed, take a moment to emphasize, *even overemphasize,* how helpful the patient was and explain where he or she should wait or what he or she should do next, *ensuring that the parent is comprehending the instructions.*

Atmosphere

3

Approach

APPROACHING THE PARENT

No discussion on dealing with children is complete without mention of how to approach the parent(s). Although children are sometimes brought for medical care by someone other than the parents, for the purposes of this discussion the caregiver is referred to as the parent.

In many cases, when performing a procedure on a child we find that we are, in fact, dealing with two patients—the parent is the second patient. The problem may then be to decide whom to speak with. The answer, however, is easy.

- If the child is capable of understanding, direct the explanation to him or her, using age-appropriate language (discussed below). The parents will listen and, consequently, understand what is expected. Communicating in this way puts the parents more at ease and increases their confidence in the radiographer's skills. They appreciate the fact that their child has been made the focus of attention.
- For children too young to comprehend, direct the explanation to the parent, explaining in simple sentences what is going to happen and what is expected of them. The importance and value of simple sentences cannot be emphasized enough. People in stress-filled situations do not think as clearly as they normally would, and many parents in this setting are under a certain amount of stress. Successful communication involves the use of short sentences, repeated once or twice in a soothing tone.

Dealing with the agitated parent

When approaching the agitated parent, the radiographer should observe the following guidelines:

- Remain calm and speak in an even tone, remembering that fear and frustration may be the cause of the agitation.
- Use phrases such as "My name is . . . . I can identify with how you must be feeling and can appreciate your concern," followed by "Let me explain to you what is happening."
- If possible, escort the parent to a nearby room or office to continue the explanation. This can avoid an unwanted scene in the waiting room.

Parent participation

The degree of parent participation is dependent on several factors:
1. The general philosophy of the department
2. The wishes of the parent and patient
3. The laws of the province or state regarding radiation protection.

For all concerned—the patient, parents, radiographers, and departmental administration—the advantages of parent participation can be many. Experience has shown that it is vital both parents have the basic procedure explained to them. However, it is advisable that only *one* parent be present in the actual imaging room. The presence of both parents often causes the room to become too crowded and is too distracting, and it can actually lengthen the procedure. Many provincial or state laws permit only one additional person in the room, and this serves nicely as the rationale when explaining this policy to parents. It is also helpful to post signs to this effect in strategic locations.

Parental participation is insisted upon by many parents and advocated by many pediatric radiographers because:
1. The parent can watch the child if the radiographer's or radiologist's attention is directed to the equipment or the fluoroscopic monitor.
2. The radiographer may need to leave the room.
3. The parent can assist with immobilization if needed (where permitted).
4. The parent who witnesses the entire procedure has little room for doubt about professional conduct.

This last point illustrates a benefit to parents as well as to medical personnel. The parent's presence ensures that no action, explanation, or question is misinterpreted by the child or adolescent. At the same time, the parent can take comfort in seeing that the child is being cared for in a professional manner. While parental participation is perhaps less controversial now than in the past, it can be put into perspective by imagining yourself in the position of the parent and asking whether or not you would want to be present. With increasing public knowledge, and the threat of litigation ever present, parents are participating in more and more procedures.

Informed parents, whether physically present in the imaging room or not, can usually help to explain the procedure to the child. Some hospitals and commercial organizations have prepared pamphlets which describe the procedure and answer many of the commonly asked questions.

It should also be noted here that in some cases parental presence is not advised (e.g., situations in which children are further agitated by their parents' presence or in which the procedures are too disturbing for the parents, such as in the angio/interventional suites).

Whenever a parent is in the room during the radiographic exposure, he/she should be protected from scatter radiation. The parent should also be given lead gloves if his/her hands will be near the primary radiation beam.

APPROACHING THE CHILD

Naturally, good communication is essential to obtaining maximum cooperation; this means speaking to a child at his or her level, using language he or she will understand. Fortunately, this is not as difficult as learning a new language and can be made even easier by keeping a few strategies in mind:

- Having prepared beforehand, greet the patient and parent in the waiting area with a smile.
- Bend down to talk to the patient at his or her eye level.
- Take a moment to *introduce yourself and ensure that you have the correct patient,* then state briefly what you are going to do.
- Suggest, rather than ask, that the child come and *help* you with some pictures. This *firm, yet gentle* approach will avoid creating the idea that the child has an option here. After all, the patient might be tempted to be emphatic and say *no.*
- Use sincere *praise.* This is a powerful motivator no matter what the age. Praise for young children (3 to 7 years old) should be immediate. Children have short attention spans and often expect to receive rewards immediately. The reward should be linked directly to the task that has been well done. Use phrases like "You sat very still for me, thank you" or "You took a nice, big breath in for that picture, and I am going to ask you do it again for the next one, OK?"

- When the outcome will be the same, *give children an option: "Would you like Mom to help lift you up on the table, or can I help you?" or "We have two pictures to do. Which would you like first—the one with you sitting down or the one with you lying down?"*
- Employ distraction techniques. As radiographers develop confidence in basic radiography skills and adapting them for children, they find themselves able to engage in *chatter* or *distraction techniques,* thus making the experience as pleasant as possible for the child. Ask the child about brothers, sisters, dogs, cats, school, or friends—the topics are limitless. As homework, watch a few popular children's cartoons. Communication is improved when one can build rapport with a child, and learning a few more distraction techniques is helpful.
- Maintaining honesty is crucial in all communication with children. Answer all questions, regardless of their nature, truthfully. All confidence and credibility built by the previous strategies can be lost if the truth is withheld. The secret is not to volunteer the information too early or dwell on unpleasantries.

A child's specific age should greatly influence your approach. Children are unique individuals with unique social styles, of course, but the following guidelines may still prove helpful.

Young infants

The basic needs of infants to the age of 6 months are warmth, security, and, of course, nourishment. They do not make an appreciable distinction among caregivers. They are often calmed by the use of a soother or pacifier, and as they get older, they become attached to familiar objects which they should be allowed to keep with them. These children are easily startled; therefore, care should be taken to minimize loud stimuli.

Children 6 months to 2 years

Children in this age group are particularly fearful of separation from their parents, pain, and limitation of their freedom of movement. This helps to explain why they are very disturbed by immobilization. Unfortunately, immobilization of these children usually requires the most assertive immobilization techniques. Experience has shown that it is less disturbing to a child to be well immobilized than to have a number of adults in lead aprons trying to hold him or her in the correct positions.

While it is necessary to be knowledgeable in the art of immobilization for this age group, particularly the challenging 2-year-olds, one of the most valuable forms of immobilization is the sleeping child. The challenge, of course, is to complete the entire radiographic sequence without waking the child. It can be done by carefully transferring the child to the table, taking care to maintain warmth, comfort, and safety.

The participation of the parents is especially valuable with this age group, as with children between the ages of 2 and 4 years. One can easily pick up tips for communicating with children by taking cues from the parents as they explain the procedure to the child. Parents are also helpful because they can act as "baby-sitters" during the procedure.

NOTE: Of necessity, chest radiography needs to be performed while children are awake. Since respirations are generally shallow during sleep, it is not possible to obtain an adequate degree of inspiration.

Children 2 to 4 years

Preschoolers can test the power of one's imagination. They are extremely curious; their favorite question is *"Why?"* They enjoy fantasy and may readily cooperate with a game-like atmosphere or with distraction techniques.

- Give explanations at their eye level by bending down or by placing children on the table.
- Take a moment to show children how the collimator light works and let them turn it on (Fig. 28-2)—this is as much fun for children as pressing the buttons in an elevator.
- Use the camera analogy to describe the x-ray tube, taking care to explain that it may move sideways but that it will never come down and touch them.
- Avoid any unnecessary equipment manipulation.
- Encourage the child gently as he or she attempts to cooperate, and praise the cooperation.

Children between 2 and 4 years of age can be verbally and physically aggressive. The child who is having a tantrum will not respond to games and distraction techniques. Making the procedure as short as possible through the use of practiced and kind, yet effective, immobilization techniques is the best approach. These young patients generally calm down quickly once they are back in their parents' arms or resuming the activity they were involved in prior to the examination.

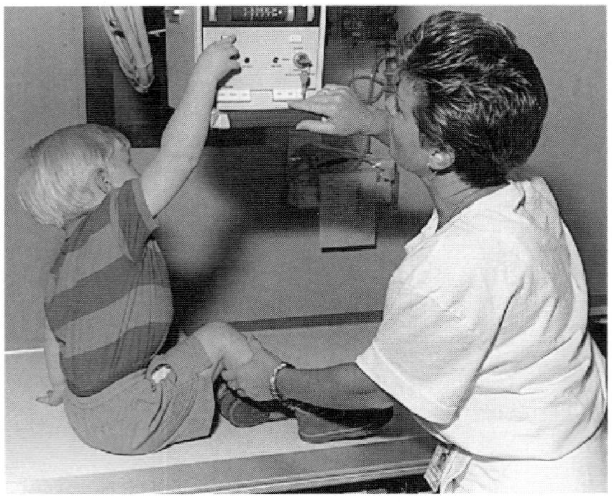

The 5-year-old

The 5-year-old has typically reached a time rich in new experiences. Reactions can differ widely, depending on how at ease the child is feeling with a given environment. Generally, children in this age group want to do things correctly and enjoy mimicking adults. When a 5-year-old feels confident he or she will act like the 6-, 7-, or 8-year-old; however, when afraid or worried, this same child may cling to parents and become reticent and uncooperative. Constant reassurance and simple explanations will help in such moments.

School-age children 6 to 8 years

For people unaccustomed to working with children, this age group is the perfect place to start. These children are generally accommodating and eager to please. They are modest and embarrass easily, making it important to protect their privacy. These children represent the easiest age group to communicate with; they appreciate being talked through the procedure, which gives them less time to worry about the surroundings or procedure. For positioning, anatomical landmarks are easy to locate and body habitus evens out nicely; the "big belly" of the toddler disappears. From an imaging standpoint, the bones are maturing with increased calcium content, which enhances subject contrast.

Adolescents

Image is important to pre-teens and adolescents. While they are better able to understand the need for hospitalization, they are upset by interference in their social and school activities. They are particularly concerned that as a result of the injury they may not be able to return to their pre-injury state. These patients require, and often demand, explicit explanations. Health care workers should not be surprised by the frankness of their questions and should be prepared for some discussion.[1]

Adolescents want to be treated as adults, and judgment is called for on the part of the radiographer in assessing the patient's degree of maturity. Radiographers should familiarize themselves with the local statutes regarding consent to understand when the child is deemed to be responsible for himself or herself.[2]

Sensitive issues, such as the possibility of pregnancy in the post-pubescent girl, must be approached discreetly. Honest responses are more likely to be elicited when the girl is alone with the radiographer (i.e., the patient's parent is not present), and the following guidelines are observed:

- Preface the questioning by stating that you need to gain information of a sensitive nature which pertains to radiation safety.
- Ask the 10-, 11-, 12-, or 13-year-old girl if she has started menstruating. To an affirmative response, continue by saying there is a slightly more sensitive question to ask; follow by asking if there is any possibility of pregnancy.
- Simply, but tactfully, ask girls 14 years old and up if there is any chance of pregnancy. Judging from the patient's expression and response, decide how to continue.
- Differing levels of maturity call for different explanations. If necessary, apologize for the need to ask sensitive questions while assuring the patient that the same questions are asked of all girls her age.
- Follow the questioning with an explanation that it is unsafe for unborn babies to receive radiation.
- If possible, have the questioning performed by a female.

Fig. 28-2. Take a moment to introduce yourself to the child and to show him or her how the collimator light will be used. Let the child turn it on.

[1]Please refer to the Wilmot and Sharko publication listed in the Selected Bibliography at the end of this chapter.
[2]Please refer to the Torres publication listed in the Selected Bibliography at the end of this chapter.

APPROACHING PATIENTS WITH SPECIAL NEEDS

Children with physical and mental disabilities

Once again, the child's age should be considered when approaching these patients. Children over the age of eight with disabilities strive to achieve as much autonomy and independence as possible. They are sensitive to the fact that they are less independent than their peers. The radiographer should observe the following guidelines:

- Direct communication toward the child first. All children appreciate being given the opportunity to listen and respond. Like any patient, these children also want to be talked to rather than talked about.
- Should this approach prove ineffective, turn to the parents. As a general rule, the parents of these patients are present and can be very helpful. It is possible that in strange environments younger children may trust only one person—the parent. In that case, the medical team can gain cooperation from the child by communicating through the parent. Parents often know the best way to lift and transfer the child from the wheelchair or stretcher to the table. Children with physical disabilities often have a fear of falling, and may want only a parent's assistance.
- After introducing yourself, give the child a brief explanation of procedure.
- Place the wheelchair or stretcher parallel to the imaging table, taking care to explain that you have locked the wheelchair or stretcher and will be getting help for the transfer. These patients often know how they should be lifted—*ask them*. They can tell you which areas to support and which actions they prefer to do themselves.

Finally, children with spastic contractions are often frustrated by muscle movements that are counterproductive to the intended action. Use gentle massage to help relax the muscle, followed by a compression band to maintain the position.

When a child has a mental disability, depending on the severity of the disability, communication can be difficult. It is important to remember that some types of patients react to verbal stimuli. Loud or abrupt phrases can startle and consequently agitate them.

Patient Care: General Concerns

PSYCHOLOGICAL CONSIDERATIONS

While many psychological characteristics of pediatric patients are the same as those of adults, some factors are worthy of mention to better prepare the radiographer for interactions with children and their parents.

The emergency patient

When an accident happens, emotions run high, thought processes are clouded, and the ability to rationalize is often lost. For the parents of the child who has been injured, there is often another powerful factor involved—guilt. As parents try to absorb information about the child's condition, they also ask themselves how they could have let this happen. Dealing with these questions often prevents parents from hearing or understanding all that is being explained. Also, fearing that permanent damage has been done, the pediatric emergency patient can feel extremely traumatized by a relatively minor injury. The radiographer should observe the following guidelines in dealing with emergency patients and their parents:

- Greet the patient and parents and proceed with short, simple, and often repeated sentences to describe the procedure.
- Remember that when patients and parents speak with a tone of urgency and frustration, it usually stems from fear. Maintaining a calm perspective in these situations can make for a smooth examination.
- Increase the level of confidence the parents and child have in the radiographer's abilities with frequent reassurance presented in a calming tone. (It should be noted that the reassurance being referred to here is reassurance that the radiographer knows how to approach the situation, not reassurance that all will be well with respect to the injury.)
- In emergency examinations, as well as any other examination ensure that only one caregiver is giving the child instructions and explanations. (Caregivers include parents, nurses, doctors, and radiographers, all of whom may be present.) Much greater success will be achieved when only one

person is speaking to the child.
- Upon completion of the procedure, ensure that you have the parents' attention and speaking slowly give clear instructions as to where to wait and what to expect.

The outpatient

Generally speaking, outpatients and their parents are easier to approach. For the radiographer who has had little experience with children, these are the best patients with whom to begin. The purpose of the outpatient visit is frequently a form of progress report, and the patients are usually ambulatory and relatively healthy. Parents, for the most part, are calm because they are not dealing with the emotions of an emergency situation or perhaps the tension or fear that the parents of the inpatient can experience. They can become agitated if kept waiting too long, which unfortunately happens often in the outpatient clinical setting.

The inpatient

For a child to be admitted to a hospital, usually he or she must be very sick. Children often become acutely ill in a much shorter period than adults. However, they generally heal more quickly than adults, which decreases the length of the child's hospital stay. The stresses the child experiences involve fear and separation from the parents, family, and friends. It is also a stressful time for the parents who, while worrying about their child's health, must often juggle time for work and for caring for other family members. By understanding that these responsibilities might be weighing heavily on parent's minds and by remembering to provide reassurance and simple explanations, the radiographer can make the child's visit to the imaging department easier.

PHYSICAL CONSIDERATIONS

Depending on the level of care being provided, children may arrive in the imaging department with chest tubes, intravenous infusions (including central venous lines), colostomies, ileostomies, or urine collection systems. Usually these children are inpatients, but in many instances outpatients present with various tubes *in situ,* particularly the interventional cases (e.g., gastrostomy or gastro-jejunostomy tube placements). Radiographers must be aware of the purpose and significance of these medical adjuncts and know how to care for the patient presenting with them.

The competent and caring radiographer takes note of the following: Are there specific instructions regarding the care and management of the patient during his or her stay in the department? Will a nurse be accompanying the child? Are there physical limitations that will influence how the examination is done? Many inpatients are on a 24-hour urine and stool collection routine. Therefore, when changing diapers on these patients, it is good practice to save the old diaper for the ward/floor personnel to weigh or assess.

Availability of nursing staff within the imaging department, along with hospital policy, can determine the amount of involvement the radiographer will have with the management of intravenous lines. The radiographer must be able to assess the integrity of the line and know what measures to take in the event of problems.[1]

[1]Please refer to the Torres publication listed in the Selected Bibliography at the end of this chapter.

Isolation protocols and universal blood and body fluid precautions

The prevention of the spread of contagious disease is of prime importance in a children's facility. Microorganisms are most commonly spread from one person to another by human hands. *Careful hand washing* is the single most important precaution, but unfortunately, it is often the most neglected. In addition, all equipment that has come in contact with the radiographer and patient during isloation cases must be washed with an appropriate cleanser.

The premise of universal blood and body fluid precautions is that *all blood and body fluids* are to be considered *infected.* The Centers for Disease Control and Prevention recommend that health care workers practice blood and body fluid precautions when caring for all patients. These precautions are designed to protect both patients and medical personnel from the diseases spread by infected blood and body fluids. All blood and body fluids, including secretions and excretions, must be treated as if they contain infective microorganisms. Working under this assumption, workers can protect themselves not only from cases where a known infective organism is present, but also from the unknown. Fig. 28-3 outlines the protective precautions the worker should observe while performing particular tasks.

The management of isolated patients varies according to the type of organism and/or pre-existing conditions, the procedure itself (some can be performed with a mobile unit), and hospital/departmental policies. The decision of when to bring an infectious patient to the department also often depends on the condition of other patients who may be in the vicinity. For example, patients with *multi-resistant organisms* should not be close to immunocompromised patients.

Radiographers should follow all precautions outlined by the physician and/or nursing unit responsible for the child. Placing a patient in respiratory, enteric or wound precautions is usually done for the protection of staff and other patients. Placing a patient in protective isolation (such as burn victims or patients with immunologic disorders) is done to protect the patient from infection. The protective clothing worn by staff may be the same in either case, but the method of discarding it will be different.[1]

[1]Please refer to the Torres publication listed in the Selected Bibliography at the end of this chapter.

UNIVERSAL BLOOD PRECAUTIONS						
PROCEDURE	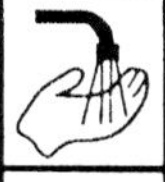	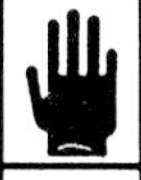	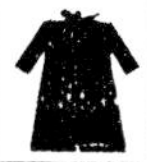	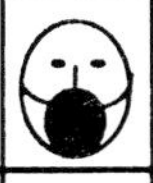	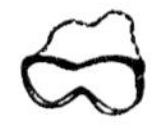	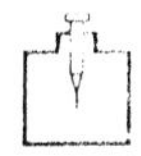
Talking to patient						
Adjusting IV rate or non-invasive equipment; food tray delivery						
Sharps disposal	X					X
Examining patient without touching blood, body fluids, mucous membranes, or non-intact skin	X					
Examining patient including contact with blood, bloody body fluids, mucous membranes, or non-intact skin	X	X				
Intravenous catheter insertion, drawing blood, heel sticks	X	X				
Suctioning - oral, nasal, tracheal Manually cleaning airway	X	X	Use gown, mask, eyewear if body fluid spattering likely			
Handling materials soiled with blood or body fluids: e.g. plumbing repairs	X	X	Use gown, mask, eyewear only if waste or linen are extensively contaminated and splattering likely			
Inserting arterial access; endoscopy; operative and other procedures which produce extensive splattering of blood and body fluids	X	X	X	X	X	
Changing diapers Emptying bedpans	X	X	X Use gloves only if visible blood present in stool or urine			

COPYRIGHT HSC 1990

Fig. 28-3. Universal Blood Precautions chart, designed as a quick reference guide showing which precautions are necessary for the various procedures.

(Reproduced with permission from The Hospital for Sick Children, Toronto.)

Patient Care: Special Concerns

As with most pediatric examinations, a team approach produces the best results. Cooperation between all caregivers and the child provides for a smooth examination. Outlined below are a few special cases which deserve individual mention.

THE PREMATURE INFANT

One of the greatest dangers facing the premature and sometimes the full-term neonate is *hypothermia*. Thermoregulation, the balance of heat losses and gains, is critical to the care and survival of the premature infant. The sources of heat loss—evaporation, convection, conduction, and radiation—are greater in the preterm infant. Premature babies have a greater surface area in comparison to body mass. They are also not capable of storing the fat needed for warmth, and they have increased metabolic rates.

To prevent hypothermia, these infants should be examined within the infant warmer or isolette whenever possible. This requires that the general radiography be done with a portable or mobile unit. Care should be taken to prevent the infant's skin from coming in contact with cassettes. Covering the cassette with one layer of a cloth diaper (or equivalent) works well; however, caution should be exercised to prevent folds or creases in the material because these will produce significant artifacts on neonatal radiographs.

When the premature patient is brought to the imaging department for gastrointestinal procedures, various types of scans, etc., the radiographer should observe the following guidelines:

- Elevate the temperature in the room 20 to 30 minutes before the arrival of the child. With the use of modern computer-controlled equipment, the ambient temperature of the imaging room may be cool compared with the temperature of the neonatal nursery.
- When it is not possible to raise the temperature, prepare the infant for the procedure while he or she is still in the isolette and remove the infant for as brief a period as possible.
- Use heating pads and radiant heaters to help maintain body temperature; however, they are often of limited usefulness because of necessary obstructions such as the image intensifier. If used, position them at least 3 feet from the infant.
- Place large bags of intravenous solutions, pre-warmed by soaking in a sink of warm water, beside the infant to serve as small hot water bottles.
- Monitor the patient's temperature throughout the procedure, and keep the isolette plugged in to maintain the appropriate temperature.

Because the risk of infection is critical to any infant in the Neonatal Intensive Care Unit (NICU), most units insist on adherence to isolation protocols such as gowning and hand-washing. (Premature and full-term infants requiring special care are often cared for in the NICU.)

Care must also be taken when positioning the NICU patient because many can tolerate only minimal handling without their heart rates slowing dramatically. The conscientious radiographer is careful when moving intravenous tubing and other equipment.

MYELOMENINGOCELE

A *myelomeningocele* is a *congenital* defect characterized by a cystic protrusion of meninges and spinal cord tissue and fluid. It occurs as a result of *spina bifida,* a cleft in the neural arches of a vertebra. It can be recognized at the 17th or 18th week of gestation by fetal ultrasonography. Myelomeningoceles may cause varying degrees of paralysis and hydrocephalus. The higher the location of the myelomeningocele, the worse the neurological symptoms.

Since myelomeningocele patients are cared for in the prone position, good patient care suggests that these patients be imaged, whenever possible, in the prone position until the defect has been surgically repaired and the wound healed. The primary imaging modalities used in the investigation and follow-up care of myelomeningoceles include ultrasound, myelography, CT, and MRI.

OMPHALOCELES AND GASTROSCHISIS

An *omphalocele* is a congenital defect which resembles an enormous umbilical hernia. Omphaloceles are covered in a thin, lucent membranous sac of peritoneum, and their contents include bowel and perhaps liver. *Gastroschisis* is a similar condition in which a portion of bowel herniates through a defect near the naval. The difference is that the bowel, in gastroschisis, is not included within a sac.

In both cases the herniated abdominal contents must be kept warm and moist; this is especially important with gastroschisis. It is wise for a responsible physician or nurse to be present when these patients are imaged, because they become rapidly hypothermic.

EPIGLOTTITIS

Epiglottitis is one of the most *dangerous causes of acute upper airway obstruction* in children and must be treated as an EMERGENCY. Its peak incidence occurs in children between the ages of 3 and 6 years. It is usually caused by Haemophilus influenzae, and the symptoms include acute respiratory obstruction, high fever, and *dysphasia*. When epiglottitis is clinically suspected, the radiographer observes the following steps:

- Transport the patient to the department on a stretcher. He or she must be supported in the upright position with an emergency physician monitoring the airway at all times.
- Do *not* proceed with the necessary lateral radiograph of the nasopharynx or soft tissues of the neck *without* the presence of the physician.
- Perform the single upright lateral image *without moving the patient's head or neck*.
- Take extreme care to ensure the child does not panic, cry, or become agitated.

OSTEOGENESIS IMPERFECTA

Osteogenesis imperfecta, a disease characterized by brittle bones, is often abbreviated OI. Children with this condition are prone to spontaneous fractures or fractures that occur with minimal trauma. Because the approach and management need to be significantly altered to accommodate these patients, radiographers should be aware of this commonly used abbreviation. While this condition can vary in severity, all patients need to be handled with *extreme care* by an experienced radiographer.

Children with OI are almost always accompanied by a key caregiver—usually a parent. Experience has shown that these patients are best handled with a team approach, in an unhurried atmosphere. The team is comprised of patient, parent (caregiver), and radiographer, with the radiographer observing the following guidelines:

- Constantly reassure the parent and the patient that everything will be explained before it is attempted.
- For the best results, explain the desired position to the parent and allow the parent to do the positioning.
- Ask older children for advice on how they should be moved or lifted.
- If possible, take the radiographs with the patient in the bed or stretcher. This is often possible, given the patient's small physical stature.

An introduction and a few moments of explanation and reassurance that the films will be done using this team approach can be all that is needed for a smooth examination. *Practical tip:* It is also wise to evaluate the technical factors by checking the first radiograph before proceeding with the remainder. (Generally speaking, the technical factors can be halved.)

CHILD ABUSE

Although there is no *universal* agreement on the definition of child abuse, it is important that the radiographer have an appreciation of the all-encompassing nature of this problem. *Child abuse* has been defined as "the involvement of physical injury, sexual abuse or deprivation of nutrition, care or affection in circumstances which indicate that injury or deprivation may not be accidental or may have occurred through neglect."[1] While diagnostic imaging staff are usually involved only in cases where physical abuse is a possibility, it is important to realize that sexual abuse and nutritional neglect are also prevalent. Legal statutes in all provinces and states in North America require health care professionals to *report suspected cases* of abuse or neglect. The radiographer, while preparing the patient or while positioning the patient, may be the first person to suspect abuse or neglect. The first course of action for the radiographer should be to consult a radiologist (when available) or the attending/responsible physician. Following this consultation the radiographer may no longer have cause for suspicion as some naturally occurring skin markings mimic bruising. However, if the radiographer's doubts persist, the suspicions must be reported to the proper authority, regardless of the physician's opinion. Recognizing the complexity of child abuse issues, many hospitals have developed a multidisciplinary team of health care workers to respond to these issues. Radiographers working in hospitals can access this team of physicians, social workers, and psychologists for the purposes of reporting their concerns, while others are advised to work through the local Children's Aid Society.

All imaging modalities can, and do, play a role in the investigation of suspected child abuse. Plain film radiography, often the initial imaging tool, can reveal characteristic radiologic patterns of skeletal injury. Corner fractures and "bucket handle" fractures (or lesions) are considered *classic indicators* of physical abuse (Fig. 28-4). The presence of numerous fracture sites at varied or multiple stages of healing can also be indicative of long-term or ongoing abuse. These cases are often interpreted by non-radiological staff (e.g., lawyers); therefore, evidence

of injury must be readily apparent. The radiographer's role is to provide physicians with diagnostic radiographs that *demonstrate bone and soft tissue equally well.* Referring physicians are dependent on the expertise of the diagnostic imaging service both for the detection of physical abuse and for the "dating" of the injuries. Radiologists are able to determine this based on the degree of callous formation or the amount of healing.

The radiographer observes the following guidelines when dealing with a case of possible child abuse:

- Give careful attention to exposure factors and film-screen combinations used for limb radiography. Film-screen combinations yielding high detail are recommended for cases of suspected child abuse.

- Perform *skeletal surveys* with *multiple images of individual areas* using appropriate centering points, collimation, and technical factors. Doing a *"babygram"* (a 14 × 17 film of the entire baby) should *be avoided* because the resultant images are of reduced diagnostic quality. Distortion (because of improper centering), scatter, and under- and overexposure of various parts all play a part in the degradation of the image. Babygrams are no longer considered an acceptable imaging protocol for the investigation of child abuse.

- While it may be difficult to do, give the parents of these children the same courtesy as any other parent. Remember that the parent who is present may not be responsible for the injuries. Deal with the parent in a non-judgmental manner aimed at not jeopardizing further relations between them and health care providers.

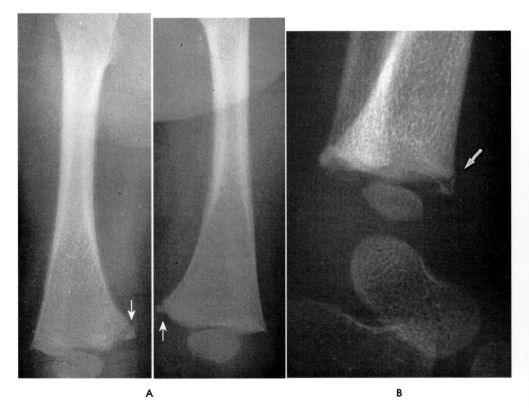

A   **B**

Fig. 28-4. Physical abuse radiographs. **A,** L and R corner fracture *(arrow)* and **B,** "Bucket handle" fractures or lesions are considered classic indicators of physical abuse in children. The "bucket handle" appearance is very subtle and demonstrated only if the "ring" is seen on profile *(arrow).*

[1]Robinson MJ: Practical pediatrics, ed 2, New York, 1990, Churchill Livingstone.

Protection of the Child
PROTECTION FROM INJURY

It is the responsibility of the diagnostic imaging department to ensure that the child neither injuries himself or herself nor is injured during the stay in the department. Emphasis on quality assurance and risk management dictates that many hospitals, and thus departments, perform routine safety inspections to take a proactive stance in minimizing the potential for harm. These are often performed by a team of two: the supervising or charge-radiographer and a front-line worker whose input is vital because he or she works with the equipment on a daily basis. The following guidelines are observed:

- To *avoid the possibility of injury,* supervise children while they are in the department or being transported to and from the department. Some departments clearly delineate, in their policy and procedure manuals, safety precautions to be carried out while the patient is in the imaging room. Such policies relate to the use of Velcro or compression bands designed to prevent patients from rolling from the imaging table.
- Regularly inspect all immobilization tools to ensure that they are maintained in working order. Experienced radiographers should instruct all novice pediatric radiographers in proper immobilization techniques, and novice radiographers' practices should be observed by senior or supervising radiographers.
- In the event of an injury, however minor, file a report documenting the specifics of the incident and the actions taken. Some departments will require that reports be filed even in the event that there was *potential* for a risk to occur.

PROTECTION FROM UNNECESSARY RADIATION

The conscientious radiographer can do much to prevent the child from exposure to unnecessary radiation. Radiographers should remember that bone marrow, active in the formation of blood cells, is distributed throughout the pediatric skeleton and that tissue damage is associated with ionizing radiation. Radiographers should observe the following steps:

- Direct efforts toward *proper centering and selection of exposure factors, precise collimation,* and *appropriate use of filters* (where required), which all contribute to safe practice.
- Use *strategic placement of gonadal and breast shielding* and the *employment of effective immobilization techniques* to reduce the need for repeat examinations.
- Use the PA, instead of the AP, projection of the thorax and skull to reduce the amount of radiation reaching the breast tissue and lens of the eye respectively. Generally speaking, all these factors are well within the control of the radiographer and are important for the protection of the patient from unnecessary scatter radiation.
- *Protect the upper torso of all children* during radiography of the upper limbs.
- Employ diagonal placement of small gonadal aprons along the thorax and abdomen to protect the sternum and gonads of the baby and toddler during supine radiography..
- Have older children wear child-size full lead aprons or adult aprons. (See Common Pediatric Examinations, Limb Radiography.)

Radiographers in supervisory and management positions have added responsibilities. In addition to ensuring that the above practices are followed, supervising radiographers should take into account the clinical needs of the radiologist and follow the ALARA principle (As Low As Reasonably Achievable) when developing technique charts. Pediatric imaging poses conflicting demands on imaging protocols. High kilovoltage is desired to keep the mAs low (thereby reducing the absorbed dose), but low mAs values can present *quantum mottle* problems when imaging small body parts, specifically pediatric limbs and neonatal chests. To be of acceptable diagnostic quality for the radiologist, relatively high resolution is needed. Practically speaking, these needs are often met by the development of a multi-speed film-screen combination. Slow speed systems are used to demonstrate small parts (limbs and neonatal chests), and faster speeds are used for spine, abdomen, and gastrointestinal procedures. The least confusing procedure is to purchase one type of film and *screens of varying speeds.* The cassettes are then color-coded along their outer edges, and the user can be directed to a corresponding color-coded chart to select the appropriate combination.

Computed radiography (CR) (see Chapter 34), used judiciously by experienced and knowledgeable personnel, can reduce radiation dose from 33% to 50%. This significantly shortens the time needed to perform the procedure, and optimizes or tailors the images to suit individual patient requirements. With the increased familiarity with the power of window level and width adjustments in CT and MRI, radiologists have developed a deeper appreciation and acceptance of the digital format. Automatic, laser-printed spot films in gastrointestinal barium studies are a common general application of *image intensifier-based digital radiography.* Pulsed fluoroscopy with "last image hold" serves to reduce patient dose and length of examination. The ability to transmit the digital image directly to a laser printer to produce hard copies saves valuable radiographer time. This often allows the radiographer to spend more time with the patient or to assist the next child sooner. *A cautionary note:* The fact that these digitally acquired images can be "post-processed," thereby correcting some exposure errors, does not negate an important truth—images of proper density are achieved by proper positioning. The anatomy to be demonstrated must be in proper alignment with the photocells; no amount of post-processing will correct this error.

Immobilization: Principles and Tools

Perhaps the two most successful tools for pediatric radiography are effective immobilization and good communication skills. Respected pediatric radiographers approach patients and parents with kindness and take care to maintain patient comfort throughout the procedure.

Naturally, a willingness to cooperate on the child's part allows for more *passive*, less aggressive immobilization techniques to be employed. Constant reassurance, the use of praise, and conversational distraction are the three ingredients of successful communication. Reassurance is the best passive immobilization technique, second only, perhaps, to sleep. A sleeping child who is moved gently, kept comfortable and warm, and not startled by sudden or loud noises will often remain asleep throughout the procedure. (It is recalled, however, that all chest images must be taken while the child is awake, as the rate of respiration is too shallow during sleep to provide full inspiration radiographs.)

Despite effective communication, it is often necessary to restrain children during radiography. If immobilization is not handled appropriately, difficulties can arise for the radiographer, patient, and parent. Immobilization should never become a traumatic, torturous event for the child, nor should any immobilization technique cause harm to the child. Experienced radiographers should teach novice pediatric radiographers how to *carefully* restrain a child. A radiographer's lack of experience, coupled with the parent's and child's fear, can often lead to frustration on *everybody's* part. With practice it is possible to achieve patient comfort as well as immobilization with a minimum of frustration.

Using the communication strategies described at the beginning of this chapter combined with the application of some *practiced* immobilization techniques, the radiographer can prevent much of this frustration. It is important to remember that the parent (presuming one is present) can do only one job. For example, a parent who assists with radiographs of her 2-year-old's forearm can help only by holding the humerus and the hand, leaving the radiographer to immobilize the other arm and legs.

Aside from the regular sponges and sandbags, three tools frequently used in pediatric immobilization deserve mention. They are the Velcro compression band (sometimes referred to as a Bucky or Body band), a strip of reusable Velcro, and a "bookend" (Fig. 28-5). These devices are effective for immobilization of children, although the application of these tools is not limited to pediatric radiography.

Other tools, such as the Pigg-o-stat and the octagonal infant immobilization cradle, are described in the following sections.

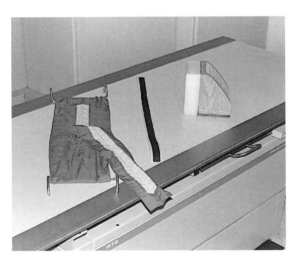

Fig. 28-5. Three tools frequently used in pediatric immobilization include (From L-R) Velcro band (often called Bucky or Body band), strip of reusable Velcro, and a "bookend."

Common Pediatric Examinations

CHEST RADIOGRAPHY

Without a doubt the most common radiographic procedure in hospitals/clinics is the chest x-ray. Radiologists agree that for most diagnostic chest radiographs in pediatric patients, upright images yield a great deal more information than supine radiographs. It is, however, important to know how to achieve diagnostic quality in both positions. Regardless of body position, accurate diagnosis depends on high quality images made with short exposure times to reduce motion. Expiratory films can lead to erroneous radiological interpretations. Therefore, images acquired *on maximum inspiration* are critically important for accurate diagnosis. Well-positioned, non-rotated radiographs are also essential for proper diagnosis because even minor degrees of rotation can significantly distort the normal anatomy.

The upright chest on the newborn to 3-year-old

The challenges of the upright images are many: preventing motion and rotation, freeing the lung fields of superimposition of humeri and scapulae, and obtaining a good inspiratory radiograph. Various methods of immobilization are used to achieve these images but often with somewhat mixed results. Fortunately, these challenges are easily met with the use of a pediatric positioner and immobilization tool called the Pigg-o-stat (Fig. 28-6). While the Pigg-o-stat is primarily used for chest radiography, other applications include upright abdominal images and radiography of the thoracic and lumbar spine.

The Pigg-o-stat is composed of a large support base on wheels, a small adjustable seat, and Plexiglas supports called *sleeves*. These sleeves come in two sizes. The seat, sleeves, and "turntable" base rotate as a unit to facilitate quick positioning from the PA to the lateral projection. Although some physicians do not favor use of the Pigg-o-stat (for aesthetic reasons and because of the possibility of sleeve artifacts), it has been shown to be one of the safest and most versatile restraining methods available for chest and upright abdominal radiography.

Communication with parents. The Pigg-o-stat requires explanation for parents unfamiliar with its use. The radiographer should offer an explanation similar to this: "Doctors prefer chest x-rays to be performed with the child in the upright position. To help your child remain still we have the child sit on this little seat. These plastic supports will fit snugly around the sides and keep the arms raised. It looks funny and your child will probably cry, but this is usually an expression of frustration with being confined. The crying actually helps to obtain a good x-ray image because, at the end of a cry, your child will take a big gasp of air, and at that moment the exposure will be taken." A complete explanation is worthwhile and essential. Show the parent that he or she can help place the child on the seat by guiding the feet in and then assist by holding the arms above the child's head. It is important for radiographers to realize that positioning a child in a Pigg-o-stat is a *two-person job*. Radiographers can safely take children out of the Pigg-o-stat without assistance, but an extra pair of hands is needed in the initial positioning. The properly instructed parent is generally willing and able to assist.

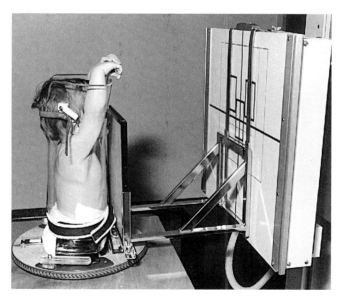

Fig. 28-6. Position for a PA chest radiograph. The Pigg-o-stat is a pediatric positioner and immobilization tool.

Method. The following steps are observed:

- Have patients undress completely from the waist up, so that once the patient is positioned, the ribs are visible on inspiration.
- Choose appropriate sleeve size. Sleeves should fit snugly, which often requires a Velcro strip or adhesive tape wrapped around the base of the sleeves (Fig. 28-6).
- Adjust seat height to approximately the correct level. The seat is at the correct height when the patient is sitting up straight and the face fits in the contours or cut-out portions of the sleeves.

This one-step positioning, with the child sitting straight on the seat and the arms raised evenly above the head, will ensure motionless and non-rotated images (Fig. 28-7). The orientation of the room (i.e., where the chest stand or film holder is located relative to the control panel) and the image requested determine how well the radiographer can see the child's thorax to ensure the exposure is made during inspiration. Listed in decreasing order of reliability, inspiration can be detected by:

1. Waiting for the end of a cry; child will take a big gasp of air
2. Watching the abdomen; a child's abdomen extends on inspiration
3. Watching the chest wall; the ribs will be outlined on inspiration
4. Watching the rise and fall of the sternum

Centering and collimation. The central ray for both PA and lateral projections is directed to the level of T6-T7, but the collimated field should extend from, and include, the mastoid tips to just above the iliac crests. Including the mastoid tips demonstrates the upper airway; narrowed or stenotic airways are a common source of respiratory problems in the pediatric patient. By collimating just above the crests of the ilia, the inferior costal margins will be included. A significant number of children present with long lung fields due to hyperinflation. Noted examples include cardiac and asthmatic patients.

The upright radiograph on the 3- to 10-year-old

These images are easily obtained by observing the following steps:

- Help the child sit on a large wooden box, a wide-based trolley with brakes, or a stool with the cassette supported using a metal extension stand. Children at this age are very curious and have short attention spans. By having them sit, one can prevent them from wiggling from the waist down.
- For the PA radiograph, have the patient hold onto the side supports of the extension stand, with the chin on top of or next to the cassette.
- When positioning for the lateral radiograph, have the parent (if he or she is permitted) assist by raising the child's arms above the head and holding the head between the arms (Fig. 28-8). Fig. 28-9 shows PA and lateral chest images of a 6-year-old patient.

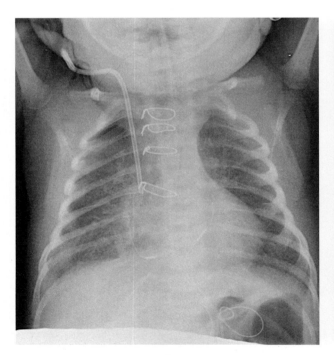
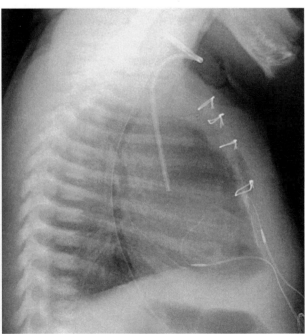

A
B

Fig. 28-7. PA and lateral chest images of a 10-day-old cardiac patient produced using the Pigg-o-stat provide motionless, non-rotated radiographs of good inspiration. Presence of sternal wires, cardiac pacing wires, and a central venous line. Nasogastric (NG) tube is seen on the lateral image.

(Courtesy Colleen Harty, M.R.T.(R).)

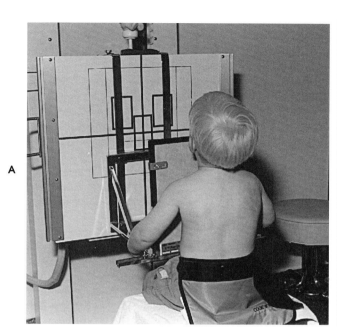

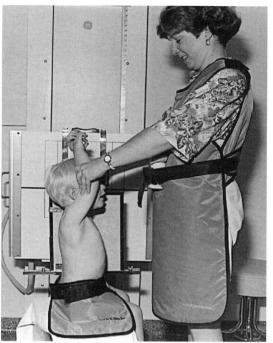

Fig. 28-8. A, PA chest radiographs should be performed on the 3- to 10-year-old with the child sitting. **B,** The parent, if present, can assist with immobilization for the lateral image by holding the head between the arms.

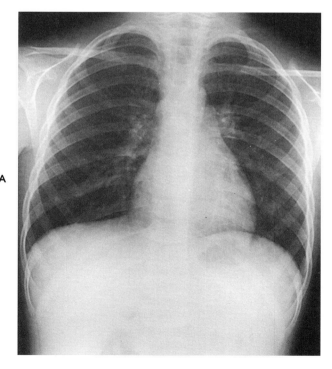

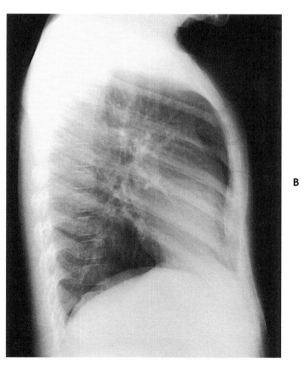

Fig. 28-9. PA and lateral radiographs of a seated 6-year-old boy. Large wooden boxes have the advantage of being sturdier than stools or trolleys, which often have wheels.

(Courtesy Colleen Harty, M.R.T.(R).)

The supine radiograph (infant immobilizer method)

Infants needing supine and cross-table lateral radiographs can be immobilized with the immobilization device pictured in Fig. 28-10. This tool is particularly useful for patients with chest tubes, delicately positioned gastrostomy tubes, or soft tissue swellings or protrusions which could be compromised by the sleeves of the Pigg-o-stat. Similar to the Pigg-o-stat, the infant immobilizer is a one-step positioning and immobilization tool.

Evaluating the image

As in adult chest radiography, the use of high kVp is also desirable in pediatric chest work; however, this is relative. High kVp in adult work generally ranges between 110 and 130, whereas the kVp for pediatric PA projections ranges between 80 and 90 kVp. Practically speaking, it is not possible to use a higher kVp because the corresponding mAs would be too low to produce a diagnostic image. The relatively high kVp helps to provide images with long scale contrast. The criteria used to evaluate recorded detail would be resolution of peripheral lung markings. Evaluating any film for adequate density involves assessment of most and least dense areas of the demonstrated anatomy. In the PA chest image, the ideal technical factors would be a selection that permits visualization of the intervertebral disc spaces through the heart (the most dense area) while still demonstrating the peripheral lung markings (the least dense area). Rotation should be assessed by evaluating the position of midline structures. Posterior and anterior midline structures should be superimposed, i.e., the sternum, airway, and vertebral bodies. The anatomical structures to be demonstrated include the airway (trachea) to costophrenic angles. Similar to chest radiography in adults, the visualization of 9 to 10 posterior ribs is a reliable indicator of a radiograph taken with a good inspiration. (see Table 28-1).

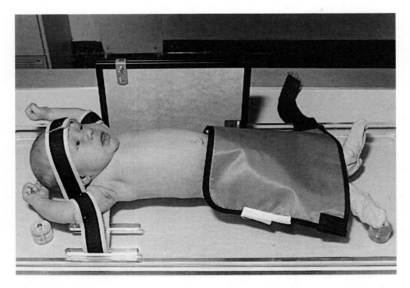

Fig. 28-10. Supine infant immobilizer, a one-step immobilization device useful when upright positioning is contraindicated. This 6-week-old baby is positioned with the arms, head, and legs immobilized with foam-lined Velcro strips. The cassette is in place for the horizontal beam lateral (cross-table lateral).

Table 28-1. Quick reference guide for film assessment

	Density		Detail	Contrast		Anatomy to be demonstrated	Rotation check
	Most dense	Least dense		Long scale >3 shades	Short scale <3 shades		
PA chest	Midline; intervertebral disc spaces; heart	Peripheral lung markings	Peripheral lung markings	Airway; heart; apices; bases mediastinum; lung markings behind diaphragm and heart		Airway to bases	Airway position; S-C joints; lung field measurement; cardiac silhouette
Lateral chest	Heart	Retrocardiac space	Peripheral lung markings	Airway; heart; apices; bases		Airway to bases; spinous processes to sternum	Superimposition of ribs; spinous processes on profile
Abdomen	Lumbar spine	Peripheral edges; soft tissue above crests of the ilia	Organ silhouettes	Diaphragm; liver; kidneys; spine; gas shadows		Right and left hemidiaphragm; symphysis pubis right and left skin edges	
Limbs	Bone	Soft tissue	Bony trabecular pattern		Bone; muscle; soft tissue	Joints above and below injury; all soft tissue	AP and lateral images must not resemble obliques
Hips	Hip joints	Crests of the ilia	Bony trabecular pattern		Bone; soft tissue	Crests of the ilia; lesser trochanter	Symmetrical crests of the ilia
Lateral lumbar spine	L5-S1	Spinous processes	Bony trabecular pattern		Bone	T12 to coccyx; spinous processes to vertebral bodies	Alignment of posterior surfaces of vertebral bodies

Table 28-1. Evaluating the radiograph to determine its diagnostic quality is a practiced skill. This chart, designed as a quick reference guide, outlines the five important technical criteria and the related anatomical indicators used in critiquing radiographs.

Common pediatric examinations

HIP RADIOGRAPHY

The hip and pelvis are areas commonly examined in both the pediatric and adult population. However, the clinical rationale for ordering these examinations varies tremendously. The informed radiographer with an understanding of these differences can be of great assistance. With a basic comprehension of some of the common pediatric pathologies and disease processes, one is better able to appreciate the skills required of the radiologist to make an accurate diagnosis.

General principles

Both hips are examined using the same projection for comparison. The common reasons clinicians order hip examinations on children include Legg Perthes disease, congenital dislocation of the hip, and nonspecific hip pain. Because these conditions require evaluation of the symmetry of the acetabula, the joint spaces, and the soft tissue, symmetrical positioning is critical.

Given its importance, it is somewhat ironic that there is little written literature to guide radiographers on the placement of gonadal shields and when, or when not, to use shielding. Radiographers should observe the following guidelines:

- *Always use* gonadal shielding on *boys.* However, take care to prevent potential lesions of the symphysis pubis from being obscured.
- In *girls,* use gonadal protection on all radiographs with the *exception* of the first AP projection of the *initial* examination of the hips and pelvis.
- Once sacral abnormality or sacral involvement has been ruled out, use shielding on subsequent images in females.
- Check the child's records or seek clarification from the parents as to whether this is the girl's first examination prior to proceeding.
- Since the female reproductive organs are located in the mid pelvis, with their exact position varying, ensure that the shield covers the sacrum and part or all of the sacroiliac joints.

NOTE: Many children have been taught that no one should touch their "private parts." Radiographers need to be sensitive and use discretion when explaining and carrying out the procedure.

- *Never touch the symphysis pubis in a child,* regardless of whether one is positioning the patient or placing the gonadal shield.
- Remembering that the superior border of the symphysis pubis is *always* at the level of the greater trochanters, use the trochanters as a guide for both positioning and shield placement.
- In the male, keep the gonadal shield from touching the scrotum by laying a 15-degree sponge or a cloth over the top of the femora. The top of the shield can be placed level with the trochanters and the bottom half of the shield can rest on top of the sponge or cloth (Fig. 28-11).
- In the female, place the top and/or widest part of the shield in the midline, level with the anterior superior iliac spine (ASIS).

Initial images

The preliminary examination of the hips and pelvis on children includes a well-collimated AP projection and what is commonly referred to as the "frog leg" position. This position is more correctly described as a coronal image of the pelvis with the thighs in abduction and external rotation, or the frog (Lauenstein) lateral projection (see Volume 1, Chapter 7).

Preparation and communication

All images of the abdomen and pelvic girdle should be performed with the diaper completely removed. This is a MUST for radiography of the hips and pelvis. Diapers, especially wet diapers, produce significant artifacts on radiographs, often rendering them undiagnostic. Sponges, gonadal shielding, a Velcro strip, and a Velcro restraining band should all be on the table before commencing the examination.

Children are usually familiar with Kermit the Frog. Explaining to the child that he or she will pretend to be Kermit serves nicely.

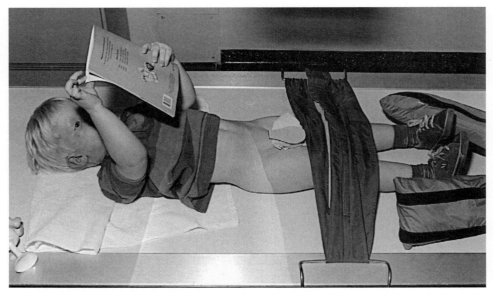

Fig. 28-11. The male gonad shield should cover the scrotum without obscuring the symphysis pubis. The greater trochanters indicate the upper border of the symphysis pubis; the top of the shield should be placed approximately ½-1 inch below this level.

Positioning and immobilization

As described previously, *symmetrical positioning* is of great importance. However, as is common in many examinations, the positions that are the most uncomfortable for the patient are often the most crucial. When a child suffers from hip pain or dislocation, symmetrical positioning is difficult to achieve because the patient often tries to compensate for the discomfort by rotating the pelvis. The radiographer should observe the following steps when positioning the patient:

- As with hip examinations on any patient, check that the ASIS are equidistant from the table.
- With careful observation of and/or communication with the patient to discover the location of pain, the use of sponges is recommended to compensate for rotation. Sponges should routinely be used to support the thighs in the frog leg position.
- Do not accept poorly positioned images. Expend considerable effort in attempting to achieve optimum positioning. This effort may include giving instruction, or re-instruction, to the novice pediatric radiographer.

Because *immobilization techniques* should vary according to the aggressiveness of the patient, the radiographer can follow these additional guidelines:

- Make every effort to use explanation and reassurance as part of the immobilization method. The patient may require only that a Velcro band be placed across the legs as a safety precaution, as shown in Fig. 28-11.
- For the active (or potentially active) patient, wrap a Velcro strip around the knees and place large sandbags over the arms (Fig. 28-12).
- If the child has enough strength to free his or her arms from the sandbags, ask a parent to stand on the opposite side of the table from the radiographer and hold the patient's humeri. The parent's thumbs should be placed directly over the child's shoulders (Fig. 28-13). This method of immobilization is used extensively. It works well for supine abdominal images, IVUs (or IVPs), overhead GI procedures, and spinal radiography.

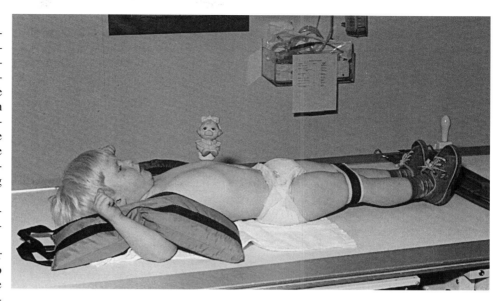

Fig. 28-12. Immobilization of the active child. Sandbags over the arms, velcro strip around the knees and a velcro band beside the patient's feet to be secured over the legs as in Fig. 28-13.

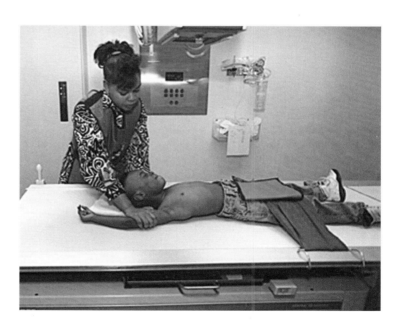

Fig. 28-13. When the child is strong enough or aggressive enough to remove the sandbags, the parent can hold the child's humeri by placing his or her thumbs directly over the shoulders, as shown above.

Evaluating the images

Rotation or symmetry can be evaluated by ensuring midline structures are, in fact, in the midline and that the ilia appear symmetrical. Depending on the degree of skeletal maturation, visualization of the trochanters can indicate the position of the legs when the radiograph was taken. Symmetry in the skin folds is also an important evaluation criterion for the diagnostician. The anatomy to be demonstrated includes the crests of the ilia to the upper quarter of the femora. The density should be such that the bony trabecular pattern is visible in the hip joints, the thickest and most dense area within the region. The visualization of the bony trabecular pattern is used as an indicator that sufficient recorded detail has been demonstrated. This, of course, should not be at the expense of demonstrating the soft tissues—the muscles and skin folds (Please see Table 28-1: Quick Reference Guide).

SKULL RADIOGRAPHY

Along with radiography of the limbs, skull radiography presents some of the greatest challenges to the radiographer. This is understandable when one considers that cranial radiography is usually one of the last areas students become comfortable with during their clinical training. The reasons are twofold: anatomically speaking the skull is complex, and the frequency of skull examinations has steadily decreased with increased availability of CT and MRI. It is easy to appreciate why the pediatric patient, such as the 3-year-old in Fig. 28-14, is perceived as an even greater challenge.

The problems associated with cranial radiography on children can be lessened by *preparing the room* before the patient and parent enter (Fig. 28-15) and avoiding *two common pitfalls:* (1) ineffective immobilization and (2) forgetting (or not taking the time) to check the first radiograph of a skull series. The first image should be treated as scout film, an image which permits assessment of the exposure factors and allows the radiographer to tailor the remaining images to suit the peculiarities of the individual patient. The clinical rationale for performing skull radiography differs tremendously between the pediatric and adult patient. Children present with many congenital abnormalities which significantly alter the bone density. Their age and consequent degree of skeletal maturation also affect the density. These factors need to be considered as the technical factors are selected, making viewing of the initial image very important.

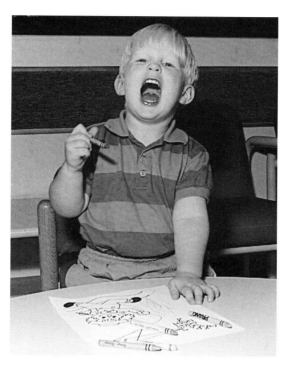

Fig. 28-14. This little boy's face spells "challenge" for skull radiography.

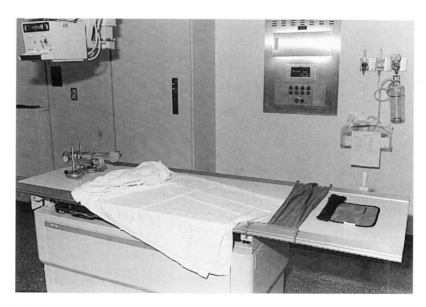

Fig. 28-15. The well-prepared radiographer can make a potentially difficult examination go smoothly. Note the gonadal shield, Velcro band, and head clamps in place. The standard hospital sheet has been unfolded and placed on the table to prepare for immobilization using the "bunny" technique.

Immobilization

All patients 3 years old and younger should be immobilized using the "bunny" technique illustrated in Fig. 28-16 (exception: the sleeping child). A well-wrapped child will remain that way through 5 to 7 images. Mastering this technique is clearly one of the secrets to successful immobilization. A few words of explanation to describe the need for wrapping the child, along with some instruction as to how the parent can help, are also very beneficial. Experience has shown that while children initially do not like being wrapped up using this technique, after their initial frustration and perhaps the use of a soother or pacifier, they often settle down and occasionally fall asleep. If it is beneficial, the soother or pacifier can be left in the patient's mouth for every image with the exception of the reverse PA projection. The parent must be cautioned not to unwrap the child until all radiographs have been checked for diagnostic quality.

Fig. 28-16. The "bunny" method used to immobilize the patient for cranial radiography. **A** to **D** focus on immobilization of the shoulders, **E** to **G** concentrate on the humeri, and **H** to **K** illustrate how the sheet is folded and wrapped to immobilize the legs. **A,** Begin with a standard hospital sheet folded in half lengthwise. Make a 6-inch fold at the top and lay child down about 2 feet from the end of the sheet. **B,** Wrap the end of the sheet over the left shoulder and pass the sheet under the child. **C,** This step makes use of the 6-inch fold. Reach under, undo the fold, and wrap it over the right shoulder. (Steps **B** and **C** are *critical* to the success of this immobilization technique because they prevent the child from wiggling the shoulders free.) **D,** After wrapping the right shoulder, pass the end of the sheet under the child. Pull it through to keep right arm snug against the body. **E,** Begin wrapping, keeping the sheet snug over the upper body to immobilize the humeri. **F,** Lift the lower body and pass the sheet underneath, keeping the child's head on the table. Repeat steps **E** and **F** when material permits. **G,** Make sure the material is evenly wrapped around the upper body (extra rolls around the shoulder and neck area will produce artifacts on 30-degree fronto-occipital and submentovertical radiographs. **H,** Make a diagonal fold with the remaining material (approx. 2 feet). **I,** Roll together. **J,** Snugly wrap this over the child's *femora*. (Tendency to misjudge location of femora and thus wrap too snugly around lower legs should be avoided). **K,** Tuck the end in front. (Should there not be enough material to tuck in, use a Velcro strip or tape to secure.)

(Reproduced with permission from The Michener Institute for Applied Health Sciences, Toronto.)

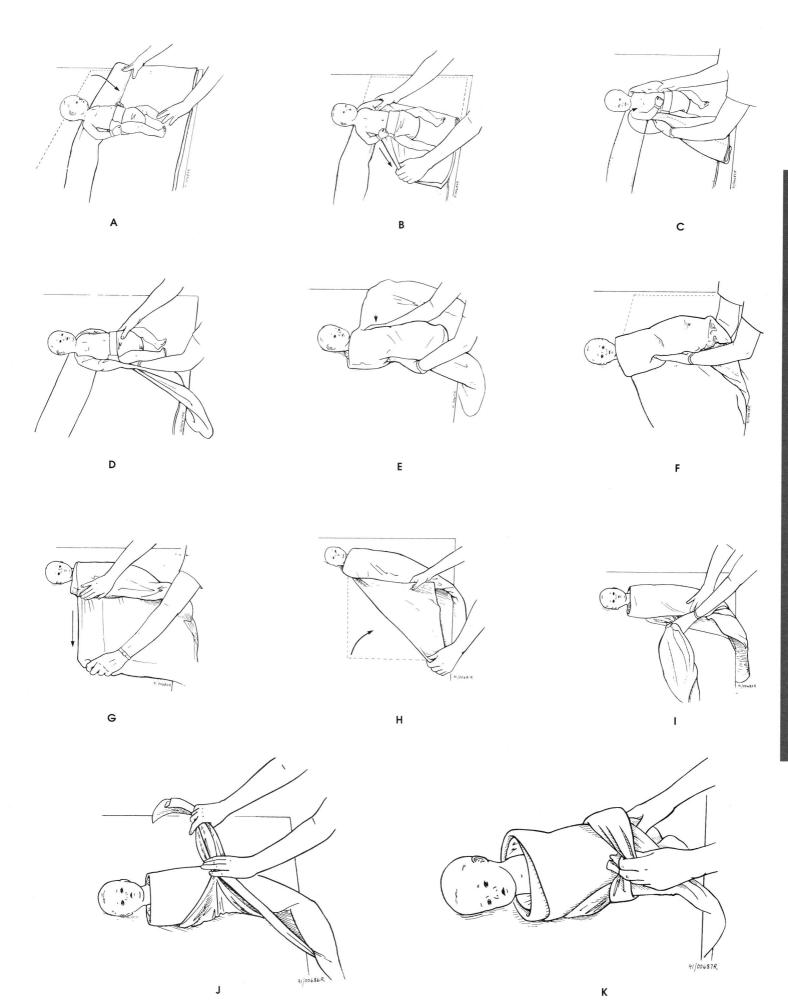

A

B

C

D

E

F

G

H

I

J

K

Fig. 28-16. For legend see opposite page.

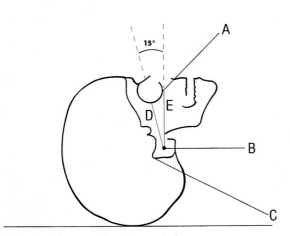

Fig. 28-17. Established tube angles and positions modified to suit the pediatric patient. **A,** Infraorbital margin, **B,** External acoustic meatus (EAM), **C,** Petrous ridge, **D,** Orbitomeatal base line (OML), **E,** Infraorbital base line (IOML). Note: In the young child the OML and IOML are 15 degrees apart (in contrast to older children and adults, where the difference is 70 degrees). It follows that this difference is also reflected in the modification of established tube angles to suit children.

(Courtesy K. Edgell, Cook (Canada) Inc.)

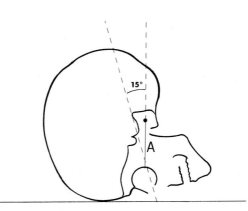

Fig. 28-18. PA projection with the OML perpendicular to the table. In the older child, teenager, and adult, a 15- to 20-degree caudal angulation would result in the petrous ridges being projected in the lower third of the orbits. In babies and young children, a 10- to 15-degree caudal angulation will achieve the same result.

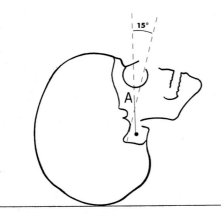

Fig. 28-19. AP projection with the OML perpendicular to the table requiring a 15-degree cephalad angulation to project the petrous ridges in the lower third of the orbits.

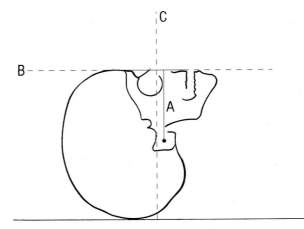

Fig. 28-20. The IOML **A,** positioned perpendicular to the table with the patient in a *comfortable** position, one the head and neck naturally assume as the patient lies down. With the patient positioned this way, there is no longer a need to angle the tube cephalad to project the petrous ridges in the lower third of the orbits (represented by dotted line **C**). With the necessary head clamps positioned, it becomes possible to ensure that the IOML remains perpendicular to the film. However, one can see from this diagram that with the IOML perpendicular to the film, the forehead and chin are parallel to the film (dotted line **B**).

*A comfortable patient is more likely to remain still.

Positioning

The growth of the skull is rapid in the first 2½ years of life, approaching the 75th percentile of adult size by that age. It is important to understand how this growth and the rate at which the cranium grows relative to the facial bones alter the position of the various radiographic landmarks and angles. Practical tip: The established cranial angulations (described in Volume 2, Chapter 21 of this atlas) can be adapted to suit young children by decreasing the angulation of the central ray by 5 degrees. The line diagrams in Figs. 28-17 to 28-20 put this in perspective. The PA projection is used as the basis for these diagrams because this image projects the petrous ridges in the lower ⅓ of the orbits which is a common baseline radiograph for many departments.

Head clamps should be used on all children, even the sleeping child. While motion is not a factor, the sleeping child's head will need some support to maintain the required positions, the exception being perhaps the lateral image where the child has fallen asleep on his or her back with the head turned to the side. Many radiographers believe that the use of head clamps further agitates some children. As with any form of immobilization, the acceptance of the method depends greatly on how it was introduced to the patient and parent. With the room prepared prior to the patient entering, the head clamps should already be in position. Attention need not be drawn to the head clamps until they are about to be used, and they can then be referred to as "ear muffs" (Fig. 28-21). This avoids the unnecessary anxiety that would otherwise be experienced. The degree to which the clamps are tightened depends on the situation. Some children need them only as a reminder to keep still, while others need to have them adjusted more tightly. Although various kinds of head clamps are available, the suction cup type is particularly effective and versatile. (The problem some users experience with the suction cups not sticking to the table is often eliminated by lightly wetting the rubber cups.)

Routines and protocols

Clinicians order skull radiographs either to assess a neurological problem or to evaluate the extent of trauma or injury. For these reasons many departments develop two routines: neurological and trauma (see Table 28-2 on next page).

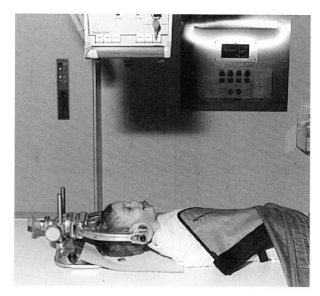

Fig. 28-21. AP projection; head clamps in place.

Neurological routine	Trauma routine
PA or reverse PA projection (Fig. 28-21)	PA or reverse PA projection (Fig. 28-21)
30-degree fronto-occipital projection	30-degree fronto-occipital projection
Lateral with vertical beam (Fig. 28-22)	Lateral with horizontal beam (Fig. 23-23A)
Submentovertical projection (Fig. 28-24)	

Table 28-2. Note: Trauma, in this instance, refers to injury. The important differences between the two are the inclusion of a submentovertical projection in the neurological routine and the need for the lateral image to be performed using a horizontal beam in the trauma routine. This lateral image with a horizontal beam is often referred to as a "cross-table lateral" and is performed to assess possible air/fluid levels which may occur as a result of the injury.

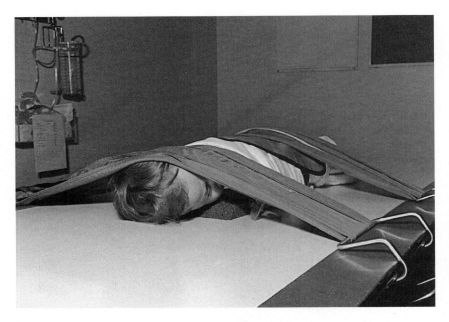

Fig. 28-22. When other methods prove unsuccessful, effective immobilization for a lateral skull radiograph with a vertical beam can be achieved with the use of a second Velcro band, *and some additional explanation to the parent.* (Some radiographers question this technique because it covers the child's eyes. Turning the head and placing the Velcro band should be the last step (apart from a quick collimation check) before the exposure is made. Anxiousness can be alleviated if the parent bends down facing the child and talks to him or her for the few seconds the radiographer needs to make the exposure.)

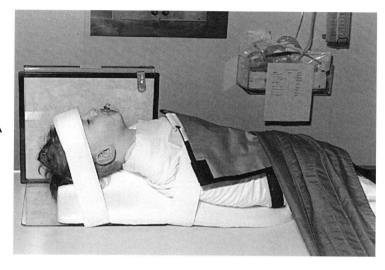 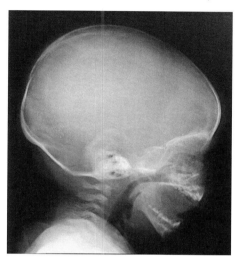

A **B**

Fig. 28-23. A, Effective immobilization for lateral skull radiographs with a horizontal beam can be achieved by using the Infant Head and Neck Immobilizer for positioning and immobilization. **B,** The resultant radiograph reveals a well-positioned, non-rotated lateral skull including the upper cervical spine.

(Courtesy Carmela Kvas, M.R.T.(R.).)

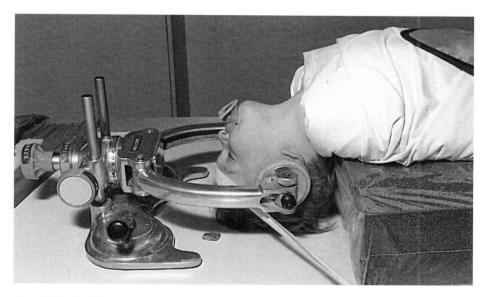

Fig. 28-24. Positioning for a submentovertical projection. Note the use of tape over the forehead to help maintain extension. (Tape is flipped over so the non-sticky surface is in contact with child's forehead.)

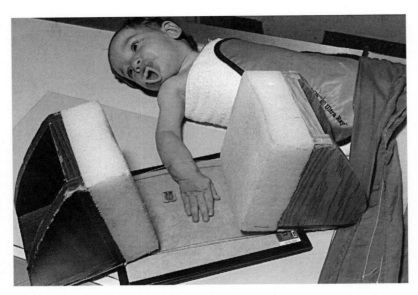

Fig. 28-25. With simple modification of the "bunny" technique using a towel (or pillow case), the child can be immobilized for upper limb radiography. Plexiglas and "book-ends" can be used to immobilize hands on children 2 years old and younger. Note that after the child is wrapped, a Velcro band is used for safety and a small apron is placed diagonally over the body to protect the sternum and gonads. The cassette is placed on a lead mat, which prevents it from sliding on the table.

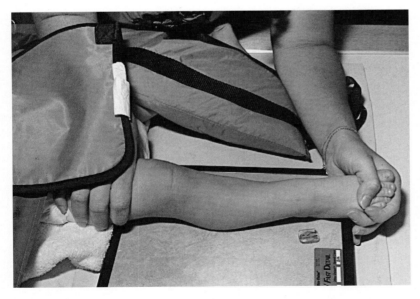

Fig. 28-26. The challenges of immobilizing lower limbs are greater than those of immobilizing upper limbs. With both of the patient's arms wrapped in a towel and a Velcro band over the abdomen, the radiographer can place a large sandbag over the unaffected leg. With careful collimation and proper instruction, the parent can hold the limb as demonstrated. (Parent's hands not shown in lead gloves or with lead draped over the hands for illustration purposes.)

LIMB RADIOGRAPHY

Accounting for a high percentage of pediatric general radiography in most clinics and hospitals, limb radiography requires some explanation. The child's age (or demeanor) determines which method of immobilization should be employed. The immobilization methods are described here according to age group. In planning the approach, the radiographer will need to consider the chronological age and psychological outlook of the patient. For example, a very active 3-year-old may be better managed using the newborn to 2-year-old approach.

Immobilization

Newborn to 2-year-old. Limb radiography on the newborn to 2-year-old is probably the most challenging; however, it is made easier when the baby is wrapped in a towel (a pillow case will suffice if a towel is not available). This wrapping technique, a modification of the "bunny" method described earlier, keeps the baby warm and allows the radiographer (and parent if assisting) to concentrate on immobilizing the injured arm. Fig. 28-25 demonstrates how a piece of Plexiglas and "bookends" can be used to immobilize the hand.

Lower limbs on patients in this age group pose the greatest challenge in all pediatric limb work. In general, both arms should be wrapped in the towel and a Velcro band should be placed across the abdomen; a large sandbag is then placed over the unaffected leg (Fig. 28-26).

Preschoolers. Upper limbs on preschoolers are best managed with the child sitting on the parents' lap as shown in Fig. 28-27. (Should the parent be unable to participate, these children can be immobilized as described previously.)

With parental participation, radiography of the lower limbs can be accomplished with the child sitting or lying on the table. Preventing the patient from falling from the table is always a prime concern with preschoolers. The parent must be instructed to remain by the child's side if the child is seated on the table. Children who lie on the table should have a Velcro band placed over them.

School-age children. These children can generally be managed in the same way adult patients would be for both upper and lower limb examinations.

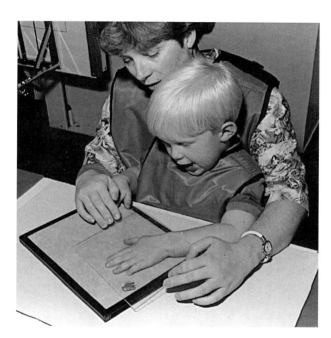

Fig. 28-27. Preschoolers are best managed with the child sitting on the parent's lap. Lead mat is used to prevent cassette from sliding.

Radiation protection

The upper body should be protected in all examinations of the upper limbs, given the close proximity of the thymus, sternum, and breast tissue to the scatter of the primary beam. Child-sized lead aprons with cartoon characters are both popular and practical (Fig. 28-28).

Management of fractures

As with adult patients who arrive in the imaging department with obvious fractures, the child with an obvious fracture *must* have the limb properly splinted by educated personnel before the radiographer commences. (This protects both the patient and the radiographer, because the radiographer could cause further injury by manipulating an unsplinted limb.) Fracture patients often arrive in the imaging department on a stretcher; the radiographer skilled at adapting routines will obtain the necessary radiographs without moving the patient onto the table.

Readers are referred back to the section on Patient Care: Special Concerns, which describes how to manage the patient with osteogenesis imperfecta while remembering that these patient are prone to fractures.

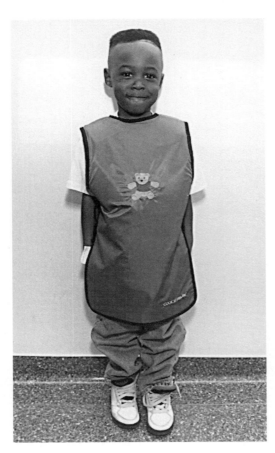

Fig. 28-28. A full-length apron, its teddy bear character making it appropriate for young children.

Evaluating the image

One of the most striking differences between adult and pediatric patients is that of the radiographic appearance of the limb. An appreciation for these differences, which are caused by the presence of epiphyseal lines, develops as one gains experience in evaluating the pediatric image. In departments where the patient mix includes children and adults, preliminary limb work may require the *contralateral* side to be examined for comparison purposes. To the untrained eye, a normally developing epiphysis may mimic a fracture. For this reason, and because fractures can occur through the epiphyseal plate, physicians must learn to recognize epiphyseal lines and their appearance at various stages of ossification. Fractures which occur through the epiphysis are called growth plate fractures. Fig. 28-29 illustrates five types of epiphyseal fractures, referred to as Salter-Harris type fractures, the most widely used form of classification.

With the growth plates comprised of cartilaginous tissue, the *density* must be such that soft tissue is demonstrated in addition to bone (See Table 28-1). As previously described for radiography of the hip, the visualization of the bony trabecular pattern is used as an indicator that sufficient *detail* has been demonstrated. Given how small the pediatric limb can be, a film-screen combination which provides better resolution power than that used for larger body parts is usually required. As a general rule, the speed of the film-screen combination for limb radiography should be half of that used for spines and abdomens.

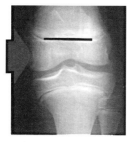 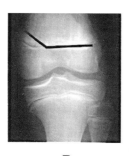 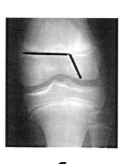 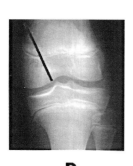 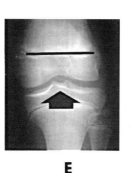

A   **B**   **C**   **D**   **E**

Fig. 28-29. Salter-Harris fractures. The black lines represent the fracture lines. **A,** In Type 1 the fracture is directly through the growth plate. **B,** In type 2 the fracture extends through the growth plate and into the metaphyses. **C,** In type 3 the fracture line extends through the growth plate and into the epiphyses. **D,** In type 4 the fracture line extends through the metaphyses, across or sometimes along the growth plate, and continues through the epiphyses. **E,** Type 5 involves a crushing of all or part of the growth plate. Fractures which occur through the epiphyses are significant injuries because they can, if not recognized and treated properly, affect the growth. Proper radiographic technique is required for the demonstration of both soft tissue and bone. This is especially important with type 1, where the growth plate is separated due to a lateral blow, and type 5, where the growth plate has sustained a compression injury. With types 1 and 5, there are no fractures through the bone.

(Knee radiograph courtesy Carmela Kvas, M.R.T.(R.).)

ABDOMINAL RADIOGRAPHY

Abdominal radiography for children is requested for different reasons than it is for adults. Consequently, the initial procedure or protocol differs significantly. In addition to the supine and upright images, the acute abdomen or abdominal series in adult radiography usually includes radiographs obtained in the left lateral decubitis position. Often the series is not considered complete without a PA projection of the chest. In the interest of keeping the radiation exposure to a minimum, the pediatric abdominal series need only include two images, the supine abdomen and an image to demonstrate air fluid levels. The upright image is preferred over the lateral decubitus in patients under 2 or 3 years because, from an immobilization and patient comfort perspective, it is much easier to perform an upright examination. [The upright can be obtained with a slight modification of the Pigg-o-stat (described below), whereas the lateral decubitus position requires significant modification of the Pigg-o-stat.]

Positioning and immobilization

Young children can be immobilized for the supine abdomen using the same methods described for radiography of the hips and pelvis (Fig. 28-13), a technique which uses basic immobilization of a patient for supine, table radiography. The radiographer should observe the following guidelines for upright abdominal imaging:

- Effectively immobilize newborns through children the age of 2½ or 3 years for the upright image using the Pigg-o-stat.
- Raise the seat of the Pigg-o-stat to avoid projecting artifacts from the bases of the sleeves over the lower abdomen (Fig. 28-30).
- Achieve the best results with older children by having them sit on a large box or trolley (or stool) with their legs spread apart to prevent superimposition of the upper femora over the pelvis.

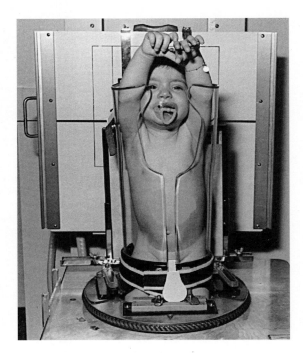

Fig. 28-30. The Pigg-o-stat, modified with seat raised to suit upright abdominal radiography. The diaper has been removed to avoid artifacts over the lower abdomen. The sleeves and seat have been cleaned and the seat has been covered with a cloth diaper or thick tissue prior to positioning the baby.

Lateral images of the abdomen are occasionally required in children, generally for the purposes of localization of something in an anteroposterior plane. Immobilization for this image is quite challenging; given this, and the fact that the immobilization is identical for immobilization of lateral spines, makes it worthy of mention here. The parent can be helpful with this radiograph if he or she is instructed properly. The radiographer then observes the following steps:

- Remember that the *parent can do only one job*.
- Ask the parent to stand on the opposite side of the table from the radiographer and to hold the child's head and arms.
- Immobilize the rest of the body using available immobilization tools. These tools include large 45-degree sponges, sandbags (large and small), a "bookend," and a Velcro band.
- Accomplish immobilization by rolling the child on his or her side and placing a small sponge or sandbag between the knees.
- Snugly wrap the Velcro band over the hips, and to prevent backward arching, position the "bookend" against the child's back with the 45-degree sponge and sandbag positioned anteriorly (Fig. 28-31).

Practical tip: It is common for pediatric clinicians to request simply "two views of the abdomen." The accompanying clinical information should support his or her request, and if it does not, the radiographer should *seek clarification before proceeding*. Depending on the physician's question, the "two views" may perhaps need to be supine and lateral images. Abdominal images requested for babies in the NICU well illustrate this point. The patient with *necrotizing enterocolitis* (NEC) will need supine and left lateral decubitus radiographs to rule out air fluid levels. However, the patient with an umbilical catheter will need a supine and a lateral image to verify location and position of the catheter.

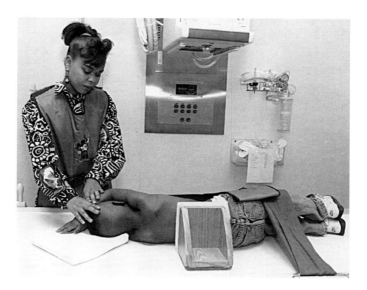

Fig. 28-31. Immobilization for the lateral abdomen also very effective for lateral thoracic and lumbosacral spines. A 45-degree sponge and sandbag are used anteriorly with a "bookend" posteriorly.

GASTROINTESTINAL AND GENITOURINARY PROCEDURES

In the interest of limiting radiation exposure to the child's gastrointestinal and genitourinary systems, examinations are tailored to each individual patient. Following introduction of oneself, the radiographer should explain the procedure and check that the patient has undergone proper bowel preparation. The radiographer can then proceed with preparation (e.g., enema tip insertion) and immobilization of the patient.

Most procedures are performed by the radiologist (exception: IVUs); however, the radiographer has an integral role in the success of the examinations. Optimum hard-copy images require a thorough understanding of the equipment, its capabilities, and its limitations. Good patient care and organizational skills can also make the examination proceed more smoothly.

Immobilization for gastrointestinal procedures

As with other immobilization techniques, there are various beliefs regarding immobilization methods for the fluoroscopic portion of gastrointestinal procedures; two methods are described. (The child may be immobilized for the "overhead" images as per the method outlined for the supine abdomen.

The modified "bunny" method. The child's torso and legs are wrapped in a small blanket or towel and secured with a Velcro strip or tape. The arms are left free, raised above the head, and held by the parent (if present) (Fig. 28-32). The radiologist can then operate the carriage with one hand, holding the child's legs with the other to rotate the patient, thus obtaining the necessary coating of barium. This technique, thought by many to be more comfortable for the child, is often preferred by radiologists because small blankets are more readily available than the octagonal infant immobilization device. Success with this technique is dependent on someone (often a parent) assisting.

The octagonal infant immobilization method This method, while effective, is less comfortable and appears more traumatic. However, with some creativity on the part of the staff, much of the child's fear can be averted by playing the "rocket ship game." The 3-year-old in Fig. 28-33 was told he would be dressed in a space suit (the hospital gown) and would go for a ride in the rocket ship.

By virtue of its construction, the octagonal immobilizer provides immobilization of the child in a variety of positions. As with the Pigg-o-stat, initial positioning of the child is a two-person process. (The additional person need not be another radiographer; a well-instructed parent can assist.) This immobilization technique, because it serves to immobilize the head and arms, is the method of choice should a parent be unable to assist.

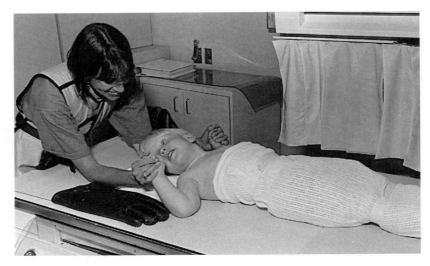

Fig. 28-32. A modification of the "bunny" technique. The arms are left free and raised above the head to prevent superimposition over the esophagus.

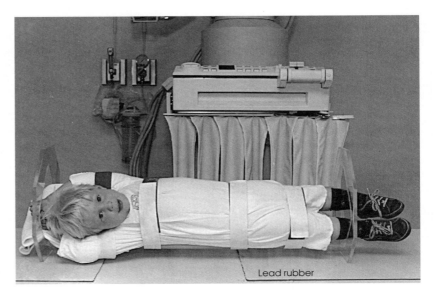

Fig. 28-33. The octagonal immobilizer (or for this child, a "rocket ship") is an eight-sided immobilization tool which permits immobilization in a variety of positions.

Radiation protection for gastrointestinal procedures

It is good practice to cover most of the table top of conventional fluoroscopic units with large mats of lead rubber (the equivalent of 0.5 mm of lead is recommended) (Fig. 28-33). Effective protection for operators and patients can be achieved by positioning the mats so that only the areas being examined are exposed.

The voiding cystourethrogram (VCUG) for genitourinary procedures

A primary purpose of the voiding cystourethrogram is to assess vesicoureteral reflux (reflux from the bladder to the ureters). In addition, VCUG on males can determine the presence of or evaluate urethral strictures. Radiation protection for the fluoroscopic portion should be the same as outlined above for gastrointestinal procedures. The VCUG assesses bladder function and demonstrates ureteral and urethral anatomy.

Method. The patient is catheterized, a procedure which often requires two people, one to perform the catheterization and one to immobilize the legs in a frog leg position. The catheter is connected, via tubing, to a 500 ml bottle of contrast media hung about 3 feet above the table. Under fluoroscopic guidance, contrast media is dripped into the bladder until the bladder is full. Images are then taken while the patient is voiding in order to demonstrate reflux.

Positioning. The female patient remains in the supine position, but the male patient must be obliqued during voiding to prevent the urethra from being superimposed over the symphysis pubis. Once obliqued, care should be taken to ensure the urethra is not superimposed over the femur.

The intravenous urogram (IVU) for genitourinary procedures

Most pathology identified on an IVU (or IVP) can also be identified with ultrasound, a noninvasive, radiation-free examination. IVUs continue to be requested by urologists despite these advantages. However, most radiologists make a conscious effort to keep the number of exposures to a minimum; indeed, many cases are completed with one preliminary radiograph and a late-stage filling radiography (between 5 and 15 minutes). Radiologists find it helpful to review previous radiographs at the time of the study to tailor the imaging sequence, thereby keeping the radiation dose as low as possible.

Examinations Unique to the Pediatric Patient

BONE AGE

Children can present with either retarded skeletal development or advanced skeletal maturation. In either case, the degree of skeletal maturation is determined by the appearance, size, and differentiation of various ossification centers. The most commonly used assessment technique, developed by Greulich and Pyle, compares an anteroposterior radiograph of the left hand and wrist with standards developed in the 1930s and 1940s. While these standards recognize the differing degrees of skeletal maturation between males and females by the use of separate standards for each sex, there are limitations in their applications. Variations can also occur due to genetic diversity, nutritional status, and race.

Radiologists evaluate the differentiation and degree of fusion between the epiphyses and shafts of the bones of the hand and wrist by comparing the patient's radiograph with the standards printed in the atlas to determine the best match. The Greulich and Pyle method is considered extremely useful for most ages. Little change occurs in the ossification centers of the hand and wrist in the first 1 to 2 years of life, while the ossification of the knee and foot develop rapidly during this time. It is for this reason that bone age protocols for 1- and 2-year-olds often include an anteroposterior radiograph of the left knee. Some department protocols specify that the knee radiograph be included on all children under the age of 2 years. Others have found it more practical to specify that if, upon reviewing the radiograph, the radiographer notes there is an apparent lack of ossification in the metacarpal epiphyses, he or she should proceed with the necessary radiograph of the left knee.

RADIOGRAPHY FOR SUSPECTED FOREIGN BODIES

The aspirated foreign body

A significant number of patients examined in emergency departments present with a history that leads the physician to suspect a foreign body has been aspirated in the bronchial tree. This is a common cause of respiratory distress in children between the ages of 6 months and 3 years, and in many cases, the foreign body is non-opaque.

The foreign body, if slightly opaque and lodged in the *trachea,* may be demonstrated with filtered, high kVp radiography of the *soft tissues of the neck.* From a radiologist's perspective, it is critical that these images be performed with the child's neck adequately extended and the shoulders lowered as much as possible. From the radiographer's perspective, this can be difficult to accomplish on the 6-month-old to 3-year-old. This challenge, however, is made easier with the use of the Infant Head and Neck Immobilizer.

Method. The radiographer observes the following guidelines:

- With the child undressed from the waist up, position him or her with the head in the contoured/cut out portion, the neck over the raised portion, and the chest on the sloped portion (Fig. 28-34).

- Lower and immobilize the shoulders using the provided towelette, and immobilize the head and upper thorax using the foam-lined Velcro strips. The extension of the neck helps to prevent the trachea from appearing "buckled," while the towelette and foam-lined Velcro shoulder straps prevent the shoulders from being superimposed on the airway. This commercially available immobilizer is especially designed for radiography of the soft tissue of the neck. However, if the radiographer does not have access to one, improvisation can be made with a 45-degree sponge and some Velcro strips.

Aspirated foreign bodies, however, are *more commonly lodged in the bronchial tree* and, more often, in the right side than in the left side. Air will become trapped on the affected side because the lodged foreign body acts like a ball valve, permitting air to enter on inspiration while preventing it from being exhaled on expiration. The result is a relatively normal-appearing inspiratory PA chest image but an abnormal appearance on the expiratory radiograph. Consequently, the *routine or protocol* for chest examinations on patients with suspected aspirated foreign bodies should be *inspiratory and expiratory PA projections and also a lateral*. It should be noted that when satisfactory inspiration and expiration images cannot be obtained bilateral lateral decubitus radiographs should be obtained. (The unaffected lung will show that the heart has migrated towards the dependent lung. The affected dependent lung will remain fully inflated, preventing any downward migration of the heart.)

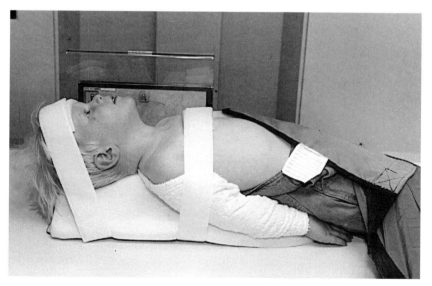

Fig. 28-34. Using the mc Infant Head and Neck Immobilizer for radiography of the soft tissue of the neck provides the necessary extension of the neck. The shoulders are kept low with the use of a towelette.

The ingested foreign body

Children frequently put objects in their mouths, and if swallowed, these objects can cause obstruction and/or respiratory distress. Coins are the most commonly ingested foreign body, and being radiopaque, they are easily identified. The first imaging examination in these cases should be radiographs either of the neck and chest or of the nasopharynx, chest, and abdomen.

Practical tip: On small children (approximately 1 year of age), this examination can be performed using a 14 × 17 cassette (Fig. 28-35). The radiographer needs to understand that the foreign body could be lodged anywhere between the nasopharynx and the anal canal. The presence of a foreign body cannot be ruled out if these areas are not well-demonstrated. Esophageal studies are often required to demonstrate non-opaque foreign bodies.

By virtue of the anatomy of the esophagus and trachea, coins identified in the coronal plane at the level of the thoracic inlet generally are lodged in the esophagus, whereas a coin found along the saggittal plane will generally be lodged in the trachea.

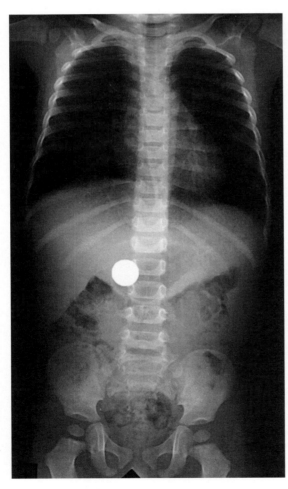

Fig. 28-35. A radiograph of the nasopharynx, chest, and abdomen is necessary to rule out presence of a foreign body. Had the coin that this child ingested not been visible, a separate radiograph of the nasopharynx would have been performed. Note that *diagonal* placement of gonadal shield (distal to symphysis pubis) prevents the lower rectum from being obscured by lead.

(Courtesy Carmela Kvas, M.R.T.(R.).)

SCOLIOSIS

Scoliosis has been defined as "the presence of one or more lateral-rotatory curvatures of the spine." Lateral means toward the side, and rotary refers to the fact that the vertebral column rotates around its axis. Scoliosis can be a congenital or an acquired (e.g., post-trauma) condition. Scoliosis, when initially suspected, is evaluated using a PA or AP projection (preferably PA) on a 3-foot long film of the entire spine. Once progression of the curve is such that the physician feels further intervention is needed, a full scoliosis series will be requested. The *full scoliosis series* should consist of 3-foot PA and lateral projections of the spine and probably right and left bending images (Fig. 28-36). (See also Volume 1, Chapter 8, Figs. 8-149 and 8-150). A PA chest radiograph is included when the series is requested preoperatively. The purpose of the bending films is to assess or predict the degree of correction that can be obtained. The follow-up radiographic examination usually includes upright PA and lateral images.

The radiographer should observe the following guidelines for the easiest and potentially most accurate method of accomplishing the bending images:

- Place the patient in the supine position on the table.
- Ask the patient to bend sideways as if he or she is reaching for the knees.
- Ensure that the anterior superior iliac spines (ASIS) remain equidistant to the table as the patient bends.
- Collimation and centering are critical because the resultant image must include the first "normal" shaped (i.e., non–wedge-shaped) cervical or thoracic vertebra, down to the crests of the ilia (Fig. 28-36). (Experience has shown that curve progression usually stops coincident with the fusing of the epiphyses of the crests of the ilia.) The geometric measurements determine the degree of curvature. The selected method of treatment will be determined in part by the measurement of the angles outlined.

Radiation protection

Since scoliosis images are performed relatively frequently to assess progression of the curves, it is important that effective methods of radiation protection be used.

- Take the 3-foot AP projection using breast shields; alternatively, position the patient for the PA projection, making the use of breast shields optional.
- Ensure that lead is draped over the patient's right breast tissue for the AP left bending image, and vice versa.
- Protect gonads by placing a small lead apron at the level of the ASIS.

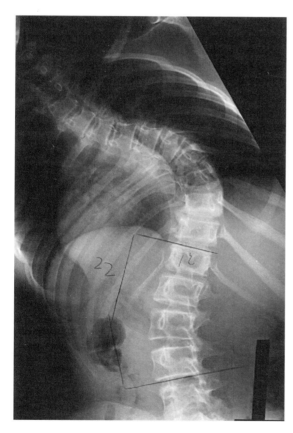

Fig. 28-36. Orthopedic surgeons, in planning corrective surgery, generally observe the bending images as if looking at the patient's back. The structures which must be demonstrated include the uppermost non–wedge-shaped vertebrae and the crests of the ilia.

(Courtesy Nancy Patfield, M.R.T.(R.).)

Imaging Advances

It is beyond the scope of this chapter to discuss *all* imaging advances having a recent impact on pediatric imaging. For this reason, the following sections highlight some advances which have directly impacted previously established protocols or routines in general radiography.

MAGNETIC RESONANCE IMAGING (MRI)

Magnetic resonance imaging is perhaps the most dramatic and widespread area of advancement. The role of MRI quickly gained acceptance in the evaluation of most organ systems in the adult population; however, its acceptance has been slower in pediatrics. This is somewhat ironic, considering that some of the advantages of MRI (enhanced contrast resolution, multi-planar capabilities, and lack of ionizing radiation) are critical considerations in pediatric imaging. Since it is reported that the successful radiologist of the 1990s must be proficient at MRI, the radiographer must similarly be proficient at providing high quality diagnostic MR images.

MRI is documented as the method of choice for evaluating such pediatric spinal cord abnormalities as *tethered cords, lipomyelomeningoceles* and *neoplasms, myelination,* and *congenital anomalies.* MRI has also proved advantageous to the cardiologist and cardiac surgeon. Diagnoses previously suggested on radiographs of the chest are now confirmed for the cardiologist. Cardiac surgeons are better able to plan corrective surgeries because MR images demonstrate the sites and full extent of collateral vessels necessary for grafting procedures. As the radiographer's experience with pediatric limb radiography increases, he or she can appreciate the difficulties the physician has in diagnosing certain types of fractures of the epiphyseal plates (Salter fractures). MRI can demonstrate fractures through cartilaginous structures which would otherwise be missed since these areas appear lucent on the standard radiograph. Elbow surgery can be less complex for the orthopedic surgeon who can first rule out additional Salter fractures with the use of multi-planar MR images. These multi-planar images include coronal, axial, and sagittal images.

COMPUTED TOMOGRAPHY (CT)

CT scanography has come to replace conventional radiographic examinations done to assess leg length discrepancy (LLD). Spot scanography, one of the relatively common conventional methods, is a technique wherein three exposures of the lower limbs (centered over the hips, knees, and ankles in turn) are made on a single 14 × 17 film (see Volume 1, Chapter 11). A radiopaque rule is included for the purpose of calculating the discrepancy on the resulting image.

Studies have shown that CT digital radiography is an accurate technique for measuring limb length discrepancy. It is reproducible, and positioning and centering errors are less likely to occur. More importantly, studies also report radiation dose to be less than that of conventional techniques, leading researchers to recommend that the CT Scoutview type option be used particularly in young patients having serial examinations.[1]

NUCLEAR MEDICINE

When bladder function is the *only* question to be answered for the physician who requests a voiding cystourethrogram (VCUG), a nuclear medicine *direct radionuclide cystogram (DRC)* can be performed. With the DRC, emphasis is on bladder function, recognizing that nuclear medicine studies assess function rather than demonstrate anatomy. The DRC permits observation of reflux during imaging over a longer period; in addition, the DRC allows for accurate quantification of post-voiding residual volume. The radiation dose to the patient is less with this procedure, making it an attractive option for the pediatric patient.

[1]Readers are referred to the Selected Bibliography at the end of this chapter for technical detail beyond the scope of this text.

Conclusion

While no one can prevent a child from experiencing the fear that a visit to the hospital can create, much can be done to allay the fear. Children's direct questions such as, "Am I going to have a needle?" require a truthful response. However, the manner in which the response is delivered can make all the difference. While children are impressionable and dependent on their caregivers, they are also often our best teachers. We need to watch and listen to these small patients, using their body language and facial expressions, as well as their questions and reactions, as cues for how we should respond to them. Our rewards, a child's smile or trust, are often shown more frequently than one might expect.

SELECTED BIBLIOGRAPHY

Aitken AGF et al: Leg Length Determination by CT Digital Radiography, AJR 144:613-615, 1985.

Dietrich RB: The Raven MRI teaching file, Pediatric MRI, New York, 1991, Raven Press.

Green M: Tech-Tips. Can J Med Rad Tech 22:119, 1991.

Green RE and Oestman JW: Computed digital radiography in clinical practice, New York, 1992, Thieme Med Publishers.

Jester JR and Scanlan BE: Fast, informative, low in dose: the digital instant image. Initial Clinical Experience (Reprint from electromedica 56 (1988) no. 4, pp 134-140, 1987, Erlangen, Germany.

Jones D, Gleason CA, and Lipstein SU: Hospital care of the recovering NICU infant, Baltimore, 1991, Williams & Wilkins.

Kleinman PK: Diagnostic imaging of child abuse, Baltimore, 1987, Williams & Wilkins.

Laudicina P: Applied pathology for radiographers, Philadelphia, 1989, WB Saunders.

Milne DA et al: Hospital for Sick Children diagnostic imaging—procedure manual, Toronto, 1993.

Nelson WE, Behrman RE, and Vaughan III VC: Textbook of pediatrics, ed 12, Philadelphia, 1983, WB Saudners.

Ozonoff MB: Pediatric orthopedic radiology, Philadelphia, 1992, WB Saunders.

Reed ME: Pediatric skeletal radiology, Baltimore, 1992, Williams & Wilkins.

Robinson MJ: Practical prediatrics, 3d 2, New York, 1990, Churchill Livingstone.

Silverman FN and Kuhn JP: Essentials of Caffey's pediatric x-ray diagnosis, St Louis, 1990, Mosby.

Silverman FN and Kuhn UP: Caffey's pediatric x-ray diagnosis—an integrated imaging approach, St Louis, 1993, Mosby.

Torres LS: Basic medical technqiues and patient care for radiologic technologists, ed 3, Philadelphia, 1989, JB Lippincott.

Wilmot DM and Sharko GA: Pediatric imaging for the technologist, New York, 1987, Springer-Verlag.

Chapter 29

TOMOGRAPHY

JEFFREY A. BOOKS

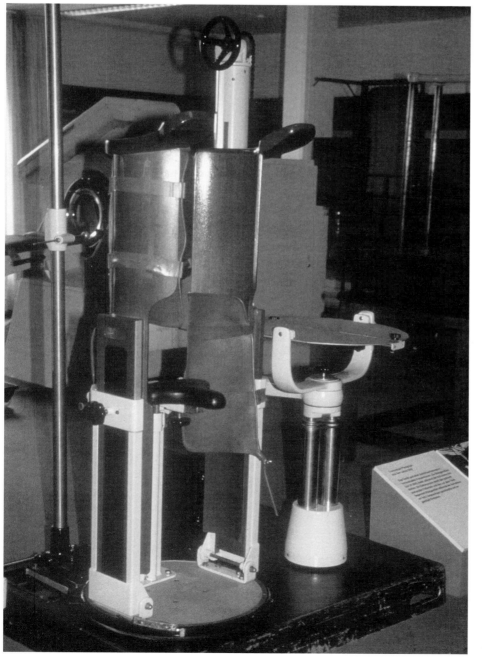

A tomographic unit. The patient sat on the seat while the film and x-ray tube moved.

Historical Development

Since its inception in the 1890s, radiography has presented the problem of trying to accurately record three-dimensional body structures on two-dimensional films. This unavoidably results in the superimposition of structures, which often obscures important diagnostic information. One attempt to overcome this problem is the use of right-angle images. Over the years many other techniques have been developed that partially circumvent the problem of superimposition, such as multiple radiographs, stereoscopic images, and subtraction techniques in angiography.

The partial or complete elimination of obscuring shadows by the effect of motion on shadow formation is a common technique used in radiography. This effect is frequently used with conventional projections. For example, in conjunction with a long exposure time, breathing motion is used to reduce rib and pulmonary shadows to a background blur on frontal images of the sternum and on lateral radiographs of the thoracic spine.

Body-section radiography, or more appropriately tomography, is a term used to designate the radiographic technique with which most of the problems of superimposed images are overcome.

*Tomography** is the term used to designate the technique whereby a predetermined plane of the body is demonstrated in focus on the radiograph. Other body structures above or below the plane of interest are eliminated from the image or are rendered as a low-density blur caused by motion.

The origin of tomography cannot be attributed to any one person; in fact, tomography was developed by several different gifted individuals experimenting in different countries at about the same time without any knowledge of each other's work.

In 1921 one of the early pioneers in tomography, a French dermatologist, Dr. André-Edmund-Marie Bocage, described in an application for a patent many of the principles used in modern tomographic equipment. Many other early investigators made significant contributions to the field of tomography. Each of these pioneers applied a different name to his particular device or process of body-section radiography. Bocage (1922) termed the result of his process *moving film roentgenograms;* the Italian Vallebona (1930) chose the term *stratigraphy;* the Dutch physician Ziedses des Plantes (1932), who made several significant contributions, called his process *planigraphy.* The term *tomography* came from the German investigator Grossman, as does the *Grossman principle,* which is discussed later in this section. Tomography was invented in the United States in 1928 by Jean Kieffer, a radiographer, who developed the special radiographic technique to demonstrate a form of tuberculosis that he had. His process was termed *laminagraphy* by another American, J. Robert Andrews, who assisted Kieffer in the construction of his first tomographic device, the laminagraph.[1]

A great deal of confusion arose over the many different names given to the general process of body-section radiography. To eliminate this confusion the International Commission of Radiological Units and Standards appointed a committee in 1962 to select a single term to represent all of the processes. *Tomography* is the term that the committee chose, and it is this term that is now recognized throughout the medical community as the single appropriate term for all forms of body-section radiography.[2]

---

*All italicized words are defined at the end of this chapter.

[1]Littleton JT: Tomography: physical principles and clinical application, Baltimore, 1976, Williams & Wilkins, pp 1-13.
[2]Vallebona A and Bistolfi F: Modern thin-section tomography, Springfield, Ill, 1973, Charles C Thomas, Publisher.

Physical Principles

In tomography, as in conventional radiography, there are three basic requirements: an x-ray source, an object, and a recording medium (film). However, to create an image of a single plane of tissue in tomography, a fourth requirement must be met—synchronous movement of two of the three essential elements during the x-ray exposure. This is achieved by moving the x-ray source and film in opposing directions about the stationary patient. Because of the end effects, tomography may be thought of as a process of controlled blurring.

The basic tomographic blurring principle is demonstrated in Fig. 29-1. At the beginning of the exposure, the tube and film are at positions T_1 and F_1, respectively. During the exposure the tube and film travel in opposite directions, and their movements are terminated at the end of the exposure at positions T_2 and F_2. The *focal plane* is at the level of the axis of rotation, or the *fulcrum*, and is considered parallel with the tabletop. Structures at the same level of the focal plane remain in focus, whereas structures in other planes above and below this level are blurred across the image. Note that the star located above the level of the fulcrum is projected to the right side of the film at the beginning of the exposure. Next observe that at the end of the exposure the relative position of the star has now moved to the left of the film. Since this is not a static image but a dynamic one, this structure is now nothing more than a blurred density on the film. The round structure located at the level of the focal plane, however, is projected at the same place on the film throughout the entire exposure and therefore is not blurred but remains in focus.

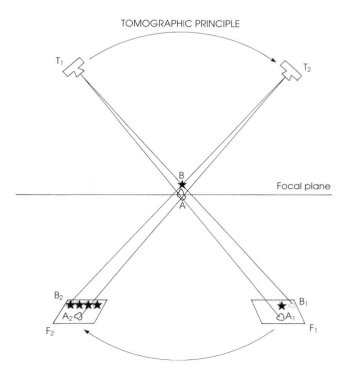

TOMOGRAPHIC PRINCIPLE

Fig. 29-1. X-ray tube *(T)*, focal plane (patient), and x-ray film *(F)*.

Tomographic sections at different fulcrum heights may be obtained by altering the level of the focal plane. This may be accomplished by one of two methods, depending on the principle utilized in the design of the tomographic device. These two principles, the *planigraphic principle* and the *Grossman principle,* are the basis of all modern tomographic equipment. The Grossman principle uses a fixed fulcrum system in which the axis of rotation, or the fulcrum, remains at a fixed height (Fig. 29-2). The focal plane level is changed by raising and lowering the tabletop and patient through this fixed point to the desired height. In contrast, the planigraphic principle uses an adjustable fulcrum system (Fig. 29-3). The actual fulcrum or pivot point is raised or lowered to the height of the desired focal plane level, whereas the tabletop and patient remain stationary at a fixed height.

The *exposure angle* (tomographic angle) is that angle of arc that is described by the movement of the tube and film during the tomographic exposure (Fig. 29-4). The width of the focal plane or the plane of tissue that is in maximum focus is called the *section thickness* (Fig. 29-5). The thickness of the tomographic section may be changed by altering the exposure angle. Since there would be no blurring in a tomogram employing a stationary x-ray tube (an exposure angle of 0 degrees), the resulting image would yield a conventional radiograph. Both would demonstrate all planes of tissue contained within the part being imaged (an infinite section thickness). In tomography, as the exposure angle increases from 0 degrees, the section thickness decreases. Tomograms using wide exposure angles will demonstrate thin sections; conversely, smaller exposure angles will demonstrate comparatively thicker sections.

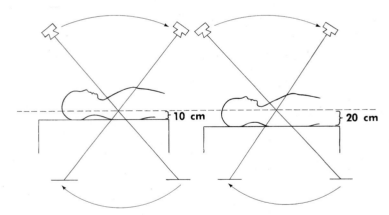

Fig. 29-2. Grossman principle (fixed fulcrum). Tabletop height is changed to alter fulcrum level.

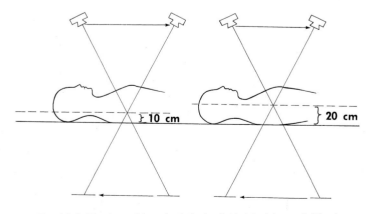

Fig. 29-3. Planigraphic principle (adjustable fulcrum). Pivot point height is changed to alter fulcrum level.

The range of section thickness produced by wide-angle tomography is approximately from 1 to 5 mm, and that produced by narrow-angle tomography, or zonography, is from slightly less than 1 cm to about 2.5 cm. *Zonography,* the tomographic technique used to demonstrate relatively thick sections or zones of tissue, was first described by des Plantes, who recommended it for examining sections of the cranium and the spinal column.

Zonography is now used in a number of other regions of the body. The blurring characteristics make it ideally suited to demonstrate structures that are low in contrast relative to adjacent structures. Zonography is frequently employed in the abdomen where the structures that comprise the soft tissue organs are extremely low in contrast relative to each other and therefore difficult to differentiate on conventional radiographs.

The degree to which definition decreases with distance from the focal plane is dependent on the width of the angle described by the tube motion. Wide angles of tube movement provide excellent blurring of structures close to the focal plane, as well as of those remote from it. Narrow angles of tube movement provide excellent blurring of structures remote from the focal plane but only moderate to slight blurring of structures close to the focal zone.

Although visibility of the objective area is greatly enhanced by the partial or complete elimination of obscuring shadows, the appearance of the tomogram is quite different from that of a conventional radiograph. The customary sharp definition and clear contrast are diminished, and the contours of all but the thinnest structures are absent. The contrast is reduced because of the way the blurring action diffuses elements in other planes over the focal plane image. This creates an overall increase in the density on the tomogram, which, in turn, results in an overall decrease in contrast in the structures demonstrated.

The formation of the tomographic image is a cumulative process. The shadows of structures in the plane of focus accumulate on the film as the area traversed by the beam of radiation swings over the arc. The images are not sharp, since the radiation traverses structures from many angles, outlining clearly only those boundaries to which it is momentarily tangential in its passage.

Zonograms are comparable in appearance to conventional radiographs, because (1) the cuts are thick enough to show structural contours; (2) the narrow arc described by the tube directs the radiation at only slightly oblique angles, so that it projects structural contours more nearly true to shape; and (3) with the reduced effects of less blurring, the contrast and detail produced are superior to those possible in wide-angle tomography. However, this is not to say that there is more diagnostic information in a zonogram than in a wide-angle tomogram; each has its place in tomography. The choice between using a wide or a narrow exposure angle primarily depends on the thickness of the structure or structures to be in the tomogram and their proximity to other structures outside the focal plane.

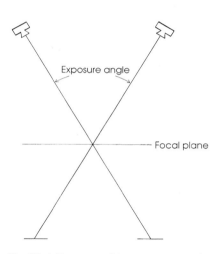

Fig. 29-4. Tomographic exposure angle.

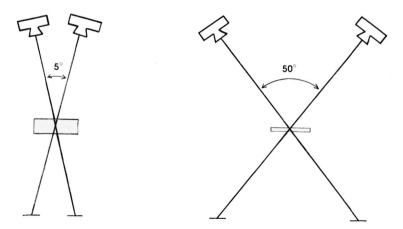

Fig. 29-5. Narrow exposure angles yield thick tomographic sections; wide exposure angles yield thin tomographic sections.

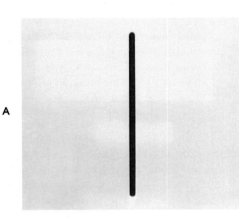

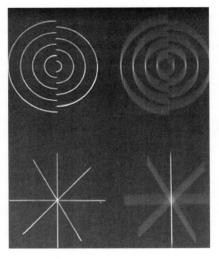

Fig. 29-6. A, Pinhole tracing of 45-degree longitudinal linear motion. **B,** Tomogram of test object at 45-degree longitudinal linear motion. Left pattern is at level of focal plane. Right pattern is 5 mm above level of focal plane. With linear motion the best blurring occurs to elements of test object oriented perpendicular to movement of tube and the least blurring to elements oriented parallel.

Blurring Motions

Modern tomographic equipment offers a variety of different blurring patterns. These blurring motions fall under two categories: *unidirectional (linear)* and *pluridirectional (complex) tomographic motions,* which include circular, elliptical, hypocycloidal, and spiral motions. A basic understanding of the characteristics of these blurring patterns is necessary for understanding their advantages as well as their limitations.

UNIDIRECTIONAL MOTION

The basic tomographic blurring pattern is the unidirectional, or linear, motion. The blurring action of linear motion is provided by elongation of structures outside of the focal plane so that they become indistinguishable linear streaks or blurs over the focal plane image. Maximum blurring occurs to those elements of structures outside the focal plane that are oriented perpendicular to the relative motion of the tube (Figs. 29-6 to 29-8). In linear tomography, therefore, elements of structures oriented parallel to the motion of the tube are incompletely blurred and can form false shadows, *phantom images,* over the focal plane image. This results in an inaccurate representation of the focal plane because of the summation of the focal

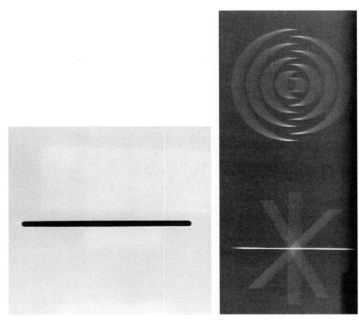

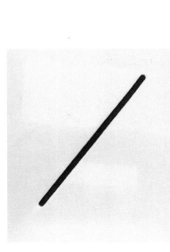

Fig. 29-7. A, Pinhole tracing of 45-degree transverse linear motion. **B,** Tomogram of test object at 45-degree transverse linear motion.

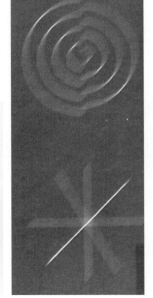

Fig. 29-8. A, Pinhole tracing of 45-degree oblique linear motion. **B,** Tomogram of test object at 45-degree oblique linear motion.

plane image and images of some structures outside the plane of focus. This characteristic is demonstrated in the tomogram of a test object.

The test object consists of two wire patterns: pattern 1 is located at the level of the focal plane (left-hand image in Fig. 29-6, *B*); pattern 2 (right-hand image) is 5 mm away from the level of the focal plane and therefore exhibits the effects of the blurring motion used.

The best blurring occurs to those elements of the patterns that are perpendicular to the tube movement, and the least occurs to those parallel. In linear tomography it is important to orient those structures to be blurred at right angles to the tube movement. For example, in tomography of the chest the tube movement is oriented perpendicularly to the ribs for maximum blurring of those structures.

A more efficient blurring motion would be one in which all of the elements of an object would be perpendicular to the movement of the tube at some time during the exposure. This is the principle of the second type of blurring motion, the pluridirectional, or complex, motion.

PLURIDIRECTIONAL MOTIONS

Circular Motion

The basic pluridirectional motion is the circular pattern (Fig. 29-9). The circular motion does not blur by mere elongation as in linear motion but by evenly diffusing the densities of those structures outside the focal plane over the focal plane image. Tomograms using a circular or any other complex motion therefore exhibit more even contrast but less contrast than do linear tomograms with their characteristic linear streaking. Note that all elements of the test pattern are equally blurred regardless of their orientation. The circular motion maintains a constant radius and angle throughout the exposure, which results in a sharp cutoff margin of the blurred structures. This in turn may result in the formation of phantom images superimposed over the focal plane image.

The phenomenon of phantom images occurs more often in circular tomography using small angles as in circular zonography. The phantom images are created by the fusion of the margins of the blurred shadows of structures slightly outside the focal plane or by annular (circular) shadows of dense structures again slightly outside the focal plane.

These phantom images are usually less dense and distinct than the actual focal plane images. They can be identified as such on successive tomograms as the real structure or structures come into focus.

The characteristics of wide-angle circular tomography are identical to small-angle circular tomography, with one exception. The wider angle results in greater displacement of the blurred shadows, reducing the possibility of phantom image formation.

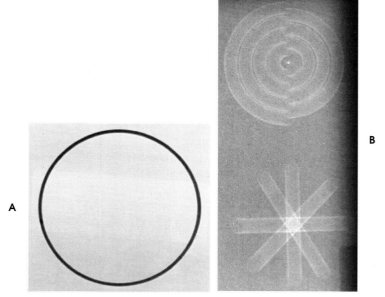

Fig. 29-9. Circular motion of 45 degrees. **A,** Pinhole tracing. **B,** Tomogram of test object demonstrating annular shadow formation and fusion of marginal blur pattern—characteristics of circular motion.

Elliptical Motion

The elliptical motion, having both linear and circular aspects to the pattern, exhibits blurring characteristics of both (Fig. 29-10). It requires the same perpendicular orientation as the linear motion and exhibits similar phantom shadow characteristics to both the linear and circular motions. Although it is a more efficient blurring motion than the simple linear motion, the quality of blur is much less than in the circular motion or the more complex motions, hypocycloidal and spiral motion.

Hypocycloidal Motion

The hypocycloidal motion offers excellent displacement of the marginal blur pattern, nearly eliminating the possibility of phantom image formation (Fig. 29-11). It provides excellent blurring of structures both close to and remote from the focal plane and has a focal plane thickness of slightly less than 1 mm.

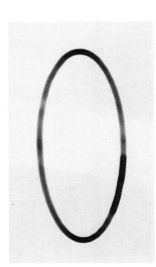

A

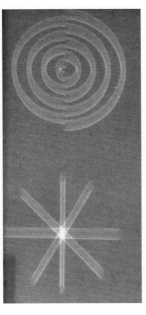

B

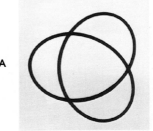

A

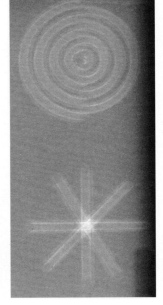

B

Fig. 29-10. Elliptical motion. **A,** Pinhole tracing. **B,** Tomogram of test object demonstrating characteristics of both linear and circular motions.

Fig. 29-11. Hypocycloidal motion. **A,** Pinhole tracing. **B,** Tomogram of test object demonstrating excellent blurring characteristics.

Spiral Motion

Tomographic equipment capable of producing a spiral motion is usually designed for a three-spired (trispiral) motion or a five-spired motion (Fig. 29-12). The spiral motion, although different in pattern from the hypocycloidal motion, also offers excellent displacement of the marginal blur pattern, exceptional resolving power, and an extremely thin section thickness of less than 1 mm.

These excellent blurring characteristics make both the hypocycloidal and spiral motion useful in examinations of any area of the body, and they are especially useful in tomographic examinations of the skull, where structures are very small and compact and require greater separation of tissue planes (Fig. 29-13).

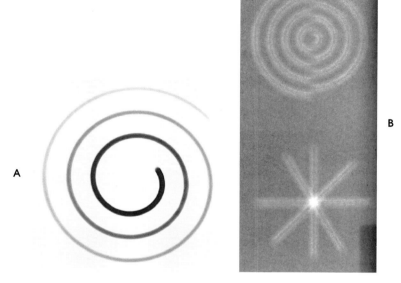

Fig. 29-12. Trispiral motion. **A,** Pinhole tracing. **B,** Tomogram of test object demonstrating excellent blurring characteristics.

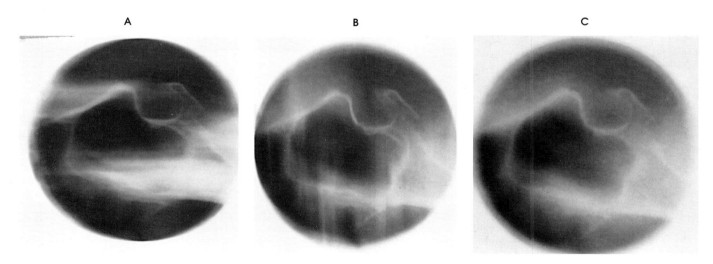

Fig. 29-13. Tomograms of sella turcica in lateral position through midplane. **A,** Transverse linear motion. **B,** Longitudinal linear motion. **C,** Trispiral motion demonstrating the sella turcica much more clearly and without parasitic linear streaking that is found in **A** or **B.**

Factors Affecting Tomographic Image

"The difference between a high quality tomogram and a poor one is very slight; hence, it is extremely important that attention be given to all the parameters which contribute to the focal plane image."[1] The factors that affect the tomographic image can be divided into two categories: (1) patient variables and (2) equipment variables.

PATIENT VARIABLES

As in conventional radiography, proper positioning of the patient and centering of the central ray are of critical importance. An equally important factor that must be considered in tomography is the selection of the proper focal plane level. The part must be adequately immobilized because any motion will add unwanted blur to the focal plane image. Object size and the relative density of structures will affect density and contrast of the image.

---

[1]Littleton JT: Tomography: physical principles and clinical application, Baltimore, 1976, Williams & Wilkins, pp 13.

EQUIPMENT VARIABLES

The tomographic principle used will affect several different properties of the image, with magnification being the most affected. Tomographic machines utilizing the *fixed fulcrum,* or Grossman, principle will maintain a constant magnification factor at any focal plane level, because the distance between the focal plane and the film remains the same at any level. Conversely, with the *adjustable fulcrum,* or planigraphic, system, the focal plane–film distance changes as the fulcrum height is varied, resulting in different magnification of the focal plane image at different fulcrum heights. This magnification is, however, at most working levels, less than the fixed rate of magnification of the fixed fulcrum machines.

The degree to which structures outside the focal plane are blurred is a function of the geometry of the blurring pattern and the angle of the tomographic arc. The more complex the blurring pattern, the greater the effacement of those structures outside the focal plane. Wide exposure angles provide greater blurring of structures close to the focal plane as well as those that are remote. The exposure angle also determines the thickness of the focal plane image. As previously mentioned, the wider the exposure angle, the thinner the section thickness, and, conversely, the narrower the exposure angle, the thicker the section thickness.

Each blurring pattern requires a specific amount of time to complete its motion. Therefore the exposure time must be sufficient to allow completion of the motion before terminating the exposure. Linear motions generally take less time to complete than do the more complex pluridirectional movements. Exposure time is one half of the mAs formula, but, since there are restrictions for certain exposure times for each different pattern, the mA and kVp must be altered to change the density. Since contrast levels are inherently low in tomography, high mAs and relatively low kVp techniques are used in most examinations to enhance the contrast between structures. Collimating to the smallest possible field size also improves the contrast of the image.

The focal spot size will affect the recorded detail of the focal plane image. In areas in which great recorded detail is required, such as the skull, cervical spine, and limbs (extremities), the smallest available focal spot should be used. In other areas, fine recorded detail may not be required; therefore, to prolong the life of the x-ray tube, the large focal spot may be used when possible. Extreme care must be taken not to exceed the recommended tube limits or cooling rate.

Tomographic machines must provide synchronous, vibration-free movement of the tube and film, because any mechanical instability may transmit unwanted motion and create additional blur to the focal plane image. For this reason, most manufacturers have designed tomographic equipment to begin the exposure after the motion has begun, allowing enough time for any unwanted motion and vibration to be stabilized that may have been caused by the rapid acceleration of the tube and film. The exposure is then terminated just before the end of the movement to avoid any motion that may occur during the rapid deceleration of the tube and film.

Since the thicknesses of cassettes vary with each manufacturer, one type of cassette should be used throughout the entire examination. Otherwise, the focal plane images will not be successively consistent from level to level because the height of the film and therefore the focal plane image will vary with each cassette used.

The film-screen combination will greatly affect the tomographic image. Very low speed film-screen combinations will produce images with very good recorded detail, but they require a greater amount of radiation. A faster combination produces images with good recorded detail and contrast with much less radiation. Other combinations using rare earth screens are available that produce radiographs with excellent detail but slightly lower contrast.

Equipment

Tomography machines may be varied in appearance and function, but all have three common requirements. Aside from the usual features of any radiographic machine, such as an x-ray source, timer, and mA and kVp selector, any x-ray machine capable of producing a tomographic image must have the following additional features: (1) the machine must have some type of linkage connecting the x-ray source and film carriage that will provide synchronous, vibration-free movement of the tube and film in opposite directions during the tomographic exposure; (2) there must be a means of imparting motion to the tube and film carriage for each different tomographic movement; and (3) there must be a means of adjusting the fulcrum height for tomograms at different levels.

As the x-ray tube moves in one direction, the film carriage will always move in the opposite direction, as shown in Fig. 29-1. The film will move synchronously with the movement of the tube, maintaining a constant relationship with each other as they move. This mechanical type of linkage is the basic type of linkage that most tomographic machines utilize, from the simplest machines to the highly sophisticated pluridirectional units. The major difference between the two is that in the pluridirectional machines the simple metal rod is replaced by a heavier metal beam or a parallelogram of thick rods that attach at either end to the x-ray tube and film carriage. The heavier material used for the linkage is required to withstand the great centrifugal force created by the tube and film carriage as it swings rapidly through the complex motions.

There is another type of linkage that has been made possible by advances in computer technology. One manufacturer developed a radiographic machine capable of linear tomography with no direct mechanical linkage between the tube and film carriage. The x-ray tube is mounted on the ceiling and is electronically linked to the film carriage through a microcomputer. The microcomputer controls separate drive motors that maintain the tube and film in alignment throughout the linear motion. This design allows for greater mobility of the x-ray tube for radiographic examinations since it is free floating when not in the tomographic mode, which makes it much more versatile than the standard radiographic/tomographic unit.

The second requirement is that there must be a means of imparting motion to the tube and film carriage for each tomographic motion. Modern machines employ motors that drive the tube and film for the blurring movement. The motor drive and the linkage mechanism must provide stable, vibration-free movement of the tube and film. Any unwanted motion may cause additional blurring of the focal plane image.

All tomographic machines must also have some means of adjusting the height of the fulcrum. In machines utilizing the adjustable or planigraphic principle, the motor drive alters the actual pivot point of the tube-film carriage assembly by raising and lowering the axis of rotation. Tomographic machines utilizing the fixed fulcrum, or Grossman, principle have a tabletop that is raised or lowered by a motor to the desired height.

Tomographic equipment has changed considerably since the early days of Vallebona and des Plantes. Their first machines were crude although ingeniously designed contrivances operated with ropes, pulleys, and hand cranks. Present-day equipment is motor driven and ranges from simple radiographic tables that can change into linear tomography devices to highly sophisticated machines designed primarily for pluridirectional tomography. The more elaborate tomographic machines offer several automatic functions, such as automatic fulcrum height adjustment and motorized cassette shift for multiple exposures on one film. The pluridirectional machines are capable of several complex motions as well as the simple linear movement.

TESTING OF TOMOGRAPHIC EQUIPMENT

Tomographic equipment is carefully checked and calibrated by the manufacturer's service representative when it is installed. The tube-film movement must be stable and exactly balanced, and there must be synchronization of the travel time and exposure time at each of the exposure angles and tomographic movements. These are checked with a pinhole test device. The pinhole test device is a lead plate with a very small beveled hole in the middle, which is positioned on the tabletop directly in line with the central ray. Pinholes must be placed either above or below the focal plane. The tomographic exposure is made, tracing on film the actual pattern of the tomographic motion used. Any mechanical instability or aberration in the correct exposure time can be noted on the pinhole tracing. Examples of pinhole tracings can be found in the section on blurring motions.

Another test device called a tomographic test phantom is used to determine the accuracy of the fulcrum height indicator and the section thickness of the different exposure angles and blurring motions. The blurring characteristics of the different motions may be determined with the phantom also (Figs. 29-6 and 29-13). Different phantoms are available, but most manufacturers of tomographic equipment recommend the test phantom developed by Dr. J.T. Littleton. This is the type of device used in Figs. 29-6 to 29-12.

Clinical Applications

Tomography is a proven diagnostic tool that can be of significant value when a definitive diagnosis cannot be made from conventional radiographs, because confusing shadows can be removed from the point of interest. Tomography may be used in any part of the body but is most effective in areas of high contrast, such as bone and lung. Body-section radiography is used to demonstrate and evaluate a number of different pathologic processes, traumatic injuries, and congenital abnormalities. A basic familiarization with the clinical applications of tomography will help the tomographer to be more effective. Some of the major areas of clinical application are described below, although the versatility of tomography lends itself to other applications.

PATHOLOGIC PROCESSES IN SOFT TISSUES

One of the most frequent uses of tomography is to demonstrate and evaluate benign processes and malignant neoplasms in the lungs. Differentiation between benign lesions and malignancies cannot always be made with conventional chest radiography. With tomography it is possible to define the location, size, shape, and marginal contours of the lesion. Differentiation between benign and malignant tumors depends on the characteristics of the lesion itself. Benign lesions characteristically have smooth, well-marginated contours and frequently contain bits of calcium. The presence of calcium in a chest lesion usually confirms it as being benign. The benign lesions most commonly found in the lungs are granulomas, which form as a tissue reaction to a chronic infectious process that has healed.

Conversely, carcinogenic neoplasms characteristically have ill-defined margins that feather or streak into the surrounding tissue and rarely contain calcium (Figs. 29-14 and 29-15). Lung cancers may originate in the lung, in which case the neoplasm would be termed a primary malignancy. Bronchogenic carcinoma is an example of a primary malignancy that may develop in the chest. Lung cancers may develop as the result of the spread of cancer from another area of the body to the lungs. These malignancies are termed secondary or metastatic tumors. Breast cancer and testicular cancer, as well as others, may metastasize to the lungs.

When there is an apparent solitary nodule noted on a conventional chest radiograph, the presence or exclusion of other lesions may be determined with general tomographic surveys of both lungs. These "whole lung" or "full lung" tomograms are used to exclude the possibility of metastatic disease from other organs. Frequently these lesions cannot be visualized by conventional radiographic techniques, and tomography is one means to identify these occult nodules. The demonstration of the number of tumors and their location, size, and relationship to other pulmonary structures is crucial to the physician's plan of treatment and the prognosis for the patient. Reexamination by tomography may be performed at a later date to check on the progress of the disease and the effectiveness of the therapy.

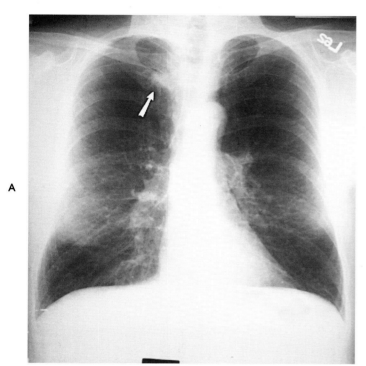

A

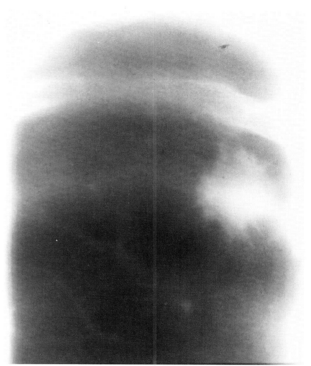

B

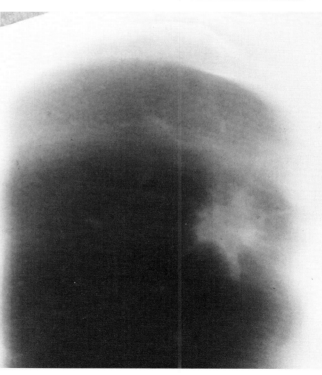

C

Fig. 29-14. A, PA chest demonstrating ill-defined density *(arrow)* in right upper chest; **B** and **C,** Collimated AP tomograms of patient in **A** demonstrating lesion in posterior chest plane with ill-defined margins that feather or streak into surrounding lung tissue, characteristic of malignant chest lesion.

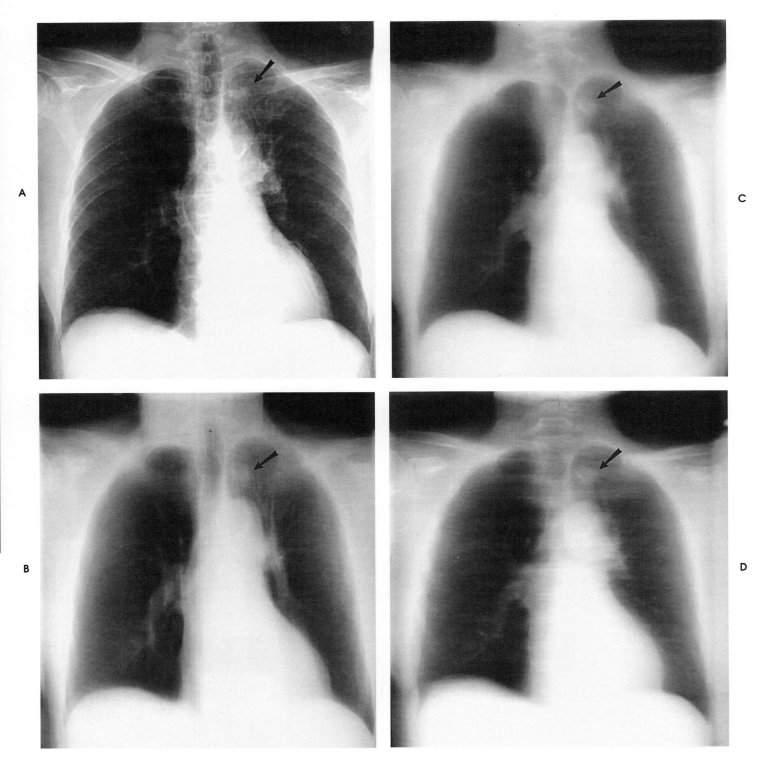

Fig. 29-15. A, AP chest with vague density *(arrow)* over medial end of left clavicle. **B** to **D,** AP full lung tomograms of patient in **A** taken to exclude possibility of other occult lesions. **B,** Trispiral tomogram 1 cm anterior to hilar plane at level of tumor. Radiographic appearance of lesion *(arrow)* is consistent with malignant chest neoplasm. **C,** Longitudinal linear tomogram of 40 degrees at same fulcrum level as **B.** Visualization of lesion *(arrow)* is decreased because of linear streaking and incomplete blurring of other structures outside focal plane. **D,** 40-degree transverse linear tomogram at same level as **B** and **C,** again demonstrating poor visualization of lesion *(arrow)* Because of linear blurring characteristics. Blurring of anterior ribs is incomplete.

PULMONARY HILA

Neoplasms involving the pulmonary hila are very effectively evaluated by tomography. It is possible with tomography to determine if and to what degree the individual bronchi are patent or obstructed. This partial or complete obstruction may occur when a neoplasm develops within the bronchus and bulges into the bronchial airspace or if a tumor grows adjacent to the bronchus. As the lesion grows, it may press against the bronchus, causing a reduction in the size of the lumen and thus restricting or obstructing the airflow to that part of the lung. Pneumonia, atelectasis, and other inflammatory or reactive changes that may occur with the obstruction may further hinder conventional imaging of this area. Demonstration of bronchial patency through a density is strong evidence that the lesion is inflammatory and not malignant (Fig. 29-16).

SOFT TISSUE LESIONS AFFECTING BONY STRUCTURES

Another major application of tomography is to demonstrate and evaluate soft tissue neoplasms in the presence of bony structures. Because of the high density of bone and the relatively low density of the soft tissue neoplasms, it is usually not possible to demonstrate the actual lesion, but it is possible to demonstrate with great clarity the bony destruction caused by the presence of the tumor.

For example, neoplasms involving the pituitary gland usually cause bony changes or destruction of the floor of the sella turcica, which would indicate the presence of a pituitary adenoma. In addition to demonstrating destruction caused by the tumor, it is possible with tomography to demonstrate the bony septations in the sphenoidal sinus, which aids the surgeon in removal of the tumor (Fig. 29-17).

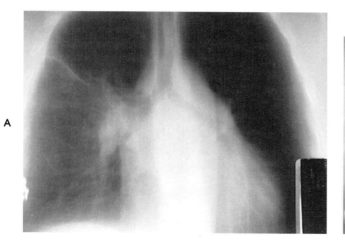
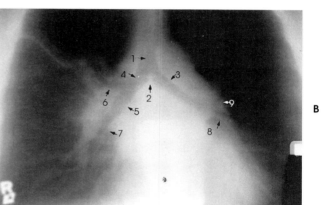

Fig. 29-16. Normal branchotomogram through midplane of hilum. **A,** Linear tomogram. **B,** Trispiral tomogram demonstrating more clearly the hilar structures: *1,* trachea; *2,* carina; *3,* left main bronchus; *4,* right main bronchus; *5,* intermediate bronchus; *6,* right upper lobe bronchus; *7,* right lower lobe bronchus; *8,* left lower lobe bronchus; *9,* left upper lobe bronchus.

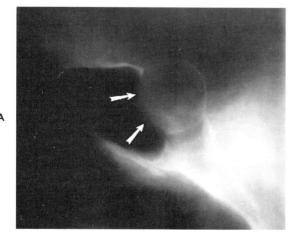
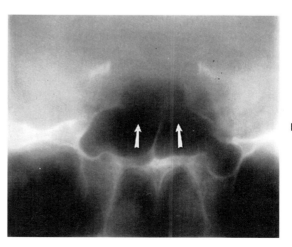

Fig. 29-17. Tomograms through midplane of sella turcica demonstrating destruction of floor *(arrows)* caused by presence of pituitary adenoma. **A,** Lateral tomogram. **B,** AP tomogram.

LESIONS IN BONE

Subtle changes that may occur as a result of a pathologic process in bone tissue may be noted on conventional radiographs, but in many instances only with the aid of tomography can the true nature and extent of the involvement be determined (Fig. 29-18). Pathologic processes involving bony structures are normally characterized by bone destruction and/or changes in the bone tissue or the surface margins. More specifically, in tomography the attempt is made to identify the extent of bone destruction, the status of the cortex of the bone (i.e., whether destruction extends through the cortical bone), the presence of any periosteal reaction to the lesion, changes in the bone matrix, new bone formation, and the status of the zone of the bone between the diseased and normal bone.

Destruction of bone or other alterations in the bone may be the result of a multitude of different benign or malignant processes that manifest themselves in different ways. Some benign processes such as osteomyelitis are presented as areas of bone destruction, whereas others such as osteomas are presented as abnormal growths of bone from bone tissue. Some processes may exhibit a combination of bone destruction and new growth, as occurs in Paget's disease and rheumatoid arthritis.

Malignant neoplasms in bone tissue may occur in the form of primary lesions or secondary lesions resulting from the metastatic spread of cancer from another area of the body.

Some forms of cancer occurring in bone will exhibit areas of both destruction and new growth, whereas others exhibit only areas of extensive destruction.

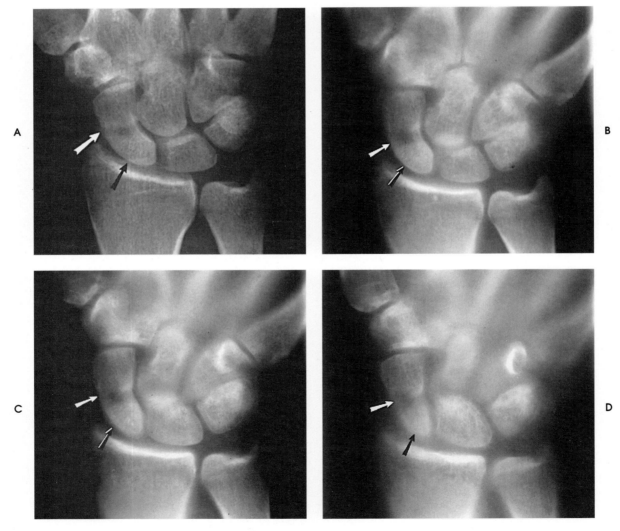

Fig. 29-18. A, PA wrist demonstrating healing fracture *(White arrow)* of scaphoid bone and increased density *(black arrow)* of proximal end. **B, C,** and **D,** Tomograms at 3 mm intervals demonstrating fracture site *(white arrows)* with dense area *(black arrows)* or sclerotic bone at proximal end of scaphoid bone, consistent with aseptic necrosis.

FRACTURES

The three major clinical applications for tomography when dealing with known and suspected fractures are (1) identification and evaluation of occult fractures, (2) better evaluation of known fractures, and (3) evaluation of the healing process of fractures.

If a fracture is suspected clinically but cannot be ruled out or identified by conventional imaging techniques, tomography may be indicated. Tomography is often used when fractures are suspected in areas of complex bone structures such as the cervical spine. The cervical spine projects a myriad of confusing shadows, often hiding fracture lines, making an accurate diagnosis impossible. With tomography it is possible to identify and evaluate these occult fractures (Fig. 29-19). Knowledge of these fractures can be crucial to the patient's plan of treatment and prognosis. Another area that frequently requires tomographic evaluation for occult fractures is the skull. The skull has many complicated bone structures that often make identification and evaluation of fractures in some areas extremely difficult without the use of tomography. The facial nerve canal that courses through the temporal bone is just one of many areas in the skull that are difficult to evaluate for fractures without tomography. Blowout fractures of the orbital floor also frequently require tomographic evaluation because of the difficulty in identifying and evaluating fractures and fragments of the thin bone of which the floor and medial wall of the orbit are composed (Fig. 29-20).

Tomography may also be used to evaluate known fractures with greater efficiency than is possible with conventional radiography. In some instances a fracture may be visualized on a conventional radiograph, but, because of the complex nature of the fracture or superimposition of shadows from adjacent structures, the fracture site cannot be adequately evaluated without the use of tomography. This often is the case in fractures of the hip involving the acetabulum. In acetabular fractures, portions of the acetabulum are often broken into many fragments. These fragments may be difficult to identify, but with tomography the fragments and any possible femoral fracture can be evaluated before any attempt is made to reduce the fracture.

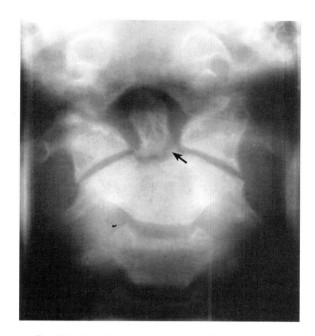

Fig. 29-19. AP tomogram of C1-3 demonstrating complete fracture at base of dens *(arrow).*

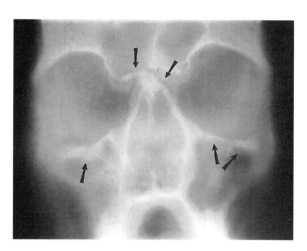

Fig. 29-20. Frontal tomogram in reverse Caldwell method demonstrating multiple facial fractures *(arrows).*

HEALING FRACTURES

Tomography may also be used to evaluate the healing process of fractures when, because of overlying shadows of fixation devices, adjacent structures, or the bone callus, conventional imaging techniques may prove inadequate. In these cases it may be impossible to tell if the bone is healing properly throughout the fracture site without the use of tomography. With tomography it is possible to identify the areas of the fracture when incomplete healing exists (Fig. 29-21).

ABDOMINAL STRUCTURES

Because of the relatively homogeneous densities of abdominal structures, both radiographic imaging and tomographic imaging of this area are most effectively performed in conjunction with the use of contrast materials. Zonography is usually preferred for tomographic evaluation of these organs. As previously stated, zonography produces focal plane images of greater contrast than is possible with thin-section tomography. This increased level of contrast aids in the visualization of the relatively low-density organs of the abdomen. The extensive blurring of remote structures that occurs with wide-angle tomography is not necessary in the abdomen since there are relatively few high-density structures in this area that would compromise the zonographic imaging of the abdominal structures. Thick sections of organs are depicted with each zonogram, and entire organs can be demonstrated in a small number of tomographic sections.

A circular motion with an exposure angle of 8 or 10 degrees is recommended for use in the abdomen. Occasionally, an angle of 15 degrees may be necessary to eliminate bowel gas shadows if the smaller angle does not provide adequate effacement (blurring) of the bowel.

Zonography using a linear movement is not recommended because it does not provide adequate blurring of structures outside the focal plane. If a linear movement is used, an exposure angle of 15 degrees should be used to provide adequate blurring. It should be remembered that linear tomography does not produce accurate focal plane images because of the incomplete blurring effect of structures oriented parallel to the tube movement. Although the possibility of false image formation does exist with circular tomography, the image of the focal plane is far more accurate than with linear tomography. Linear tomograms are higher in contrast than circular tomograms, but this is actually due to the linear streaking caused by the incomplete blurring characteristics of the linear motion. The circular motion, on the other hand, will produce an accurate focal plane image with slightly less but even contrast.

The most common tomographic examinations of the abdomen are of the kidneys and biliary tract. These examinations are normally performed with contrast material.

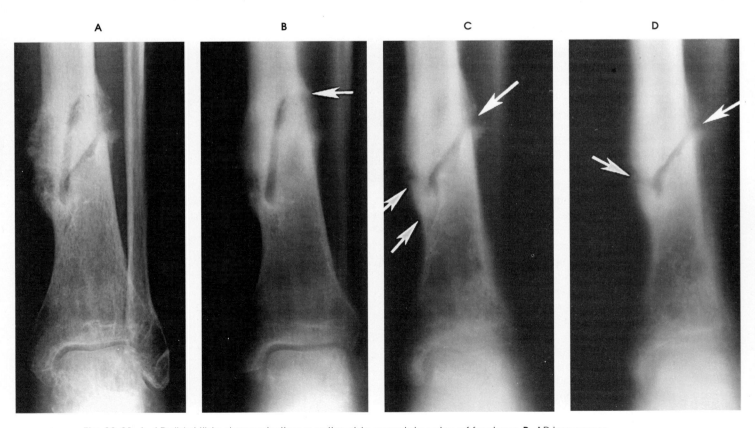

Fig. 29-21. A, AP distal tibia demonstrating questionable complete union of fractures. **B,** AP tomogram of same patient as in **A,** demonstrating incomplete union of longitudinal fracture *(arrow)*. **C** and **D,** Tomograms demonstrating incomplete union of oblique fractures *(arrows)* through shaft of tibia of same patient as in **A** and **B. C,** 0.5 cm and, **D,** 1 cm posterior to **B.**

RENAL TOMOGRAPHY

Many institutions include tomography of the kidneys as part of the intravenous urography (IVU) procedure (Fig. 29-22). The tomograms are usually taken immediately following the bolus injection of the contrast material. At this time the kidney is entering the nephrogram phase of the IVU in which the nephrons of the kidney begin to absorb the contrast material, causing the parenchyma of the kidney to become fairly radiopaque. It is then possible to demonstrate, using zonography, lesions in the kidney that may have been overlooked with conventional radiography alone.

Another typical renal tomographic examination is the nephrotomogram. The major difference between this and the IVU is the method of introduction of the contrast material. In nephrotomography the contrast material is drip-infused throughout the examination instead of introduced in a single bolus injection. This method allows for a considerably longer nephrographic effect, since the nephrons opacify the kidney as they continuously absorb and excrete the contrast material as it is being infused.

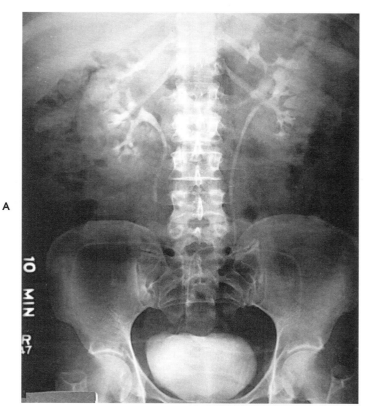

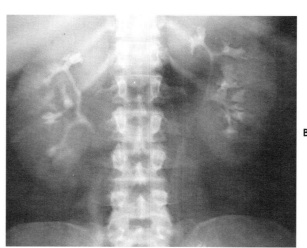

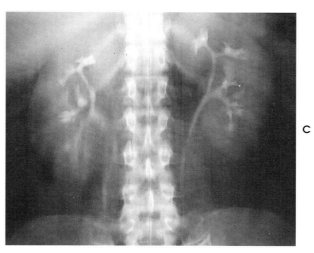

Fig. 29-22. A, Intravenous urogram, AP abdomen. Bowel shadows obscure kidneys. **B,** AP tomogram of same patient as in **A** through midplane of kidneys using 8-degree circular motion. Bowel shadows are absent, and visualization of kidneys is improved over **C. C,** AP tomogram of same patients as in **A** and **B** and at same levels as in **B,** but employing 20-degree linear motion. Note linear streaking and loss of detail of collecting systems and kidney borders.

INTRAVENOUS CHOLANGIOGRAMS

The biliary tract is another organ system that may require tomography for adequate evaluation. If an oral cholecystogram does not yield sufficient information for a diagnosis or if biliary ductal disease is suspected in a cholecystectomized patient, then an intravenous cholangiogram (IVC) may be indicated. The IVC is performed by infusing a solution of the contrast material Cholegrafin into the bloodstream, where it is first absorbed into and then excreted by the liver into the biliary ducts. The drip infusion should be administered slowly over approximately 20 to 30 minutes to reduce the possibility of anaphylactic shock. Opacification of the ducts is generally not dense enough for adequate evaluation with conventional radiography alone. The ducts may also be partially or completely obscured by the superimposition of structures in the abdomen. Even though the ducts may be well opacified on conventional radiographs, tomography should be performed to provide additional information not available with conventional radiography (Fig. 29-23). Zonography is normally used for IVCs; however, there may be instances in which more blurring or a thinner tomographic section is desired. For those instances, a trispiral or hypocycloidal motion may be preferred. If a linear motion is to be employed, an exposure angle of 15 to 20 degrees should be used.

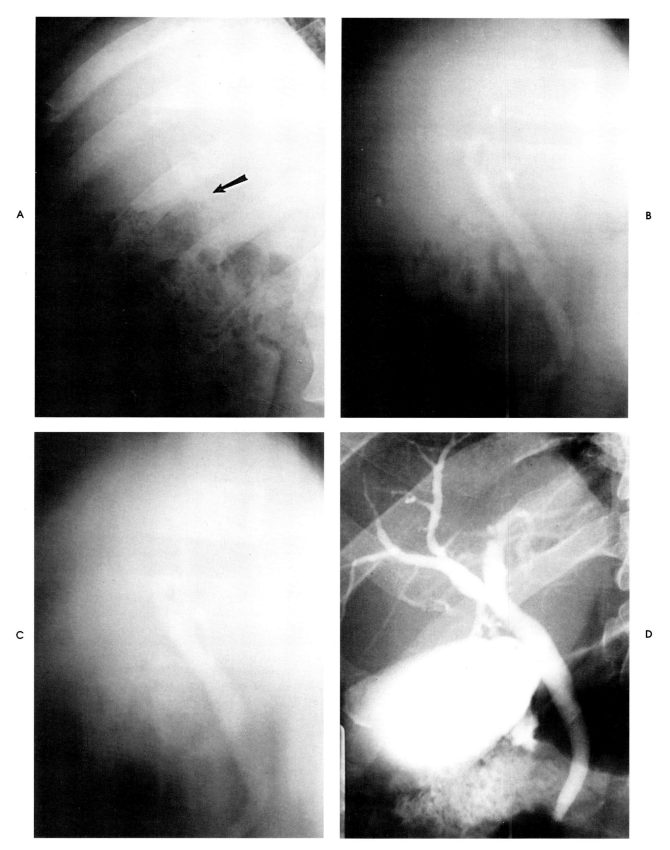

Fig. 29-23. A, Intravenous cholangiogram, AP oblique projection, RPO position. Faintly opacified common bile duct *(arrow)* is obscured by bowel gas and liver. **B** and **C,** RPO tomograms of same patients as in **A** through level of common bile duct. Visualization of duct is improved over plain film study **(A). D,** Transhepatic cholangiogram of same patient as in **A** to **C.**

Basic Principles of Positioning

In conventional radiography rarely does one single radiographic image contain all the diagnostic information necessary to make an accurate diagnosis. This is also true in tomography; one series of tomograms in a single plane usually does not contain enough information to make an accurate diagnosis. As in radiography, two or more image planes are usually required for most tomographic examinations. In the case of bilateral structures, such as the internal acoustic (auditory) canals, only one radiograph may be used. In such cases, tomograms of the contralateral side are made for comparison.

Many fundamental radiographic body positions are used in tomography. The AP and lateral projections are basic to most tomographic examinations. Occasionally, a special oblique projection may be necessary to optimally visualize the part under investigation. The following positioning guidelines are observed.

- In tomography, orient the structures basically either parallel or perpendicular to the tomographic plane. For example, when evaluating structures in the base of the skull, position the patient's head in a basal projection so that the base of the skull will be oriented parallel to the section plane. This parallel position not only produces images that are more anatomically correct but also reduces the total number of tomograms necessary to cover the area of interest. If the base of the skull is not parallel but is slightly obliqued, more tomograms are required to adequately evaluate the area of interest. This also pertains to other areas of the body in which large, relatively flat surfaces occur, such as in long bones.
- When making tomograms of long bones such as the femur, adjust the long axis of the bone to be parallel to the tomographic plane.
- For some structures, such as the sella turcica, use a perpendicular orientation for tomography. Since the presence of a pituitary adenoma usually affects the floor of the sella, orient it perpendicular to the section plane. The AP and lateral radiographs are routinely used for this examination, and in both images the floor will remain perpendicular to the tomographic plane.

There are very few areas in radiology in which the demand placed on the knowledge and ability of the radiographer are as great as in the field of tomography. The tomographer must possess a strong background and understanding of anatomy and of the spatial relationships of the structures of the body. Tomographic radiographers must know where certain structures of the general body parts are located, how to best position those structures for tomographic examination, at what depth the particular structures are located, and how the tomographic image should look. There are many occasions when even the experienced tomographer must rely heavily on the knowledge and instruction of the radiologist monitoring the examination. A close working relationship between the radiographer and the radiologist should exist because no two tomographic examinations are exactly alike and each case must be considered individually. The radiographer should observe the following guidelines when assisting with the tomographic examination:

- Provide the radiologist with an adequate clinical history of the patient.
- Obtain this information from the patient's medical records if it is not provided on the examination requisition or by interviewing the patient.
- Review and discuss this clinical information and any pertinent radiographs with the radiologist before beginning the examination. After reviewing this information the radiologist and radiographer can then decide on the area of interest, the optimum position, the size of the field of exposure, the type of blurring motion and exposure angle to be used, the separation intervals between tomographic sections, and the parameters for the fulcrum height. It is recommended that the most complex motion available be used whenever possible.

- Complete all equipment preparation before positioning the patient. This will reduce the amount of time that the patient is required to maintain an often uncomfortable position.
- Briefly and simply explain the procedure to the patient and offer a rough estimate of the expected length of the examination. Many patients are under the mistaken impression that the procedure consists of a few radiographs taken in a matter of minutes and that they will then be permitted to leave. They are not aware that they will be required to maintain a certain position throughout the procedure. The patient who knows beforehand what to expect will be better able to cooperate throughout the lengthy examination.
- Ensure the patient's comfort, which is extremely important. The use of a suitable table pad is recommended for tomographic examinations. A table pad that is 4 cm thick will add an insignificant amount of distance to the overall patient thickness and will greatly increase the patient's comfort. If the patient is not comfortable, even the most cooperative patient will not be able to hold still for the examination.
- Use angle sponges and foam blocks to assist the patient in maintaining the correct position wherever applicable.
- Do not, however, use foam sponges for use in tomographic examinations of the head. Section intervals of 1 or 2 mm are often employed in this area, and foam sponges do not give firm enough support of the head. With little change in pressure the head may move, drastically altering the desired focal plane levels.
- Use folded towels to support the head if needed; they offer greater resistance to any downward pressure of the head.

Immobilization Techniques

The most effective immobilization technique is the radiographer's instructions to the patient. No amount of physical restraint will keep a patient from moving if he or she does not fully understand the importance of holding still from the first preliminary film to the end of the tomographic series. The radiographer should observe the following guidelines:

- Because suspension of respiration is mandatory in examinations of the chest and abdomen, give explicit breathing instructions to the patient for examinations of these areas.

- In chest tomography instruct the patient to take a consistant, uniform deep breath for each tomogram.

- Caution the patient not to strain to take in the maximum breath since the patient may have difficulty in holding the breath during the exposure.

- Tell the patient to take in a moderately deep breath that can be comfortably held for the duration of the tomographic exposure. This not only allows for optimum inflation of the lungs but also provides consistency between the focal plane levels throughout the tomographic series. This consistency in inspirations is vitally important if the area of interest is located near the diaphragm. Slight variations in the amount of air taken in may result in obscuring the area of interest by the elevated diaphragm. Suspension of respiration is also necessary to prevent blurring of structures by the breathing motion.

- Have the patient suspend respiration in the expiratory phase in examinations of the abdomen to elevate the diaphragm and visualize more of the abdomen. As in chest tomography, the suspension of respiration will assist in maintaining consistency in tissue planes and reduce motion artifacts.

- Use suspended respiration techniques in tomographic examinations of the head if needed. Unwanted motion of the head may occur when obese people or women with large breasts are positioned in the RAO position for lateral skull tomography. This problem may be resolved by having the patient suspend respiration during the exposure or by turning the patient over into an LPO position.

- Mark the entrance point of the central ray on the patient's skin. If the patient does happen to move, he or she can easily be repositioned using this mark as a reference point. This will eliminate the need to take another scout film to recheck the position. If the mark is made with a grease pencil, it can easily be removed at the completion of the examination.

- When performing tomographic examination of the skull in the lateral position, place a small midline mark on the patient's nasion to facilitate measuring for the midline tomogram and to recheck the position between the scout films and the actual tomographic series. By ensuring that this mark is still at the same level from the tabletop, that the interpupillary line is still perpendicular to the tabletop, and that the central ray is still entering at the reference mark, the correct position can be maintained throughout the entire examination.

Scout Tomograms

Three preliminary tomograms are usually taken to locate the correct levels for the tomographic series. One tomogram is taken at the level presumed to be at the middle of the structure or area to be examined. The other two scout tomograms are taken at levels higher and lower than this midline tomogram. The separation interval between these tomograms depends on the thickness of the structure. Tomograms of small structures, such as those found in the skull, may be made at 5 mm or 1 cm intervals for the preliminary films. Once the correct planes have been determined, the tomographic series will be taken at smaller intervals. When the total depth of the area of interest is several centimeters thick, the separation interval for these scout tomograms is increased to 2 cm or more. Table 29-1 includes separation intervals for the preliminary tomograms and the tomographic series. The following guidelines are observed:

- Use external landmarks as reference points to assist in the determination of the proper fulcrum level.
- In some cases, such as chest lesions that can be identified on a PA and lateral chest radiograph, take measurements from these radiographs to aid in the selection of the scout tomogram levels.
- For example, to determine the proper level to a chest lesion for AP tomography, measure the distance on the conventional lateral chest radiograph from the posterior chest wall to the middle of the lesion.
- Then add this distance to the thickness of the table pad.
- Ensure that a scout tomogram taken at this fulcrum height is in the middle of the lesion.
- Use a similar process for tomography in the lateral position taking the measurements from the AP chest radiograph.
- If the area of interest is not localized on the scout films, take a plain radiograph centered exactly as the preliminary tomograms were if necessary. This is done to confirm that the area of interest is actually in the collimated field of interest and recentering is not required.

Table 29-1. Positioning for tomography

Examination part	Projection	Central ray position	Preliminary tomographic levels	Separation intervals	Comments
Sella turcica	AP	Glabella	1.5, 2.5, and 3.5 cm anterior to tragus	2 mm	Shield eyes.
	Lateral	2.5 cm anterior and superior to tragus	−1, 0, and +1 cm to midline of skull	2 mm	Place water bag under patient's chin for support.
Middle ear (internal acoustic canal, facial nerve canal, etc.)	AP	Midpoint between inner and outer canthi	−0.5, 0, and +.5 mm to tip of tragus	1 or 2 mm	Shield eyes.
	Lateral	5 mm posterior and superior to external acoustic canal	At level of outer canthus and 1 and 2 cm medial	1 or 2 mm	Place water bag under patient's chin for support.
Paranasal sinuses (general survey) and orbital floors	Reverse Caldwell	Intersection of median sagittal plane and infra-orbital rims	−2, 0, and +2 cm to level of outer canthus	3 or 5 mm	Infraorbitomeatal line should be perpendicular to tabletop.
	Lateral	2 cm posterior to outer canthus	−3 and +3 cm to midline of skull	3 or 5 mm	Place water bag under patient's chin for support.
Base of skull	Submentovertex	Midpoint between angles of mandible	+1, 0, and −1 cm	2 or 3 mm	Orbitomeatal line should be parallel to tabletop.
Cervical spine	AP	To vertebral body(ies) of interest	0, −2, and −4 cm to external acoustic meatus	3 or 5 mm	
	Lateral	To vertebral body(ies) of interest	−2, 0, and +2 cm from midline of back	3 or 5 mm	Place water bag under patient's chin for support and two or more on neck to equalize density for entire cervical spine.

Table 29-1. Positioning for tomography—cont'd

Examination part	Projection	Central ray position	Preliminary tomographic levels	Separation intervals	Comments
Thoracic spine	AP	To vertebral body(ies) of interest	3, 5, and 7 cm from tabletop	5 mm	Flex knees slightly to straighten spine.
	Lateral	To vertebral body(ies) of interest	−2 and +2 cm from midline of back	5 mm	Flex knees and place sponge against patient's back for support.
Lumbar spine	AP	To vertebral body(ies) of interest	4, 7, and 10 cm from tabletop	5 mm	Flex knees slightly to straightne spine.
	Lateral	To vertebral body(ies) of interest	−2, 0, and +2 cm from midline of back	5 mm	Flex knees and place sponge against patient's back for support.
Hip	AP	Head of femur	−2, 0, and +2 cm from greater trochanter	5 mm	Place water bag over area of greater trochanter to equalize density in hip.
	Lateral (frog leg)	Head of femur	5, 7, and 9 cm from tabletop	5 mm	Place water bag over area of femoral neck to equalize density
Limbs	AP and lateral	At area of interest	5 mm to 1.5 cm depending on size of limb	2-5 mm	Adjust limb to be parallel to tabletop.
Chest (whole lung and hila)	AP	9-12 cm below sternal notch	10, 11, and 12 cm above tabletop	1 cm	Use trough filter (80-90 kVP).
	Lateral	Midchest at level of pulmonary hila	−5, 0, and +5 cm from midline of back	1 cm	Place sponge against patient's back for support.
Chest (localized lesion)	AP and lateral	Measure distance to lesion from chest wall on plain radiographs and center at this point on patient	Measure distance to lesion on lateral chest image and and thickness of table pad; −2, 0, and +2 cm from measurement	2, 3, or 5 cm	Use low kVP (50-65) for high contrast.
Nephrotomogram	AP	Midpoint between xiphoid process and top of crests of the ilia	7 cm for small patient; 9 cm for average patient; 11 cm for large patient	1 cm	Use 8-10° of circular movement or 15-20° of linear movement.
Intravenous cholangiogram	AP oblique, 20 degree RPO	10 cm lateral to lumbar spine	10, 12, and 14 cm for small patient; 12, 14, and 16 cm for average patient; 13, 16, and 19 cm for large patient	5 mm to 1 cm	Use 8-10° of circular movement or 15-20° of linear movement.

General Rules for Tomography

- Know the anatomy involved.
- Position the patient as precisely as possible.
- Utilize proper immobilization techniques.
- Use a small focal spot for tomography of the head and neck and limbs.
- Use a large focal spot for other areas of the body where fine detail is not critical.
- Use low kVp when high contrast is desired.
- Use high kVp when it is necessary to reduce contrast differences between structures; for example, whole lung tomography requires high kVp (80-90) in conjunction with a trough filter.
- Use water or flour bags in other areas when necessary to absorb primary or secondary radiation; for example, in lateral cervical spine tomography place the filter bags on the upper cervical spine area to reduce the density difference between the spine and dense shoulders.
- Collimate the beam as tightly as possible to reduce patient exposure and improve contrast.
- Shield the patient, especially the eyes, in examinations of the skull and upper cervical spine.
- Use the proper blurring motion. In general, use the most complex blurring motion available. Where zonography is required, use a circular motion. If linear motion is the only one available, take care to orient the part correctly to the direction of the tube.
- Mark each tomogram with the correct layer height. This may be done by directly exposing lead numbers on each tomogram or by marking each tomogram after it is processed. Another technique is to vertically shift the right or left marker used on each successive film. By knowing the level of the first film the radiographer can determine the correct level for each successive film. If multiple tomograms are taken on one film, follow the same shift sequence to avoid confusion in marking the layer heights.

TOMOGRAPHY OF SKULL

Strict immobilization techniques must be utilized for any tomographic examination of the skull. Reference points should be marked on the patient for rechecking the position.

The basic skull positions are outlined in the following sections and are to be used in conjunction with Table 29-1.

AP projection

- Adjust the patient's head to align the orbitomeatal line and the median sagittal plane perpendicular to the tabletop.
- Ensure that the distances from the tabletop to each tragus (the tonguelike projection of the ear just in front of the external acoustic meatus) is equal, which indicates that the head is positioned perfectly straight.

AP projection, reverse Caldwell method

- Position the infraorbitomeatal line and the median sagittal plane perpendicular to the tabletop.
- Ensure that the tragi are equidistant from the tabletop.

Lateral projection

- Position the median sagittal plane parallel to the tabletop.
- Ensure that the interpupillary line is perpendicular to the tabletop.
- Check that the orbitomeatal line is approximately parallel to the lower border of the film.

TOMOGRAPHY OF OTHER BODY PARTS

Standard radiographic projections (AP, lateral, and oblique) are utilized for most areas of the body. The same general rules of tomography apply to all areas. In general, the projection that best demonstrates the area of interest in a conventional radiograph is usually the best for tomography. Selected tomograms are shown in Figs. 29-24 to 29-29.

For information on panoramic tomography, which is used to radiographically demonstrate the entire mandible and temporomandibular joint on one film, see Volume 2, Chapter 21 of this atlas.

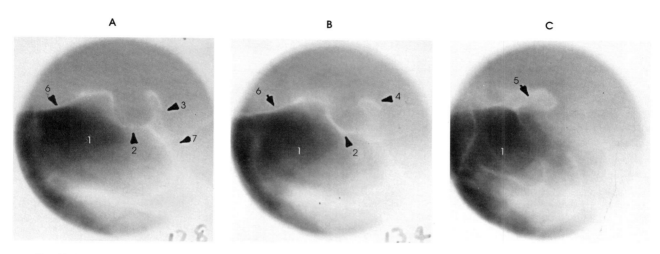

Fig. 29-24. Tomograms of lateral sella turcica. **A,** Through midplane of sella. **B,** 5 mm lateral to **A. C,** 1 cm lateral to **A.** *1,* Sphenoidal sinus; *2,* floor of sella; *3,* dorsum sellae; *4,* posterior clinoid process; *5,* anterior clinoid process; *6,* planum sphenoidale; *7,* clivus.

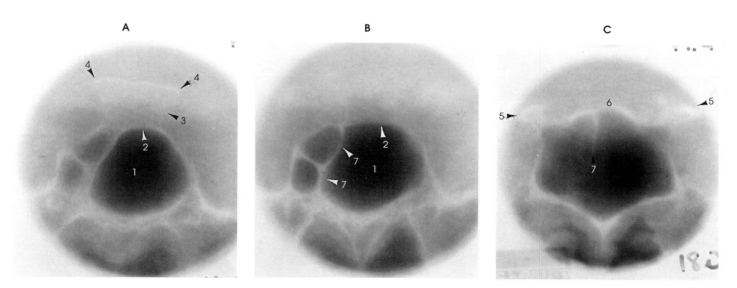

Fig. 29-25. Tomograms of AP sella turcica **A,** Posterior plane of sella turcica. **B,** 1 cm anterior to **A** demonstrating floor of sella. **C,** 2 cm anterior to **A** demonstrating anterior clinoid processes. *1,* Sphenoidal sinus; *2,* floor of sella; *3,* dorsum sellae; *4,* posterior clinoid processes; *5,* anterior clinoid processes; *6,* planum sphenoidale; *7,* septations of sphenoidal sinus.

A

B

C

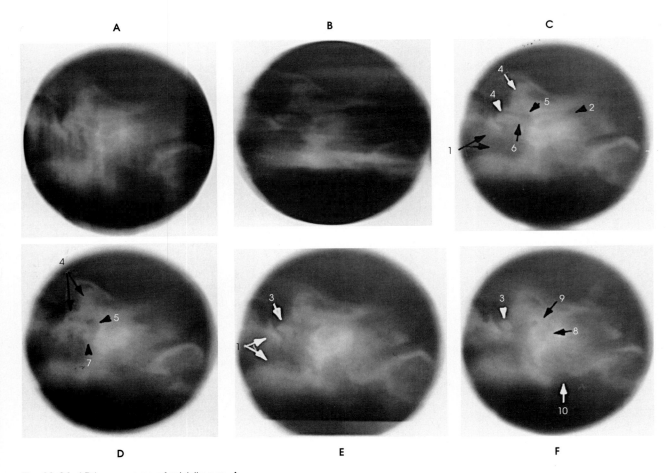

D

E

F

Fig. 29-26. AP tomograms of middle ear. **A,** Longitudinal linear; **B,** transverse linear; and **C,** trispiral motion are at same posterior level of middle ear. Note improved visualization of structures with trispiral motion **(C)**. **D** to **F,** Anterior to level of **C** by 2, 4, and 6 mm, respectively. *1,* External acoustic canal; *2,* internal acoustic canal; *3,* ossicular mass including malleus, incus, and lateral and superior semicular canals *4,* acoustic ossicles; *5,* vestibule; *6,* fenestra vestibuli; *7,* fenestra cochlea; *8,* cochlea; *9,* cochlear portion of facial nerve canal; *10,* carotid canal.

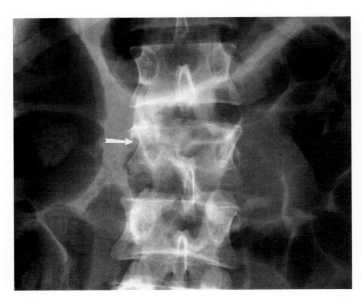

Fig. 29-27. AP lumbar spine showing suspected fracture *(arrow)* of L2 (see Fig. 29-28).

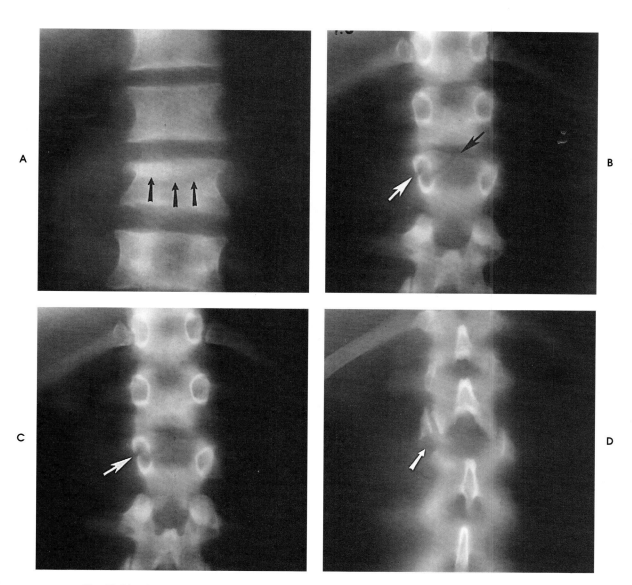

Fig. 29-28. AP tomograms **A** to **D** further delineate fracture site shown in AP radiograph in Fig. 29-27. **A,** AP tomogram through anterior plane of vertebral body. *Arrows,* Wedging of vertebral body of L2. **B,** AP tomogram 2 cm posterior to **A** through plane of pedicles. Fracture line extends through right pedicle *(white arrow)* and vertebral body *(black arrow).* **C,** AP tomogram 3 cm posterior to **A** demonstrating displacement of fracture fragment *(arrow).* **D,** AP tomogram 4 cm posterior to **A** demonstrating displaced fracture *(arrow)* of superior articular process of L3.

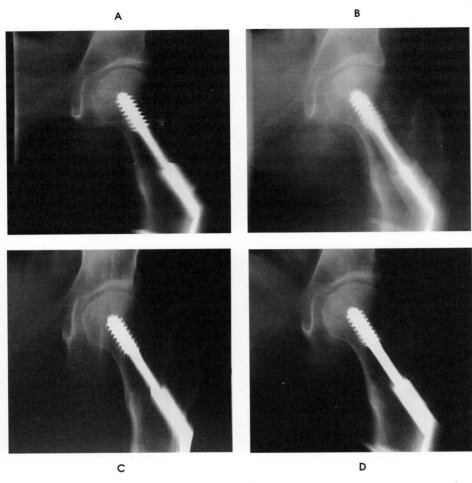

Fig. 29-29. AP tomograms of hip with fixation device at same level comparing different blurring motions; **A,** trispiral; **B,** circular; **C,** longitudinal linear; **D,** oblique linear.

Summary

Tomography has changed dramatically since the early days of Bocage and des Plantes. Their crude devices bear little resemblance to today's modern tomographic machines. Tomography has been widely accepted as an extremely useful diagnostic tool. Linear tomographic machines can now usually be found in even the smallest hospitals. Many large hospitals have one or more linear units in addition to a pluridirectional machine.

Computed tomography (CT) and magnetic resonance imaging (MRI) have certainly proven themselves as extremely valuable diagnostic tools, and in most cases their images are far superior to those of conventional tomography. There are, however, many instances in which tomography can provide sufficient information for an accurate diagnosis, at a cost far less than that of the more sophisticated imaging modalities. Also, most MRI and CT scanners are extremely busy, and many cannot handle the high workload. Conventional tomography can often answer the question satisfactorily or at least screen the patient for further evaluation by the other, more sophisticated imaging modalities.

Although many equipment manufacturers still market a variety of x-ray machines capable of performing linear tomography, the more expensive complex motion tomography units have been dropped from their product lines. Many companies now offer a line of very basic CT scanners at prices comparable to that of a good tomography unit in years past. This has allowed many smaller facilities that would have once opted for a complex motion tomography machine to now purchase CT scanners. Even top-of-the-line scanners are more affordable, making it more feasible to add a second CT scanner than to replace a worn tomography unit with another. In this cost-conscious era, it is likely that tomography will remain for many years a valuable diagnostic imaging tool for large hospitals as well as small.

Definition of Terms

adjustable fulcrum Tomographic fulcrum that is either raised or lowered to achieve the desired fulcrum height. (See planigraphic principle.)

complex tomographic motion (See pluridirectional tomographic motion.)

exposure angle Degree of arc angulation described by the movement of the x-ray tube and film during a tomographic motion.

fixed fulcrum Tomographic fulcrum remains at a fixed height. (See Grossman principle.)

focal plane That plane of tissue that is in "focus" on a tomogram.

fulcrum The point of axis of rotation for a tomographic motion.

Grossman principle Tomographic principle in which the fulcrum or axis of rotation remains at a fixed height. The focal plane level is changed by raising or lowering the tabletop through this fixed point to the desired height.

laminagraphy (See tomography.)

linear tomographic motion Basic tomographic movement that occurs when x-ray tube and film movement occurs with the longitudinal axis of the tomographic table.

phantom images False tomographic images that appear but do not represent an actual object or structure within the focal plane. These images are created by the incomplete blurring or the fusion of the blurred margins of some structures characteristic to the type of tomographic motion used.

planigraphic principle Tomographic principle in which the fulcrum or axis of rotation is raised or lowered to alter the level of the focal plane; the tabletop height remains constant.

planigraphy Synonymous with tomography.

pluridirectional tomographic motion Tomographic motion that moves in many different directions.

section thickness The tomographic plane that is in maximum focus.

stratigraphy Synonym for tomography.

tomographic angle (See exposure angle.)

tomography A radiographic technique that depicts a single plane of tissue by blurring images of structures above and below the plane of interest.

unidirectional tomographic motion Tomographic motion that moves in only a linear direction.

zonography Tomography that uses exposure angles of 10 degrees or less depicting thick sections or zones of tissue.

SELECTED BIBLIOGRAPHY

Andrews JR: Planigraphy. I. Introduction and history, AJR 36:575, 587, 1936.

Berrett A: Modern thin-section tomography, Springfield, Ill, 1973, Charles C Thomas, Publisher.

Bocage AEM: French patent no. 536464, 1922.

Bosniak MA: Nephrotomography: a relatively unappreciated but extremely valuable diagnostic tool, Radiology 113:313-321, 1974.

Chasen MH et al: Tomography of the pulmonary hila: anatomical reassessment of the conventional 55 posterior oblique view, Radiology 149:365, 1983.

Durizch ML: Technical aspects of tomography, Baltimore, 1978, Williams & Wilkins.

Ho C, Sartoris DJ, and Resnick D: Conventional tomography in musculoskeletal trauma, Radiol Clin North Am 27:929, 1989.

Holder JC et al: Metrizamide myelography with complex motion tomography, Radiology 145:201, 1982.

Kieffer J: United States patent, 1934.

Littleton JT: Tomography: physical principles and clinical applications, Baltimore, 1976, Williams & Wilkins.

Littleton JT et al: Adjustable versus fixed-fulcrum tomographic systems, AJR 117:910-929, 1973.

Littleton JT et al: Linear vs. pluridirectional tomography of the chest: correlative radiographic anatomic study, AJR 134:241-248, 1980.

Maravilla KR et al: Digital tomosynthesis: technique for electronic reconstructive tomography, AJR 141:497, 1983.

Older RA et al: Importance of routine vascular nephrotomography in excretory urography, Radiology 136:282, 1980.

Potter GD et al: Tomography of the optic canal, AJR 106:530-535, 1969.

Sone S et al: Digital image processing to remove blur from linear tomography of the lung, Acta Radiol 32(5):421-425, 1991.

Stanson AW et al: Routine tomography of the temporomandibular joint, Radiol Clin North Am 14:105-127, 1976.

Valvasori GE: Laminagraphy of the ear: normal roentgenographic anatomy, AJR 89:1155-1167, 1963.

Chapter 30

THERMOGRAPHY AND DIAPHANOGRAPHY

JACK C. MALOTT

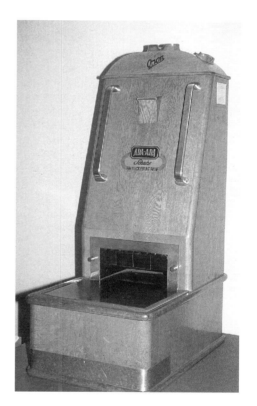

A foot fluoroscope used to fit shoes. Foot fluoroscopes have been illegal in the United States since the 1950s.

THERMOGRAPHY

The use of thermography has declined rapidly in the last 20 years. It is used infrequently today. However, some institutions find this procedure quite useful. We therefore give it our full attention here.

Thermography is the procedure by which the heat naturally emitted by the body is detected, measured, and imaged. The resultant image—the *thermogram**—is a visualization of the distribution of the heat patterns of the body surface. This heat is naturally emitted as a result of normal body function, disease, or injury.

In infrared thermography (the most widely used method of thermography), the heat (infrared) radiation emanating from the skin is detected by a camera in a manner similar to that used in light photography. The infrared radiation is then electronically changed into a signal used to generate an image on a cathode ray tube (typically, a television monitor). This image is then viewed in real time, and the observations are used to properly adjust the equipment. The real-time image can then be recorded electronically but is most commonly recorded photographically (Fig. 30-1). Polaroid film or another photographic paper is often used to record the image. Recording on transparent film in a manner similar to that used for gamma camera, computed tomography, or ultrasound images may also be used. These images are then used for viewing and interpreting the diagnostic findings.

---

*All italicized terms are defined at the end of this chapter.

The above method, in comparison with the following methods, may properly be called *telethermography* because the body heat patterns are detected at some distance (usually a few feet or 1 to 2 meters from the patient's body surface). However, the current practice is to call this method simply *thermography*.

Liquid crystal thermography uses certain chemical substances that are painted or otherwise applied to the body surface. These substances change color depending on the local temperature. These color changes can be either observed or photographed.

Computer-assisted thermography (judged by some as an inappropriate term since computer assistance may be used in any of these applications) is a method that consists of obtaining multiple local temperature measurements over the body surface. A computer program is then used to determine the likelihood of disease by attempting to recognize specific temperature patterns. Microwave thermography measures and images microwave wavelength radiation emanating from the body. Microwave radiations penetrate better through tissues and thus are thought to give a more in-depth representation of the changes in body heat than the more superficial measurements used in infrared thermography.

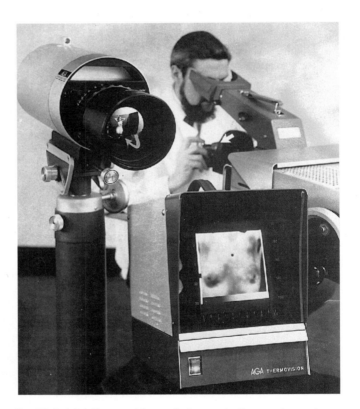

Fig. 30-1. AGA Thermovision unit demonstrating equipment components necessary in thermography. Patient is out of photograph but can be seen reflected in mirror lens of camera *(Curved arrow)*. In foreground is "slave unit" that provides enlargement of conventional cathode ray image, which operator is viewing on control panel in background while adjusting controls *(straight arrow)* of camera. Camera attached to control panel records real-time image on cathode ray tube. Larger slave unit shown here is not in general medical use. This arrangement is for direct scan.

(Courtesy AGA Corp.)

Physics

Infrared radiation is a form of electromagnetic radiation. It is part of the same wide spectrum of wavelike radiations that include radio and light waves, ultraviolet rays, x rays, and cosmic rays. Infrared lies just beyond the red end of the visible spectrum of light and thus has a somewhat longer wavelength and lower energy than light rays. Infrared energy, or heat radiation, is emitted as a function of local temperature. All objects in nature seek to acquire or remain in thermal equilibrium with their surroundings. Thus areas of the skin that are warmer than the surroundings will radiate more infrared rays.

Metabolism generates heat. Local metabolism is often increased in areas of malignant tumor, inflammation, or injury. Circulation and some other body mechanisms contribute to the maintenance of human thermal equilibrium. In the course of these processes, some areas of the skin will be warmer and others cooler. Although heretofore invisible, this spontaneously emitted radiant energy, which is fundamental to all nature, is the physical basis for thermography.

The relationship of temperature to disease has long been recognized as an important factor in medical diagnosis and treatment. The birth of thermal imaging occurred in the early 1950s.

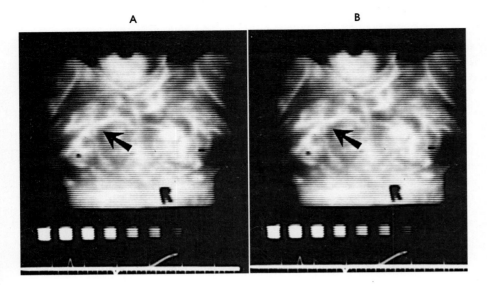

Fig. 30-2. Thermograms made with both types of polarity. **A,** Warmer veins appear white. **B,** Same veins appear black.

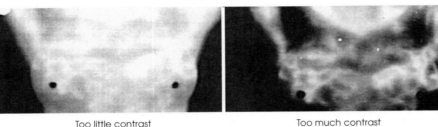

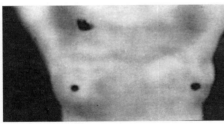

Too little contrast
Range, 6.5°C

Too much contrast
Range, 4°C

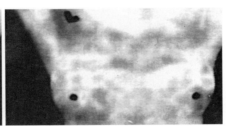

Out of focus
Range, 5.5°C, near correct

Properly exposed
Range, 5°C

Fig. 30-3. Four thermograms of breasts of same patient illustrate importance of proper focus, contrast, and brightness in obtaining thermal image.

Equipment and Methodology

Thermographic technology developed steadily after the introduction of the medical thermogram. Development has slowed since about 1970 as a result of difficulties in establishing the real value of this procedure and the extremely vigorous development of competing imaging diagnostic methods (diagnostic ultrasound, computed tomography, magnetic resonance imaging, and others). Minor advances have been made in the detection systems and the video display chains; since 1970, liquid crystal thermography, microwave thermography, and computer-assisted thermography have all been developed.

An excellent historical summary is provided by Gershon-Cohen,[1] one of the early pioneers of thermography. A description and a categorization of the thermographic instruments have been presented by Curcio and Haberman.[2]

The input of an infrared imaging system is the radiant energy spontaneously emitted by the patient. The output is the image generated by the resulting electronic signal. The detector converts the heat (infrared) radiation received by the camera into an electronic signal that is then further amplified and processed to eventually produce the image. This image must be sufficiently clear to reveal details of temperature differences and must portray the smallest such differences that might have clinical significance.

[1]Gershon-Cohen J: A short history of medical thermometry, Ann NY Acad Sci 121:4-11, 1964.
[2]Curcio B and Haberman J: Infrared thermography: a review of current medical application, instrumentation and technique, Radiol Technol 42:233-247, 1971.

In a typical thermogram, temperature is represented in shades of gray. The most frequently used method represents warmer levels of temperature in lighter shades of gray (whiter areas) and cooler levels in darker shades, although some physicians favor a reversal of this polarity (Fig. 30-2). Most designs provide both types of polarity at the option of the user. In thermographic imaging, focus, contrast, and brightness must be controlled and adjusted (Fig. 30-3). *Focus* refers to the proper distance of the patient from the sensing device and proper adjustment of the lens. *Contrast,* which may also be termed the sensitivity of the particular thermogram, consists of the gradients of tones between black and saturated white displayed on the thermogram. Contrast depicts the range of temperatures, and the sensitivity setting of the instrument should depend on the temperature ranges being emitted by the part examined. *Brightness* relates to the overall lightness or darkness of the thermal image and to the ease with which it can be studied. The most satisfactory brightness for a thermogram is reached when the warmest temperature of the subject approaches, but does not reach, saturated white.

The emitted radiation must be allowed to flow unhampered and unrestricted to the sensing device. The environment in which the patient is examined must be significantly cooler than the surface temperatures of the patient's skin to prevent interference from heat radiation from nearby objects or walls. The patient's clothing must be removed, and the patient is normally required to wait some time for the unclothed area of interest to cool to normal skin temperature. This is because clothing acts as an insulator and allows the temperature of the skin to warm in a more uniform pattern. Additionally, rubbing or scratching of the skin by clothing or other body parts will produce localized elevation of the skin's temperature.

Because infrared radiation travels in a straight line, the patient may be examined by direct scanning, in which case the patient is directly in front of the instrument, or by the use of an angled mirror that will reflect the radiation into the system when the patient is examined in the recumbent position (Fig. 30-4). A body part whose total surface cannot be evaluated in one position must be arranged in several positions to allow evaluation of the entire surface.

In summary, the following steps are observed:

- Uncover the patient's skin and allow it to come to a normal state of temperature distribution.
- Arrange the patient to allow optimum reception of the radiation by the infrared sensing device.
- Adjust the instrument to receive all temperature information being emitted by the source.
- Finally, ensure that the recording method accurately records the thermal image demonstrated at the moment (the real time) of the examination.

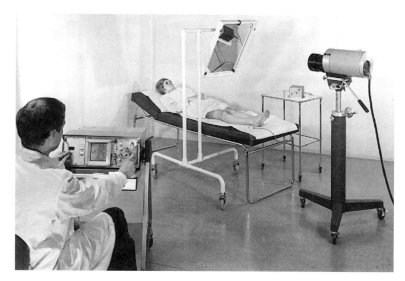

Fig. 30-4. Position of AGA Thermovision for use with reflection mirror. This method is employed when patient can be more conveniently examined in recumbent position. Thermal "real-time" image is displayed on cathode ray tube on control panel.

Selected Clinical Applications

Skin temperatures are the result of normal physiologic processes and disease. They are also influenced by external conditions, such as the temperature of the surroundings, humidity, and evaporation.

BREAST DISEASE

One of the most widely used applications of thermography has been in the detection of breast cancer. It was once widely believed that a detailed qualitative as well as quantitative study of the thermograms was essential. Comparison of the breast image with that of the opposite side breast, with previous thermograms, and with known normal patterns were all considered in evaluation of the thermographic images (Fig. 30-5). The basic principle of the search for malignant tumor was to search for areas of elevated temperature and for disturbances of the heat distribution pattern.

The features favoring the use of thermography for this purpose are that (1) the procedure is totally noninvasive; (2) no ionizing radiation is used; (3) it is fairly fast, convenient, and, compared with other imaging procedures, inexpensive; and (4) because of the above features, it may be readily repeated for comparison purposes and performed without concern for patient safety.

Unfortunately, and despite this promise, efforts to establish thermography as a tool for breast cancer detection have been unsuccessful.[1,2,3] Even now, after nearly 2

decades of investigation, the majority opinion is that thermography is not reliable as a tool in screening for early breast cancer. One reason is that it is relatively insensitive in recording some small tumors. In addition, its inability to achieve reliable and consistent interpretation of the images has not been surmounted. In view of the anticipated advantages, the thermographic method's lack of diagnostic value has been a disappointment. It cannot be recommended today as a reliable tool for breast cancer detection. Except for continuing investigative work and occasional use in special circumstances, thermography is seldom used. The same conclusions apply to liquid crystal thermography, microwave thermography, and other thermographic methods. When any of these procedures are used in detecting breast disease, one has to constantly guard against the false security brought about by an apparently negative thermogram.

The accuracy of thermography for breast cancer detection has been reported to be only 42%, compared with 57% for physical examination and 91% for mammography.[1] Clearly, x-ray mammography is a diagnostically superior tool compared with thermography. The radiation exposure from mammography has been decreasing, and with up-to-date techniques, mammography has a very good risk-versus-benefit ratio (see Chapter 24) and is the recommended imaging procedure of choice for breast cancer detection.[1-4]

[1]Gold RH et al: Breast imaging: state of the art, Invest Radiol 4:298-303, 1988.
[2]Pera A and Freimanis AK: The choice of radiologic procedures in the diagnosis of breast disease, Clin Obstet Gynecol 14(3):635-649, 1987.
[3]Dodd GD: Heat sensing devices and breast cancer detection. In Feig AS and McLelland R, editors: Breast carcinoma: current diagnosis and treatment, New York, 1983, Masson Publishing USA, pp 207-225.
[4]Sickles EA: Breast thermography. In Feig AS and McLelland R, editors: Breast carcinoma: current diagnosis and treatment, New York, 1983, Masson Publishing USA, pp 227-231.

[1]Gold RH et al: Breast imaging: state of the art, Invest Radiol 4:298-303, 1988.
[2]Pera A and Freimanis AK: The choice of radiologic procedures in the diagnosis of breast disease, Clin Obstet Gynecol 14(3):635-649, 1987.
[3]Medicare Program: Withdrawal of coverage for thermography, Federal Register, vol 57, no. 2, pp 54, 798-99, 825, 1992.

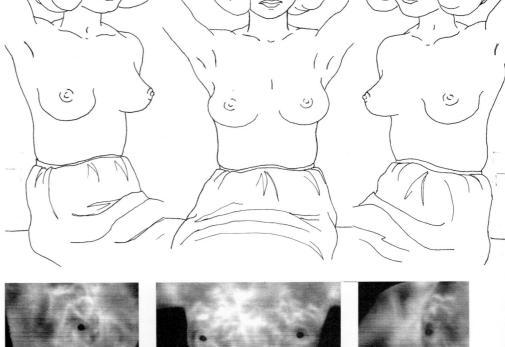

Fig. 30-5. Frontal and oblique positions and corresponding images for routine breast thermography. Frontal position is not sufficient to scan all breast tissue, so that, in addition to frontal surface, the lateral surface of each breast must be turned to sensing device and evaluated separately.

OBSTETRIC APPLICATIONS

Since the placenta is a site of great biologic activity, it is considerably warmer than the surrounding tissues, and thermography has been used for its localization. The advantages of using thermography for localization of the placenta are that it employs no ionizing radiation, it can be used with complete safety to the fetus, and it is not difficult to perform unless the patient is in hard labor.

The patient may be examined in the upright or recumbent position. Scanning is performed under conditions of constant temperature and humidity. All clothing must be removed, and *cross-radiation* must be eliminated by moving the arms well away from the body. Placental studies usually include thermograms made in the frontal and right and left lateral positions.

The placenta, being a warm region, will appear as a light area on the thermogram. Thermography is most accurate in identifying vertical and anteriorly placed placentas (Figs. 30-6 and 30-7). Posteriorly placed placentas are usually so deeply seated that they cannot be imaged by thermography. Thermal scanning does not yield fetal measurements or other details.

Thermography does not provide exact contours; thus ultrasound, which is precise and widely available in hospitals throughout the United States, has become the diagnostic modality of choice for placental localization.

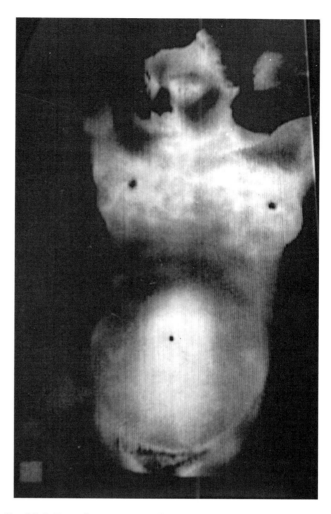

Fig. 30-6. Torso thermogram of a pregnant woman shows large area of increased temperature related to placenta. Breasts also show typically warm appearance associated with increased vascularity and hormonally stimulated physiologic activity of breasts in pregnant state.

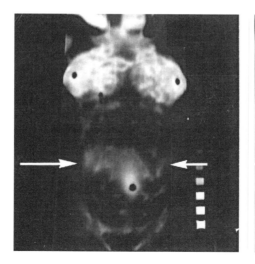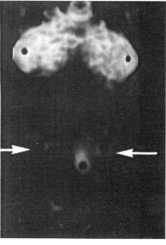

Fig. 30-7. Supine thermogram of 26-year-old woman in last trimester of pregnancy. *White arrows,* high anterior placenta.

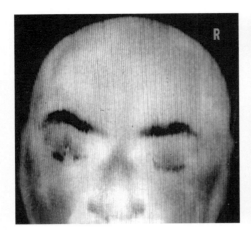

Fig. 30-8. Thermogram of forehead of normal skull shows typical homogeneous appearance.

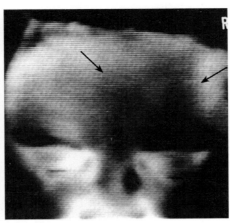

Fig. 30-9. Thermogram of patient with thrombus in right carotid artery. Drop in temperature in right side *(arrows)* reflects decreased right internal carotid artery circulation.

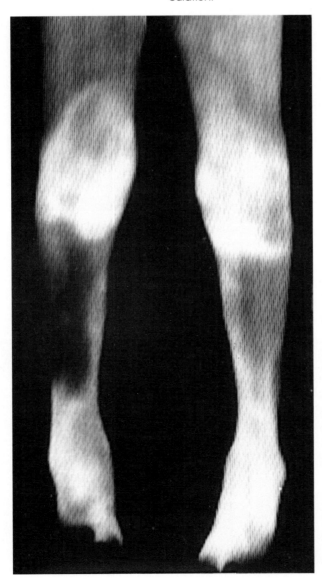

Fig. 30-10. Frontal thermogram of lower limbs of patient with rheumatoid arthritis. Heat is greater over joints. Effects of various therapeutic measures in treatment of arthritis can be monitored by serial thermography.

OTHER MEDICAL APPLICATIONS

Thermography is employed to study rheumatic and other orthopedic diseases, vascular and cerebrovascular diseases, ophthalmologic diseases, and dermatologic diseases (Figs. 30-8 to 30-10). For evaluation of small details, standard roentgenography, angiography, computed tomography, magnetic resonance imaging, and ultrasound are superior. Because of the simplicity of the method, thermography as a study of impairment of circulation or innervation is still used by some medical practitioners. Emphasis was placed on the use of thermography to objectively confirm an organic basis for pain as recently as 1990. Although a normal thermogram does not exclude organic disease as a cause for pain, a positive (abnormal) thermogram is said to confirm an organic cause for the pain. However, there are no well-documented, controlled studies to prove that these findings are indeed reliable.

Summary

The noninvasive and simple diagnostic thermographic procedure created much hope that it would prove to be a useful screening and diagnostic tool. However, other imaging procedures have presently passed thermography in their reliability in producing diagnostic results, as well as in having better sensitivity and specificity. The use of medical thermography declined rapidly in the late 1970s and 1980s as more scientific articles reported on its lack of diagnostic accuracy. In 1984, Medicare discontinued reimbursement for thermography used in the diagnosis of breast disease. In 1992, Medicare discontinued reimbursement for thermography for all indications, stating that while thermography might be a useful screening tool, it has not proven to be a reliable diagnostic test.[1]

In 1993, the American College of Radiology made a similar pronouncement, stating that thermography is not a reliable diagnostic test.

The future of thermography in diagnostic imaging appears to be nonexistent. It may continue to be investigated for screening purposes, but its widespread use in diagnostic imaging is probably doomed by the lack of scientific evidence of its usefulness.

[1]Medicare Program: Withdrawal of coverage for thermography, Federal Register, vol 57, no. 2, pp 54, 798-99, 825, 1992.

Diaphanography is an imaging modality that uses light to examine the breast. Although similar to transillumination, *diaphanography* uses selected wavelengths of light and special imaging equipment. Diaphanography appears to have a place in the screening and diagnosis of breast disease, but it is still under clinical evaluation. Further studies comparing the efficacy of this modality with traditional methods are necessary to define the role of diaphanography in breast examination.

Transillumination is a technique that permits the inspection of a structure's interior by directing light through its exterior wall. Visualization of a structure is dependent on the clarity of the fluids contained, the thickness of the overlying tissue, and the intensity of the transillumination light source, as well as the adaptation of the examiner's eyes. The clinical use of transillumination was first recorded in 1831 by Richard Bright, who used the sun and candles as light sources while reporting an apparent hydrocephalus.

In adults, transillumination has been used to diagnose conditions of the maxillary and frontal sinuses, the breast, and the scrotum. Transillumination has also found uses in the operative suite, including transventricular illumination for the detection of septal defects, vascular visualization to ensure blood supply, and dacryotransillumination during a dacryocystectomy or dacryocystorhinostomy procedure. Fiberoptic transillumination has also been used in dentistry for the detection of decay and cracks in teeth.

These applications have all used light in the visible spectrum. More recently, transillumination techniques of the breast have used other wavelengths of light. This contemporary transillumination technique has been termed *diaphanoscopy* (likened to fluoroscopy for the real-time observation of the image) and diaphanography (likened to radiography for the still-framed recorded images). Both terms are derived from the Greek term "dia," meaning through or across, and "phane," meaning shining, thus translating into "shining through." Diaphanography has also been referred to as "transmission spectroscopy" because it is a combination of transillumination light scanning and spectroscopy. The use of light in the visible and infrared spectra coupled with new electronic and sensing systems is responsible for a renaissance in transillumination. Use of these light spectra is said to allow for the differential absorption of infrared and other wavelengths. Recording can be done with infrared-sensitive film and preferably electronic recording devices. Digital recording of the information allows for computerized reconstruction and image analysis.

The efficacy of diaphanography remains under investigation. Since no ionizing radiation is used, transillumination of the breast is an attractive, but as yet unproven, modality for screening for breast cancer. However, transillumination is not without potential complications. Heat from the light source can cause burns, although this problem can be avoided through careful use and appropriate design of the equipment.[1, 2]

Historical Development

Diaphanography, later termed "breast transillumination," was first reported in 1928; however, early instrumentation was plagued with problems in providing enough light intensity. Differentiation between variations in tissues and the ability to distinguish between solid tumors and cysts without producing extreme heat at the patient's skin were not possible. The low-light intensity used required dark adaptation of the operator's eyes and made photography extremely difficult. Additionally, poor contrast made image interpretation subjective and ultimately led to the short-term abandonment of the technique in the 1940s.

In France, from 1950 to 1970, improved instrumentation was developed, eliminating the problem of heat from the light source; this allowed improved penetration of the breast and photography of the images. The efficacy of this system was still dependent on the operator's ability, and it appeared that the human eye alone was unable to differentiate the various grades of light absorption needed to distinguish between benign and malignant tumors. This posed problems, because the film required special developing, which was available only on a limited basis.[3, 4]

In recent years new dimensions have been added to the transillumination techniques. The use of selected wavelengths to allow comparison of tissue types, coupled with real-time imaging, has made diaphanography more practical. The use of tissue samples suggests that various wavelengths of light are absorbed differently in the layers of tissue through which the light passes.

There seem to be different absorptions for light just as there are for x rays. This would mean diaphanography is more than passing light through tissue with the shadows of the internal structures appearing on the surface of the skin. Comparison of the light absorption characteristics of normal and cancerous tissue samples has shown absorption or spectral differences. Unfortunately, cysts filled with blood or another colored material may produce similar changes, and the extent to which other benign lesions produce similar changes is not known. Further, whether small lesions (less than 1 cm or 5 mm) can be regularly detected is also not substantiated.

[1]Church S et al: Transillumination in neonatal intensive care: a possible iatrogenic complication, South Med J 74:76, 1981.
[2]McArtor RD et al: Iatrogenic second-degree burn caused by a transilluminator, Pediatrics 63(3):422-423, 1979.
[3]Carlsen E: Transillumination light scanning, Diagn Imaging, p 28, April 1982.
[4]Ohlsson BS et al: Diaphanography: a method of evaluation of the female breast, World J Surg 4(6):701-706, 1980.

Diaphanography Equipment

The contemporary instrumentation needed for transillumination includes a light source, a light transilluminator, a special electronic camera, digital processing electronics, a television monitor, and a film imaging system (Fig. 30-11). Because light in the infrared spectrum is used, the system must be capable of converting the infrared light to visible light.

The light source must meet two requirements. First, it must not be hot to the skin, and second, it must have wavelengths that penetrate the tissues. These wavelengths range from 600 nm (6000 Å) through the near infrared waves. The transilluminator functions to evenly spread the light via fiberoptics. Transilluminated light is collected by an infrared optical lens system that formats the information into an image, which is transformed into a raster-scanned or television image. The amplified signal is then available for further processing by analog-to-digital conversion.

The equipment functions by sequentially transmitting light of two different wavelengths through the tissue. Informa-tion from the two images is then digitized and stored in the computer memory. Next, it is processed to an algorithm that super-imposes the information in the two im-ages pixel by pixel. This is accomplished in real time, providing a single video im-age that displays the differential informa-tion in color and intensity brightness on the monitor. This imaging technique is ex-tremely sensitive to variations in tissue characteristics.

Optical Principles

In performing transillumination studies and viewing these images, an understand-ing of the optical principles of transillumi-nation is helpful. A lesion near the surface of the skin will show marked absorption of light at the surface of the skin. As the lesion absorbing the light moves deeper in relation to the skin surface, the image is less discernible for several reasons. First, an object farther from the surface pro-duces more light scatter interference. Sec-ond, the more distant lesion produces a larger halo around the image of the mass; this can be compared with the radi-ographic problem of geometric unsharp-ness with increased object-to-image re-ceptor distance.

These problems can be overcome when imaging deep lesions. First, several views can be obtained to bring the lesion as close to the skin as possible. Second, those wavelengths that do not help with differentiation between lesions and nor-mal tissue can be removed from the light source. This is much like filtering the x-ray beam; "white light," which contains all wavelengths, is detrimental to image quality. One last important factor: as the light's wavelength increases, the amount of scattering decreases; therefore wave-lengths further into the infrared spectrum should produce more contrast for those le-sions deeper in the tissue.

Clinical Applications

The primary application of diaphanogra-phy is in the examination of the breast, al-though other soft tissue structures can be evaluated (Figs. 30-12 to 30-14). Di-aphanography is still in the investigational stage, and further clinical evaluation of this technology is necessary before there is widespread acceptance.

Several reports on the efficacy of di-aphanography have been published. The true-positive rate for carcinoma ranges from 20% to 93%, and the rate for diag-nosing benign lesions ranges from 6% to 36%.

The future of diaphanography lies in its ability to detect an occasional cancer as small as 4 to 6 mm. The sensitivity and specificity need to be established by blinded, controlled, prospective trials be-fore the value of diaphanography can be established. Currently, the use of di-aphanography in the screening and evalu-ation of breast disease should not be sub-stituted for established methods of breast examination but used rather as an adju-vant imaging modality on a selective ba-sis.

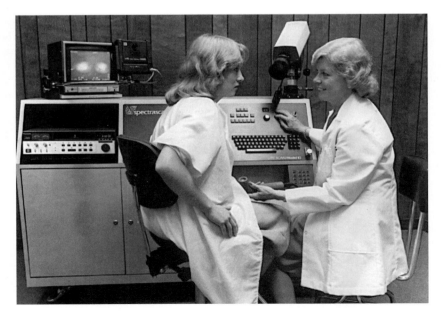

Fig. 30-11. An example of a diaphanography unit. The light source is held in the operator's hand, and the camera is mounted on the console.

(Courtesy Spectrascan Inc.)

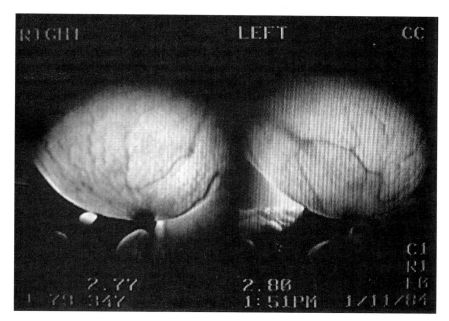

Fig. 30-12. Diaphanography. Vasculature of the breast is demonstrated; note the similar density of both breasts.

(Courtesy Spectrascan Inc.)

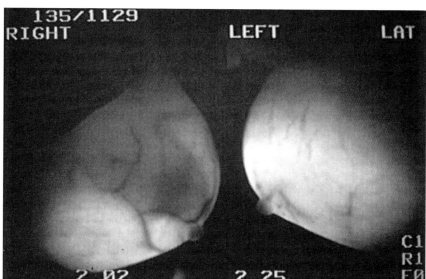

Fig. 30-13. Diaphanography. Patient with a carcinoma of the right breast. The carcinoma *(arrows)* is demonstrated as an increased density as a result of light being absorbed by the lesion.

(Courtesy Spectrascan Inc.)

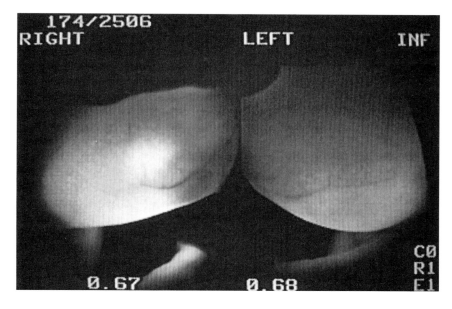

Fig. 30-14. Diaphanography. Patient with a cyst in the right breast. The cyst *(arrows)* allows increased transmission of light and appears as a decreased density.

(Courtesy Spectrascan Inc.)

Definition of Terms

brightness The degree of lightness or darkness of the thermographic image.

contrast The range of gray tones on the thermographic image.

cross-radiation Infrared radiation emanating from adjacent body structures.

diaphanography Transillumination using selected light wavelengths and special imaging equipment.

diaphanoscopy Real-time transillumination.

focus Placement of the patient at the proper distance from the sensing device and the proper adjustment of the lens.

infrared radiation Electromagnetic energy between the red visible light waves and the radio waves having wavelengths between 770 nm (7700 Å) and 12,000 nm (120,000 Å).

telethermography Thermogram made at a distance from the patient's body surface.

thermogram A graphic record of variations in body temperature (heat).

thermography Photographically recording the infrared radiation emanating from the patient's body.

transillumination The passage of light through body tissues for purposes of examination. The part being examined is placed between the light source and the examiner.

SELECTED BIBLIOGRAPHY
Thermography

Andersson I et al: Breast cancer screening and mammography: a population based randomized trial with mammography as the only screening mode, Radiology 132:273-276, 1979.

Anonymous: Comparison of thermography and electromyography, Muscle and Nerve, 14(8):785-787, 1991.

Baer MS and Hetherington: Preliminary report on the use of liquid crystal thermography in podiatry, J Foot Surg 27(5):398-403, 1988.

Baker LH: Breast cancer detection demonstration project: 5 year summary report, CA 32(4):194-225, 1982.

Brooks PG et al: Breast screening in the primary care office: a plea for early detection, J Reprod Med 27(11):685-689, 1983.

Cotton P: AMA's council on scientific affairs takes a fresh look at thermography, JAMA 267(14):1885-1887, 1992.

Curcio B and Haberman J: Infrared thermography: a review of current medical application, instrumentation and technique, Radiol Technol 42:233-247, 1971.

Dodd GD: Heat sensing devices and breast cancer detection. In Feig AS and McLelland R, editors: Breast carcinoma: current diagnosis and treatment, New York, 1983, Masson Publishing USA, pp 207-225.

Feig SA et al: Thermography, mammography and clinical examination in breast cancer screening: review of 16,000 studies, Radiology 122:123-127, 1977.

Gautherie M: Improved system for the objective evaluation of breast thermograms, Prog Clin Biol Res 107:897-905, 1982.

Gautherie M, Kotewicz A, and Gueblez P: Accurate and objective evaluation of breast thermograms: basic principles and new advances with special reference to an improved computer assisted scoring system, International Conference on Thermal Assessment of Breast Health, Washington, DC, July 1983.

Gershon-Cohen J: A short history of medical thermometry, Ann NY Acad Sci 121:4-11, 1964.

Gold RH et al: Breast imaging: state of the art, Invest Radiol 4:298-303, 1988.

Haberman JD, Love TJ, and Francis JE: Screening a rural population for breast cancer using thermography and physical examination techniques: methods and results—a preliminary report, Ann NY Acad Sci 335:492-500, 1980.

Handelsman H: Thermography for indications other than breast lesions. Health Technology Assessment Reports, 1989, US Department of Health and Human Services, no. 2, pp 1-31, 1989.

Heywang-Kobrunner SH: Nonmammographic breast imaging techniques, Curr Op Radiol 4:146-154, 1992.

Isard HJ: Thermography in breast cancer, JAMA 268(21):3074, 1992.

Jeracitano D et al: Abnormal temperature control suggesting sympathetic dysfunction in the shoulder skin of patients with frozen shoulder, Br J Rheuma 31(8):539-542, 1992.

Jones CH et al: Thermography of the female breast: a five year study in relation to the detection and prognosis of cancer, Br J Radiol 48:532-538, 1975.

Kopans DB: Nonmammographic breast imaging techniques: current status and future developments, Clin Obstet Gynecol 25(5):961-970, 1987.

LaBorde TC: Reimbursement for unproven therapies: the case of thermography, JAMA 270(21):2558-2559, 1993.

Lally J: Thermography: a prototype of failed technology, Delaware Med J 65(12):789-90, 1993 (editorial).

Lawson RN: Thermography: a new tool in the investigation of breast lesions, Can Serv Med J 13:517-521, 1957.

Lawson W et al: Infrared thermography in the detection and management of coronary artery disease, Am J Cardiol 72(12):894-896, 1993.

Moskowitz M: Screening for breast cancer: how effective are our tests? CA 33(1):26-39, 1983.

Moskowitz M et al: Lack of efficacy of thermography as a screening tool for minimal and stage 1 breast cancer, N Engl J Med 295:249-252, 1976.

Moskowitz M et al: The potential of liquid crystal thermography in detecting significant mastopathy, Radiology 140:659-662, 1981.

Nyirjesy I: Breast thermography, Clin Obstet Gynecol 25(2):401-408, 1982.

Pera A and Freimanis AK: The choice of radiologic procedures in the diagnosis of breast disease, Clin Obstet Gynecol 14(3):635-649, 1987.

Shapiro S et al: Ten to 14 year effect of screening on breast cancer mortality, JNCI 69(2):349-355, 1982.

Sickles EA: Breast thermography. In Feig AS and McLelland R, editors: Breast carcinoma: current

diagnosis and treatment, New York, 1983, Masson Publishing USA, pp 227-231.

Specchiulli F et al: Acute lesions of the lateral ligaments of the ankle: Clinical and radiographic review, Ital Ortho & Trauma 17(2):261-268, 1991.

Sterns EE et al: Thermography in breast diagnosis, Cancer 50:323-325, 1982.

Tabar L and Gad A: Screening for breast cancer: the Swedish trial, Radiology 138:219-222, 1981.

Thomas D et al: Computerized infrared thermography and isotopic bone scanning in tennis elbow, Annals Rheu Dis 51(1):103-107, 1992.

Vecchio PC et al: Thermography of frozen shoulder and rotator cuff tendinitis, Clin Rheumatol 11(3):382-384, 1992.

Wenth J and Stein MA: Efficacy of breast cancer screening by thermography, Acta Thermographica 0392-0712, pp 76-81, 1983.

Diaphanography

Angquist KA et al: Diaphonoscopy and diaphanography for breast cancer detection in clinical practice, Acta Chir Scand 147:231-238, 1981.

Bartrum RJ et al: Transillumination light scanning to diagnose breast cancer: a feasibility study, AJR 142:409-411, 1984.

Carlsen E: Transillumination light scanning, Diagn Imaging, p 28, April 1982.

Carlsen EN: Transmission spectroscopy: an improvement in light scanning, RNM Images 13(2):23-25, 1983.

Church S et al: Transillumination in neonatal intensive care: a possible iatrogenic complication, South Med J 74:76, 1981.

Cohen SW: Dacryo-transillumination, Am J Ophthalmol 63:427, 1967.

Ersek RA: Mesenteric transillumination for vascular visualization, Surg Gynecol Obstet 152:339, 1981.

Fodor J et al: Diaphanography: transillumination of the breast, Radiol Technol 55(4):97-100, 1984.

Gisvold JJ et al: Comparison of mammography and transillumination light scanning in the detection of breast lesions, AJR 147:191-194, 1986.

Gold RH et al: Breast imaging state-of-the-art, Invest Radiol 21:298-304, 1986.

Gundersen J et al: Diaphanography for assessment of breast changes, Lakartidningen 76:1425-1427, 1979.

Hedley AJ: Breast transillumination using the sinus diaphanograph, Br Med J 283(6291):618-619, 1981.

Holliday HW et al: Breast transillumination using the sinus diaphanograph, Br Med J 283:411, 1981.

Isard HJ: Diaphanography: transillumination of the breast revisited, The Society for the Study of Breast Disease Annual Meeting, Philadelphia, 1980.

Kopans DB: Nonmammographic breast imaging techniques: current status and future developments, Radiol Clin North Am 25:961-970, 1987.

Kuhns LR et al: Diagnosis of pneumothorax or pneumomediastinum in the neonate by transillumination, Pediatrics 56:355, 1975.

Martin JE: Breast imaging techniques: mammography, ultrasonography, computed tomography, thermography, and transillumination, Radiol Clin North Am 21(1):149-153, 1983.

McArtor RD et al: Iatrogenic second-degree burn caused by a transilluminator, Pediatrics 63(3):422-423, 1979.

Monsees B et al: Light scan evaluation of nonpalpable breast lesions, Radiology 163:467-470, 1987.

Morgan PP: Trial of electronic diaphanography for detecting breast cancer, Can Med Assoc J 129:686-687, 1983.

Ohlsson BS et al: Diaphanography: a method of evaluation of the female breast, World J Surg 4(6):701-706, 1980.

Pera A and Freimanis AK: The choice of radiologic procedures in the diagnosis of breast disease, Obstet Gynecol Clin North Am 14:635-649, 1987.

Profio AE et al: Scientific basis of breast diaphanography, Med Phys 16:60-65, 1989.

Shurtleff DB et al: Clinical use of transillumination, Arch Dis Child 41:183, 1966.

Sickles EA: Diaphanography. In Feig SA and Mclelland R, editors: Breast carcinoma: current diagnosis and treatment, New York, 1983, Masson Publishing USA, pp 246-250.

Sickles EA: Breast cancer detection with transillumination and mammography, AJR 142:841-844, 1984.

Spector SL et al: Comparison between transillumination and the roentgenogram in diagnosing paranasal sinus disease, J Allergy Clin Immunol 67:22, 1981.

Thomas BA: Breast transillumination using the sinus diaphanograph, Br Med J 283(6298):1057, 1981.

Watmough DJ: Diaphanography: mechanics responsible for the images, Acta Radiol (Oncol) 21(1):11-15, 1982.

Chapter 31

CARDIAC CATHETERIZATION

STEPHEN T. MONTELLI

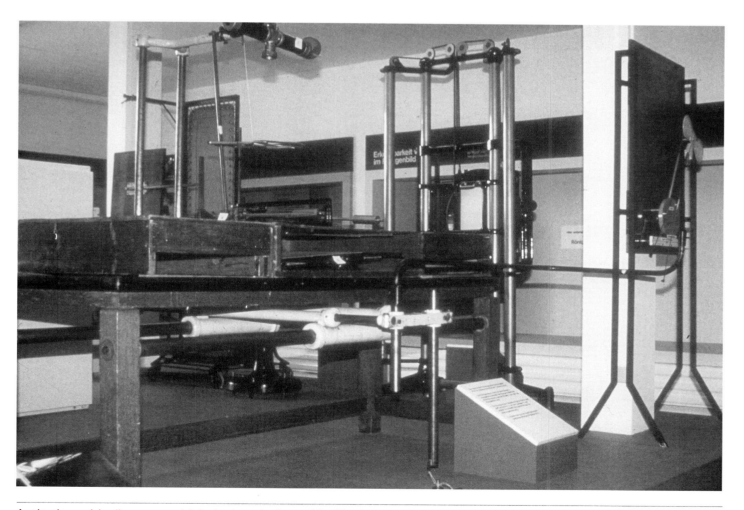

A planigraphic (tomographic) device designed by Ziedses des Plantes. The x-ray tube (top) is attached with a bar to the Bucky tray. The continuous metal bar extends downward to the front side of the Bucky tray assembly. Mounted on the floor is a peg with a string attached. One operator turned the lower bar while a colleague made the exposure. While it was turning, the string wrapped itself around the peg with a spiral movement. The result was a tomographic image.

Cardiac catheterization is a comprehensive term used to describe a minor surgical procedure that involves the introduction of a catheter into the heart and surrounding vasculature for the purpose of diagnostic evaluation and/or therapy (intervention) associated with a variety of cardiovascular-related disorders in both children and adults. National statistics have revealed that the typical adult heart catheterization patient is a male over the age of 45.

Cardiac catheterization can be classified as either a diagnostic study or an *intervention** procedure. The primary purpose for conducting diagnostic studies is to collect information or data necessary to evaluate the patient's condition. Interventional procedures involve applying therapeutic measures such as injecting cardiovascular medications (*thrombolytic* therapy) or inserting specially designed catheters used to treat or improve certain disorders.

---

*All italicized terms are defined at the end of this chapter.

Historical Development

As early as 1844, experimentation in placement of catheters into the hearts of animals led to the successful catheterization of both the right and left ventricles of a horse by French physiologist Claude Bernard. The first human cardiac catheterization was reported in 1929 by Werner Forssman, a 25-year-old surgical resident, who placed a catheter into his own heart, then walked to the radiology department where a chest radiograph was made to document this medical achievement.

Catheterization of the heart soon became a valuable tool used primarily for diagnostic purposes. Through the 1940s the basic catheterization study remained relatively uncomplicated in nature and easy for physicians to perform; however, the risk to the patient was significant.

Physician-operated catheterization methods and techniques increased in number and complexity and were refined in the years that followed. These refinements included the development of the Seldinger (see volume 2, Chapter 26) and transseptal left heart catheter-introduction approaches as well as techniques for selective catheterization of the coronary artery by Sones and Judkins during the 1950s.

During the 1960s and 1970s, tremendous advances in radiologic and cardiovascular medicine and technology occurred. Radiographic imaging and recording equipment, physiologic monitoring equipment, and cardiovascular pharmaceuticals and supplies became increasingly reliable. Since the 1970s, a major emphasis in the field of cardiac catheterization has been the increased dependency, applicability, and diversity of interventional techniques. Application of computers in the catheterization laboratory has also facilitated the development of this rapidly growing and extremely specialized subspecialty of the cardiovascular medical and surgical sciences. These advances and trends have enabled cardiac catheterization to evolve from a simple but hazardous diagnostic investigation to its current state as a sophisticated and low-risk diagnostic study or interventional procedure.

Indications, Contraindications, and Risks

There are general indications, contraindications, and risks associated with diagnostic and interventional cardiac catheterizations. These must be considered by the physician when attempting to determine the appropriateness of conducting any type of catheterization.

GENERAL INDICATIONS

Cardiac catheterization is performed to identify the anatomic and physiologic condition of the heart. Coronary *angiography* is currently the most definitive procedure for visualizing the coronary anatomy. The anatomic information gained from this procedure may include the presence and extent of obstructive atherosclerotic coronary artery disease, thrombus formation, coronary artery collateral flow, coronary anomalies, coronary artery size, aneurysms, and other coronary obstructions such as spasms.

The most common disorder necessitating catheterization of the adult heart is advanced coronary artery disease (nearly 80% of all cases). This disease is caused primarily by the accumulation of fatty intracoronary *atheromatous* plaque leading to *stenosis* and *occlusion* of the coronary arteries. Coronary artery disease is symptomatically characterized by severe chest pain *(Angina pectoris)* or by a heart attack *(myocardial infarction)*. Treatment of coronary artery disease includes both medical and surgical intervention.

One general indication for conducting diagnostic cardiac catheterization of the adult with coronary artery disease is to assess the appropriateness and feasibility of various therapeutic options. For example, cardiac catheterization is performed before open heart surgery to provide essential information such as *hemodynamic* and *angiographic* data to document the presence and severity of disease. In selected circumstances, postoperative catheterization is performed to assess the results of surgery. For relief of *arteriosclerotic* coronary artery stenosis, an interventional procedure called *percutaneous transluminal coronary angioplasty (PTCA)* may be indicated.

Diagnostic studies of the adult heart also aid in evaluating the patient who has confusing or obscure symptoms (such as chest pain of undetermined cause) and to evaluate nonsurgical disease of the heart (for example, certain *cardiomyopathies*).

In children, diagnostic heart catheterization is employed in the evaluation of congenital and valvular disease, disorders of the cardiac conduction system, and certain cardiomyopathies. Interventional techniques are also performed in children primarily to alleviate the symptoms associated with certain congenital heart defects.

"Guidelines for Coronary Angiography," a special report published in the Journal of the American College of Cardiology contains a thorough discussion of the indications for this procedure. These indications include patients with the following disease states:

- Known or suspected coronary heart disease, both symptomatic and asymptomatic
- Atypical chest pain of uncertain origin
- Acute myocardial infarction (evolving, completed, and convalescent)
- Valvular heart disease
- Known or suspected congenital heart disease
- Other conditions (such as disease affecting the aorta and the presence of dilated cardiomyopathy)

These guidelines also indicate the risks, benefits, and utilization of the procedure by placing the above disease categories into three classifications:

- Class 1: conditions for which there is general agreement that coronary angiography is justified
- Class 2: conditions for which coronary angiography is frequently performed but for which a divergence of opinion exists with respect to its justification in terms of value and appropriateness
- Class 3: conditions for which there is general agreement that coronary angiography ordinarily is not justified

CONTRAINDICATIONS AND ASSOCIATED RISKS

Cardiac catheterization, like other surgically related procedures, has associated inherent risk factors. According to Grossman,* however, the only absolute contraindication for heart catheterization is refusal by a mentally competent patient.

Contraindications to perform coronary angiography are relatively few when the appropriateness of the procedure is based on the condition of the patient. Relative contraindications may include the following:

- Active gastrointestinal bleeding
- Renal insufficiency
- Recent stroke
- Fever from infection or presence of an active infection
- Severe electrolyte imbalance
- Severe anemia
- Short life expectancy because of other illness
- Digitalis intoxication
- Patient refusal of therapeutic treatment such as PTCA or bypass surgery.

Some of these conditions could be temporary or treated and reversed before a cardiac catheterization is attempted.

The risk of cardiac catheterization varies according to the type of procedure as well as the individual patient. Variables include the anatomy to be studied, the type of catheter and approach used, history of drug allergy, the presence of basic cardiovascular disease and noncardiac disease (such as asthma and diabetes), hemodynamic status, age, and other patient characteristics.

---

*See the bibliography at the end of this chapter.

The Society for Cardiac Angiography reviewed the catheterizations for 53,581 patients performed in 66 member laboratories from October 1979 to December 1980 and found the overall mortality rate to be 0.14%. Mortality varied from 1.75% in children under 1 year of age to 0.25% in patients over 60 years of age; the vast majority of patients between 1 and 60 years of age had a mortality rate of only 0.07%. The major complication rate reported for the entire group was 1.82%. Major complications included acute myocardial infarction, cardiac arrest, emergency surgery, and death.

The risk associated with cardiac catheterization has decreased dramatically in recent years. It should be noted, however, that as the severity of the patient's disease increases, so does the risk associated with the procedure. Therefore the benefits expected to be derived from cardiac catheterization must be weighed against the associated risk.

Specialized Equipment

Cardiac catheterization has developed into a highly complex, sophisticated procedure requiring equipment and supplies with similar characteristics. Unlike earlier radiographic examinations of the intracardiac structures, modern cardiac catheterization requires more than a simple fluoroscope and a recording modality such as that used in overhead radiography.

Equipment required for cardiac catheterization can be categorized in five groups: (1) cardiovascular, (2) fluoroscopic, (3) cineangiographic, (4) digital imaging, and (5) ancillary equipment/supplies. The following are examples of equipment typically contained in each group.

CARDIOVASCULAR EQUIPMENT
Catheters

Catheters are long, very thin tubes placed into the human vasculature. They are available in various lengths, shapes, diameters, and number of holes. The decision about which catheter to use in a particular circumstance is made by the physician. Cardiac catheters are radiopaque, presterilized, preshaped, and disposable.

The catheter (or catheters) placed into the patient's vasculature can function either as a fluid column for recording pressure data or as a conduit for contrast media and/or drug infusion. Blood samples can be drawn directly from selected cardiac chambers for the purpose of *oximetry* or other laboratory analysis. To accomplish these and other tasks, a system of three or four valves (stopcocks) are combined to form a manifold attached to the proximal end of the coronary catheter (Fig. 31-1). Using a manifold does not require disconnecting the catheter to perform such functions as drawing blood samples, administering medications, or recording blood pressures.

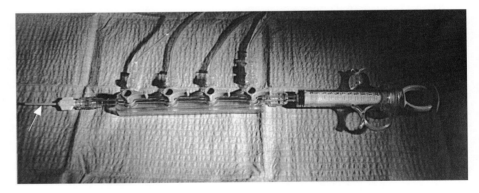

Fig. 31-1. Four-port disposable manifold. Catheter on left side *(arrow)*, three-ring syringe for injection of contrast on right.

Physiologic monitoring equipment

A major piece of equipment integral to cardiac catheterization procedures is a physiologic recorder, which is used to monitor and record vital patient functions including the electrical activity within the heart and certain hemodynamic parameters such as the pressures within various intracardiac chambers (Fig. 31-2). Patients are monitored during the entire catheterization procedure (regardless of the type performed) with periodic electrocardiographic and pressure recordings.

To collect hemodynamic data during the catheterization, it is necessary to connect the physiologic recorder (requiring information in electrical form) to the catheter (carrying information in the form of physical fluid pressure). Devices called *transducers* are interfaced between the manifold and the physiologic recorder to convert fluid (blood) pressure into an electrical signal.

For a standard cardiac catheterization, physiologic recorders usually have four channels, two for ECG recording and two for pressure recording, but can have as many as sixteen. A channel (or module) is an electrical component of the physiologic recorder capable of measuring an individual parameter such as a specific type of electrocardiogram or intravascular pressure. The number of channels required for a particular catheterization increases as the amount of detailed information required increases.

Pressure injector

The pressure injector for the administration of radiographic contrast medium is not only used during catheterization but also in general angiography, as described in Chapter 26 (Fig. 31-3). In the catheterization lab, the pressure injector is generally used for the injection of a large amount (25 to 50 cc) of contrast material into the left ventricle (the main pumping chamber of the heart) or to visualize the aortic root and pulmonary vessels. Administration of contrast medium into the coronary arteries generally does not require the use of a high-pressure injector.

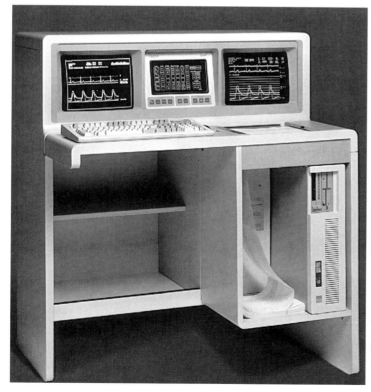

Fig. 31-2. Computer-based physiologic monitor used to monitor patient ECG and hemodynamic pressures during cardiac catheterization.

(Courtesy Quinton Instrument Co.)

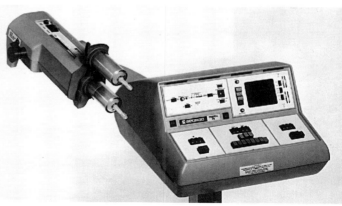

Fig. 31-3. High-pressure injector for radiographic contrast medium.

FLUOROSCOPIC IMAGING

The fluoroscopic imaging equipment found in the cardiac catheterization laboratory is essentially the same as that found in the vascular angiography suite. The goal of fluoroscopy in the catheterization lab is to have an electro-optical system capable of producing fluoroscope images with the greatest amount of recorded detail available. Maximum resolution from the optical system is crucial because of the small size of the cardiac anatomy.

Fluoroscopic tubes must be capable of producing ionizing radiation for the long periods of time associated with fluoroscopy and must therefore be designed to withstand greater heat loading. For most catheterization imaging, multifocal spot, high-speed rotating fluoroscopic tubes are desirable. Extremely short exposure times are required to accommodate the rapid exposure sequencing of the various recording systems.

Operation of a high-resolution imaging and recording system requires several pieces of equipment, including the image intensification tube. The image intensification tube should produce the maximum recorded detail necessary for cardiac catheterization. The image intensification tube used in the cardiac catheterization lab generally comes with a choice of two, three, or four magnification modes to allow for enhanced visualization of small anatomic structures. To view the "live" fluoroscopic image, a television camera is coupled to the output phosphor of the image intensifier, and its signal is fed to television monitors placed so that images can be easily observed during the procedure.

CINEANGIOGRAPHIC AND VIDEOTAPE IMAGE RECORDING

Cineangiography ("cine" meaning film) and videotape systems permanently record the images on film and at the same time allow for immediate playback and review during the procedure. Permanent recording of the cineangiographic image is made on 35 mm, black and white movie film. To accomplish this, a high-resolution motion picture camera is attached to the image intensifier and records the cine image at 30 or 60 frames per second. Cineangiographic recording and videotape recording occur simultaneously.

DIGITAL ANGIOGRAPHIC IMAGE RECORDING

Digital angiography has gained universal acceptance in the catheterization laboratory. Digital imaging now produces resolution comparable to that of the 35 mm cineangiographic film image. The resolution possible with early digital equipment was a drawback to using them in the catheterization laboratory. The obvious solution to this problem, higher matrix sizes, allowed for acceptable resolution but also created another problem: how to acquire and store large volumes of digital information.

In the late 1970s and early 1980s, the high-speed parallel transfer disk (PTD) was introduced to solve the acquisition and storage problem. This new disk acquired and stored an entire coronary angiogram and made real-time digital playback during the procedure possible.

Permanent storage of the digital images remained a problem. Floppy disk and computer tape storage was not an adequate solution because it required significant amounts of time and supplies.

Timely, long-term storage of large amounts of digital information was eventually solved by the optical disk. This relatively new data storage technology has a number of advantages:

- The optical disk holds numerous digital coronary angiograms.
- Images can be transferred at a relatively high speed.
- The optical disk has greater reliability than tape storage systems.
- The entire angiogram can be digitally stored so that there is no loss in image quality over time.

There has been speculation that digital imaging systems will someday replace cine film as the standard for cardiac catheterization laboratory imaging. This has not yet become a reality. The problem of how to easily transport and view digital images persists. While a 35 mm cine film can be viewed on any cine projector, the same is not true for the digital images. Digital images must be downloaded from the computer system to some easily accessible medium, usually ½ or ¾ -inch videotape. Although all catheterization labs have a cine projector to view 35 mm film angiograms, not every catheterization lab has the equipment needed to view these tapes. There is also the problem of reduction in an image quality with a download to videotape.

The cine versus digital question is solved through the use of "simultaneous acquisition" technology, which means that cine film and digital images are acquired at the same time. The practicality of 35 mm cine film is combined with the image manipulation and analysis capabilities (e.g., left ventricular *ejection fraction* calculations and coronary artery stenosis sizing) of digital angiograms.

Digital imaging, as used in the catheterization lab, does not generally mean "digital subtraction." In most catheterization labs, only the "raw" digital image is acquired and displayed because the motion of the heart does not allow for adequate subtractions. The subtracted digital image, except when done with extreme care on a very compliant patient, is usually found to be inferior to the non-subtracted image.

ANCILLARY EQUIPMENT AND SUPPLIES

Because of the nature of the patient's condition and the inherent risk associated with cardiac catheterization, each catheterization room requires a fully equipped emergency cart. The cart typically contains emergency medications, cardiopulmonary resuscitation equipment, defibrillator, intubation equipment, and other related supplies. Oxygen and suction must also be readily available. Oximeters are used to determine the oxygen saturations of the blood samples obtained during adult and pediatric catheterizations (Fig. 31-4).

Several iodinated radiographic contrast media are approved for intravascular, intracardiac, and intracoronary use in both adults and children. Transient (temporary) electrocardiographic changes during and immediately following the injection of contrast medium are common. Administration of nonionic contrast medium or ionic low-osmolar contrast medium is used in many cardiac catheterization laboratories and has gained acceptance because of the properties associated with these media. Unfortunately, the newer contrast media are considerably more expensive. Nonionic contrast media have some definite advantages over ionic high-osmolar contrast media. They display a reduced incidence of cardiovascular reactions and side effects as a result of their lower osmotic pressure. Most catheterization laboratories now use these newer contrast media.

Patient Positioning for Cardiac Catheterization

Procedures such as selective coronary arteriography and certain pediatric catheterizations require that the patient be carefully positioned to reduce the superimposition created by the cardiac vasculature. Moving the patient is not desirable during the catheterization, particularly when catheters have been carefully positioned to demonstrate specific anatomic structures or to record certain data. To obtain optimal images, it becomes necessary to rotate the fluoroscopic equipment (image intensifier and fluoroscopy tube) around the patient.

Normal and pathologic variations in the adult coronary anatomy and pediatric heart exist; therefore, positioning of the patient cannot be specified for each type of catheterization procedure. Each patient's anatomy must be fluoroscopically evaluated to ascertain the optimal degree of rotation and cranial or caudal angulation necessary to visualize each structure of interest.

In many catheterization laboratories, the image intensifier and fluoroscopic tube are mechanically suspended in a C-arm configuration to allow for equipment rotation around the patient and to provide cephalic/caudal angulations as well. In some interventional procedures, biplane C arms prove advantageous because they allow simultaneous imaging of cardiac structures in two different planes (Fig. 31-5).

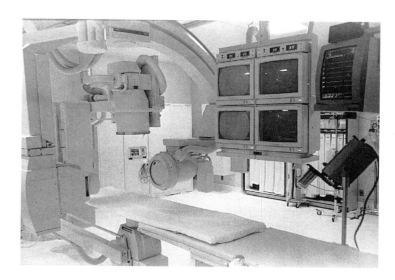

Fig. 31-5. Biplane radiology equipment used in the cardiac cath lab.

(Photo of USC University Hospital Cardiac Cath Lab.)

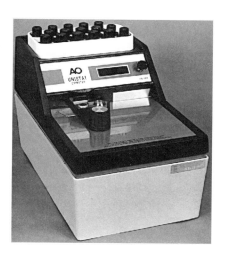

Fig. 31-4. Oximeter used to measure oxygen saturations in blood.

Catheterization Methods and Techniques

Different cardiac catheterizations require various combinations of methods and techniques to allow for precise data acquisition or the application of therapeutic interventions. Some of the methods and techniques common to most cardiac catheterizations are presented.

PRECATHETERIZATION CARE

Patient history, physical examination, chest radiograph, basic blood work, and an electrocardiogram, and other noninvasive cardiology procedures (e.g., echocardiography) are usually performed before cardiac catheterization. Various premedications are frequently administered for sedation and for control of nausea.

Patients brought to the catheterization laboratory are typically not allowed anything to eat or drink for 4 to 6 hours before the procedure. During all catheterizations a protocol or detailed record of the procedure, including fluoroscopy time, medications administered, and supplies used, is maintained.

CATHETER INTRODUCTION

After the patient has been transported to the catheterization laboratory, electrocardiographic (ECG) monitoring is initiated. The appropriate site for catheter introduction must be prepared using aseptic technique to minimize the risk of subsequent infection. Specific sites for catheter introduction are numerous and vary according to patient's age and habitus, physician's preference, and procedure attempted.

For catheterization of the femoral artery or vein, the percutaneous approach is employed (see Seldinger technique detailed in Chapter 26). In the Seldinger technique, the skin is aseptically prepared and infiltrated with local anesthetic. A special angiography needle is used to puncture the skin and is placed into the desired vessel. A guidewire is then advanced through the needle into the artery or vein and the needle removed, leaving the guidewire in the vessel. An introducer, essentially a one-way valve, is placed over the guidewire and slid into place in the vessel. This creates a controlled access into which the catheters may be introduced with very little loss of blood. The catheter is placed over the guidewire and advanced toward the heart. The guidewire may be removed or temporarily left in place to facilitate further placement of the catheter. When the catheter is in the proper position, the guidewire is removed, the catheter is connected to the manifold, and the coronary angiogram may begin.

If the percutaneous approach cannot be used, a cut-down is sometimes employed. The cut-down approach requires that a small incision be made in the skin to allow for the direct visualization of the artery or vein the physician wants to catheterize. The skin is aseptically prepared and infiltrated with local anesthetic, and the vessel or vessels are bluntly dissected and exposed. After an opening is created in the desired vessel (*arteriotomy* or *venotomy*), the catheter is introduced and advanced toward the heart. Cut-downs are frequently performed in the right antecubital fossa to access the basilic or other large medial arm vein or the brachial artery.

Data Collection

The acquisition of certain data is essential regardless of the type of catheterization performed. Physiologic data typically collected include hemodynamic parameters and electrocardiogram and oximetry readings.

Hemodynamic parameters include blood pressure and *cardiac output*. The monitoring and recording of intracardiac (within the heart) as well as extracardiac (outside the heart) vascular pressures require use of the catheter-manifold-*transducer*-physiologic apparatus system described earlier in this chapter. Cardiac output, an important indicator of the heart's overall ability to pump blood, can be measured in the catheterization laboratory. There are several methods used to obtain estimates of the patient's cardiac output. The electrocardiogram is continuously monitored during catheterizations and can be simultaneously recorded with intracardiac or extracardiac pressures (Fig. 31-6). Blood oxygen saturations are determined in various locations.

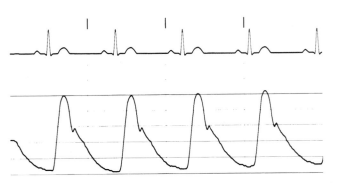

Fig. 31-6. Simulated normal electrocardiogram (top) and simultaneous aortic pressure (bottom).

Catheterization Studies and Procedures

The primary purpose of a diagnostic cardiac catheterization is data collection, and the primary purpose of the interventional procedure is therapy. The following section briefly describes some of the more commonly performed diagnostic and interventional heart catheterizations.

BASIC DIAGNOSTIC STUDIES

Adult

Catheterization of the left side of the heart is a widely performed, basic diagnostic cardiac catheterization study. The catheter may be introduced through the brachial or femoral artery, advanced to the ascending aorta, and passed through the aortic valve into the left ventricle. Arterial oximetry is performed, and pressures are taken in the left ventricle; these measurements are repeated as the catheter is withdrawn across the aortic valve. Selective angiography of the right and left coronary arteries is performed, using different images to allow for the evaluation of the extent of intracoronary stenosis (Figs. 31-7 and 31-8). Coronary arteriograms are obtained in nearly all catheterizations of the left side of the heart.

Selective angiography of the left ventricle is performed in approximately 94% of catheterization studies of the left side of the heart (Fig. 31-9). Left ventriculography provides information related to wall motion that can be used to estimate the ejection fraction.

Catheterization of the right side of the heart is another commonly performed study. A venous catheter is inserted in the groin or antecubital fossa and advanced to the vena cava, into the right atrium, across the atrioventricular (tricuspid) valve, to the right ventricle, and through the pulmonary valve to the pulmonary artery, until wedged distally in the pulmonary artery. Oximetry is performed and pressures are recorded in various locations. Selective cineangiography is performed as appropriate.

It frequently becomes necessary to perform simultaneous catheterization of the right and left sides of the heart. The same limb can be used for catheterization of both sides of the heart. The right-side pulmonary wedge pressure can then be superimposed on the left ventricular pressure and oximetry performed on both sides of the heart.

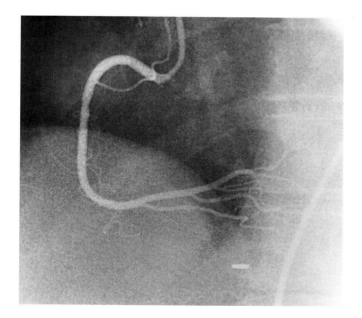

Fig. 31-7. Normal right coronary artery.

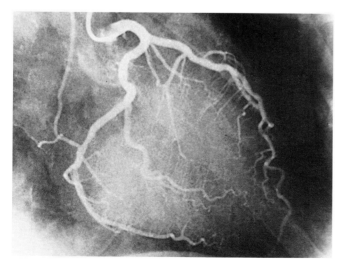

Fig. 31-8. Normal left coronary artery.

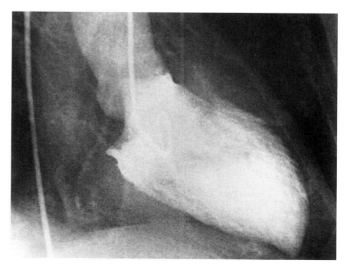

Fig. 31-9. Normal left ventirculogram during diastole.

Pediatric

A primary indication for diagnostic catheterization studies in children is the evaluation and documentation of specific anatomy, hemodynamic data, and selected aspects of cardiac function associated with congenital heart defects. Methods and techniques used for catheterization of the pediatric heart vary depending on the patient's age, heart size, type and extent of defect, and other coincident pathophysiologic conditions.

Pediatric cardiac catheters are often introduced percutaneously into the femoral vein and, sometimes in older children, into the femoral artery. In very young patients, it may be possible to pass a catheter from the right atrium to the left atrium (thereby allowing access to the left side of the heart) through either a *patient foramen ovale* or a pre-existing atrial septal defect. Should the atrial septum be intact, temporary access to the left atrium may be obtained by using a transseptal catheter system. The transseptal catheter system involves the use of a long introducer and needle to puncture that right atrial septum of the heart to gain access to the left atrium when access cannot be attained as previously described.

ADVANCED DIAGNOSTIC STUDIES

Exercise hemodynamics are sometimes required in the evaluation of valvular heart disease, especially mitral stenosis. In such cases a simultaneous catheterization of both sides of the heart is performed including right and left pressures taken at rest, after the legs are raised, and during and after exercise. Exercise often consists of pedaling a stationary bicycle ergometer that is placed on top of the examination table.

Electrophysiology studies, performed on either adult or pediatric patients, involve the collection of sophisticated data that will subsequently allow a detailed mapping of the electrical impulse routes within the heart itself (used in determining the origin and site of heart rhythms and blocks). This technique is employed principally to define and localize disorders of the conduction system of the heart that produce dysrhthmias. After characterization of the precise defect, an appropriate course of therapy can be undertaken.

INTERVENTIONAL PHARMACOLOGIC PROCEDURES

Adult

Interventional pharmacologic procedures in the adult consist of therapeutic intravascular administration of a medication during heart catheterization. An example is the intracoronary infusion of thrombolytic agents such as streptokinase and urokinase, in the catheterization laboratory, during the early hours of an acute myocardial infarction in an effort to modify its course. It is estimated that thrombotic coronary artery occlusion is present in 75% to 85% of patients with acute myocardial infarction. When *reperfusion* of the *ischemic* myocardium is effective, the scarring is reduced. Reperfusion in the early stages of myocardial infarction offers higher potential for heart muscle salvage.

Another thrombolytic agent used in this type of procedure is a somewhat new medication called tissue-type plasminogen activator (t-PA). The research and results associated with this medication have indicated a decreased morbidity and mortality for those receiving the agent during the first 2 hours after the onset of acute myocardial infarction symptoms; thus administration of the medication occurs before the patient is brought to the catheterization laboratory.

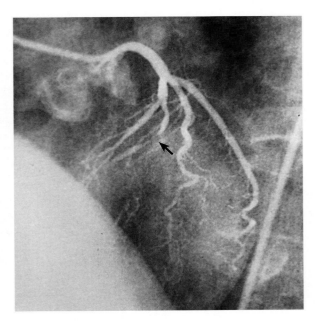

Fig. 31-10. Stenotic coronary artery, pre-PTCA. (*Arrow* indicates the stenotic area estimated at 95% with minimum blood flow distal to the lesion.)

INTERVENTIONAL MANIPULATIVE PROCEDURES

Adult

Interventional manipulative cardiac catheterization techniques requiring special purpose catheters have expanded significantly since the late 1970s. One such technique, percutaneous transluminal coronary angioplasty (PTCA), employs balloon dilation of a discrete coronary artery stenosis. The first successful PTCA was performed in 1977 by Andreas Greuntzig, a Swiss cardiologist.

Following catheterization of the left side of the heart, a specially designed guiding catheter is placed into the orifice of the stenosed coronary artery (Fig. 31-10). Next, a special balloon tip catheter is advanced through the guiding catheter until the balloon section is centered within the stenotic area (Fig. 31-11).

In some cases an over-the-wire balloon system is used. If this type of system is utilized, the wire is first advanced through the balloon catheter and across the stenotic area. The balloon catheter is then advanced over the wire across the stenotic area and inflated. A fixed-wire system allows only a specific amount of wire movement through the lumen of the balloon catheter. The over-the-wire system will allow the wire to cross the lesion first and continue to advance until the balloon portion of the catheter is centered in the stenotic area. Some newer systems employ a balloon attached only to a hollow-core wire. Each of these systems has advantages when used in the proper situation and within the proper vessel. Once the proper balloon is across the stenotic area, slow, precise inflation of the balloon portion of the catheter fractures or compresses the fatty deposits in the muscular wall of the artery. This is documented by the concurrent injection of contrast medium. The catheter is then deflated to allow for the rapid return of perfusing blood to the distal heart muscle. The inflation procedure, followed by arteriography, may be repeated several times until a satisfactory degree of patency is observed (Fig. 31-12). More than one lesion may be dilated during the same procedure. Approximately 70% to 80% of the single-lesion vessels dilated with the PTCA technique remain patent for 1 year after the initial procedure.

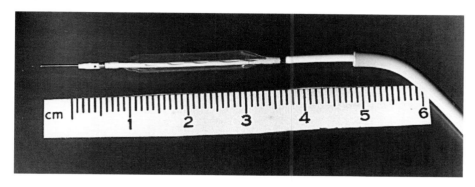

Fig. 31-11. Catheter system for PTCA. The three sections of the system are the outer guiding catheter (right), central balloon catheter (middle), and internal steerable guidewire (left).

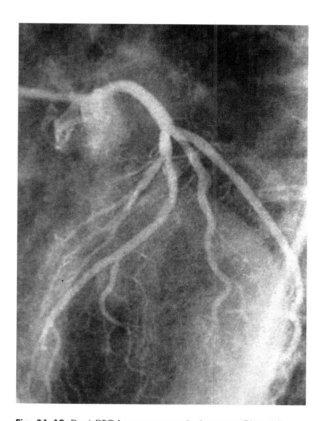

Fig. 31-12. Post-PTCA coronary arteriogram (Blood flow estimated to be 100%). Same patient as in Fig. 31-10.

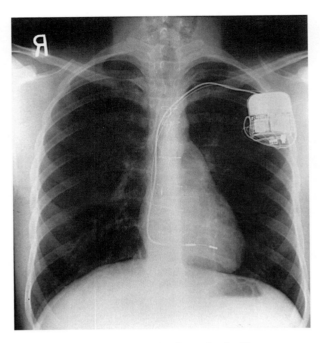

Fig. 31-13. Chest radiograph of a patient with a permanent pacemaker implanted. (Note pacemaker location in the superior and anterior chest wall with distal leads located in both the right ventricle and the right atrium of the heart.)

Because of the inherent risks associated with coronary artery dilation, open heart surgical facilities must be immediately available. Coronary occlusion, for example, is a major complication requiring emergency surgery for the PTCA patient.

Another manipulative interventional procedure being performed with greater frequency in cardiac catheterization laboratories, rather than in operating rooms, is permanent pacemaker implantation (insertion). The procedure can be successfully performed on selected adult and pediatric patients without general anesthesia. Permanent pacemakers are typically used to treat patients with cardiac conduction disorders that are not responsive to medications.

The insertion of a permanent pacemaker usually involves puncture of the subclavian vein and introduction of pacemaker leads that are electrically insulated wires with distal electrodes. The leads are manipulated so that the tip is in direct contact with the right ventricular or right atrial endocardium, or both. The proximal end of the pacemaker lead is then attached to a battery pack implanted in a subcutaneous pocket created in the anterior chest wall (Fig. 31-13). Modern lithium-type batteries can last from 5 to 10 years.

Endomyocardial biopsy provides tissue for direct pathologic evaluation of cardiac muscle. A special biopsy catheter with a bioptome tip is advanced to the right ventricle under fluoroscopy (Fig. 31-14). The instrument is then used to obtain myocardial tissue samples from the septal wall which are submitted for pathologic evaluation. Endomyocardial biopsy is frequently used to monitor cardiac transplantation patients for early signs of tissue rejection.

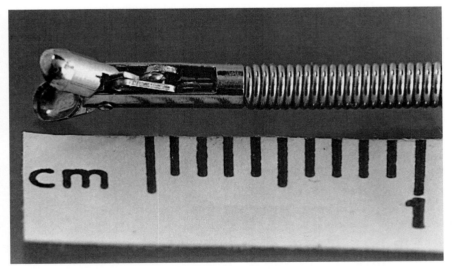

Fig. 31-14. Bioptome catheter tip used for myocardial biopsy. (The jaws on the tip close and take a "bite" from the inside of the heart muscle.)

Pediatric

A number of congenital cardiac defects in children are amenable to interventional procedures that can be performed in the catheterization laboratory. As with PTCA procedures, cardiovascular surgical support services must be readily available.

Certain pediatric interventional procedures, when successful, negate the need for surgical correction of defects. Some procedures, however, are performed for palliative purposes to allow the child to grow to a size and weight at which subsequent open heart surgery is feasible.

One such technique, balloon atrial septostomy, may be used to enlarge a patent foramen ovale or pre-existing atrial septal defect. Enlargement of the opening enhances the mixing of right and left atrial blood, resulting in an improved level of systemic arterial oxygenation. *Transposition of the great arteries* is one condition for which atrial septostomy is performed.

Balloon septostomy requires a catheter similar to the type used in PTCA. The balloon is passed through the atrial septal opening into the left atrium, inflated with contrast media, then snapped back through the septal orifice, causing the septum to tear. It is often necessary to repeat this technique until the septal opening is sufficiently enlarged to allow for the desired level of blood mixing, as documented by oximetry, intracardiac pressures, and angiography.

In cases where the atrial septum does not contain a pre-existing opening, an artificial defect can be created. A special catheter containing an internal folding knifelike blade is advanced into the left atrium employing a transseptal system approach (Fig. 31-15). Once inside the left atrium, the blade is advanced out of its protective outer housing and pulled back to the right atrium, creating an incision in the septal wall. This blading technique may be repeated. A balloon septostomy is then performed to widen the new opening and is monitored by oximetry, pressures, and angiography.

A patent ductus arteriosus is sometimes evident in the newborn. In utero the pulmonary artery shunts its blood flow into the aorta via the ductus arteriosus, which normally closes following birth. Patent ductus arteriosus occurs when this channel fails to spontaneously close. In some instances, closure can be induced with medication. When this is unsuccessful and the residual shunt is deemed significant, surgical closure (ligation) of the vessel is appropriate.

For some patients, occlusion of the patent ductus arteriosus can be accomplished in the catheterization laboratory. A catheter containing an occlusion device (such as an umbrella) is advanced to the ductus. After confirmation of proper positioning in the lesion by angiography, the occluder is released. Subsequent clotting and fibrous infiltration permanently stop the flow and subsequent mixing of blood.

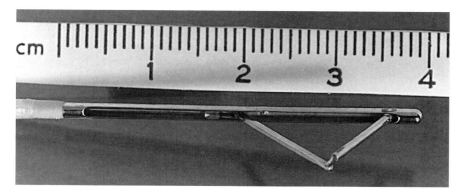

Fig. 31-15. Blading catheter tip used to incise septal walls in pediatric interventional procedures.

Postcatheterization Care

On completion of the catheterization procedure, all catheters are removed. If the cut-down approach was used, the arteriotomy or venotomy is repaired as appropriate. If the percutaneous approach was used, pressure is held on the puncture site until the bleeding in controlled. Wound sites are cleaned and dressed to minimize risk of infection. Elastic dressing are often used to encourage *hematostasis*.

Postcatheterization medications are prescribed by the physician. The puncture site must be observed for hemorrhage, and the status of the distal pulse is recorded on the protocol record before the patient leaves the catheterization laboratory. Vital signs should be monitored on a regular schedule for at least 24 hours after the catheterization. Oral fluids should be encouraged, and pain medication may be indicated. Cardiac catheterization may also be performed on an outpatient or day-treatment basis. In these cases the patient is monitored for 4 to 8 hours in a recovery area and then allowed to go home. Instructions for home care recovery procedures are usually given to the patient or a family member before the patient leaves the recovery area.

Cardiac Catheterization Trends

Techniques and methods for cardiac catheterization will continue to advance at an increasing rate. Angiographic imaging and recording equipment will become even more sophisticated, yielding greater resolution and detail. Development and clinical use of intravascular ultrasonic imaging and other improved computerized image enhancements will allow for more precise data collection and catheter manipulation.

Many experts feel that the greatest area for growth in the field of cardiac catheterization is interventional procedures. Many procedures classified as experimental or investigational in the early 1980s are now being performed with regular frequency. Application of laser technology combined with fiber optic direct visualization of intraluminal pathologic conditions is evolving as a new therapeutic modality for coronary artery disease patients. For example, laser angioplasty of the coronary anatomy is already being performed. In addition, atherectomy devices have also been employed in the treatment of coronary artery disease. The *directed coronary atherectomy (DCA)* procedure uses a specially designed cutting device to shave the plaque out of the lumen of the coronary artery (Fig. 31-16). It is anticipated that many existing and new interventional procedures will provide patients with viable, relatively low-risk, and financially reasonable alternatives to open heart surgery. Current trends indicate that the number and variety of outpatient cardiac catheterizations will continue to increase. It is expected that the equipment used and procedures performed in cardiac catheterization laboratories of the future will be significantly different from those associated with existing facilities. However, despite changes in cardiovascular technology and medical techniques, cardiac catheterization laboratories will continue to provide essential patient care services necessary for the diagnosis and treatment of a vast number of cardiovascular-related diseases.

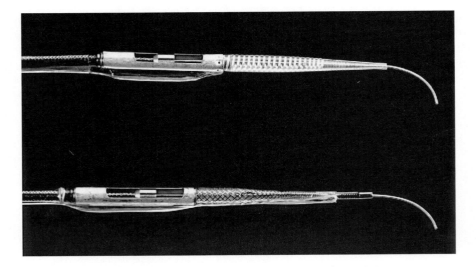

Fig. 31-16. Coronary atherectomy device. (Balloon on the bottom is inflated inside the coronary artery; plaque is forced into the opening, then shaved off and collected in the tip.)

(Courtesy Devices for Vascular Intervention, Inc.)

Definition of Terms

angina pectoris A severe form of chest pain and constriction near the heart usually caused by a decrease in the blood supply to the cardiac tissue. This decrease is most often associated with stenosis of a coronary artery as a result of atherosclerotic accumulations or spasm. Incidence of pain generally lasts for a few minutes and is more likely to occur after stress, exercise, or other activity resulting in an increased heart rate.

angiography The radiographic demonstration of blood vessels following introduction of a contrast material.

arteriosclerotic General pathologic condition characterized by thickening and hardening of arterial walls leading to a general loss of elasticity.

arteriotomy Surgical opening of an artery.

atheromatous Degenerative change in the inner lining of arteries caused by deposition of fatty tissue and subsequent thickening of arterial walls occurring in atherosclerosis.

cardiac output The amount of blood pumped from the heart per given unit of time. The cardiac output can be calculated by multiplying the stroke volume (amount of blood in milliliters ejected from the left ventricle each heart beat) by the heart rate (number of heart beats per minute). A normal, resting adult with a stroke volume of 70 ml and a heart rate of 72 beats per minute would therefore have a cardiac output of approximately 5.0 liters per minute.

cardiomyopathies A relatively serious group of heart diseases typically characterized by enlargement of the myocardial layer of the left ventricle, resulting in decreased cardiac output. Hypertrophic cardiomyopathy is a condition often studied in the catheterization laboratory.

cineangiography High-speed, 35 mm motion picture film recording of a fluoroscopic image while structures contain radiographic contrast medium.

directed coronary atherectomy (DCA) The excision of atheroma via percutaneous transcatheter approach using a rotating cutting device supported by a balloon positioned on the backside of the catheter.

ejection fraction Measurement of ventricular contractility expressed as the percentage of blood pumped out of the left ventricle during contraction. The ejection fraction can be estimated by evaluation of the left ventriculogram. The normal ejection fraction range is between 57% and 73% with an average of 65%. A low ejection fraction indicates failure of the left ventricle to pump effectively.

hematostasis The arrest of blood flow in a hemorrhage.

hemodynamics The study of those factors involved in the circulation of blood. Hemodynamic data typically collected during heart catheterization are cardiac output and intracardiac pressures.

intervention A therapeutic modality, mechanical or pharmacologic, used to reestablish blood flow through a previously occluded artery.

ischemic A local decrease of blood supply to myocardial tissue associated with temporary obstruction of a coronary vessel, typically as a result of a thrombus (blood clot).

myocardial infarction An acute ischemic episode resulting in myocardial damage and pain (commonly referred to as a "heart attack").

occlusion Obstruction or closure of a vessel, such as a coronary vessel, as a result of foreign material, thrombus, or spasm.

oximetry The measurement of oxygen saturation in the blood.

patent foramen ovale An opening between the right atria and left atria that normally exists in fetal life to allow for the essential mixing of blood. The opening normally closes shortly before or after birth.

percutaneous transluminal coronary angioplasty (PTCA) Manipulative interventional procedure involving the placement and inflation of a balloon catheter in the lumen of a stenosed coronary artery for the purpose of compressing/fracturing the diseased material, thereby allowing for subsequent increased distal blood flow to the myocardium.

reperfusion Reestablishment of blood flow to the heart muscle through a previously occluded artery.

stenosis The narrowing or constriction of a vessel, orifice, or other type of passageway.

thrombolytic An agent such as a drug that causes the breakup of a thrombus.

transducer A device used to convert one form of energy into a different form of energy. Transducers used in cardiac catheterization convert fluid (blood) pressure into an electrical signal that is fed into the physiologic recorder.

transposition of the great arteries A congenital heart defect in which the aorta arises from the right side of the heart and the pulmonary artery arises from the left side of the heart. This condition requires interventional therapy.

venotomy Surgical opening of a vein.

SELECTED BIBLIOGRAPHY

Berne R and Levy M: Cardiovascular physiology, ed 4, St Louis, 1981, The CV Mosby Co.

Braunwald E: Heart disease: a textbook of cardiovascular medicine, vols 1 and 2, Philadelphia, 1980, WB Saunders Co.

Daily E and Schroeder J: Hemodynamic waveforms—exercises in identification and analysis, St Louis, 1983, The CV Mosby Co.

Ford RD: Cardiovascular disorders, Ed 4, Philadelphia, 1984, Springhouse Corp.

Freed M and Griles C: Manual of interventional cardiology, Birmingham, 1992, Physicians Press Limited.

Grossman W: Cardiac catheterization and angiography, ed 2, Philadelphia, 1980, Lea & Febiger.

Hurst JW: The heart, ed 5, vols I and II, New York, 1976, McGraw-Hill Book Co.

Topol E: Textbook of interventional cardiology ed 1, Philadelphia, 1990, WB Saunders Co.

Verel D and Grainger RG: Cardiac catheterization and angiography, ed 3, New York, 1978, Churchill Livingstone, Inc.

Zimmerman HA: Intravascular catheterization, ed 2, Springfield, HA: Charles C Thomas, Publisher.

Chapter 32

COMPUTER FUNDAMENTALS AND APPLICATIONS IN RADIOLOGY

JANE A. VAN VALKENBURG

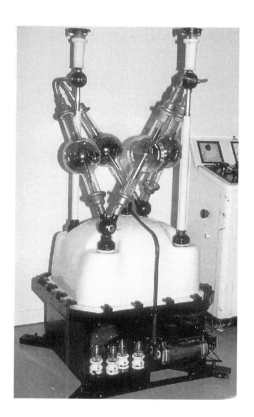

A four valve tube rectifier unit from approximately 1940.

The progressive and evolutionary growth in medicine would not be possible without the aid of computers. As a result of the applications of the computer in the storage, analysis, and manipulation of data, pathologic conditions can be diagnosed more accurately and earlier in the disease process, resulting in an increased patient cure rate. The increasing use of computers in medical science clearly demonstrates the need for qualified personnel who can understand and operate computerized equipment. This chapter is designed to introduce the fundamental concepts and principles of computer technology and to briefly discuss the application of the computer in diagnostic imaging, management utilization, and education.

Definition

The computer is a fast, computational, electronic machine that receives input data, processes the data by performing arithmetic or logical operations using a program stored in its memory, and then generates output data that are displayed on the appropriate equipment. As a machine, the computer is limited to performing arithmetic or logical operations and cannot make rational, diagnostic judgments. However, the development of medical artificial intelligence–based expert computer systems, such as ICON (see below), provides the capability to compare the observations of the radiologist with clinical information and compare this information with similar cases, allowing the radiologist and/or physician to make more informed judgments.

Artificial intelligence may be defined as comparing computer function with human judgment. In medicine, artificial intelligence has been concentrated on developing computer systems that contain detailed data about specific medical subjects. In contrast, the expert computer systems contain vast amounts of data used for making decisions about a specific problem. Expert systems are designed to duplicate the human reasoning process, thereby providing a differential diagnosis or critique of the diagnosis. When the artificial intelligence system and the expert system are integrated, the information generated aids in analytical reasoning and decision making. The artificial intelligence–based expert system used in radiology is known as the IMAGE/ICON system.

Historical Development

The abacus is known as the first "digital" calculator; it was used as early as the 6th century B.C. The abacus is a device with beads strung on parallel wires or sticks, that are attached to a frame.

In 1642 a young Frenchman, Blaise Pascal, built a small mechanical adding device to aid him in his work as an accountant. The device consisted of cogwheels in a box; each cogwheel had ten teeth, and each tooth represented one digit from 0 through 9. As one of the wheels passed from the position of 9 to 0, a small sprocket on the wheel would interdigitate with the next wheel and provide an automatic carry-over. This was the first mechanical adding machine and was known as the "arithmetic machine." The concept is used today in the mechanical paper-tape adding machines and was the forerunner of the clock industry.

In 1694 Gottfried Wilhelm von Leibnitz, using Pascal's "arithmetic machine" concept, developed a mechanism that used step-cylinders instead of cogwheels. The machine could add, multiply, and divide and was known as a "calculating machine." The machines developed by Pascal and Leibnitz, improved by further developments, are the predecessors of the modern keyboard adding machines.

A French inventor, Joseph Jacquard, displayed an automatic weaving loom at the Paris Industrial Exhibition in 1801. The sequence of the loom's operations was based on coded information punched into thick paper cards. The pattern of the tapestry woven on this loom was produced by the holes in the punched cards. The positioning of the threads was determined by the presence and position of the holes on the card. To produce a single tapestry, approximately 24,000 punched cards were used.

In 1822 Charles Babbage, considered the originator of the modern computer, presented an outline for a machine that could calculate celestial tables used to aid in the navigation of ships. Errors in calculating these tables had caused ships to go off course and often resulted in shipwrecks. The machine's calculations were based on the constant variation, or difference, in a series of multiplications, additions, divisions, or squares and could tabulate up to 20 decimals with seven differences. Because this "difference machine," as it was called, required accurate precision in the positioning of the cogs, wheels, shafts, and sprockets, the engineering technology was not available to accurately construct it, although the design was sound (Fig. 32-1). Although he spent 20 years attempting to build this machine, Babbage was never able to complete it.

Meanwhile, Babbage had been presented with one of Jacquard's tapestries and was intrigued by Jacquard's idea of a punched card and its application to constructing a machine to do calculations. In 1834, Babbage presented the principle of what he called an "analytic engine," from which today's computer was developed. Babbage divided the construction of this machine into two main components: the "store," which is comparable to the *memory,** and the "mill," which is similar to the *central processing unit (CPU)* in modern computers. The mill performed the calculations and was controlled by a punched card. The store held the numbers for use as the calculation proceeded. Babbage devoted years of his life to the development of this analytic engine, but unfortunately he never finished it. After his death, the analytic machine was constructed using his complete and detailed drawings.

---

*All italicized terms are defined at the end of this chapter.

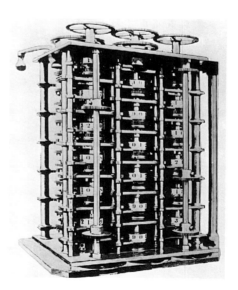

Fig. 32-1. The idea for a "difference machine" that would compute mathematical tables, such as logarithms, was first conceived by Babbage in 1812. After 20 years of labor, financial difficulties compelled him to stop work and the machine was never completed.

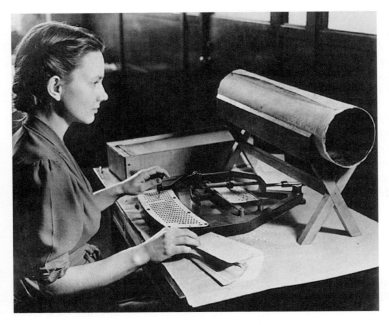

Fig. 32-2. Device used by Hollerith to punch programs, single and manually, in cards.

(Courtesy IBM Corp.)

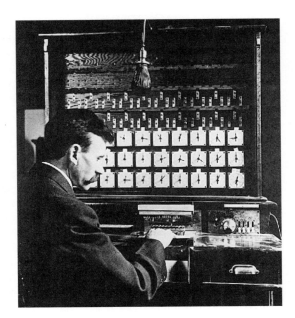

Fig. 32-3. The dial cabinet used by Hollerith to count the holes in the punched cards. The properly punched cards were then filed for future use.

(Courtesy IBM Corp.)

Table 32-1. Important events in computer development

Date	Developer	Event
1937-1944	Howard Aiken, Harvard University	Using Babbage's mechanical design, IBM joined Aiken in the development of Mark 1, an electromechanical, automatic, sequenced-controlled calculator; program sequencing was done with paper tape.
1943-1946	John Mauchley and J. Presper Eckert, University of Pennsylvania	A high-speed electronic calculator, the Electronic Numeric Integrator and Calculator (ENIAC); first machine to use vacuum tubes, which allowed faster switching functions.
1946-1952	John Von Neumann, University of Pennsylvania	Designed a machine with a stored memory, Electronic Discrete Variable Automatic Computer (EDVAC); capable of reading instructions from memory and executing them in proper sequence that allowed programming.
1951	Eckert-Mauchley	The first commercially available computer, Universal Automatic Computer I (UNIVAC), using a stored memory; used by the U.S. Census Bureau-; company later bought by Sperry-Rand Corporation.
1954	Bell Telephone Laboratories	First computer to use solid-state transistors and diodes, Transistor Digital Computer (TRADIC); allowed development of much smaller machines.
1963-1964	Numerous researchers	Integrated circuits and semiconductors; development based on principles presented by Wilhelm Schottky.
1973	Numerous researchers	Miniaturization of electronic circuits or microchips; marketing of the minicomputer to general public.

During the 1880s, Herman Hollerith and James Powers, who worked with the U.S. Bureau of Census, were concerned about tabulating the census for the growing American population and decided that an automatic process for counting the census must be developed. Working independently, they each constructed versions of punched-card tabulating machines, and the 1890 census was tabulated using these machines. Hollerith obtained a patent on his machine and founded a company to further develop his ideas (Figs. 32-2 and 32-3). In 1911 this company merged with two other companies to form the Computer Tabulating Recording Company; and in 1924 this company became the International Business Machine Corporation, IBM, a leader in the development of computer technology.

After 1920 computer development progressed at a rapid rate. For a summary of the important events in the advancement of computer development see Table 32-1.

The significant changes in the development of computers are referred to as *generations*. The notable changes that signify the evolution of computer development are listed in Table 32-2.

Table 32-2. Evolution of computer development

Generation	Development	Date
First	Vacuum tubes	1943-1946
Second	Solid-state transistors	1954
Third	Integrated circuits and semiconductors	1963-1964
Fourth	Silicon chips or microchips	1973

Types of Computers

There are three categories of computers: the microcomputer, the minicomputer, and the mainframe computer. The smallest computer, the microcomputer, usually contains the circuitry or central processing unit (CPU) on a single integrated-circuit chip. The main limitation of this system is that it is typically a one-person or one-function system.

Minicomputers usually have faster responding CPUs and more memory and storage. Unlike most microcomputers, minicomputers are multiuser or *multitasking* systems; several people (2 to 30) may use the system at one time. They are capable of more tasks and can use various programs because they contain several chips or one or more printed circuit boards filled with many integrated circuits.

Mainframe computers are used when there is an increased need for data storage, processing speed, and memory requirements and when the number of users increases. The distinction between the mainframe computer and the minicomputer is becoming less distinct as a result of innovative technology and miniaturization of computer components. Tasks that were once performed only by mainframe computers are now being handled by minicomputers. The advantage of the large mainframe system is its ability to process large amounts of data efficiently (Fig. 32-4). Mainframe computers are used by the U.S. Census Bureau, Internal Revenue Service, large corporations, research libraries, universities, and other organizations requiring the processing, acquisition, and storage of large amounts of information.

The supercomputer is a type of mainframe computer developed to process mathematically intense operations, such as rapid processing of deep-space images for NASA, astronomical projections, and real-time national weather forecasting; this type of computer is currently used by the U.S. Census Bureau. These supercomputers, or maxicomputers, claim to have computing speeds approaching ten billion floating point operations per second, have one billion bytes of memory, and can switch from one transmission state to another in one-thousandth of a billionth second, or one picosecond. The supercomputer will become the fifth generation of computers and incorporate artificial intelligence. The next decade promises revolutionary changes in the development of computer circuitry, resulting in future minicomputers that have the capabilities of maxicomputers and making obsolete the supercomputers presently being used.

The computers used in radiology departments are usually microcomputers and minicomputers. Applications of these computers are divided into two categories: *control* and *data management*. Microcomputers are typically used to control operations in radiographic/fluoroscopic rooms, automatic processing regulation, and rapid film changers. Minicomputers are found in computed tomography units or in any equipment where image reconstruction is performed. Both microcomputers and minicomputers are used for word processing, billing systems, and inventory management. *Real-time* imaging, which is used in ultrasound and digital radiography where immediate data manipulation is important, requires special purpose hardware interfaced with a minicomputer.

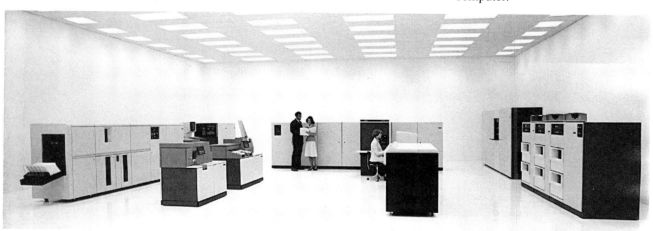

Fig. 32-4. Mainframe computer system with disk drives and magnetic tape memory systems.

(Courtesy IBM Corp.)

Functional Components of a Computer

The term *hardware* is used to describe the functional equipment components of a computer and is everything concerning the computer that is visible. *Software* designates the parts of the computer system that are invisible, such as the *machine language* and the programs. A computer program is a clearly defined set of *instructions* that gives the computer specific tasks to perform. Programs are written in *high-level languages* that are intelligible to the user and translated into machine languages that are then intelligible to the computer.

The computer hardware consists of four functionally independent components (Fig. 32-5): (1) the *input* devices; (2) the CPU, which houses (a) the *control unit* and (b) the *arithmetic/logic unit (ALU);* (3) the *primary memory;* and (4) the *output* devices.

INPUT DEVICES

Input devices are the units that "read" the instructions represented on the input medium (such as a keyboard), transform this information into *binary* digits, and then feed this information to the CPU for processing.

Input media used in the past were punched cards and punched paper tape. Today keyboards (similar to a typewriter) and video *terminals* are common devices used to give instructions to the CPU. The input device reads the coded instructions represented by the holes punched in the cards or paper tape, typed on a keyboard, or drawn directly on a video terminal by means of a light pen attachment. The coded instructions enable the input device to translate the external data into binary representations that can then be handled by the CPU.

Other forms of input devices are magnetic ink readers, *optical scanners,* and magnetic *disks* or tapes. Magnetic ink, made from iron oxide particles, is used to provide direct instructions to the input device. Optical scanners are frequently used by testing agencies to score examinations by using a light or lens system to scan a sheet of paper for information that is then converted to digital information by the input device. Magnetic disks and tapes may contain information or data to be screened and changed to binary representations by the input device (Fig. 32-6).

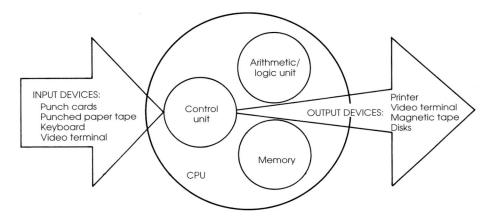

Fig. 32-5. Fundamentals of a computer. Central processing unit (CPU) or operating system.

INPUT DEVICES:
Punch cards
Punched paper tape
Keyboard
Video terminal

Arithmetic/logic unit

Control unit

Memory

CPU

OUTPUT DEVICES:
Printer
Video terminal
Magnetic tape
Disks

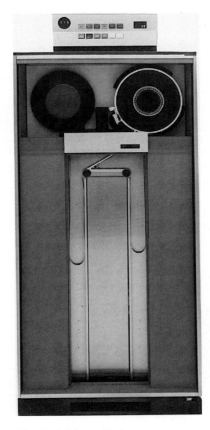

Fig. 32-6. Magnetic tape memory system. The tape loops in the lower center area, and is suspended in vacuum compartment to facilitate the tape passage at high speeds.

(Courtesy IBM Corp.)

CONTROL UNIT

The sequence of events or tasks performed by the computer is regulated and coordinated by the control unit housed within the CPU. The control unit retrieves information from the memory and sends it to the arithmetic/logic unit (ALU) to be processed; after this processing, the control unit then sends that data back to the memory for storage or to the appropriate output device. The function of the control unit is similar to a police officer stationed at a busy intersection preventing mass confusion by directing traffic into the proper lanes in an orderly fashion.

On initiation of a specified program by the operator, the control unit retrieves the information from the memory and sends it to the ALU for processing. On completion of the tasks by the ALU, the control unit transmits the processed information or data back to the memory or to an output device, as instructed by the operator. These functions occur in microseconds, milliseconds, and nanoseconds, depending on the circuitry of the machine, which determines the speed of the functions.

ARITHMETIC/LOGIC UNIT

The arithmetic/logic unit (ALU) does all of the computations, comparisons, and logical operations using binary numbers for additions, subtractions, multiplications, and/or divisions. The control unit determines the numbers to be acted on and what the operation will be. Following the calculations, the information can be displayed immediately or placed in the memory for future use.

The calculations take place within the ALU in areas known as *registers* or "accumulators." To combine two numbers, for instance, the numbers would be called from the memory by the control unit and placed in two separate registers. The control unit passes control to the ALU to perform the computation. When completed, the result is displayed on an output device or sent back to the memory for future use.

MEMORY

There are two types of memory storage: primary and secondary. The primary memory is an integral part of the circuitry and can store data for immediate retrieval when needed. Data contained in the primary memory can be transferred back and forth to the CPU for further calculations. The primary memory is described according to the *storage capacity* and is quantified by the letter K. The letter K is derived from the metric system and denotes the quantity of 1000. However, because 1024 rather than an even 1000 is a mathematical integral power of 2, K stands for 1024 when applied to computer technology. For example, a 256K memory means that approximately 256,000 locations exist within the primary memory for data storage; however, the more accurate figure is 262,144 locations. The memory is divided into small sections called locations, with each location having a storage *address*. The address is usually represented by a number or numbers that the CPU uses to find the information for further processing or display.

Within the primary memory of a computer, there are two types of addressable memory: the *random access memory (RAM)* and the *read only memory (ROM)*. One may read, change, delete, and store on the RAM with immediate access to data; but if the voltage to the computer should suddenly drop or fluctuate, the information is lost unless it has been stored in secondary or auxiliary storage areas, such as magnetic tapes or disks. To correct this deficiency in the primary memory and to prevent the loss of important instructions that are needed to operate the computer without reprogramming for each usage, the ROM was developed; its contents are generally imprinted at the factory. Instructions and information within the ROM are nonvolatile; and whether the computer is on or off, it is not affected. Although the CPU can retrieve the information on the ROM, the information or instructions cannot be changed or deleted or new instructions stored. The ROM is used primarily to secure programs that are used frequently and need to be accessible as soon as the power is turned on.

In computers with a smaller capacity, the ROM may be removed by the operator and changed; for example, the cartridges used for video games. The computers used in a radiology department have a ROM as an integral part of the circuitry that is "burned in" at the factory. When performing diagnostic imaging studies, a very fast transmission of data must occur between the CPU and the ROM; therefore, in these computers the ROM is often located within the CPU. The ROM is a program and is usually considered software. In the types of computers where the ROM is part of the circuitry and is purchased as an integral part of the computer and not separately, it is then referred to as firmware. The ROM can be changed in these special types of computers, but a person skilled in computer circuitry is needed to do the task.

The primary memory, consisting of the RAM and the ROM, is limited in storage capacity; it is relatively expensive to add circuitry for storage purposes. Use of less expensive and mass capacity storage areas is necessary to keep records for long periods of time. The secondary memory storage areas, such as magnetic tapes, disks, and magnetic drums, fill this need. These secondary or auxiliary storage mediums can be removed from the computer and stored separately. When needed, they can then be inserted into a device that is interfaced with the computer, and information can be retrieved from them by use of the storage address.

OPERATING SYSTEM

An operating system is a set of programs to help other programs use the computer and its peripheral devices; for example, printers and video terminals. These sets of programs serve four basic functions: (1) they request programs and cause the computer to execute the instructions in the program; (2) they manage the input and output and use of peripheral devices; (3) they manage the information within the files and the priority of processing; and (4) they manage the information stored in the RAM.

The control unit within the CPU directs the functions of the operating system and sees that the correct programs are performed. The CPU responds to the request for a program, locates the program in the operating system, copies it into a workspace in the primary memory, and begins execution of the program's instructions. An operating system eliminates the need to *write* instructions into every program the operator wishes to perform.

Contained within each operating system are three management systems for instructions, sometimes called "managers." The input/output (I/O) manager coordinates all transfers of information between devices connected to the computer. This manager also knows which peripheral device is connected to what other devices in the computer. This permits each peripheral device to send and receive information in different ways from different locations. The file manager handles all the information that is to be stored in auxiliary storage areas by packing the information into indexed groups. The file manager also keeps track of where individual files are located in order to retrieve the information when it is needed by recording the file name and location with the indexed information groups. When a storage disk or magnetic tape is inserted into the computer, the file manager reads where the file is stored, locates it, and loads (copies) it into a waiting area called a *buffer*. The third manager handles all of the computer's immediate records stored in the RAM.

In an operating system, when a program is requested from an input device such as a video terminal, the CPU monitors the terminal, interprets the request for a program, and then requests the file manager to retrieve the data from the files, unless it is stored in the RAM where it can be immediately found.

The file manager searches its directory for the file needed and loads the file onto a buffer. The file manager reports the file's status to the CPU. If the file is not found, the file manager reports that the file is "not found." If the file is found, the manager informs the CPU that the file is in the buffer.

The CPU then requests that the memory manager reserve a portion of the primary memory for the program. The program moves from the buffer to the designated space and the CPU starts operation of the program.

If the program should need additional memory, or to use a peripheral device, a request is transmitted to the CPU, which then refers this request to the memory manager, I/O manager, or file manager. When the program is completed, the CPU gains control of the system and waits for additional commands.

OUTPUT DEVICES

Output devices display the results of the computations or tasks the computer has been instructed to complete. The most common devices are the video terminal and/or *cathode ray tube (CRT)*, the high-speed printer, and magnetic tapes or *disk drives*. Other types are the card punch and paper-tape punch. These output devices will respond only when directed by the control unit of the CPU.

The copies made by high-speed printers and the information recorded on magnetic tapes or disks provide permanent records of the tasks completed. The printers are usually used when visual data are required, whereas magnetic tape drives and disk drives are used when data need to be stored for records or possible further computations and usage (Fig. 32-7). The data stored on magnetic tapes or disks can be retrieved and displayed on a video screen (CRT) when desired and further data added or deleted.

Mass information is usually stored on magnetic tapes, which are inexpensive and can store millions of pieces of information. The reel-to-reel magnetic tape drives are rather large and the initial cost is quite expensive; therefore, this output device is used when large amounts of information are to be stored.

Magnetic disk drives are the most popular output devices and are called either a "hard" disk drive or a "floppy" disk drive. The hard disks are rigid and larger, can store megabytes (M-bytes) of information, and range in size from a long-playing phonograph record to a compact disk. In 1972 when IBM introduced these "hard" disks, they were called "30-30" disks, or *Winchester disk* drives, because each disk would hold 30 M-bytes of information, now considered a small storage capacity.

Floppy disk drives range in size from 3 1\2 to 8 inches in diameter and are made of a flexible plastic material. These disks or diskettes are lightweight and relatively inexpensive. They are used primarily in microcomputers and minicomputers; however, they have a slower access time and lower storage capacity than other recording media.

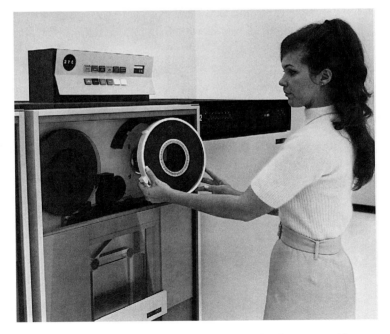

Fig. 32-7. Magnetic tapes may be removed for storage and then retrieved for use at a future date.

(Courtesy IBM Corp.)

Computer Operations
ANALOG COMPUTERS

Unaltered electricity, demonstrated in the form of a continuous sine wave, can be used to run a computer. A computer designed to operate directly from unaltered or continuous electricity is called an *analog computer*. The tasks performed by this type of computer depend on the ability to measure distinctions in the various voltages and the precision of the circuitry. Because the electricity is in an unbroken or continuous sine wave, discrete values are difficult to measure; and if a new or different function needed to be performed, the circuit would have to be rewired.

DIGITAL COMPUTERS

To overcome the inherent problems with analog computers, *digital computers* were developed. Digital computers break up the electricity sine wave into distinct, measurable values (Fig. 32-8). A familiar example of this would be the digital electronic timing system used in sporting events that breaks the time or sine wave into hundredths of a second. A computer is capable of breaking the sine wave into millionths of a second. With this finer digitization, the sine wave would approach an almost smooth-looking curve.

Because digital computers are faster and more accurate, most modern computers are digital. Much of the information from examinations performed in a radiology department is initially in the form of raw or unaltered electricity; therefore, to obtain more uniform and consistent results, the computers contain an *analog-to-digital converter (ADC)* that changes the sine wave into digital form and discrete values.

BINARY SYSTEM

A digital computer operates on a binary system that is similar to the Morse code, but instead of dots and dashes, two digits are used—the 1 and the 0. The American Standard Code for Information Interchange (ASCII) established a standard code consisting of a string of eight zeros and ones referred to as a *byte*. Each individual digit is called a *bit* or *binary digit*. The coded instructions contained in the first four bits tell the computer if the information is a number, letter, or symbol. For example, a prefix of 1011 signifies a number, and 1100 or 1101 a letter, depending on its placement within the alphabet. A different set of instructions represents a method of encoding four bits of memory into a binary representation of one decimal digit or number and is known as a binary coded decimal, or BCD. An example of a binary coded decimal method is $0 = 0000$; $1 = 0001$; $2 = 0010$; $3 = 0011$; $4 = 0100$; $5 = 0101$; $6 = 0110$; $7 = 0111$; $8 = 1000$; $9 = 1001$.

The binary system forms the basis for digital electronics by allowing only two voltage levels. Information is stored by activating electronic switches or "logic gates" to an "off" position, represented by 0, and to the "on" position, represented by 1. By stringing these zeros and ones together, coded instructions are received by the computer as to which function or task to perform.

Integrated, microscopic circuits are etched onto wafer-thin layers of silicon. Each of these silicon layers or chips contains a circuit that has a carefully and specifically designed maze of logic gates or switches. These integrated circuits, or transistors, on each of the silicon chips are then assembled into a larger circuit on a board with the output of one circuit, or transistor, interfacing with the input of another. The circuit boards are designed to enable the computer to perform specialized functions.

Although the complexity of a computer can become enormous as a result of the number of circuit boards involved, the basic circuitry or electronics using the binary system and logic gates remains the same.

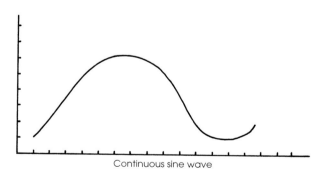
Continuous sine wave

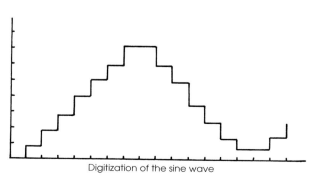
Digitization of the sine wave

Fig. 32-8. A continuous sine wave is used in analog computers. Digital computers use a sine wave broken into distinct time increments.

PROGRAMMING

A computer program is a series of simple arithmetic steps in the binary system that occurs in a millionth of a second in the circuitry of the computer. The construction of the transistors and circuit boards within a computer determines the machine language that must be used to operate a specific computer; therefore, a certain type or brand of computer will operate only on the machine language designed for it.

Computer programs stored within the primary memory or inserted in the secondary memory are known as computer software. When coded instructions are received by the control unit, data are retrieved from the memory and transferred to the ALU in the order of their memory location for computations.

Since the development of computer programs is time-consuming, tedious, and prone to programming errors that can become costly, the computer industry devised what are known as high-level *languages*. These high-level languages can be translated into a specific machine language by special programs called *compilers* or interpreters. Some of the high-level languages developed to perform specific types of tasks that are relevant to a certain field or discipline are listed in Table 32-3.

The use of high-level languages, such as FORTRAN (which is used in imaging processing), has allowed the formation of sophisticated computer systems that can process the large amounts of data generated by the equipment used in a radiology department. The explosive growth of digital imaging modalities has resulted in the development of an integrated medical image management system known as "picture archiving and communication system," or PACS. The PACS system is a group of computer programs that allows a radiology department to electronically acquire images on a terminal or CRT, transport them to various places, store the images, and catalog them on magnetic tapes or optical disks.

Table 32-3. High-level computer languages

BASIC	Beginner's all-purpose symbolic instruction code; the standard language provided with most personal computers.
COBOL	Common business-oriented language; used for financial applications; sometimes used for medical information systems.
ALGOL or PASCAL	Algorithmic language; language used by mathematicians.
FORTRAN	Formula translation; language for scientific programs that performs calculations based on complex formulas.
PL/1	Programming language, verison 1; developed by IBM to replace COBOL, FORTRAN, and ALGOL; used as a literary searcher for filer.
MUMPS	Massachusetts General Hospital utility multiprogramming system; originally developed for medical information–processing applications; most radiology information management systems have been developed from this language.

Applications in Radiology

Although the CPU of a computer system defines the processing of data, the *interface* with the *peripheral* input/output devices is important in radiology. The various imaging modalities depend on specific peripheral imaging devices that interface with a computer; therefore, in the purchase of a computer system, an important consideration is the ability to upgrade the system to accommodate the newer peripherals.

BASICS OF INTERFACING PERIPHERAL DEVICES

The transfer of data between the CPU, memory, and input/output devices must occur rapidly when an examination is performed in a radiology department. To enable computers to process this rapid influx of data, a "bus" structure was developed to provide standardization and flexibility in the operating system. The bus consists of parallel conductors on a circuit board, known as a "mother" board. The circuit boards that contain the CPU, memory, and the interface to the peripheral input/output devices are plugged into the mother board, allowing communication with each other by way of the bus.

The parallel conductors on the bus serve in three definite capacities: (1) as address lines, which select a memory location or a specific input/output interface; (2) as data lines, which carry a specified number of data bits; and (3) as control lines, which carry the timing, status, and initiation of signals from one device to another. Because the bus communicates the data to and from the CPU by means of these parallel circuits instead of a string of serial bits, the processing is many times faster (Fig. 32-9).

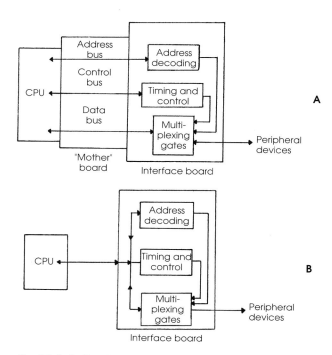

Fig. 32-9. A, Simplified diagram of bus system. Allows rapid data transfer, up to 32 bits at a time. **B,** Data transferred to CPU in a serial or single string of bits; takes much longer for transmission.

ANALOG-TO-DIGITAL CONVERTERS AND VIDEO IMAGE PROCESSORS

Devices that produce images of real objects, such as patients, produce an analog rather than digital signal. The electrical signal being emitted from the output phosphor of an image intensifier on a fluoroscopic unit, the scintillation crystal of a nuclear medicine detector, the ionization chamber or scintillation detector of a computed tomography (CT) unit, or the piezoelectric crystal of an ultrasound machine is in analog form with a variance in voltage. For these signals to be read as data by the computer, they must be digitized and converted into the binary number system. The peripheral device that performs this task is the analog-to-digital converter, which transforms the sine wave into discrete increments with binary numbers assigned to each increment. The assignment of the binary numbers depends on output voltage, which in turn represents the degree of attenuation of the various tissue densities within the patient.

The basic component of an analog-to-digital converter (ADC) is the "comparator" that outputs a "1" when the voltage equals or exceeds a precise analog voltage and a "0" if the voltage does not equal or exceed this predetermined level. The most significant parameters of an ADC are (1) *digitization depth* (the number of bits in the resultant binary number); (2) *dynamic range* (the range of voltage or input signals that result in a digital output); and (3) *digitization rate* (the rate that digitization takes place). Achieving the optimal digitization depth is necessary for resolution quality and flexibility in image manipulation. Digitization depth and dynamic range are analogous to producing optimal contrast and latitude in a radiograph.

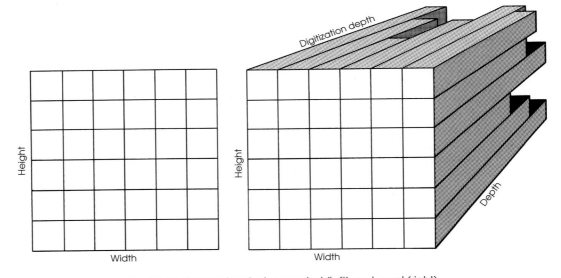

Fig. 32-10. Comparison between pixel (left) and voxel (right).

To produce a video image, the field size of the image is divided into many cubes or a matrix, with each cube assigned a binary number proportional to the degree of the attenuation of the x-ray beam or intensity of the incoming signal. The individual three-dimensional cubes with length, width, and depth are called *voxels* (*vol*ume *el*ement), with the degree of attenuation or intensity of the incoming voltage determining their composition and thickness (Fig. 32-10). For example, the contrast media used in a CT or digital fluoroscopy examination would produce voxels with less digitization depth than the surrounding tissues, as a result of the attenuation of the x-ray beam. Digitization depth allows flexibility in the manipulation of the image.

Because the technology for displaying three-dimensional objects has not been fully developed, a two-dimensional square or *pixel* (*pic*ture *el*ement) represents the voxel on the television display monitor or cathode ray tube. The matrix is an array of pixels arranged in two dimensions, length and width, or in rows and columns. The more pixels contained in an image, the larger the matrix becomes, with the resolution quality of the image improving. For instance, a matrix containing 256×256 pixels has a total of 65,536 pixels or pieces of data; whereas a matrix of 512×512 pixels contains 262,144 pieces of data. One should not confuse field size with matrix size. You can have a small field size and a large matrix size, or vice versa, depending on the equipment. The larger matrix also allows for more manipulation of the data or the image displayed on the television monitor and is very beneficial and useful in the imaging modalities, such as digital subtraction fluoroscopy, CT, nuclear medicine, and ultrasound.

After the image has been produced on the video display unit, *hard copies* are then made on single-emulsion film, using a multiformat camera, or a laser camera that directs a laser beam onto a single-emulsion film. The laser camera also permits the images to be reproduced on paper. The images may also be stored on magnetic tape or on a disk for future reference. A computer system that has one or more peripherals included in the system, like the one described above, is called a *multiprogramming* system (Fig. 32-11).

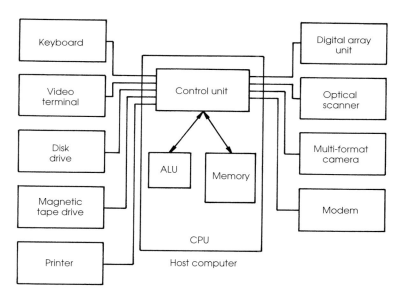

Fig. 32-11. Host computer with various input/output devices.

ARRAY PROCESSORS AND OTHER SPECIAL PURPOSE PROCESSORS

To acquire a 512×512 pixel matrix at 30 television frames per second, an analog-to-digital converter must be able to process 10^7 digitizations per second, with each pixel being eight to ten digits deep to allow for satisfactory image manipulation. The hardware developed to handle this mass amount of data is the "array processor" or "special purpose processor." The array processor was initially designed to calculate arithmetic operations at speeds ten to 1000 times faster than the CPU and has since progressed to the point that it has become a specialized small computer but is still considered peripheral to the host computer. Its function is to speed the processing of the matrices and other array of numbers by means of highly repetitive arithmetic operations.

The arithmetic operations performed within the array processor are aided by fast Fourier transforms that reduce the amplitude and increase the frequency of the sine wave through mathematic manipulation to allow faster processing. Because sine waves are not of equal intensity, Fourier transformation is a complex mathematical summation and/or multiplication of the sine waves that depict a spatial location within the body to provide a more accurate analysis and manipulation of the data. Other methods that speed up the processing are matrix multiplication, inversion, and convolution. Mathematic operations achieve speeds of up to 14 *million floating-point operations per second* (megaflops); because of the special design of the array processor, many of the different operations are performed simultaneously. One definition given of an array processor is this:

It has at least one adder and one multiplier that can run simultaneously and do floating-point arithmetic; it can be programmed; and it achieves high performance through parallel processing or "pipelining."

The alternatives to the array processor for arithmetic operations are the dedicated "single component" microprocessor and the "bit-slice" microprocessor. These two special processors are less expensive but have considerably slower *response time* than the array processor.

Array processors are designed to handle massive amounts of data. Therefore they are justified for use where vast amounts of photons or signals are being emitted, as in several radiologic procedures (e.g., from the output phosphor of an image intensifier, an ionization chamber, scintillation detector of a CT unit, or the antenna of a magnetic resonance imaging device). All of these units require an array processor to "crunch the numbers" so that they may be handled by the host computer (Fig. 32-12). For a 512×512 matrix image, the reconstruction process, without the use of an array processor, can take several minutes; whereas with an array processor, the task can be completed in less than 5 seconds (some in less than 1 second), with each rotation of an image requiring at least 5 million operations.

GRAPHIC DISPLAY DEVICES

Although many graphic display systems are available, they have not been used extensively in the medical imaging field. True graphic display is used extensively in the designing-type industries; for example, automobiles and architecture. Gray level mapping is used in computed tomography, MRI, sonography, and nuclear medicine and is referred to as graphs. However, radiation therapy departments have used graphic display devices to demonstrate two-dimensional representations of tumors or even three-dimensional representations of tumors, with shading within the graphic.

A graphic display system houses a display processing unit (DPU) and a dedicated computer with its own set of commands, data formats, and memory. The display processing unit creates an image on a display monitor and then regenerates this image 30 to 60 times a second to avoid a flicker in the image. For image display and regeneration of the image, the "raster-scan" or television-type system is used, dividing the picture into horizontal lines. The regeneration of the image takes place one line at a time.

A display list processor, which is housed in the host computer, transmits instructions to the display processing unit to create a graphic picture. The DPU then executes these instructions from 30 to 60 times per second to maintain the image on the television screen.

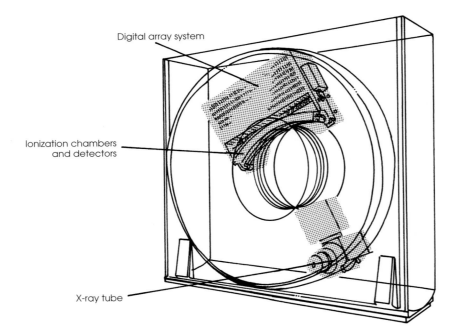

Digital array system

Ionization chambers and detectors

X-ray tube

Fig. 32-12. Gantry of a third-generation CT unit. The digital array system contains the ionization chambers and detectors, an analog-to-digital converter, and a digital array unit. The attenuated x-rays are converted to an electrical signal, digitized, and transmitted to the array processor for image reconstruction.

Many graphic display systems use the "frame buffer" display technology, where the digitization depth of each voxel is written into the display processing unit's memory. There is less flexibility in the manipulation of the image with this system, but it allows for "selective erasure" of background intensity levels or anatomic structures. Another advantage of this system is that the host computer can perform contrast stretching, windowing, and other functions without disturbing the image data stored in the display processing unit's memory.

Gray level mapping may be thought of as a graph of the gray levels within an image, and it is sometimes referred to as histogram stretching, windowing, or contrast enhancement. A histogram of the image is produced using gray level mapping and represents a bar chart of the number of pixels versus gray levels (Fig. 32-13). The capability of producing a gray scale histogram or graph is made possible by having a scan conversion memory tube within the computer system that uses a logarithmic transformation of the image into relative exposure values. The histogram is then easily changed into a graph representing the gray levels within an image. A low-contrast histogram (Fig. 32-13,*A*) representing an image has a wide histogram or a long scale of contrast, whereas a high-contrast histogram (Fig. 32-13,*B*) has a narrower histogram or a short scale of contrast.

In medical imaging equipment, *window width* refers to the width of the steep part of the curve, or the contrast within the image; *window level* refers to the location of the steep part of the curve within the gray levels and is analogous to image brightness or darkness (Fig. 32-14). The gray level map or graph can be thought of as analogous to the density scale of a radiographic film, an H & D, or a characteristic curve. A windowing operation is the selection of a certain range of the gray scale displayed as an image and the use of the full brightness scale of the television equipment to display only a specific preselected range of gray levels. The remainder of the gray scale outside of the window is subtracted from the gray scale map, leaving only the desired portion of the image displayed, as illustrated in Fig. 32-14.

Machine language is coded in binary numbers (0 and 1; "on" or "off") and the shortest possible *word* is a *bit*. Each voxel depicts an individual depth level of grayness and is represented by a bit, or two characters, 0 and 1. The number of shades of gray in an image, representing depth, that can be present is determined by a formula, 2 raised to the power of the number of bits, or 2^n. A gray scale with discrete values is assigned to the bits of voxel depth. For example, 2^2 equals 4 gray levels; 2^8 equals 256 gray levels; 2^{10} equals 1024 gray levels; and 2^{16} equals 65,536 gray levels. Bytes, or longer words, are necessary in digital imaging for faster processing. An 8-bit word is known as a *byte;* however, by convention, the computer system is referred to as an 8-bit system, a 10-bit system, or a 16-bit system. Gray levels are conceptualized as being parallel to contrast latitude: the more levels or shades of gray, the more contrast latitude. Discrete values assigned to the brightness of the levels of gray are known as Hounsfield units in computed tomography; however, this concept is used by computer systems in digital radiography, nuclear medicine, magnetic resonance imaging, and sonography.

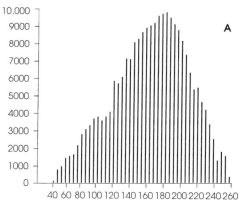

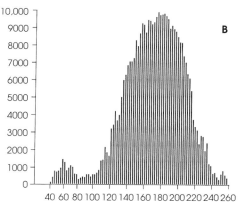

Fig. 32-13. A, Histogram demonstrating low (long scale) contrast in an image, and **B,** histogram demonstrating high (short scale) contrast in an image.

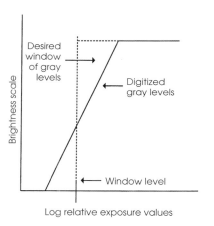

Fig. 32-14. Gray level windowing.

Digital Imaging Processing

Within the computer system, digital images are represented as groups of numbers. Therefore these numbers can be changed through applying mathematic operations, and as a result the image is altered. This important concept has provided extraordinary control in contrast enhancement, image enhancement, subtraction techniques, and magnification without losing the original image data.

CONTRAST ENHANCEMENT

Contrast enhancement is accomplished by windowing, which was explained in the previous section of this chapter (see graphic display devices). Window width encompasses the range of densities within an image. A narrow window is comparable to the use of a high-contrast radiographic film. As a result, image contrast is increased. Increasing the width of the window allows more of the gray scale to be visualized or more latitude in the densities of the image visualized (Fig. 32-15). A narrow window is valuable when subtle differences in subject density need to be better visualized. However, the use of a narrow window increases image noise, and the densities outside of the narrow window are not visualized.

IMAGE ENHANCEMENT OR RECONSTRUCTION

Image enhancement or reconstruction is accomplished by the use of digital processing or filtering, which can be defined as accenting or attenuating selected frequencies in the image. The filtration methods used in medical imaging are classified as (1) convolution; (2) low-pass filtering, or smoothing; (3) band-pass filtering; and (4) high-pass filtering, or edge enhancement. The background intensities within a medical image consist mainly of low spatial frequencies, whereas an edge, typifying a sudden change in intensities, is composed of mainly high spatial frequencies; for example, the bone-to-air interface on the skull when using computed tomography. Spatial noise originating from within the computer system is usually high spatial frequencies. Filtration reduces the amount of high spatial frequencies inherent in the object. The percentage of transmission versus spatial frequency, if plotted on a graph, is called modulation transfer function (MTF). One effort of continuing research in medical imaging is to develop systems with higher modulation transfer function.

Fig. 32-15. Lateral cervical spine image using different window settings. Window widths of: **A,** 381; **B,** 658; and **C,** 2544. Notice as the window width increases in numeric value, the scale of contrast increases (more long scale).

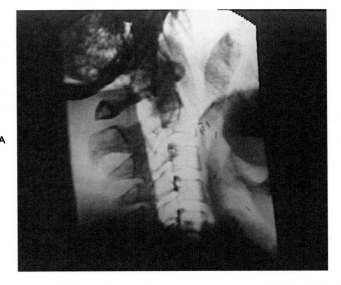

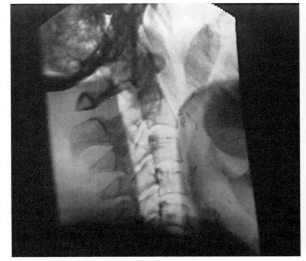

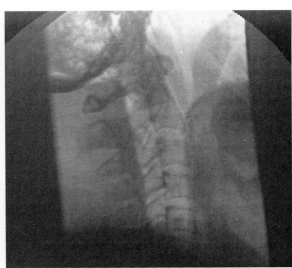

Convolution is accomplished automatically with computer systems that are equipped with fast Fourier transforms. In the systems that do have fast Fourier transforms, the convolution process is implemented by placing a filter mask array, or matrix, over the image array, or matrix, in the memory. A filter mask is a square array or section with numbers, usually consisting of an area of 3×3 elements. The size of the filter mask is determined by the manufacturer of the equipment, although larger masks are not often used because they take longer to process. The convolution filtering process can be conceptualized as placing the filter mask over an area of the image matrix, multiplying each element value of the filter mask by the image value directly beneath it, obtaining a sum of these values, and then placing that sum within the output image in the exact location as it was in the original image (Fig. 32-16). Convolution filtering is performed primarily to attenuate the higher frequencies within the image. The result of the convolution process is a blurring of the higher frequencies or intensities within the image.

Smoothing, or low-pass filtering, can also be used to remove the high-frequency noise within an image. Smoothing is accomplished by replacing the individual pixel values in the output image by gaining an average of the pixel values around each pixel. To clarify the concept, each pixel's value in the output image is replaced by gaining the simple average of it and eight neighboring pixels (Fig. 32-17). The averaging of the pixels is completed for each pixel within the matrix. The smoothing process smooths or attenuates the sudden differences in intensities or densities in the image by attenuating the higher frequencies within the image matrix (Fig. 32-18).

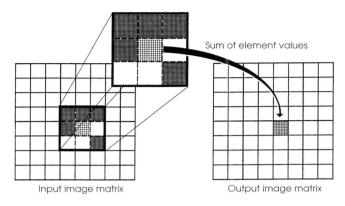

Fig. 32-16. Convolution filtering.

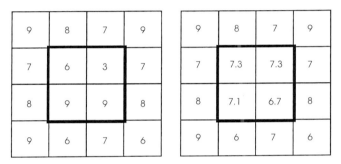

Fig. 32-17. Smoothing, or low-pass, filtering.

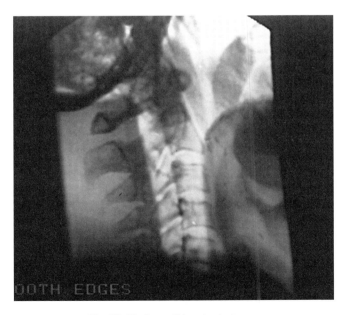

Fig. 32-18. Smoothing technique.

Band-pass filtration removes or attenuates all frequencies or intensities within the image except those in a preselected range. Band-pass filtering corresponds to the windowing process previously discussed.

High-pass filtration, or edge enhancement, uses a special edge filter to produce an edge-sharpening effect. If a standard high-pass filter were to be used in medical imaging, a remarkably high-contrast image would be produced. An edge filter provides a more diagnostic image by averaging the gray levels similarly to the convolution process and then establishing a threshold within the gray level scale. Thresholding allows saturation to black of all the gray levels below the threshold value and saturation to white of all the levels above the threshold. The thresholding process generates a higher contrast image of the anatomic area of interest and is particularly useful in demonstrating small structures. Research is being conducted with mammography equipment using high-pass filtration to accentuate the structural fine details within the breast and to minimize the background of the breast tissue. Digital subtraction angiography is well known for using high-pass filtration or edge enhancement to accentuate smaller vessels filled with contrast media (Fig. 32-19).

SUBTRACTION TECHNIQUES

The advantages of using digital subtraction include the ability to visualize small anatomic structures and to perform the examination via venous injection of contrast media. The most common digital subtraction techniques are temporal subtraction and dual energy subtraction. Hybrid subtraction is a combination of these two methods.

Temporal subtraction may be defined as a digital imaging process based on time intervals or limited by time, and in its simplest form it is produced by obtaining a mask (similar to a scout radiograph) and subtracting the pixel values of the mask from the pixel values of a postinjection image (see Chapter 35, digital subtraction). There should be no change in the images except for the contrast media–filled vasculature, and the subtracted image should primarily demonstrate the opacified blood vessels. However, a serious problem with this technique is the probability of patient motion between exposures. To correct the motion problem, a time interval difference (TID) mode is used for the digital processing. The TID technique involves obtaining a series of mask images and storing the images in adjacent memory locations. When the contrast medium is injected, a series of exposures is made at a very rapid rate; for

example, 15 images per second for 4 seconds. The postinjection images are identified as frame numbers and stored in adjacent memory locations. The frames, or postinjection data, are then subtracted from the masks, or original data, by allowing the computer to follow a set, programmed procedure. Examples of this set procedure are subtracting mask #1 from frame #2, mask #2 from frame #4, and so on.

Dual energy subtraction does not require the acquisition of images before the injection of contrast media. After an iodinated contrast medium is injected, a series of rapid exposures is made at a high kVp setting above the K-edge of iodine, 35 keV; and another series of exposures is made at a low kVp setting, below the 35 keV attenuation coefficient of iodine. The high kVp setting will diminish the bone contrast in the image, whereas the low kVp setting will enhance the less dense anatomic structures (e.g., the small vessels). A subtraction process of the two sets of images is then performed, with the outcome being increased contrast of the opacified vessels. To digitally perform the dual subtraction technique after the images have been acquired, the densities of the straight line portion of the film's H & D curve are correlated to the desired window level to produce the image. Advantages of dual subtraction are (1) patient motion is not as much of a problem as in the temporal subtraction method and (2) the high kVp and low kVp images allow the display of bone only or soft tissue only, or a combination of the tissues.

Hybrid subtraction is a combination of the temporal subtraction, TID, and the dual energy subtraction methods. When using the hybrid subtraction method, a set of masks is obtained for the high kVp setting and for the low kVp setting. Therefore, two sets of masks and two sets of frames with iodinated contrast media are acquired. The low kVp masks are subtracted from the frames with contrast media, and the high kVp masks are subtracted from the high kVp frames. The hybrid subtraction procedure eliminates bone, leaving only the contrast-filled vessels.

Mask registration is a procedure that is useful when patient motion occurs between the time of the mask exposures and the time of the contrast media frames. To correct the motion problem, the absolute density value of each pixel within the ma-

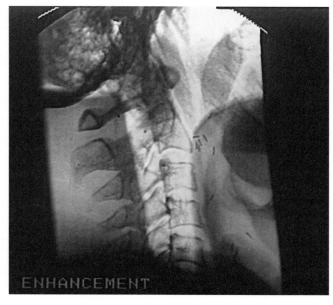

Fig. 32-19. Edge enhancement.

trix of each mask and each frame is calculated and portrayed as a reregistration of the image. The calculation of the absolute values of the pixels is similar to the smoothing filtration method described previously.

MAGNIFICATION

Magnification, sometimes called zooming, is a process of selecting an area of interest and copying each pixel within the area an integer number of times. Large magnifications may give the image an appearance of being constructed of blocks. To provide a more diagnostic image, a smoothing or low-pass filter operation can be done to smooth out the distinct intensities between the blocks.

THREE-DIMENSIONAL IMAGING

When three-dimensional imaging was first introduced, the images were less than optimal because of the resolution being too low to adequately visualize anatomic structures deeper within the body. The images often adequately displayed only the more dense structures closer to the body surface, or surface boundaries, which appeared blocky and jagged; therefore, the soft tissue or less dense structures were not visualized. By using fast Fourier transforms (3DFT), new *algorithms* for mathematic calculations, and the development of computers with faster processing time, three-dimensional images have become smooth, sharply focused, and realistically shaded to demonstrate soft tissue. The ability to demonstrate soft tissue in three-dimensional imaging is referred to as a volumetric rendering technique.

Volumetric rendering is a computer program whereby "stacks" of sequential images are processed as a volume with the gray scale intensity information in each pixel being interpolated in the z axis (perpendicular to the x and y axes). Interpolation is necessary because the field of view of the scan (the x and y axes) is not the same as the z axis because of interscan spacing. Following this computer process, new data are generated by interpolation, resulting in each new voxel having all the same dimensions. The volumetric rendering technique enables definition of the object's thickness, a crucial factor in three-dimensional imaging and in visualizing subtle densities.

Generation of three-dimensional imaging typically requires a stack of 50 scans with a resolution of 256×256, for a total

of 6 megabytes of information and the processing capability of 5 million instructions per second. An average examination takes approximately 25 to 40 minutes of scan time to complete. The entire examination, from the time the patient enters until he or she exits the department, would more than likely be more than an hour.

OPTICAL STORAGE AND RETRIEVAL SYSTEMS

Because of the storage and retrieval problems within a radiology department, there is currently a trend to develop optical storage technology. Optical storage technology embraces the concept of using some form of optical device to record and retrieve information from a light-sensitive medium. The optical devices currently being used are either gas or diode lasers. The media being used for recording are rectangular plates or disks resembling long-playing phonograph records.

Manufacturers of optical disk systems use minute holes made in the disk by the laser beam for the recording of information. The pits made in the media surface range in size from 1 to 2 micromillimeters in size, with the spacing between the rows 1.5 to 2 micromillimeters. Using a matrix of $1,024 \times 1,024 \times 8$ bits per image, a laser optical disk can store approximately 3,000 images; a matrix of $2,048 \times 2,048 \times 12$ bits per image allows approximately 400 images to be stored. Research currently being conducted will significantly increase the storage capability of optical disks in the near future.

Digital computer imaging systems using the binary system can send instructions to the optical laser system to encode the disk. The length of the pits and the distance between them made by the laser beam on the disk represent a digital coding scheme that can be retrieved. The advantages of this system are that, unlike radiographs, a disk does not deteriorate and requires very little storage space.

To retrieve the information on the disk, a reading laser produces a light source on the surface of the disk. If no information is on the portion of the disk where the laser is focused, the light is reflected back. When the reading laser is focused on an area that has been encoded, or where there is a pit, the light is partially refracted, according to the length and depth of the pit. The refraction of the light is then transmitted to the surface where a photodetector is excited, produces a lower voltage, and is

processed through digitization of the sine wave.

Digital optical systems can be used throughout the radiology department for the processing, storage, and retrieval of data; they can be used not only in the area of image processing but also for management services. As the technology develops, the cost of this system will be reduced. The radiology department of the future may not use radiographic films. A radiologist will be able to correlate, integrate, and evaluate images with the medical records of a single patient by use of a digital optical system.

Another form of image processing that was developed primarily by NASA and that will have an impact on the practice of radiology is the use of a digitizing camera for the analysis of data. A radiograph exposed and processed using current methods can be digitized by placing the film or a microdensitometer on a lightbox in front of a digitizing camera that operates in a fashion similar to that of the optical laser devices. The image is then digitized and processed by the computer system, which allows for the manipulation of the image. Such a system would obviate repeat radiographs.

An innovative application of the digitizing camera and special image processors, called "teleradiography," uses the digitizing camera to digitize the radiographic images of examinations on patients in rural areas for transmission by means of a *modem* over conventional telephone lines to a remote facility. The images are then processed by a special image processor and displayed on video terminals for diagnosis by physicians in prominent medical centers. This system would enable small, rural hospitals to provide improved medical care without the great expense of obtaining sophisticated computer equipment. It is predicted that networks will be established among large medical research centers and smaller hospitals and clinics through the use of teleradiography, for the purpose of providing more accurate diagnosis in pathologic conditions and trauma situations.

INFORMATION AND MANAGEMENT SYSTEMS

Most of the information and management computer systems used in radiology have been developed from the MUMPS programming languages. The modules contained in the majority of information management systems are registration, scheduling, process control, film file management, and reporting. The use of these modules also contributes to the quality control of the department.

The function of the registration module is to record the information typically found typed on a card file in the department—the dates and types of examinations a patient has had. Use of a computer file provides more accurate recording of information and much faster retrieval of the file.

Combined with the registration program is the scheduling module that makes the patient's appointment. This program aids in smoothing out the department's workload, thus making better use of equipment and personnel. Another function of this program is to check the patient's file for previous examinations and to sequence the examinations in the proper order. This module can also check to see what rooms are available for the study, calculate the average time it takes to complete the examination, print workloads for the entire department or a particular room, and produce schedules for the nursing stations, outpatient clinics, and physicians.

The process module tracks the process of performing and interpreting the examination. This process starts with the arrival of the patient in the department and includes the examinations performed, the rooms used, the radiographer who performed the examination, the number of radiographs per examination, whether retakes were done and the reason for the retakes, and whether any medications or contrast media were used. Before the patient leaves, a computer check is done to determine whether the patient needs any pending examinations and whether all examinations have been completed. The program will also record the time the report was dictated, transcribed, and signed by the radiologist. Use of this module or program can provide a very detailed repeat analysis that can be used to justify repair of equipment, new equipment purchases, or inservice education or further education of the radiographers.

Computer management of the film file provides a library system that records the files within the department and their location or individual radiographs loaned to outside departments, doctors, clinics, and medical facilities. The system can provide lists of files or radiographs that are overdue, which helps in the recovery of these

medical records before they are lost. Used with a scheduling module, a list of patients and the previous examinations completed on each patient can be produced so that they may be retrieved from the file archives the day before the scheduled examinations. Lastly, this program will also print adhesive labels that can be attached to the file jacket to record the date and type of examination performed.

A reporting program assists in the preparation and interpretation of the examinations. This module usually includes a word processing program used by the transcriptionist. Using CRTs in transcription and proofreading can save clerical time and improve the accuracy of the reports. Some systems even allow the radiologist to electronically sign the reports. A teaching file can also be developed with this system by having the radiologist dictate a code to be included with the transcription. The code enables the computer to identify the more interesting cases to be used for educational purposes.

All of these modules can be used on a time-sharing basis. *Time sharing* is a computer system in which each person using the system is given, for a small fraction of time, the total use or resources of the larger, multiprogram computer. The use of the large computer is rotated among the users under the direction of the operating programs and is determined by priorities. A time-sharing computer system makes a computerized information management system cost effective, even for small hospitals and clinics.

The other modules that can be included in an information management system contain administrative and financial programs. The most common of these is the billing system that can provide accurate and detailed itemized lists of expenses.

An overall benefit of all of these modules and the data or information generated is the potential to enhance quality control throughout the entire department and hospital. Management decisions, based on the statistics provided by such a system, will promote efficiency and improve operations, thereby providing quality patient care.

APPLICATIONS IN EDUCATION

Computers have been used to facilitate learning for the past 20 years. The development of miniaturized transistors and semiconductors allowed the mass distribution of microcomputers and minicomputers that has resulted in the adoption of computer-assisted instruction at all educational levels.

One must distinguish between computer-assisted instruction (CAI) and computer-managed instruction (CMI). CAI programs involve the learning of new information and actually assist in the teaching process. Methods incorporated in CAI are the presentation of new material, reinforcement through immediate feedback, questioning, and graphics. To ensure that learning has occurred, the students can be tested for knowledge and repeat the training if necessary. CMI uses testing procedures and then directs the student to reference material for further information or help, with no initial instruction being performed by the computer. Many CMI programs often serve as nothing more than electronic bookkeepers, because their function is to grade tests, provide test scores, and provide statistical data on the tests.

Instruction using a CAI system is concentrated on the presentation and learning of concepts, principles, and rules, or what is known as the "cognitive domain" of learning. Its effectiveness is limited in the teaching of psychomotor skills, such as radiographic positioning, and in the "affective domain," the learning of professional attitudes and empathy. Learning in these latter two domains may be enhanced by adding a video disk system to the computer system.

Although CAI has a high potential for the enhancement of learning, it will not replace the instructor in the classroom or in the clinical setting, just as the computer will not replace human judgment in making a diagnosis. A distinct advantage of CAI is that students exposed to this method of instruction will have the opportunity to become familiar with computers and their operation, and therefore will more readily adapt to the computerized equipment in the clinical setting.

Summary

Radiology departments in the future will become more reliant on the computer for imaging, therapeutic purposes, file management, billing, quality assurance, patient monitoring, education, and research. Radiologists will find their time absorbed and divided among the various imaging and therapeutic procedures. As this occurs, radiographers will gain additional responsibility and be required to possess the knowledge and skills necessary to understand and operate the computerized equipment and systems. Therefore, it is essential that radiographers know how to operate a computer, just as they must know how radiation is produced.

Definition of Terms

address The label, name, or number identifying a register, location, or unit where data are stored; in most cases, address refers to the location in the computer memory.

algorithm A defined set of instructions that will lead to the logical conclusion of a task.

analog computer Computer that performs operations on continuous signals.

analog-to-digital converter (ADC) An input device for changing continuous (analog) signals into digital form (i.e., discrete numbers).

arithmetic/logic unit (ALU) That part of the computer that performs computations, comparisons, and logical operations.

assembler A computer program used to assemble machine code from symbolic code.

assembly language A computer programming language that is machine-oriented and can be translated directly into machine instructions.

baud rate The rate at which information is transmitted serially from a computer; expressed in bits per second.

binary A numbering system based on twos rather than tens (decimals); the individual element can have a value of 0 or 1 and in computer memory is known as a bit.

bit Constructed from the words *BI*nary digi*T*. The term refers to a single digit of a binary number. For example, the binary number of 101 is composed of three bits.

boot The process of initializing a computer operating system; also referred to as "booting up."

buffer An auxiliary storage area for data input in order to match the speed differences between machines.

bug A common term used to describe an error in operation or in a program.

byte A term used to define a group of bits, usually eight, being treated as a unit by the computer.

cathode ray tube (CRT) An electronic tube (like the familiar television tube) that makes the computer output visible; sometimes called a VDU (visual display unit).

central processing unit (CPU) The brain of the computer; it is the circuitry that actually processes the information and controls the storage, movement, and manipulation of the data.

character Any letter, digit, or punctuation mark; characters are usually represented by a binary code composed of eight bits, or one byte.

command A portion of code that represents an instruction for the computer.

compiler A set of programs that compiles or converts a program into the machine language instructions for a particular computer.

console Usually the front panel of the CPU by which the operator supervises and controls the machine.

control unit That part of the CPU that directs the sequence of operations, such as which instruction is to be executed next.

cursor A character, usually an underline or a graphics block, that indicates position on a display screen.

data acquisition unit A peripheral device that acquires signals from equipment and transmits them to the computer.

data base A large file of organized information that is produced, updated, and manipulated by one or more programs.

data management system A group of commands that create, update, and reference a data base.

digital computer A computer in which discrete numbers are used to express data and instructions.

digitization depth The dimension of depth within a matrix, represented by a number of pixels, which, in turn, signifies the levels or shades of gray available within an image.

digitization rate The amount of time needed to change data from analog form to digital form.

direct access Access to data independent of the previously obtained data; it may also be called "random access."

disk A circular plate coated with magnetic material and used to store data.

disk drive A device used to read data from and to write data onto disks.

downtime The time a computer system is out of operation, usually for repairs and/or maintenance; often expressed as a percentage of the normal operating hours.

dynamic range The range of voltage or input signals that result in a digital output.

file A collection of related data or information kept as a unit.

generation A group of computers produced within the same period, based on the model of an earlier product.

hard copy Any readable output from a computer; it is usually on paper, but in radiology the output of images is usually on radiographic film.

hardware The physical devices and/or equipment of a computer system.

high-level language A computer language in which each user instruction corresponds to multiple instructions when converted to machine code; examples: FORTRAN, FOCAL, COBOL, and ALGOL.

hybrid computer A computer with both analog and digital computing capability.

input The information the computer receives via media; for example, magnetic tape, disks, punched cards, or keyboard.

input/output terminal (I/O terminal) A machine or device capable of both feeding information into and retrieving information from the computer.

instruction A program step that tells the computer exactly what to do for a single operation in a program.

interface A device that serves as a common boundary between two other devices; a connection between two pieces of computer hardware.

interrupt A temporary suspension of processing by the computer; caused by input from another part of the computer or by an auxiliary device or machine.

K A symbol for 1000; in computer language, it means 2^{10} or 1024 and denotes the number of units a computer can store in its memory; example: $32 \times 1024 = 32{,}768$ or 32K.

language A defined set of characters that, when used alone or in combinations, form a meaningful set of words and symbols; used to write instructions for a computer; examples: ALGOL, COBOL, BASIC, and FORTRAN.

machine language A programming language consisting only of numbers or symbols that the computer can understand without translation.

magnetic memory Any memory device using magnetic fields as a means of storing data; for example, magnetic tape or disks.

memory The storage of information and data by the computer.

modem (*MO*dulator/*DEM*odulator) A device that allows data to be transmitted long distances, usually over telephone lines, by impressing digital pulses onto an analog carrier wave.

125

multiprogramming The ability of a computer system to permit execution of more than one separate task at a time; is used in time-sharing and/or multiuser systems.

multitasking A computer system or a single machine that can process several programs.

off-line Portions of the computer that are not under the direct control of the CPU or the operator.

on-line Portions of the computer that are directly under the control of the CPU and the operator.

optical scanner A device that scans the light either reflected or transmitted through a surface and then converts the signal into a machine-readable input.

output The results generated when the computer has performed the requested combinations of tasks.

peripheral A device that is separate but connected to the computer for the purpose of supplying input and/or output capability.

pixel (picture element) One individual cell surface within an image matrix used for CRT image display.

primary memory A portion of a computer that is used to store information, either data or programs; the size of a computer may be referred to by the amount of user memory; usually measured in kilobytes.

random access The ability to access locations of data without regard to sequential data; access may be accomplished by going directly to the location.

random access memory (RAM) Pertaining to a storage device in which access time is effectively independent of the location of the data.

read only memory (ROM) A memory that is similar to the RAM except that data cannot be written into it but is capable of being read.

real time Computer operations that occur fast enough to be analyzed and used immediately for decision making.

register A device in the CPU that stores information for future use.

response time The time between the input of information into a computer and the response or output.

serial processing Digital computer processing in which programs are run sequentially, rather than simultaneously or together.

software A general term that applies to any program or set of instructions that can be loaded into a computer.

storage capacity The amount of data that can be stored in the computer memory, usually expressed in terms of kilobytes.

terminal An input/output device, usually consisting of a keyboard and display screen.

time sharing The process of accomplishing two or more tasks at (apparently) the same time; the computer will process one task at a time, but only a small portion, before switching to the next; because the computer can process a large amount of data in a short period of time, the switching between tasks is not noticed by human observation.

voxel (volume element) An individual pixel with the associated volume of tissue based on the slice thickness.

Winchester disk drive A smaller, less-expensive, hard disk drive capable of transferring data at an increased rate with sophisticated error detection and correction procedures.

window Arbitrary numbers used for image display based on various shades of gray; window width controls the overall gray level and affects image contrast; window center (level) controls subtle gray images within a certain width range and ultimately affects the brightness and overall density of an image.

word The number of bits processed as a single unit in an arithmetic operation.

word length The number of bits composing a word.

write To record data on a memory device.

x-y digitizer An input device that allows the motion of the cursor or pen to be transduced and fed into the computer as a series of x-y coordinates.

SELECTED BIBLIOGRAPHY

Bushong SC: Radiologic science for radiographers—physics, biology, and protection, ed 5, St Louis, 1993, Mosby.

Chandler R: PACS: applications in the modern radiology department, Admin Radiol, June, 1987.

Convey HD et al: Computers in the practice of medicine, introduction to computer concepts, vol I, 1980, Reading, Mass, Addison-Wesley Publishing Co.

Cook LT et al: Image processing: shape analysis, texture analysis, and three-dimensional display, Appl Radiol 13(3):123-134, 1984.

Curry T et al: Christensen's introduction to the physics of diagnostic radiology, ed 4, Philadelphia, 1990, Lea & Febiger.

Dwyer SJ III et al: Computer applications and digital imaging: RSNA '92 meeting notes, 186:939, 1993.

Edwards M et al: Computers in radiology—interfacing with peripheral devices, Appl Radiol 2:37-46, March/April 1984.

Enlander D: Computers in medicine—an introduction, St Louis, 1980, Mosby.

Fishman EK et al: Volumetric rendering techniques: applications for three-dimensional imaging of the hip, Radiology 163:737-738, 1987.

Gay JE, Taubel JP: Effects of ionizing radiation and magnetic fields on digital data stored on floppy disks, Radiology, 189:583, 1993.

Giger ML et al: "Intelligent" workstation for computer-aided diagnosis, Radiographics 13:647, 1993.

Gonzoley R et al: Digital image processing, Reading, Mass, 1977, Addison-Wesley Publishing Co.

Gould RG: Digital hardware in radiography and fluoroscopy, Appl Radiol 13(3):137-140, 1984.

Greenfield GB and Hubbard LB: Computers in radiology, New York, 1984, Churchill Livingstone.

Hendee WR, Ritenour E: Medical imaging physics, ed 3, St Louis, 1992, Mosby.

Honeyman JC, Dwyer SJ III: Computers for clinical practice and education in radiology: historical perspective on computer development and glossary of terms, Radiographics 13:145, 1993.

Hunter TB: The computer in radiology, Rockville, Md, 1986, Aspen Publications.

Kuni CC: Introduction to computers and digital processing in medical imaging, St Louis, 1988, Mosby.

Lehr JL: Computer languages and the operating systems, Appl Radiol 13(1):35-41, 1984.

Lehr JL, editor: Planning guide for radiologic installations: fascicle 9: computer information systems, Chicago, 1977, American College of Radiology.

Lehr JL: Software: basics and applications in radiology, Semin Ultrasound 4(4):260-269, December 1983.

Lieberman DE: Computer methods, the fundamentals of digital nuclear medicine, St Louis, 1977, Mosby.

Ney D et al: Interactive real-time multiplanar CT imaging, Radiology 170:275-276, 1989.

Novick G: Introduction to computer hardware and internal representation, Appl Radiol 12(6):51-62, 1983.

Powis RL et al: A thinker's guide to ultrasonic imaging, Baltimore, 1984, Urban & Schwarzenberg.

Richardson ML, Gillespy T II: Inexpensive computer-based digital imaging teaching file, AJR 160:1299, 1993.

Robb WL: Future advances and directions in imaging research, Am J Radiol 150:39-42, 1988.

Rowberg AH: Digital hardware in CT and NMR, Appl Radiol 13(4):71-74, 1984.

Scott R: Artificial intelligence: its use in medical diagnosis, J Nucl Med 34:510, 1993.

Seeram E: Computed tomography technology, Philadelphia, 1982, WB Saunders.

Simborg DW: Local area networks: why? what? what if?, MD Computing, Computers in Medical Practice 1(4):10-20, 1984.

Staab EV: Computers for clinical practice and education in radiology: introduction, Radiographics 13:143, 1993.

Strong HM and Cerva JR: Image storage and transmission technology, Semin Ultrasound 4(1):270-279, 1983.

Swett HA and Miller PL: ICON: a computer-based approach to differential diagnosis in radiology, Radiology 163:555-558, 1987.

Swett HA et al: Expert system-controlled image display, Radiology 172:487-493, 1989.

Trux PG: The current state of operating systems: 1983 and 1984, MD Computing, Computers in Medical Practice 1(4):58-63, 1984.

Ubaldi S et al: The use of microcomputers in radiologic technology training programs: focus on education, Radiol Technol 53(3):271-273, 1981.

Chapter 33

COMPUTED TOMOGRAPHY

STEVEN J. BOLLIN, SR.
KENNETH C. JOHNSON

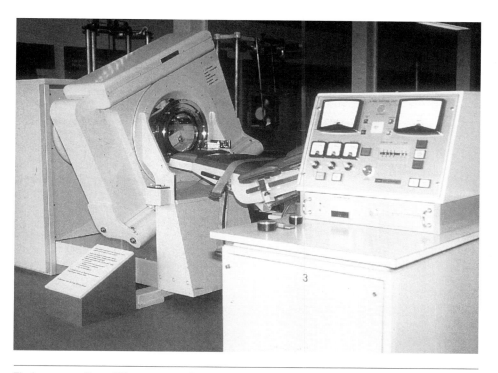

First generation CT scanner. Operator console (right) permitted little manipulation of the image. Patient couch and gantry (left rear) were used to examine the limited area of the brain extending from skull base to the top of the skull.

This chapter presents the fundamental concepts of *computed tomography (CT)*.* As seen in Fig. 33-1, CT is the process of creating a cross-sectional tomographic plane of any part of the body. A patient is *scanned* by an x-ray tube rotating about the body part being examined. A *detector assembly* detects the radiation exiting the patient and feeds back the information, referred to as *raw data,* to the host computer. Once the computer has compiled the data and calculated it according to a preselected *algorithm,* it assembles it in a *matrix* to form an *axial* image. Each image, or *slice,* is then displayed on a *cathode ray tube (CRT)* in a cross-sectional format.

*All italicized terms are defined at the end of this chapter.

CT is used for a wide variety of neurologic and somatic procedures. The most common procedures involve the brain, chest, and abdomen. Other areas of the body, such as the neck, spine, pelvis, and upper and lower extremities, are routinely scanned. Specific anatomical regions can also be examined. Within the head, the sinuses, facial bones, orbits, IACs, and sella turcica are frequently scanned. Specific body organ scans of the heart, liver, adrenal glands, kidneys, and prostate are less common; they are usually included as part of abdominal or chest examinations.

CT-guided biopsies and drainage of fluid collections offer an alternative to surgery for some patients. Although the procedures are considered invasive, they offer shorter recovery periods, no exposure to anesthesia, and less risk of infection. CT is also used in radiation oncology for radiation therapy treatment planning. CT scans taken through the treatment field, with the patient in treatment position, have drastically improved the accuracy and quality of therapy provided.

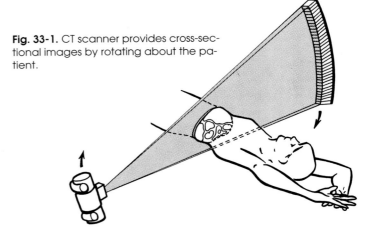

Fig. 33-1. CT scanner provides cross-sectional images by rotating about the patient.

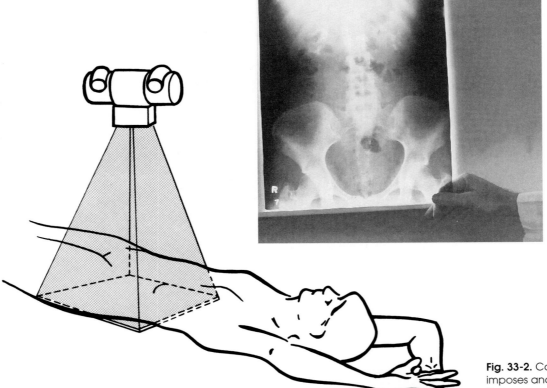

Fig. 33-2. Conventional radiograph superimposes anatomy and yields one diagnostic image with fixed density and contrast.

Comparison with Conventional Radiography

Reviewing conventional radiography helps explain the usefulness of CT. When a conventional x-ray exposure is made, the radiation passes through the patient and is recorded on radiographic film. Often body structures are superimposed over each other (Fig. 33-2); visualizing specific structures requires the use of contrast media, varied positions, and usually more than one exposure. Localization of masses or foreign bodies requires at least two exposures and a ruler calibrated for magnification.

In a CT examination, individual slices are taken through the area of the body being scanned. A typical procedure *protocol* will call for a 1 cm slice taken every 1 cm through the area of interest. Slices may be taken contiguously, be slightly overlapped, or have a small space between each scan, depending on the examination protocol. The total number of slices varies by slice thickness, *table increment,* and the size of the body part being scanned. For an abdominal CT of the area demonstrated by Fig. 33-3, *A,* 40 to 50 or more 1-cm contiguous slices may be required (Fig. 33-3, *B*), or as few as 15 to 20 slices may be required if table increments are increased.

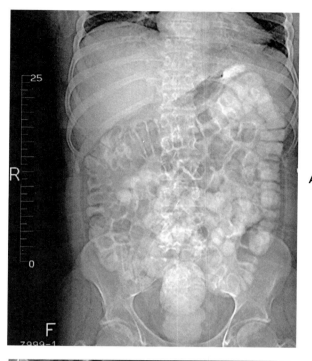

A

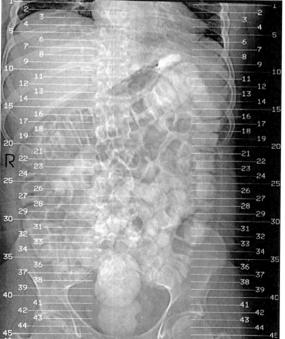

B

Fig. 33-3. A, Digital KUB (kidney, ureter, and bladder). **B,** Digital KUB demonstrating the number of 1-cm slices required for a complete CT scan of the abdomen and pelvis.

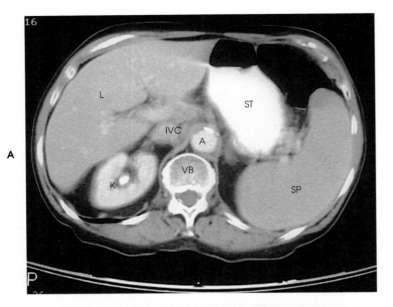

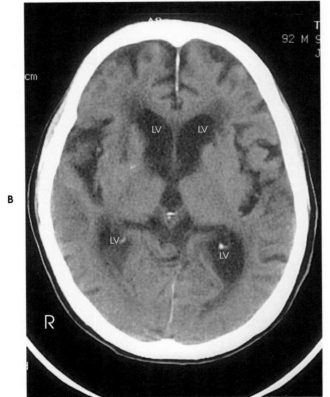

In the radiograph of the abdomen in Fig. 33-3, *A,* the high-density bone and low-density gas are seen, but many soft-tissue structures, such as the kidneys or intestines, are not clearly identified; contrast media is needed to visualize these structures. A CT examination of the abdomen would demonstrate all the structures that lie within the slice. In Fig. 33-4, *A,* the liver, stomach, kidneys, spleen, and aorta can be identified. CT has the ability to distinguish minute differences in tissue densities; this ability is referred to as *contrast resolution.* Differences as low as .25% can be demonstrated, compared with conventional radiography, which can demonstrate tissue densities as low as 2%.

CT also can resolve small objects within the body. With *spatial resolution,* objects as small as 2 mm can be identified and accurately located. In comparison, conventional radiography can resolve objects as small as .1 mm, but distortion and magnification affect the recorded size of the object relative to its actual size and position within the body.

Fig. 33-4, *B* is an axial image of the brain, which differentiates the gray from the white matter as well as shows bony structures, calcifications, and cerebrospinal fluid within the ventricles. Because CT can demonstrate subtle differences of various tissues, radiologists are able to diagnose pathologic conditions more accurately than if they were to rely on radiographs alone. Also, because the image is reconstructed by the computer, it can be reformatted into different body planes to optimize the diagnostic information available to the physicians.

Fig. 33-4. A, Axial image of abdomen demonstrating liver (L), stomach (ST), spleen (SP), aorta (A), inferior vena cava (IVC), vertebral body of thoracic spine (VB), and kidney (K). **B,** Axial image of brain demonstrating enlarged lateral ventricles (LV) and gray and white matter.

(**B,** Courtesy Kim Bailey, R.T.)

Historical Development

The first successful demonstration of CT was conducted in 1970 in England, at the Central Research Laboratory of EMI, Ltd. Dr. Godfrey Hounsfield, an engineer for EMI, and Dr. James Ambrose, a physician at Atkinson Morley's Hospital in London, England, are generally given credit for development of CT. Their research was awarded the Nobel Price in 1979. After CT was shown to be a useful clinical imaging modality, the first full-scale commercial unit, referred to as a "brain tissue scanner," was installed in Atkinson Morley's Hospital in 1971. An example of an early dedicated head CT scanner is seen in Fig. 33-5. Physicians recognized its value for providing diagnostic neurologic information, and its use became accepted rapidly. The first CT scanners in the United States were installed in June 1973 at the Mayo Clinic and later that year at Massachusetts General Hospital. Both of these early units were also dedicated head scanners. In 1974 Dr. Robert S. Ledley of Georgetown University Medical Center developed the first whole body scanner, which greatly expanded the diagnostic capabilities of CT.

After CT was accepted by physicians as a diagnostic modality, numerous companies in addition to EMI began manufacturing scanners. Although there were differences in the design of units, the basic principles of operation were the same. CT scanners have been categorized by *generation,* which is a reference to the level of technological advancement of the tube and detector assembly. There were four recognized generations of CT scanners, although newer scanners are no longer categorized by generation but by tube and detector movement.

The early units, referred to as the first generation scanners, worked by a process known as translation/rotation. The tube produced a finely collimated beam, or pencil beam. Depending on the manufacturer, one to three *detectors* were placed opposite the tube for radiation detection. The tube movement (translation) was followed by a rotation of 1 degree. Scan time was usually 3 to 5 minutes per scan, which required the patient to hold still for extended periods. Because of the slow scanning and reconstruction time, CT was limited almost exclusively to neurologic examinations; an example of a CT image from a first generation scanner is seen in Fig. 33-6.

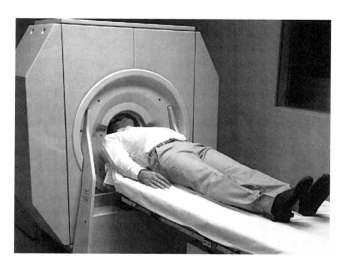

Fig. 33-5. First generation CT unit: dedicated head scanner.

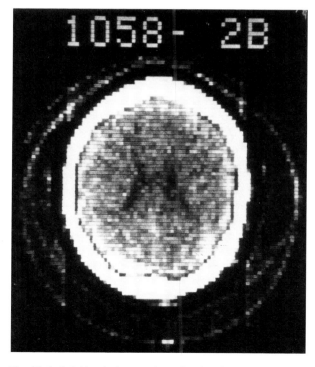

Fig. 33-6. Axial brain image from the first CT scanner placed in operation in the United States at the Mayo Clinic. The 80 × 80 matrix produced a noisy image. Examination performed July 1973.

(Courtesy Eugene D. Frank, R.T.)

When the second generation of scanners was introduced, they were considered a significant improvement over first generation scanners. The fan beam and multiple detectors were introduced by manufacturers for better radiation production and detection. Tube and detector movement was still translation/rotation, but the rotation was 10 degrees between each translation. These changes improved overall image quality and decreased scan time to about 20 seconds for a single slice. However, the time required to complete one CT examination remained relatively long.

The third generation of scanners introduced the rotate/rotate movement, in which the tube and detector assembly revolved concentrically about the body part (Fig. 33-7). Scan times were decreased to 1 to 10 seconds per slice, which made scans much easier for patients and helped to decrease motion artifact. Advancements in computer technology also decreased image reconstruction time, resulting in a substantial reduction in examination time.

The next major change in CT scanner design, the fourth generation, introduced the rotate-only movement, in which the tube rotated about the patient, but the detectors were stationary in fixed positions within the gentry (Fig. 33-8). The use of stationary detectors required greater numbers of detectors to be installed in a scanner. Fourth generation scanners tended to yield a higher patient dose per scan than previous generations.

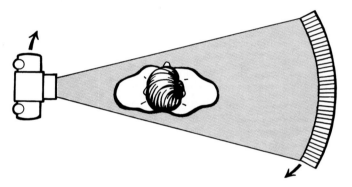

Fig. 33-7. Rotate/rotate. Tube and detector movement of a third generation scanner.

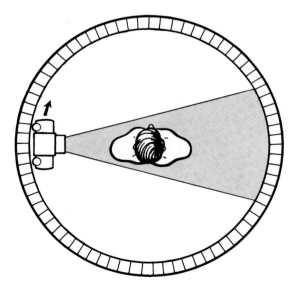

Fig. 33-8. Rotate-only. Tube movement with stationary detectors of a fourth generation scanner.

ELECTRON BEAM TOMOGRAPHY

Another type of CT technology is the electron beam tomography scanner (EBT). An electron gun generates an electron beam directed at four stationary targets to create a fan beam. Although scanning, radiation detection, and image reconstruction are basically the same as in conventional CT, there is no mechanical movement of the tube or detectors. The scanner is capable of extremely fast scan times, up to 17 scans per second, which can freeze most body motion. Facilities with EBT scanners can use them for diagnostic examinations as they do conventional CT, but EBT is primarily used for cardiac studies.

SLIP RING TECHNOLOGY

A number of companies have introduced systems utilizing *slip ring* technology. Slip ring, or continuous rotation scanners, utilize an x-ray system that continuously rotates about the patient. This continuous rotation allows routine scan times of 1 second with minimal interscan delay.

When third generation scanners were introduced, the tube/detector assembly rotated about the patient from a set starting point, rotated back to the starting point (referred to as the home position) after the scan, then repeated the sequence for each slice until the examination was completed. Manufacturers introduced the bi-directional tube movement, in which the tube rotated about the patient in one direction, then rotated in the opposite direction for the next scan. This eliminated tube rotation back to home position, which helped to reduce examination time and excessive equipment wear. Scan times were lowered to 3 to 5 seconds per slice, but average examination time still averaged 15 to 30 minutes.

Slip ring technology, by comparison, rotates continuously about the patient during the examination, averaging one 360-degree rotation per second; average scan times used are 1 to 2 seconds. This speed, combined with the latest computer technology, has decreased actual scanning time to 5 to 10 minutes for a typical CT. Using scan times as short as 1 to 2 seconds has helped to eliminate or at least substantially reduce motion artifact while allowing much more efficient use of contrast for visualizing vascular structures (Fig. 33-9). Patient motion from discomfort is also reduced because of the shortened examination time. The scanner can be programmed to scan rapidly through noncooperative patients without reconstructing images, completing an examination in as little as 2 minutes actual scanning time.

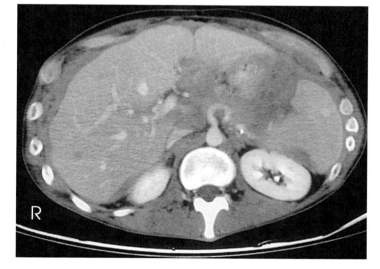

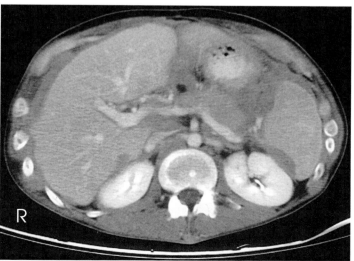

Fig. 33-9. Contiguous slices demonstrating contrast flow through blood vessels.

Technical Aspects

To obtain one axial image, a series of steps is performed by the computer. The tube rotates about the patient, radiating the area of interest. The detectors measure the remnant radiation, translate it into an *attenuation coefficient,* and relay it to the computer. When all raw data is collected, the computer analyzes it according to the algorithm selected. The CT radiographer selects the algorithm through the scan program. Algorithms are usually preprogrammed by the manufacturer in the computer's memory as part of the scan program; however, the radiographer may alter the program to a different algorithm when necessary. The algorithm is usually set for specific body areas; there are different algorithms for large and small body sections, soft tissue, and bone. The algorithm selected allows the radiographer to display the image as required for the examination protocol.

The axial image created by CT is actually made up of thousands of small squares called *pixels* (*pic*ture *el*ements), which combine to form a *matrix.* The pixels are associated with the volume of the slice, referred to as the *voxel* (*vol*ume *el*ement) (Fig. 33-10). The voxel is defined as the area of the pixel multiplied by the thickness of the slice.

When the computer receives the data from the detectors, it creates a *CT number* based on the average intensity of the remnant radiation. CT numbers are defined as a relative comparison of x-ray attenuation of each voxel of tissue with an equal volume of water. Since water is uniformly dense, it is assigned an arbitrary value of 0. Tissues that are denser than water are given positive values; tissues less dense than water are given negative values. The scale of created numbers ranges from 1000 to 4000, the numbers are also referred to as *Hounsfield units (HU).* Average Hounsfield units (CT numbers) for various tissues are listed in Table 33-1.

Once the computer has analyzed the data and assigned CT numbers according to the measured tissue densities, it assigns the numbers to individual pixels within the matrix so that an axial image can be created. The computer uses a 512 matrix (that is, 512 × 512) for image reconstruction and storage. After the information has been stored in the computer's short-term memory, it can be viewed on the CRT.

Table 33-1. Average Hounsfield units for selected substances

Substance	HU
Air	−1000
Lungs	−250 to −850
Fat	−100
Orbit	−25
Water	0
Cyst	−5 to +10
Fluid	0 to +25
Tumor	+25 to +100
Blood (fluid)	+20 to +50
Blood (clotted)	+50 to + 75
Blood (old)	+10 to +15
Brain	+20 to +40
Muscle	+35 to +50
Gall bladder	+5 to +30
Liver	+40 to +70
Aorta	+35 to +50
Bone	+150 to +1000
Metal	+2000 to +4000

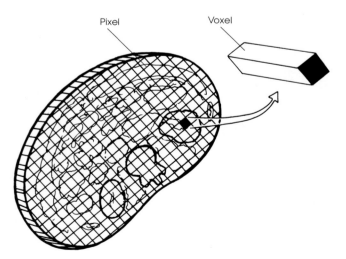

Pixel   Voxel

Fig. 33-10. CT image is composed of a matrix of pixels, each representing a volume of tissue (voxel).

Scanner Components

The major components of a CT scanner are the computer and operator's console, the gantry, and the table. Scanners will have slight variations in design and appearance according to manufacturers, but the basic components are illustrated in Fig. 33-11.

COMPUTER

The computer is included in the model in Fig. 33-11 as part of the operator's console; various scanners may have a separate cabinet for the computer. As each scan is completed, the *data acquisition system (DAS)* converts the signals from the detectors into digital data and relays it to the computer. The computer is able to integrate the information from the DAS and reconstruct images almost instantaneously. Early CT computers could do only one process at a time, which resulted in image reconstruction times from as short as 15 seconds to as long as several minutes, depending on the level of software installed. Advanced CT computers are able to scan the patient, collect the data, reconstruct the image, *archive* the image, and begin the next scan in about 2 to 5 seconds. The computer's main disk drive can provide only short-term storage for images; eventually the finished examinations must be archived, or copied, to a long-term storage device so that the patient's scan can be *retrieved* if necessary.

The computer can also accept a wide variety of software programs, such as three-dimensional (3D) and multiplanar reconstruction, which create different views of patient anatomy from axial image data; bone density measuring, which measures the density of bone in a patient, usually the spine; the cardiac scanning, which provides axial images of the heart while intravenous (IV) contrast is being injected. Several CT options are discussed later in this chapter.

The types of storage devices most commonly used are magnetic tape, cassette tape, and optical disk. Magnetic tape is a common storage device, but each tape holds a limited number of images. Retrieving images from tape can be a time-consuming process and with some CT systems it is not possible to scan a patient when images are being retrieved. Images stored on a magnetic tape are typically stored in a 256 matrix to save space and to put as many images as possible on each device. The total number of images stored per tape varies by manufacturer, but an average would be about 250 images. Cassette tapes are much faster than magnetic tapes and are capable of archiving up to 2000 images in a 256 matrix, which preserves original image quality. They are relatively inexpensive and their small size makes them easy to store. Optical disk technology has been adapted for CT image archival. The optical disk also archives image data in a 256 matrix and requires very little space for storage, but it is somewhat more expensive. Optical disks can archive up to 9000 images in a 256 matrix, which substantially reduces the number of storage devices required for image storage. CT departments keep a library of storage devices so that patient examinations can be retrieved when necessary. If the storage devices can be reused, images will be kept for about 1 year before new images are copied over the old ones.

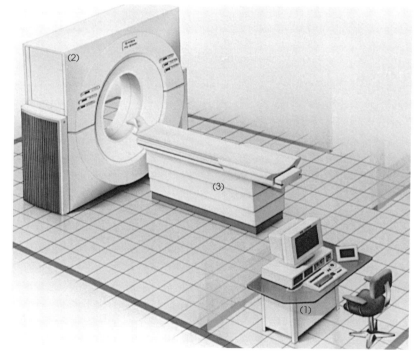

Fig. 33-11. Components of a CT scanner. **1,** Computer and operator's console, **2,** gantry, and **3,** patient table.

(Courtesy Picker International, Inc.)

GANTRY

The *gantry* houses the x-ray tube, DAS, and detectors for radiation production and detection. The x-ray tube is similar to those used for conventional radiography but is designed to handle and dissipate excessive heat units created during a CT examination. Most CT tubes can handle around 2.1 million heat units; advanced units can tolerate 4 to 5 million heat units.

The DAS and detector assembly, designed as a single unit within the gantry, provide the necessary data to the computer for image reconstruction. As previously mentioned, the DAS converts electronic signals from the detectors into digital data for processing by the CT computer. The detector assembly is constructed of either pressurized gas detectors, made of stable gases such as xenon, or dense crystal detectors, made of materials such as calcium tungstate.

Every gantry has an opening, or *aperture,* to accommodate most patients; most apertures are approximately 70 cm wide. The gantry can be tilted in either direction, up to 30 degrees depending on manufacturer, to compensate for body part angulation. Anatomic regions such as the head and spine often require that the gantry be tilted to obtain an accurate cross-sectional image. For patient positioning, a light is attached to the tube assembly to indicate where on the body the scan will be taken; this light is used not only for localization of individual slices, but also for positioning of the patient for scout views. The radiographer will use external landmarks, such as the manubrial notch, xiphoid process, or symphysis pubis, to include the entire body region being scanned, such as the chest or abdomen.

For certain head studies, such as those of facial bones, sinuses, or the sella turcica, a combination of patient positioning and gantry angulation will result in a *direct coronal* image of the body part being scanned. Fig. 33-12, *A* demonstrates a typical direct coronal image of C1-C2. Compare this image with the computer-reconstructed coronal image demonstrated in Fig. 33-12, *B,* which is created from axial scans through the body part. Notice the loss of overall image resolution and quality of the reconstructed image compared with the direct coronal image.

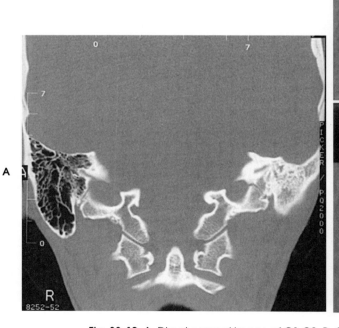
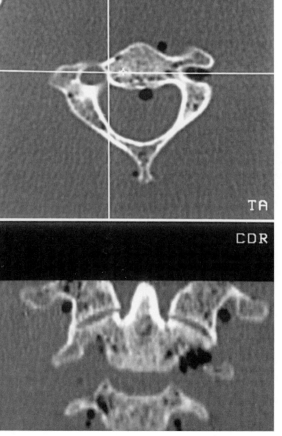

Fig. 33-12. A, Direct coronal image of C1-C2. **B,** Computer-reconstructed image of C1-C2.

(Courtesy Siemens Medical System.)

TABLE

The table is an automated device linked to the computer and gantry. It is designed to *index* after every scan according to the scan program. The table is an extremely important part of a CT scanner. Indexing must be accurate and reliable, especially when thin slices (1 or 2 mm) are taken through the area of interest. Most CT tables can be programmed to move either in or out depending on the examination protocol and the patient.

CT tables are made of either wood or low-density carbon composite, both of which will support the patient without causing image artifacts. The table must be very strong and rigid to handle patient weight and at the same time maintain consistent indexing. All CT tables have a maximum patient weight limit; this limit varies by manufacturer from 136 to 272 kg (300 to 600 lbs). Exceeding the weight limit can cause inaccurate indexing, damage to the table motor, or even possible breakage of the tabletop, which could cause serious injury to the patient.

Accessory devices can be attached to the table for a variety of uses. A special device, or cradle, is used for head CT examinations. The head cradle helps to hold the head still and, because it extends beyond the table top, minimizes artifact or attenuation from the table while scanning the brain. It can also be used for positioning the patient for direct coronal images.

OPERATOR'S CONSOLE

The operator's console (Fig. 33-13) is the point from which the radiographer controls the scanner. Originally, units were command-driven, which required that a dialogue be initiated between the radiographer and the computer. This was accomplished by typing the necessary commands on the keyboard. To start any program, the proper commands had to be entered in correct sequence for the computer to perform the scan.

As computer technology progressed, scanners became menu-driven; the computer presented a menu, or a selection of options, from which the radiographer could make a choice and type in the appropriate option. The computer would then run the program selected. Advanced models, such as the unit shown in Fig. 33-13, have operator-interactive menus, which allow the radiographer to make a menu selection by touching the display screen or using a computer mouse instead of typing in the selection.

Before starting an examination, the radiographer must enter the patient information, so a keyboard is still necessary for some functions. Usually the first scan program selected is the scout program from which the radiographer will plan the sequence of axial scans. Examples of typical scout images are seen later in the chapter. The operator's console is also the location of the CRT, where image manipulation takes place. Most scanners display the image on the CRT in a 1024 matrix, interpolated by the computer from the 512 reconstructed image.

Once an axial image is displayed on the CRT, the radiographer can view it many different ways. To properly display an image, the radiographer must select a *window,* an arbitrary set of computer numbers that can be manipulated to show various anatomical structures or tissues. The radiographer can adjust the image by changing the width or center (level) of the window.

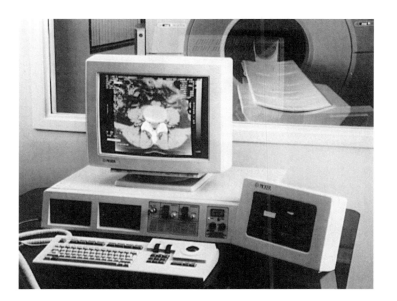

Fig. 33-13. Operator's console demonstrating image screen, menu screen, and keyboard.

(Courtesy Picker International, Inc.)

Scanner components

Window center is a representation of average CT numbers within the image seen on the CRT. Different anatomy can be demonstrated by changing the center. For example, setting the center at 30 to 50 will allow visualization of soft tissue structures in the head, chest, or abdomen. Increasing the center to 500 to 700 will provide bony detail of osseous structures within the image. The range of numbers available for adjustment vary by manufacturer, but most scanners have a range of +1000 to −1000. Center adjustments give the radiographer control over the optical density of the image displayed on the CRT.

Window width controls the range of grays within a selected center. Width is adjusted according to the anatomy demonstrated. A width setting of 300 to 450 at a center setting of 35 to 50 will demonstrate soft tissue detail of an abdominal CT image. If the radiographer wants to display the spine in the same abdominal image, a center of 500 to 700 may be selected. Adjusting the width from 2000 to 3000 allows adequate visualization of bony detail. Changing the width allows the radiographer to control the image contrast. Increasing the width will help compensate for the effects of noise or metal on image quality, although the resultant image will demonstrate a grayer, smoother appearance, as well as a decrease in overall image resolution. In Fig. 33-14, an axial image is seen in two different windows: a standard abdomen window and a bone window adjusted for the spine.

Any image can be adjusted on the CRT to compensate for differences in patient size and tissue densities or to display the image as desired for the examination protocol. Examples of typical window width and center settings are listed in Table 33-2. These settings are averages and usually vary by machine. Note how the center, although an average, is approximately the same as the CT numbers expected for the tissue densities.

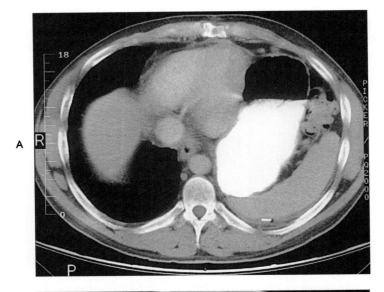
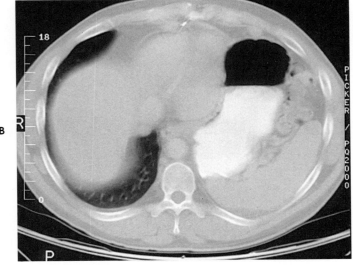

Fig. 33-14. A, Abdominal image, soft tissue window. **B,** Abdominal image, bone window.

(Courtesy of Kim Bailey, R.T.)

Table 33-2. Typical window settings

CT examination	Width	Center (level)
Brain	190	50
Skull	3500	500
Orbits	1200	50
Abdomen	400	35
Liver	175	45
Mediastinum	325	50
Lung	2000	−500
Spinal cord	400	50
Spine	2200	400

In addition to displaying axial images, radiographers can reconstruct images in coronal or sagittal body planes by manipulating the data from the axial images. Fig. 33-15, *A*, demonstrates a sagittal reconstruction of the data obtained from axial images; Fig. 33-15, *B*, demonstrates a coronal reconstruction. These images were produced without any additional radiation to the patient.

One of the most important functions of the operator's console is to produce hard copies of axial images, in the form of film. The most commonly used filming devices are the matrix camera and the laser printer, shown in Fig. 33-16 docked directly to a processor. The matrix camera had been the standard filming device used in CT. Today, the laser printer is the preferred device for filming, and it should be docked directly to a processor whenever possible.

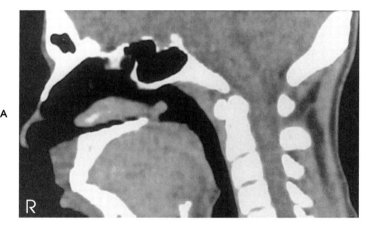

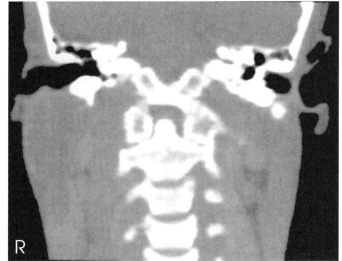

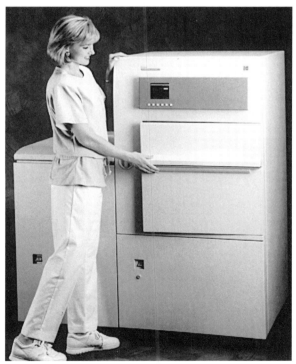

Fig. 33-15. A, Computer-reconstructed sagittal image. **B,** Computer-reconstructed coronal image.

(Courtesy Siemens Medical Systems.)

Fig. 33-16. Laser printer direct-docked to an automatic processor.

(Courtesy Eastman Kodak Company.)

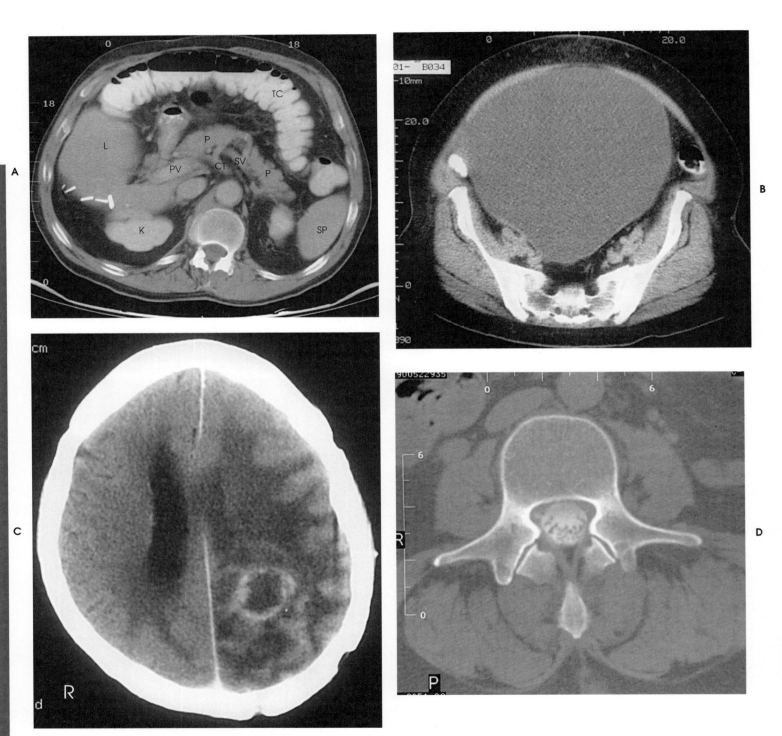

Fig. 33-17 . A, Abdominal image demonstrating transverse colon (TC) with air/fluid levels, oral contrast, liver (L), pancreas (P), spleen (SP), kidney (K), portal vein (PV), celiac trunk (CT), and splenic veins (SV); surgical clips are seen in posterior liver. **B,** Abdominal image demonstrating extremely large ovarian cyst. **C,** Brain image demonstrating parieto-occipital mass with characteristic IV contrast ring enhancement. **D,** Image of L-3 postmyelogram demonstrating contrast in thecal sac.

(**B,** Courtesy Brenda J. Rogers, R.T.)

Diagnostic Applications

CT originally was used primarily for diagnosis of neurologic disorders. As scanner technology advanced, the range of applications was extended to other areas of the body. The most commonly requested procedures are of the head, chest, and abdomen. CT is the examination of choice for head trauma; it clearly demonstrates skull fractures and associated subdural hematomas, cerebral vascular accidents (CVAs), epidural hematomas, and other pathologic conditions, such as benign and malignant tumors, hydrocephalus, and atrophy. CT of the chest and abdomen can be used to demonstrate metastatic lesions, aneurysms, abscesses, and other disease processes within the body. Fig. 33-17 demonstrates various anatomy and pathology identified by CT.

For any procedure, a protocol is required to maximize the amount of diagnostic information available. Specific examination protocols will vary according to the needs of different medical facilities and physicians; examples of protocols are listed in Table 33-3. These are generalized protocols and are by no means the only ones that can be used nor are they necessarily the protocols that will be most successful.

Table 33-3. Examination protocols*

Scout view (scanogram, topogram)	Can be programmed for an AP image (Fig. 33-18) or a lateral image (Fig. 33-19). The scout should include the entire body area being examined, so that the scans can be plotted according to the selected scan program. A pre-scan scout image, demonstrating the scans as programmed before the examination starts, is seen with the scout image in Fig. 33-18. A post-scan scout, demonstrating the actual slices taken, is seen in Fig. 33-19.
Brain scans	Without contrast (unenhanced)—1 cm × 1 cm from base of skull through cranial vault; can be modified to 5 mm × 5 mm through the posterior fossa of skull; recommended gantry angulation of 15 to 20 degrees caudad to OML. With contrast (enhanced)—Same protocol as an unenhanced brain CT after injection of IV contrast; requires patient be NPO at least 2 hours before scan. Sinus (generally done unenhanced)—Axial: 5 mm × 5 mm from bottom of maxillary sinuses through the frontal sinuses. Direct (or reverse) coronals: 5 mm × 5 mm from posterior sphenoid sinus through frontal sinuses.
Neck scans	With contrast—5 cm × 5 cm from orbits through the neck to the manubrial notch.
Body scans	Chest—1 cm × 1 cm starting just superior to apices through the bases; may be advantageous to scan through suprarenal glands; contrast can be given to highlight vessels of mediastinum, but patient must be NPO at least 2 hours before scan. Abdomen and Pelvis—1 cm × 1 cm from just above the diaphragm through the symphysis pubis; patient should be NPO at least 4 hours before scan (preferably after midnight); standard bowel prep of oral contrast; IV contrast; rectal contrast if requested by radiologist. 1 cm × 1.5 cm for general abdominal survey films for lymphoma, metastases, or abscesses.
Spine scans	Without contrast—5 mm slice × 4 mm table increment through vertebrae of interest. Overlapping slices improve quality of sagittal and coronal reconstructions. Gantry should be angled so that the beam is at a right angle to the vertebral bodies. For lumbar spine through L5-S1, the angle may be as much as 25 degrees caudad. Scan can also be done after a myelogram to demonstrate the cord, in addition to radiographs obtained during the myelogram.
Special scans	High resolution chest—1 mm × 1 mm through a specified level to evaluate nodules within the lung; done on an edge-enhancement algorithm; can be magnified to the area of interest. Suprarenal glands—5 mm × 5 mm through the suprarenal glands; usually done as part of an abdominal scan. Pancreas—5 mm × 5 mm through the pancreas; usually magnified to include the area of interest.

*Slice thickness and table increments are generally specified in the protocol but can be changed as necessary. Most scan protocols specify contiguous (adjacent) slices, to cover the entire area of interest. For better detail, or location of small objects, thinner slices and table increments can be programmed. As previously mentioned, overlapping slices over table increments improves the quality of sagittal and coronal reconstructed images.

Diagnostic applications

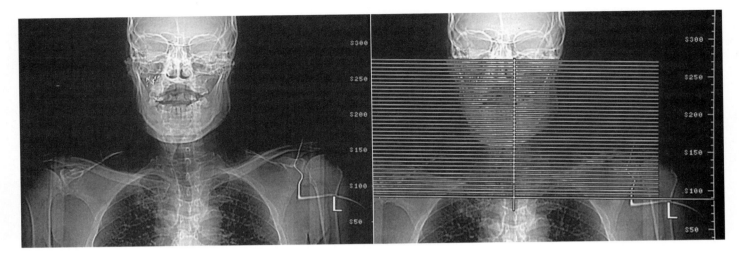

Fig. 33-18. AP scout image of neck with pre-scan slice demonstration.

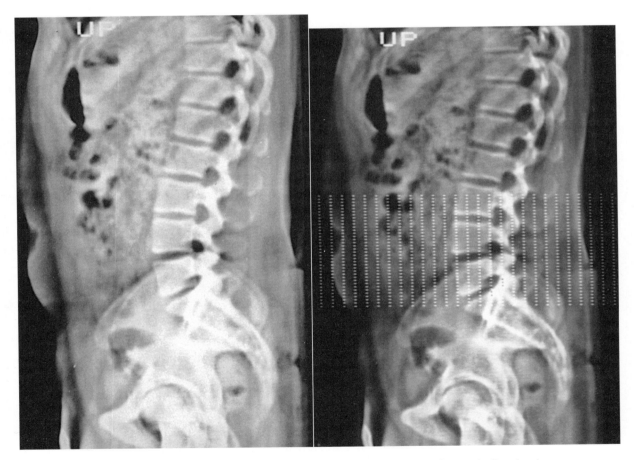

Fig. 33-19. Lateral scout image of lumbar spine with post-scan slice demonstration (post-scout view).

(Courtesy Steve Bollin, R.T.)

CONTRAST MEDIA

Contrast media may be part of a scan protocol, given either intravenously or orally (or rectally if requested by radiologist). Generally, IV contrast is the same as that used for excretory urograms. Many facilities use nonionic contrast for these studies, despite the relatively high cost, because of the low incidence of reaction and known safety factors associated with nonionic contrast. IV contrast is useful for demonstrating tumors within the head; Fig. 33-20 shows a brain scan with and without contrast. The lesion is evident in the unenhanced scan; in the enhanced scan, the tumor demonstrates characteristic ring enhancement typical of tumors seen in CT scans. IV contrast can also be used to visualize vascular structures in the chest and the abdomen. IV contrast should be used only with approval of the radiologist, after careful consideration of patient history. Many CT examinations can be done without IV contrast if necessary; however, the amount of diagnostic information available can be limited.

Oral contrast is generally a 2% barium mixture. The low concentration prevents contrast artifacts but allows good visualization of the stomach and intestinal tract. Iodinated contrast such as oral Hypaque can be used but must be mixed at low concentrations to prevent contrast artifacts. Rectal contrast is often requested as part of an abdominal or pelvic protocol. Usually mixed in the same concentration as the oral contrast, it is useful for demonstrating the distal colon relative to the bladder or other structures of the pelvic cavity.

QUALITY ASSURANCE

Any CT scanner is a complex combination of sensitive and expensive equipment. Most CT scanners require biweekly preventative maintenance to keep them operating properly and to keep the measured values within tolerance. Preventative maintenance is usually performed by the manufacturer's service department or by a third-party service company. Radiographers can perform daily test scans on a water phantom. Hounsfield unit measurements are taken of the water phantom to ensure consistency as well as to record the standard deviation. This not only enables the radiographer to assess the scanner's current operating condition, it provides service with a performance evaluation over longer periods of time. Many units are also capable of *air calibrations,* which do not require the water phantom and can be done between patients for unit self-calibration. Other tests include scanning composite phantoms, made of materials with known densities, for evaluation of *contrast resolution* and accuracy of Hounsfield units. A phantom, made with pins or wires of known measurements and spacing, is used for *spatial resolution* and table increment testing.

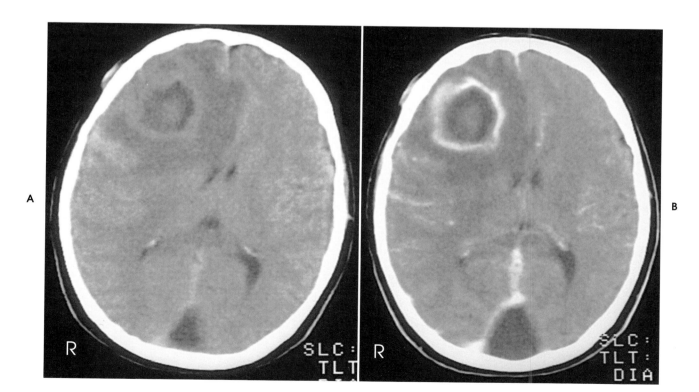

Fig. 33-20. A, Brain image without IV contrast. **B,** Brain image with IV contrast.

Factors Affecting Image Quality

The axial CT image is an electronic representation of a patient's anatomy rather than an actual image recorded on film. As with conventional radiography, a variety of factors can affect the final image produced. Some factors are beyond the radiographer's control; they include system noise, contrast resolution, spatial resolution, and certain artifacts.

System noise is a factor for any CT scanner. As previously noted, CT numbers are based on the value for water density, which is 0. When a water phantom is scanned, a *region of interest (ROI)* can be taken to measure the average CT numbers of water. Any difference between the measured values and the actual values for water is referred to as the standard deviation, which is a statistical measurement of system noise. Noise is dependent on several factors, but detector efficiency and *useful patient dose* have the greatest effect. Noise manifests itself as graininess on a finished image and detracts from overall image resolution.

Contrast resolution is the ability of the scanner to demonstrate different tissue densities. This particular ability makes CT a valuable diagnostic tool. Most scanners can demonstrate tissues with very little difference in density, often as low as .25%, depending on the level of technology. Contrast resolution is limited by the noise of the system and the area, volume, and density of tissue being scanned.

The spatial resolution of CT is not as inclusive as that of conventional radiography. Objects as small as 2 mm can be demonstrated on axial scans; however, it is not the size, but how accurately objects can be differentiated, that makes CT useful. Ultimately the size of the pixel and the efficiency of the detectors will control spatial resolution.

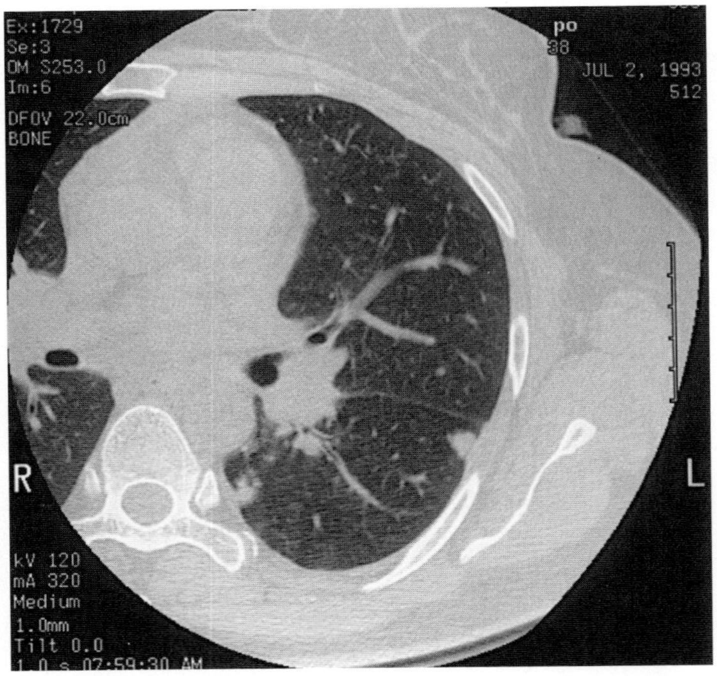

Metallic objects, such as dental fillings, pacemakers, and artificial joints, can cause starburst or streak artifacts, which can obscure diagnostic information. Dense residual barium from fluoroscopy examinations can cause artifacts similar to those caused by metallic objects. Many CT departments will perform a patient's CT examination several days after barium studies, to allow the body to eliminate the residual barium from the area of interest. Large differences in tissue densities of adjoining structures can cause artifacts that detract from image quality. Bone—soft tissue interface, such as the skull and brain, often causes streak or shadow artifacts on CT images; these are referred to as *partial volume averaging*.

Patient factors also contribute to the quality of an image. If a patient cannot or will not hold still, the scan will likely be nondiagnostic. Body size also can have an affect on image quality. Larger patients attenuate more radiation than smaller patients; this can increase image noise, detracting from overall image quality. Usually an increase in mAs is required to compensate for larger body size. Unfortunately, this results in a higher radiation dose to the patient. Factors that the radiographer can control include slice thickness, scan time, scan diameter, and patient instructions. Slice thickness is usually dictated by image protocol. As in tomography, the thinner the slice thickness, the better the image detail. Thin section CT scans, often referred to as high resolution scans, are used to better demonstrate structures (Fig. 33-21).

Scan times are usually preselected by the computer as part of the scan program, but they can be altered by the radiographer. When selecting a scan time, the radiographer must take into account possible patient motion, such as inadvertent body movements, breathing, or peristalsis. A good guideline is to choose the scan time that will minimize patient motion and at the same time provide a quality diagnostic image. When it is necessary to scan an uncooperative patient quickly, using the shortest scan time possible may allow the radiographer to complete the examination, although the quality of the images obtained will likely be somewhat compromised.

Fig. 33-21. High resolution 1-mm slice using edge enhancement algorithm, demonstrating nodule in left lung.

(Courtesy Jeannie M. Danker, R.T.)

The image that appears on the CRT is dependent on the *scan diameter*. Scan diameter can be adjusted by the radiographer to include the entire cross-section of the body part being scanned or a specified region within the part. The anatomy demonstrated is often referred to as the *field of view (FOV)*. Like scan time, scan diameter is usually preselected by the computer as part of a scan program but can be adjusted as necessary by the radiographer. For most head, chest, and abdomen examinations, the selected scan diameter includes all anatomy of the body part to just outside the skin borders. Certain examinations may require the scan diameter to be reduced to include specific anatomy, such as the sella turcica, sinuses, one lung, mediastinal vessels, suprarenal glands, one kidney, or the prostate. Decreasing the scan diameter is a way for the radiographer to magnify an image using scan data; however, as with any image magnification, some loss of resolution will occur.

Patient instructions, as in conventional radiography, are a critical part of a diagnostic examination. Explaining the procedure fully to the patient in terms he or she can understand will increase the level of compliance from almost any patient.

Special Features
DYNAMIC SCANNING

One of the advantages of CT is the ability to obtain data for image reconstruction by the computer. The scanner can be programmed to scan through an area rapidly, saving raw data but bypassing image reconstruction after each scan to shorten scan time. Known as *dynamic scanning*, this is a feature every scanner offers. Dynamic scanning is used most often for visualization of vascular structures enhanced with IV contrast. By minimizing interscan delay, the data can be obtained while a contrast *bolus* is given to the patient. Fig. 33-22 demonstrates the flow of contrast through the major vessels of the mediastinum; visualization of normal anatomy allows radiologists to diagnose mediastinal adenopathy. Dynamic scanning also gives the radiographer the ability to reduce or eliminate patient motion if the patient is unable or unwilling to hold still. This is especially helpful for trauma or pediatric cases, where patient cooperation is minimal. The primary disadvantage of dynamic scanning is that the radiographer does not see the images until after the dynamic sequence is completed.

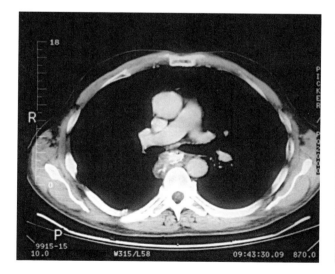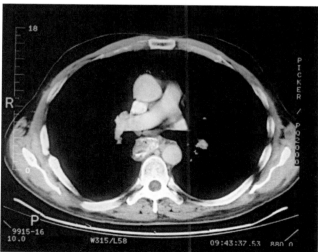

Fig. 33-22. Consecutive dynamic images demonstrating great vessels of mediastinum after bolus injection of 100 cc of IV contrast.

VOLUME SCANNING

One of the technological advancements of slip ring technology is volume scanning, also known as spiral or helical CT scanning. Spiral CT combines newer and faster computers, fast scan times, and continuous table movement and obtains a large amount of scan data in a very short time. As the patient is advanced through the gantry, the CT computer acquires and stores the vast amount of data provided continuously by the DAS. Since the tube rotates about the patient once per second, a 1-second scan time can be used. Table movement is programmed according to slice thickness desired. If a 1-cm slice

thickness is programmed, the table moves 1 cm per second through the gantry; if a 1-mm slice is needed, then the table moves 1 mm per second. It is the continuous rotation combined with the continuous table movement that forms the spiral path (hence the name spiral or helical) from which scan data is obtained.

One of the unique features of spiral CT is that it scans a volume of tissue rather than a group of individual slices. This makes it extremely useful for detection of small lesions. Because a volume of tissue can be scanned in a single breath, respiratory motion can be eliminated. In a volume scan of the chest as demonstrated in Fig. 33-23, the patient was instructed to hold

his or her breath; a tissue volume of 24 mm was then obtained in a 5-second spiral scan. Two of the resultant images demonstrate a small lung nodule without breathing interference of *image misregistration;* a 3D reconstruction of the lung clearly shows the patheology (Fig. 33-23). Spiral CT is also used to scan noncooperative or combative patients, patients who cannot tolerate lying down for long periods of time, and patients who will not hold still, such as pediatric cases or traumas. In some cases, the use of spiral CT has decreased the amount of contrast necessary to visualize structures, which is both safer and more cost-effective for the patient.

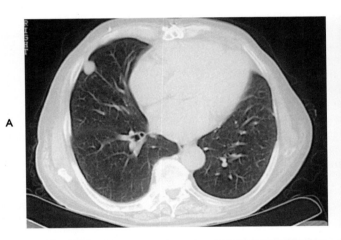

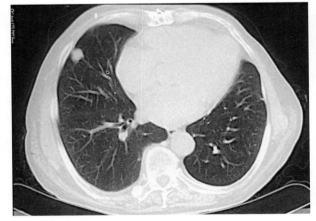

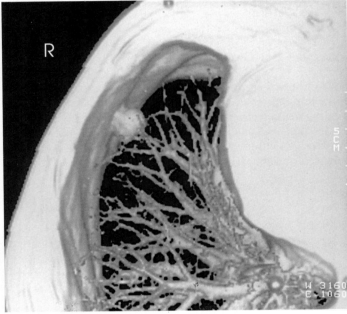

Fig. 33-23. A, and **B,** Spiral images of lung demonstrating lung nodule and associated vasculature. **C,** 3D reconstruction of lung nodule *(arrow)* following spiral scan.

(Courtesy Siemens Medical Systems.)

ANGIO CT

Once spiral CT was demonstrated as a reliable diagnostic imaging method, radiologists and radiographers attempted new ways to use it. One method is angio CT, in which contrast boluses are combined with spiral scans through vascular structures to obtain enhanced images. Angio CT is not designed to replace angiography as a diagnostic mode; rather, it is a complementary examination that allows image reconstructions of different body planes without further radiation to the patient. Fig. 33-24 demonstrates the vessels of the brain, while Fig. 33-25 highlights the great vessels of the heart in a 3D format.

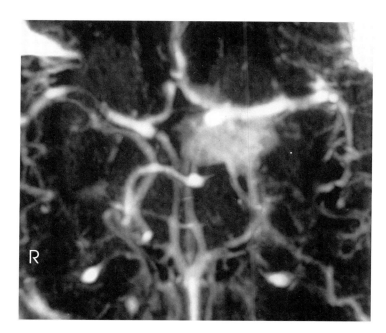

Fig. 33-24. Vessels of the brain.

(Courtesy Picker International, Inc.)

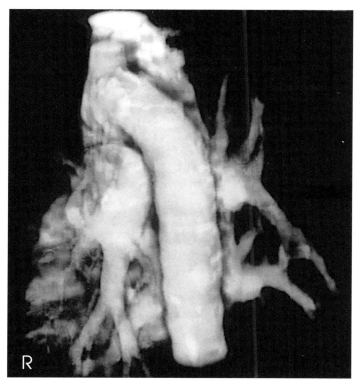

Fig. 33-25. Great vessels of heart in 3D format.

(Courtesy Picker International, Inc.)

Special features

THREE-DIMENSIONAL IMAGING (3D)

By combining all axial images of a scan, the computer is able to reconstruct a three-dimensional computer image of the patient. As previously outlined, CT detects and stores all tissue data within a given slice as CT numbers. That information is available for image reconstruction in a variety of body planes. 3D imaging allows the images to be displayed as the patient's anatomy would actually appear to the physician.

Early 3D programs were not very useful for diagnostic radiologists. Surgeons, especially those specializing in craniofacial malformations, head trauma, and facial reconstruction, found that they could clinically correlate the 3D images to the actual anatomic contours of their patients. 3D imaging was able to demonstrate the bony structure of the skull but was unable to show adequate soft tissue detail (Fig. 33-26). Bony structure of the spine and pelvis could also be demonstrated very well.

The introduction of advanced computers and faster software programs has dramatically increased the range of applications of 3D imaging. Fig. 33-27 shows various anatomical structures in 3D reconstruction. 3D reconstructions are often requested as part of patient evaluation after trauma to the head and spine and also as part of angio CT protocols.

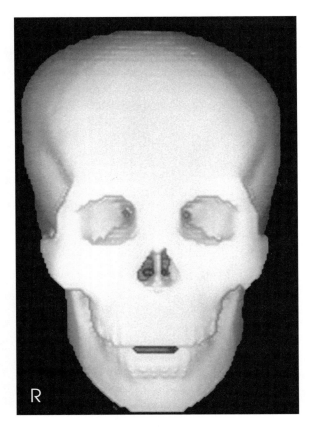

Fig. 33-26. 3D image of skull.

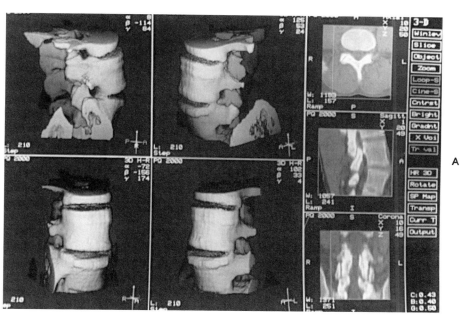

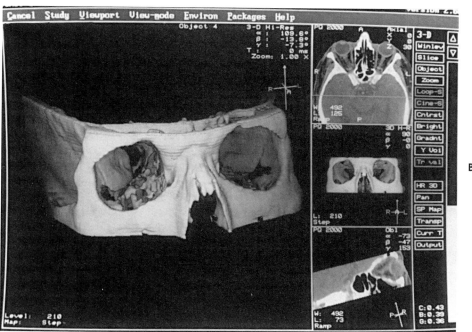

Fig. 33-27. A, 3D lumbar spine. **B,** 3D of bony orbits.

(Courtesy Picker International, Inc.)

CT-GUIDED RADIATION THERAPY TREATMENT PLANNING

Radiation therapy has been used as a form of treatment for nearly as long as radiology as a medical healing art has been in existence. The planning of a patient's radiation therapy required the use of x-rays and fluoroscopy of the treatment area, to simulate the path of the radiation. Visual interpretation of the radiographs, a thorough understanding of the anatomical structures within the treatment area, and manipulation of the information presented on the radiographs was necessary before prescribing gradiation. Even for the most skilled and careful medical dosimetrists and radiation oncologists, a margin of error existed within the treatment planning phase.

The introduction of CT has had a major impact on therapy treatment planning. A CT scan through the treatment area demonstrates the internal structures that lie within the radiation path. This helps the dosimetrist to plan the treatment so that the radiation dose to the target is maximized and the dose to normal tissue is minimized. A CT treatment planning scan is obtained under certain specific conditions. The following steps are observed:

- First, place the patient in the position used for actual treatment. This is necessary to see what anatomical structures lie in the treatment field. If a patient is placed supine with the arms up, but the treatment position calls for arms down, this not only will alter what structures appear visualized but also will change the location of the skin marks relative to the target and internal structures.

- Next, use a special flat treatment pad in place of the normal diagnostic CT table pad. This simulates the treatment machine table, which also is flat. Most CT manufacturers offer treatment pad inserts for their tables, or one can be purchased from any company marketing radiation therapy products.

- When preparing the patient for the treatment planning CT, place radiopaque markers on the skin marks to allow evaluation of the external contours of the radiation field. Demonstration of the external skin markers checks the accuracy of the treatment field and demonstrates what structures will be in the beam's path (Fig. 33-28). Measurements from the skin border to the center of the area being treated define the tissue depth, which affects the radiation. A thin radiopaque marker works best; many departments use catheters cut into small sections for markers.

- Finally, be sure to include the skin border of the patient in the field of view. When the dosimetrist plans the treatment, the CT images are magnified to true patient size so that the dose distribution can be calculated. When the skin borders are included, the dosimetrist can determine if the target volume is included in the treatment field.

Once the patient is in the treatment position on the CT table, slices are taken through the treatment field, according to the protocol specified by the radiation oncologist or medical dosimetrist. There may be only one slice required, taken through the center of the treatment field, or three, taken at the top, center, and bottom of the treatment field. Slices may also be taken at 1-cm increments through the entire field if requested, to view the target as well as surrounding tissue.

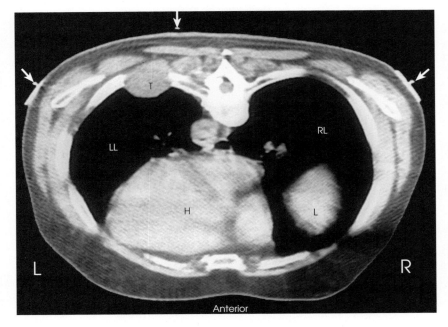

Fig. 33-28. Patient in prone position for treatment planning; radiopaque catheters *(arrows)* demonstrate location of treatment field skin marks, tumor (T), heart (H), liver (L), right lung (RL), and left lung (LL).

Comparison of CT and MRI

As CT was developing and advancing into a significant diagnostic modality, magnetic resonance imaging (MRI) was also progressing. Like CT, the first MRI scans were of the brain; the ability to do whole body scans followed shortly afterwards. As MRI advanced and quality of the images improved, it became apparent that MRI images exhibited better low-contrast resolution than CT images. A CT image of the brain does not demonstrate soft tissue detail as well as an MRI image at approximately the same level (Fig. 33-29).

The initial introduction of MRI created concerns that it would make obsolete the use of CT scanners. However, this has not occurred because each modality has unique capabilities, making them useful for different clinical applications. As previously mentioned, CT does not demonstrate soft tissue as well as MRI; however, CT demonstrates bony structures better.

Patients often have ferrous metal within the body. These patients cannot be scanned on MRI; one option is the use of CT. The CT scanner does not affect metal in the patient, although metal can cause artifacts on CT images when the metal lies within the scan plane.

Many patients are extremely claustrophic, combative, or uncooperative. CT is useful for scanning these patients quickly and easily, especially pediatric and trauma cases, because of the small gantry, relatively large aperture, and short scan times.

Because equipment costs are lower and a greater number of procedures can be accomplished per day, CT can often be a less costly examination than MRI. Physicians have found that CT and MRI can be complementary examinations; often both examinations are ordered to provide as much diagnostic information as possible.

The Future of CT

Technological advancement continue to make examinations more tolerable for patients. Higher quality images increase the accuracy of diagnosis and treatment, which ultimately improves patient care. Because of the diagnostic information it produces and its cost-effectiveness, CT will continue to be a widely used diagnostic imaging tool.

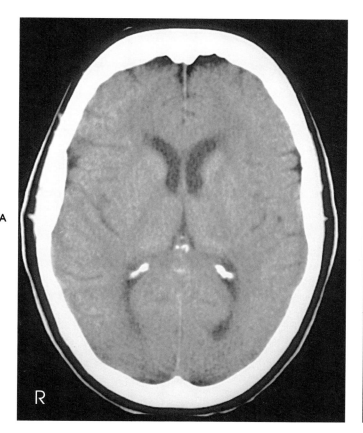
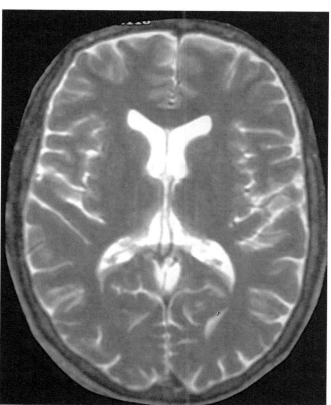

Fig. 33-29. A, CT image of brain. **B,** MRI image of brain.

(**A,** Courtesy Eric Parsels, R.T.; **B,** courtesy Daphne Smith, R.T.)

Definition of Terms

air calibration Scan of air in gantry; based on known value of −1000 for air, scanner will calibrate itself according to this density value relative to the actual density value measured.

algorithm Mathematical formula designed for computers to carry out complex calculations required for image reconstruction; designed for enhancement of soft tissue, bone, or edge resolution.

aperture Opening of the gantry through which patient passes during scan.

archive Storage of CT images onto a long-term storage device such as a cassette tape, a magnetic tape, or an optical disk.

attenuation coefficient CT number assigned to measured remnant radiation intensity after attenuation by tissue density.

axial The plane of the image as presented by a CT scan; same as transverse.

bolus Preset amount of radiopaque contrast injected rapidly per IV into patient to visualize high blood flow vascular structures, usually in conjunction with a dynamic scan; most often injected through use of a pressure injector.

cathode ray tube (CRT) Electronic monitor used for image display or scan protocol display; resolution of a CRT is dependent on the lines per inch (1pi); the greater the 1pi, the better the resolution

computed tomography (CT) Process by which a computer-reconstructed transverse (or axial) image of a patient is created by an x-ray tube and detector assembly rotating 360 degrees about a specified area of the body; also called "CAT (computed axial tomography) scan."

contrast resolution Ability of a CT scanner to demonstrate different tissue densities.

CT number Arbitrary number assigned by the computer to indicate the relative density of a given tissue; CT number varies proportionately with tissue density; high CT numbers indicate dense tissue, low CT numbers indicate less dense tissue. All CT numbers are based on the density of water, which is assigned a CT number of 0. Also referred to as a Hounsfield unit.

data acquisition system (DAS) Part of the detector assembly that converts analog signals to digital signals that can be used by the CT computer.

detector Electronic component used for radiation detection; made of either high density photoreactive crystals or pressurized stable gases.

detector assembly Electronic component of a CT scanner that measures remnant radiation exiting the patient, converting the radiation to an analog signal proportionate to the radiation intensity measured.

direct coronal Patient position used to obtain images in a coronal plane; used for head scans to provide images at right angles to axial images; patient is positioned prone for direct coronals and supine for reverse coronals.

dynamic scanning Process by which raw data is obtained by continuous scanning; images are not reconstructed but are saved for later reconstruction; most often used for visualization of high flow vascular structures; can be used to scan a noncooperative patient rapidly.

field of view (FOV) Area of anatomy displayed by the CRT; can be adjusted to include entire body section or a specific part of the patient anatomy being scanned.

gantry Part of CT scanner that houses the x-ray tube, cooling system, detector assembly, and DAS; often referred to as the "doughnut" by patients.

generation Description of significant levels of technological development of CT scanners; specifically related to tube/detector movement.

Hounsfield unit (HU) Number used to describe the average density of tissue; used interchangeably with CT number; named in honor of Godfrey Hounsfield, the man generally given credit for development of the first clinically viable CT scanner.

image misregistration Caused by combination of table indexing and respiration; table moves in specified increments, but patient movement during respiration may cause anatomy to be scanned more than once or not at all.

index Table movement; also referred to as "table increments."

matrix Mathematical formula for calculation; made up of individual cells for number assignment. CT matrix stores a CT number relative to the tissue density at that location; each cell or "address" stores one CT number for image reconstruction.

partial volume averaging A calculated linear attenuation coefficient for a pixel that is a weighted average of all densities in the pixel; the assigned CT number and ultimately the pixel appearance are affected by the average of the different densities measured within that pixel.

pixel (PIcture ELement) One individual cell surface within an image matrix used for CRT image display.

protocol Instructions for CT examination specifying slice thickness, table increments, contrast administration, scan diameter, and any other requirements specified by the radiologist.

raw data CT number assigned to the matrix by the computer; the information required to reconstruct an image.

region of interest (ROI) Measurement of CT numbers within a specified area for evaluation of average tissue density.

retrieval Reconstruction of images stored on a long-term device; can be done for extra film copies or when films are lost.

scan The actual rotation of the x-ray tube about the patient; used as a generic reference to one slice or an entire examination.

scan diameter Also referred to as "zoom" the "focal plane" of a CT scan; predetermined by the radiographer to include the anatomical area of interest; determines field of view.

slice One scan through a selected body part; also referred to as a "cut." Slice thickness can vary from 1 mm to 1 cm, depending on the examination.

slip ring Low voltage electrical contacts within the gantry designed to allow continuous rotation of an x-ray tube without the use of cables connecting internal and external components.

spatial resolution Ability of a CT scanner to demonstrate small objects within the body plane being scanned.

system noise Inherent property of a CT scanner; the difference between the measured CT number of a given tissue and the known value for that tissue; most often evaluated through the use of water phantom scans.

table increments Specific amount of table travel between scans; can be varied to move at any specified increment. Most protocols specify from 1 mm to 20 cm, depending on type of examination. It is also referred to as "indexing."

useful patient dose Radiation dose received by the patient that is actually detected and converted into an image.

voxel (VOlume ELement) An individual pixel with the associated volume of tissue based on the slice thickness.

window Arbitrary numbers used for image display based on various shades of gray; window width controls the overall gray level and affects image contrast; window center (level) controls subtle gray images within a certain width range and ultimately affects the brightness and overall density of an image.

SELECTED BIBLIOGRAPHY

Alexander J et al: Computed tomography, Berlin and Munich, 1986, Siemens Aktiengesellschaft.

Berland L: Practical CT: technology and techniques, New York, 1987, Raven Press.

Bentel GC et al: Treatment planning and dose calculation in radiation oncology, Elmsford, 1988, Pergamon Press.

Boethius J et al: CT localization in stereotaxic surgery, Appl Neurophysiol 43:164-169, 1980.

Boethius J et al: Stereotaxic computerized tomography with a GE 8800 scanner, J Neurosurg 52:794-800, 1980.

Bushong, SC: Radiologic science for technologists, St Louis, 1993, Mosby.

Chiu LC, Lipcamon JD, and Yiu-Chiu VS: Clinical computed tomography: illustrated procedural guide, Rockville, Md, 1986, Aspen Systems.

Coulam CM, et al, editors: The physical basis of medical imaging, New York, 1981, Appleton-Century-Crofts.

Curry TS et al: Christensen's introduction to the physics of diagnostic radiology, ed 3, Philadelphia, 1984, Lea & Febier.

Federle FP et al: Computed tomography in the evaluation of trauma, Baltimore, 1982, Williams & Wilkins.

Genant HK, editor: Computer tomography of the lumbar spine, San Francisco, 1982, University of California.

Godwin JD, editor: Computed tomography of the chest, Philadelphia, 1984, JB Lippincott Co.

Haaga JR et al: Computed tomography of the whole body, ed 2, vols I and II, St Louis, 1988, Mosby.

Hammerschlag SB et al: Computed tomography of the eye and orbit, Norwalk, Ct, 1983, Appleton-Century-Crofts.

Haughton V: Computed tomography of the spine, St Louis, 1982, Mosby.

Hendee WR: The physical principles of computed tomography, Boston, 1983, Little, Brown, & Co.

Kubota K et al: Some devices for computer tomography radiotherapy treatment planning, J Comput Assist Tomogr 4:697-699, 1980.

Lee JKT, Sagel SS, and Stanley RJ, editors: Computed body tomography with MRI correlation, ed 2, New York, 1989, Raven Press.

Lee SH and Rao Krishna CVG, editors: Cranial computed tomography and MRI, ed 2, New York, 1987, McGraw-Hill.

Mancuso AA et al: Computed tomography and magnetic resonance of the head and neck, ed 2, Baltimore, 1985, Williams & Wilkins.

Moss AA et al: Computed tomography of the body, Philadelphia, 1983, WB Saunders.

Naidich DP et al: Computed tomography of the thorax, New York, 1984, Raven Press.

Naidich TP et al: Superimposition reformatted CT for preoperative lesion localization and surgical planning. J Comput Assist Tomogr 4:693-696, 1980.

Newton TH et al, editors: Radiology of the skull and brain, vol 5. Technical aspects of computed tomography, St Louis, 1981, Mosby.

Newton TH et al, editors: Modern neuroradiology, vol 1. Computed tomography of the spine and spinal cord, San Anselmo, Calif, 1983, Clavadel Press.

Post MJD, editor: Radiographic evaluation of the spine, New York, 1980, Masson.

Stevens JM, Valentine AR, and Kendall BE: Computed cranial and spinal imaging: a practical introduction, Baltimore, 1988, Williams & Wilkins.

Van Maes PFGM et al: Direct coronal body computed tomography, J Comput Assist Tomogr 62:58-66, 1982.

Definition of terms

Chapter 34

COMPUTED RADIOGRAPHY

MARCUS W. HEDGCOCK, JR.
RICHARD C. PASKIET, JR.

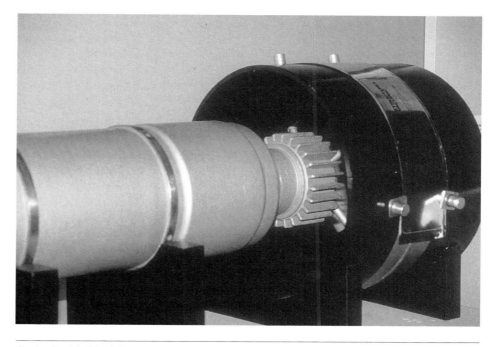

An industrial turbine with a radiographic film that is held in place by magnets (two on the top and two on the side). A radiation source was placed inside the turbine to check for flaws and faulty welds. The Roentgen Museum also exhibits industrial and molecular uses of radiation.

Since the days of Wilhelm Conrad Roentgen, radiography has been continuously improved and diversified. Even in the 1990s, the fluorescent x-ray film-screen combination remains the most widely used radiographic method. However, conventional film-screen radiography limits image manipulation to "hot-lighting" or duplication. More recent modalities, such as computed tomography (CT) and ultrasound, are *digital**; they provide cross-sectional images and allow the image to be manipulated. Conventional projection radiography (which accounts for nearly 60% of a radiology department's volume) has, until the past decade, remained an *analog* modality.

Various methods for enhancing the diagnostic capability of x-ray images have been used over the years; for example, stereoscopic radiography. In stereoscopic radiography two images of the same anatomic structure are obtained, with the x-ray tube shifted 6 degrees after the first image is obtained. The two resulting x-ray images are then placed side by side on a light box and viewed by using a stereoscope. This three-dimensional viewing helps the radiologist to some degree, but the process is operationally cumbersome.

*All italicized terms are defined at the end of this chapter.

Analog and Digital Information

Analog information is represented in a continuous fashion, whereas digital information is represented in discrete units. An analogy is the difference between oil paints and a box of crayons. The oil paints can be mixed to provide an infinite number of color shades, whereas the box of crayons can provide only the number of colors in the box. The advantage of digital information is that we know the location and nature of each digital level and can adjust each accordingly. All digital imaging systems, such as computed tomography, ultrasound, and computed radiography, acquire information by a process called *analog-to-digital conversion*. After the x-ray or ultrasound beam has passed through the patient, it is still an analog signal. This signal varies smoothly from zero (where all the radiation has been absorbed by some part of the patient) to the maximum intensity (where no radiation has been absorbed).

In a computed tomographic scanner (Chapter 33), the analog-to-digital conversion occurs when the x-ray beam strikes the detector located in the gantry. Each detector corresponds to an anatomic location that absorbed the radiation, and the detectors have a limited number of responses. The number of responses the detectors can make is called the gray level display of the system. If the system has 256 gray levels (0 being black, 256 being white), the computer assigns the gray level of these 256 shades that is closest to the intensity of the radiation striking the detector. The system then reproduces the image by combining the responses of all of the detectors. In a computed radiographic system, the analog-to-digital conversion occurs when the exposed image plate is scanned with a laser, and the emitted light pattern is then converted to digital information by the image reader, as explained on the following page.

Computed and Analog Radiography

Computed radiography, often abbreviated CR, refers to conventional projection radiography, in which the image is acquired in digital format using an imaging plate rather than film. Conventional projection radiography includes all of the radiographic procedures that are now performed using a film-screen system. These include the familiar radiographic procedures that comprise the majority performed in an imaging facility: chest, abdomen, and orthopedic radiographs and contrast-enhanced radiographic studies, such as excretory urography and barium studies examining the gastrointestinal tract.

The major obstacle to developmental changes in the field of conventional projection radiography has been that one specific medium, x-ray film, serves three distinct functions in the radiographic process; x-ray film is the sensor to acquire the diagnostic information, it is used to display the information, and it is used to store the information.

Historical Development

At the 1981 International Congress of Radiology (ICR) meeting in Brussels, Fuji Photo Film Co., Ltd., introduced the concept of computed radiography employing *photostimulable phosphor* plate technology. In 1983, the first clinical use of computed radiography was performed in Japan, and in early 1993 over 500 systems were in clinical use worldwide.

The operating principle of the phosphor plate, explained later in this chapter, has been shown to provide excellent image quality. Computed radiographic technology is digital and supports the development of a variety of computer-based diagnostic information processing systems. As such, computed radiography provides the missing link for the completely electronic radiographic imaging department and is now a practical imaging modality.

Converting conventional projection radiography into a digital format can be accomplished (1) by digitizing the standard radiographic film images, or (2) by acquiring a digital image directly by having the x rays strike an electronic sensor or an image intensifier, or by using an imaging plate that is then scanned with a laser and the emitted light read by an electronic sensor. The second technique described is currently the best option for computed radiography when a reusable imaging plate is used. In the remainder of this chapter, computed radiography refers to imaging performed using these imaging plates.

Unlike scanned projection radiography or intensifier-based systems which require that the images be acquired on dedicated equipment, the reusable photostimulable phosphor plate system can be used with any standard radiographic imaging equipment. The key to computed radiography's development is the separation of the functions of sensing, displaying, and storing information. Each function uses separate media and devices, and each function can be separately manipulated, yet central control of the final image is maintained through computer technology.

Operational Components: Separation of Image Acquisition, Display, and Storage Functions

IMAGE ACQUISITION FUNCTIONS

The image acquisition or "sensor" function served by the photostimulable phosphor imaging plate, like x-ray film, receives the portion of the x-ray beam that has passed through the patient. A computed radiography imaging plate looks physically much like an intensifying screen (Fig. 34-1), and the plate is placed in a cassette similar to an x-ray film cassette. The imaging plate (IP) is made of either a lightweight aluminum or rigid steel frame with the x-ray tube side composed of honeycombed carbon fiber to produce a low x-ray attenuation surface. These cassettes are primarily for protection of the imaging plate and not for light control due to the nature of the imaging plates. The imaging plate contains a layer of Europium-doped barium fluorohalide ($BaFX:Eu^{2+}$) crystals (the photostimulable phosphor). When x rays strike the crystals, BaFX is changed to a new semistable state. It is the distribution of these semistable molecules that forms the *latent image*. The $BaFX:Eu^{2+}$ phosphor is applied to a polyester support base and then coated with a clear protective layer. This protective layer is composed of either a polyethylene terephthalate or a fluorinated polymer material (Fig. 34-2). Below the phosphor is a supporting layer that protects the phosphor layer from external shocks. The supporting layer also prevents reflection of the laser light. Next is a backing layer that protects the imaging plate from scratches during transfer and storage. Last is a bar code label that contains a number assigned to the imaging plate. This bar code provides a mechanism for associating each imaging plate with patient identification and related examination and positioning information.

The imaging plate is flexible and less than 1 mm thick. A unique property of the phosphor material is its "memory" capability; it has the ability to maintain a latent image for a certain period of time after exposure to x rays. Although some image degradation occurs as time lapses, a plate will retain a diagnostic image for at least 6 hours.

A valuable characteristic of the imaging plate is its extreme *dynamic range*. The imaging plate demonstrates an excellent linear response to the intensity of x-ray exposure over a broad range. When the imaging plate response is compared with the characteristic, or H & D, curve of radiographic film (Fig. 34-3), the superior performance capability of the imaging plate is seen to provide far more information in the low and high exposure regions of the image.

The *image plate reader* is another important component of the image acquisition control in computed radiography (Fig. 34-4). The image reader converts the continuous analog information (latent image) on the imaging plate to a digital format. As the imaging plate is scanned by the laser in the image reader, the portion of the plate struck by a laser emits light. This emitted light is directed by high-efficiency light guides to the photomultiplier tubes where the light is converted to digital electrical signals. The first reader systems became available in 1983 and were capable of processing only 40 plates per hour. Reader systems today are more compact and are capable of processing approximately 110 plates per hour. Several image readers can be interfaced to one film recorder unit. For high-volume applications, such as chest radiography, stand-alone systems with integrated image processors are available. In any of the reader systems, the imaging plate is transported internally through all the various stages of processing, which are transparent to the operator.

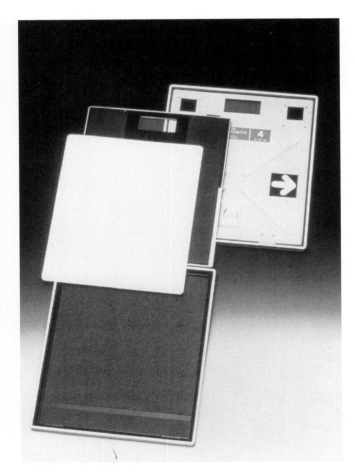

Fig. 34-1. Computed radiography photostimulable phosphor imaging plate (center left) shown lying on opened cassette. Back of closed cassette shown on upper right.

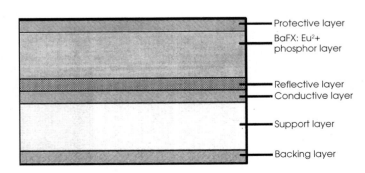

Protective layer
BaFX: Eu^{2+} phosphor layer
Reflective layer
Conductive layer
Support layer
Backing layer

Fig. 34-2. Schematic diagram showing layered composition of photostimulable imaging plate.

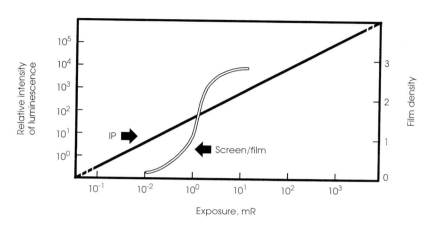

Fig. 34-3. Comparison of radiographic film H and D response curve to linear imaging plate response.

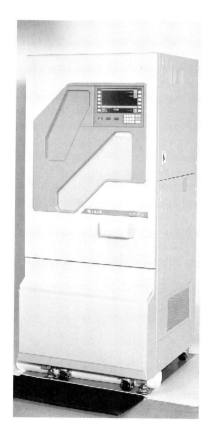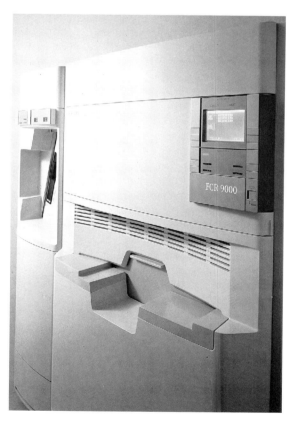

Fig. 34-4. Example of computed radiography components. The image reader device (left) processes approximately 40 imaging plates per hour. The larger system (right) is capable of processing approximately 110 imaging plates per hour.

DISPLAY FUNCTIONS

The display of computed radiography data is basically the result of *spatial frequency response processing* and *gradation processing,* which are used to control the contrast and density of the displayed image. Spatial frequency response controls the sharpness of boundaries between two structures of different densities. Gradation processing controls the range of densities used to display structures on the image; gradation processing is similar to the window settings used in computed tomography for display. These two different characteristics, contrast and density, are optimized by the digital image processor for the specific anatomic region being studied.

To produce an image for viewing, the computed radiography computer system constructs (formats) the image from the raw data as read from the photostimulable plate. Because the computed radiographic image is in digital format, the raw image data can be manipulated to accentuate or suppress various features of the image; the image can be tailored to a specific clinical task. This is similar to the operation of other digital imaging modalities such as computed tomography, where the window and level setting of the image can be changed to visualize a specific structure such as the liver or lung.

If no special parameters are specified by the user, the image is reconstructed using the *default,* or preset, settings that the specific medical center has decided produce the best-quality images. If special image characteristics are desired to highlight specific structures, the reconstruction factors can be changed by the radiographer or other user. The final image can be displayed on a monitor or produced as a hard-copy image on film or other medium. Unlike computed tomography, the computed radiography image is reconstructed each time from the raw data. If the image is displayed on a monitor, the image characteristics can be adjusted visually by the user to examine all features of the image to best advantage. To assist in the display process, various work stations with high-resolution *cathode ray tube (CRT)* monitors can be directly interfaced to the computed radiography unit.

There is little doubt that the electronic work station represents the alternator (viewbox) of the future. Work stations may be linked to a central image archive (an "electronic file room") and also to the text data in the radiology and hospital information systems, to provide a central clearing area for all information (images and text) needed by the imaging specialist. The functions for these work stations continue to be expanded (Table 34-1). These work station functions allow the user to alter the image display to best advantage for interpretation. The gradational enhancement (contrast) and spatial frequency (sharpness) enhancement can be varied on the work station, which is similar to formatting the hard-copy image. If, for example, two images have been taken sequentially, or taken using different energy characteristics (see dual energy subtraction discussed below), the images can be subtracted much like angiography with the use of radiographic film and digital subtraction systems. The image also can be "zoomed," or magnified. The density of a portion of the image can be estimated by selecting a *region of interest (ROI).* The image can also be rotated, flipped, or inverted. Statistical analyses can be performed on portions of the image, by calculating surface areas and estimated volumes or by characterizing the change in density in a part of the image. Most important for daily operations, however, the work station contains a data base that enables the user to easily locate images and create lists of images for conferences, interpretation, or teaching files.

The number of CRT monitors required for an interpretation work station is still under review. However, it is clear that at least two monitors are needed. The monitor resolution factor remains a point of contention among experts in this field. Currently, 1K × 1K (kilobyte) *matrix* monitors are generally used. The resolution is adequate for most studies, and the cost is within reason. However, 2K × 2K monitors are expected to be the norm for primary review work stations. With 2K × 2K resolution, all studies can be appropriately displayed with little or no loss of diagnostic information. The main deterrent at this time to routine use of 2K × 2K monitors is cost, which should become lower as availability increases. Finally, there is discussion concerning the use of 4K × 4K monitors. These monitors cannot be used to full potential until the computed radiographic image resolution is increased from the current 2K × 2K, which requires major changes in the system scanning architecture to acquire data at the 4K × 4K ratio. Cost will remain a major consideration for the use of these very high–resolution monitors.

Computed radiography also offers several options for film-based display. Fig. 34-5 shows a 2-on-1 format of an identical shoulder image. The image on the left demonstrates the shoulder with display factors similar to those of a conventional film-screen radiograph. An *edge enhanced* image is also automatically displayed as seen on the right image. Certain studies and pathologic conditions benefit from this enhanced image.

Table 34-1. Work station functions

Gradational enhancement	ROI display
Spatial frequency enhancement	Rotation/inversion
Subtraction/addition	Statistical analysis
Image magnification	Data base functions

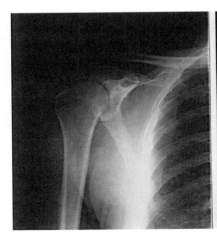
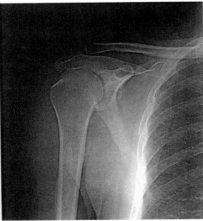

Fig. 34-5. Computed radiograph of a shoulder with conventional (left image) and edge-enhanced (right image) display parameters.

STORAGE FUNCTIONS

Computed radiography decreases image archive storage space requirements by reducing the size of films stored or by converting bulky film storage to electronic storage. Benefits include tremendous space savings, reduction in image retrieval time, and decreased film loss from nonreturns.

Several points must be considered regarding the design of electronic image archive devices. Flexibility is important. The device should interface with desired modalities and be expandable. The amount of storage on the electronic image archive should be adequate for the amount of data to be stored. Storage capacity of an electronic image archive depends on several variables, including the size of the basic storage unit (usually optical disk), the number of units on-line (jukebox size), and the ratio of data compression that is used.

An optical disk is currently the long-term storage medium of choice for computed radiography images. Computed radiography images contain more total data per individual image than any other digital modality, such as computed tomography or ultrasound (Table 34-2). Each computed radiography image contains about 5 *megabytes (M-byte)* of data. For example, a PA and a lateral chest image contain about 10 megabytes of data, which requires the same amount of electronic storage as the first four volumes of digital text found in the *Encyclopaedia Britannica*. One 12-inch dual-sided dual-density 2 *gigabyte (G-byte)* optical disk platter has the ability to store up to 800 computed radiography images with reversible 2:1 compression, or 7200 computed radiography images if 18:1 nonreversible compression is used. Such a factor alone projects the space savings benefit. By using an optical disk jukebox, approximately 200,000 radiographs can be stored in a space the size of a refrigerator.

Table 34-2. Capacities of various electronic data storage media

Medium	Capacity
Magnetic tape (2400 feet reel)	166 M-bytes
Winchester magnetic disk	700-1400 M-bytes
Optical disk	
Single optical disk	
12 inch	2 G-bytes
18 inch	6.8 G-bytes
Multiple platter optical "jukebox"	200-1000 G-bytes
Optical tape (2400 feet reel)	200 G-bytes

*1 gigabyte = 1000 megabytes.

With optical electronic storage, there is no deterioration of digital data. When such data are retrieved at a later date for image review and/or to make a copy on film, the reproduced image will be an exact duplicate of the initial image. In addition, any number of copies may be made using the original data, each being an original image. With these storage media, computed radiography image data can be searched for, retrieved, transmitted, or processed with tremendous ease.

Other large-capacity memory devices can be used for digital data storage. Magnetic tape, digital cassettes, streamer tape, or even verbatim cards can all serve these storage needs with various degrees of efficiency. Naturally, x-ray film can still be used to store visual analog patterns for image data filing purposes.

With a computed radiography system, flexibility can exist with the three primary options of (1) maintaining an active film file for display and storage purposes, (2) reviewing data on work stations and using long-term archiving devices for permanent electronic files, and (3) employing a combination of these methods to accommodate individual preferences.

Characteristics of a Computed Radiographic Image

Three factors are directly responsible for computed radiography image resolution: (1) the dimension of the crystals in the imaging plate, (2) the size of the laser beam in the reader, and (3) the image-reading matrix. Computed radiography contrast resolution is currently greater than that of conventional film, but *spatial resolution* is slightly less than that of film. Computed radiography resolution averages from 2 to 5 lp/mm (line pairs per millimeter), whereas standard film can demonstrate 3 to 6 lp/mm. With further advances in imaging plate phosphor quality, a reduction in the microbeam laser size, and an increase in matrix dimension and image, spatial resolution will become inherently superior to that of conventional film-screen parameters. Present-day diagnoses are not hampered by the current resolution factors. However, chest imaging and mammography will further benefit from the increased spatial resolution that these examinations demand.

Clinical Applications

The sequence of events in computed radiography imaging in the clinical environment is shown in Fig. 34-6. The computed radiography process begins at the reception desk, where demographic information such as patient name, birthdate, sex, ID number, and examination ordered is entered into a reception terminal. Transfer of this information to the computed radiography processor may be accomplished directly via a radiology information system (RIS) or health information system (HIS) interface, bar code, magnetic card, or optical scanner.

The radiographer exposes the imaging plate in the same manner as a conventional film-screen cassette is used. The exposure may be made using either a table-top, mobile, or table/wall Bucky technique. The exposed imaging plate cassette is taken to the control terminal of the computed radiography reader unit. Here the patient demographic and examination information is entered and the cassette is scanned with the bar code reader, linking each specific exposed imaging plate to the correct patient and image data. This replaces the typical ID camera step in film radiography.

The radiographer inserts the exposed cassette into the cassette insertion area of the reader unit (Figs. 34-6 and 34-7), and the reader door is then closed. Once inside, the cassette is automatically opened, and the imaging plate is removed and replaced with an erased plate for rapid "cassette" turnaround. If an imaging plate changer magazine (which will retain 30 imaging plates for arteriographic or mass examination studies) is used instead of a single plate cassette, the magazine is inserted into its appropriate space and the plates are automatically removed one at a time for reading. The reading process on the original plate is then initiated.

The internal functions of a computed radiography system are illustrated in Fig. 34-7. Inside the system and not apparent to the radiographer is the image plate reader assembly, which scans the imaging plate. The plate is transported through the system at right angles to a red *helium-neon (633 nm) laser* beam or aluminum gallium indium phosphorus (AlGaInP) semiconductor (680 nm) laser beam until the entire plate is sequentially scanned. When the barium fluorohalide crystals on the exposed photostimulable plate are exposed to the laser beam, the crystal layer emits the energy in the form of light, which was retained in its "memory" fol-

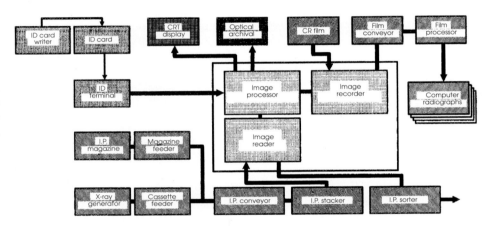

Fig. 34-6. Computed radiography sequence flow chart.

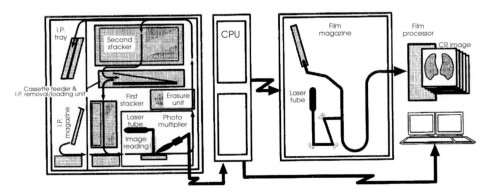

Fig. 34-7. Generalized internal functions and components of a computed radiography system.

lowing x-ray exposure. The light intensity emitted is proportional to the amount of x rays that initially excited the crystal layer. Tracking with the laser beam is a light guide, or photomultiplier pick-up tube, which collects the light emissions from all scanned areas and converts the light energy into electrical signals. Through an analog-to-digital converter, the electrical signal is converted into digital information, which is related spatially and is proportional in intensity to the original x-ray exposure in each segment of the imaging plate (Fig. 34-8).

The imaging plates offer wide exposure latitude. To make effective use of this latitude, the computed radiography system employs a sampling procedure for sensitivity adjustment during the plate reading stage. During the scanning process, a sample of the image data is acquired. These rough image data plus the entered anatomic data are examined to analyze the image characteristics and determine the best reading sensitivity and exposure latitude display parameters. By using this sampling capability, it is possible to normalize and digitize the entire luminescent area where the x-ray image exists. Errors in technical exposure factors are virtually eliminated. Exposure factors 500% greater than or 80% less than that which would normally be used to present the information aesthetically on a conventional film-screen system can be corrected by using the computed radiography system. These examples are obviously the extreme limits of correction and would rarely occur, but it must be realized that even gross technical errors are correctable when using the computed radiography system. Moreover, a general reduction in patient exposure can be realized when using computed radiography, compared with using the conventional 400-speed film-screen combination.

Technical corrections are achieved with computer-aided auto-ranging techniques. Optimized computed radiography display parameters are achieved through *histogram* analysis in proportion to the linear dynamic range of the imaging plates and tailoring the final image characteristics to an agreed-upon subjective H & D curve for best display of the anatomic structure(s) of interest.

To understand the effects of this process, consider the chest radiographs in Fig. 34-9. Analog and computed radiographic images were simultaneously obtained using a cassette containing both a radiographic film and an imaging plate. Despite technique factors that produced inadequate analog radiographs, all of the computed radiographic images are of consistent and appropriate penetration and quality. The "sampling" process normalized the image for the particular anatomic region being studied.

After the exposure of the imaging plate and its subsequent scanning by the laser beam, the image on the plate is erased. The energy remaining on the imaging plate after reading is completely eliminated by exposing the plate to a uniform and specific light source. This light source is either a bright sodium-vapor or a high-brightness fluorescent with both filtered and non-filtered ultraviolet components. The plates are reusable for thousands of times. In fact, the plate may well be mechanically destroyed or damaged before any degradation of the crystalline structure would ever be realized.

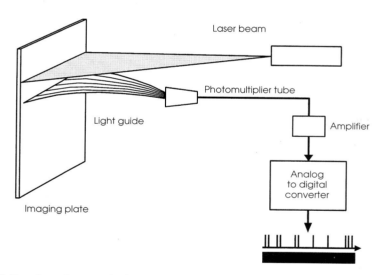

Fig. 34-8. Reading of computed radiographic imaging plate and conversion to digital information.

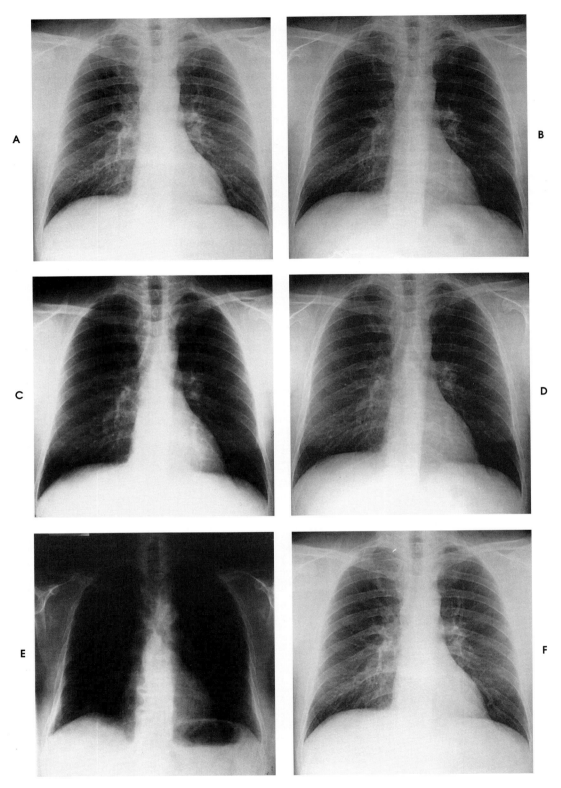

Fig. 34-9. Six images **(A** to **F)** showing pairs of analog (left images) and computed radiographs (right images) acquired simultaneously. Note that despite the widely differing exposure factors, the computed radiographic image does not vary in quality, although the analog radiographs are clearly suboptimal in quality. **A,** Analog radiograph and, **B,** CR image, both using exposure factors of 125 kVp, 1 mAs. **C,** Analog radiograph and, **D,** CR image, both using 125 kVp, 2.5 mAs. **E,** Analog radiograph and **F,** CR image, both using 125 kVp, 6.3 mAs.

Other Techniques to Improve Diagnostic Efficacy

Several other techniques (besides manipulation of the images on the work station) are available to improve the diagnostic power of computed radiography. These include acquisition techniques, such as *dual energy imaging*, higher resolution plates, analysis of computed radiography imagery by computer, and networking for review centralization. The computed radiographic systems may also use several inherent processing techniques such as dynamic range compression and unsharp masking to provide image characteristics which delineate a broad diagnostic visual range.

Image analysis by computer allows the user to extract more diagnostic information from the image. This is a relatively new technique, but it promises to open new diagnostic horizons for diagnosis using computed radiography. Fig. 34-10 shows profiles of bone mineral in the hand of a patient with rheumatoid arthritis; this image can be used to diagnose such a condition and determine improvement following therapy.

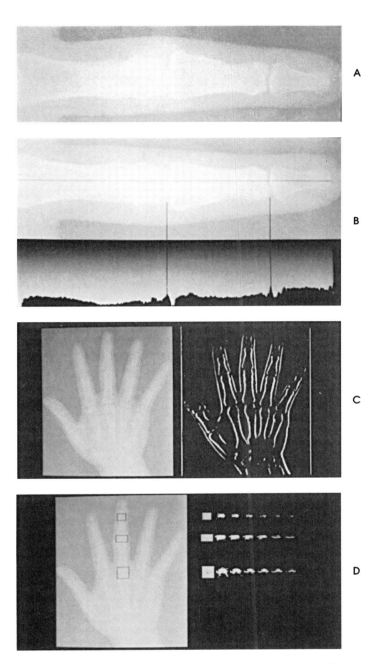

Fig. 34-10. Analytic techniques used on computed radiographic image of the hand to characterize the feature of the bones and detect abnormal variations. **A,** Computed radiographic image of third digit. **B,** Profile of density distribution of digit. **C,** Edge recognition algorithm. **D,** Transverse edge recognition of phalanx joints.

Clinical Acceptance

Computed radiography is being used at medical centers and hospitals in all applications where conventional projection radiography can be used, such as chest, bone, and mobile radiography, and contrast-enhanced examinations such as excretory urography and gastrointestinal radiography. Angiographic applications are primarily performed using digital radiography; angiographic applications are addressed in Chapter 35 in this atlas.

Quality Assurance Concerns

A positive design feature of a computed radiography system is its ability to minimize resultant image *artifacts,* whether induced from system irregularities or operator errors. Periodic failures in these safeguards, however, are inevitable and will affect image quality.

System noise, artifacts, and unevenness in an image are determined by the noise inherent in the imaging plate (structure noise) and reader system (quantum noise). Digital processing errors can create artifacts and density irregularities.

Several artifacts can be controlled by the operator. Dust on the imaging plate can be seen on the resulting image. It is, therefore, important to maintain a periodic schedule of cleaning the imaging plate surfaces for quality assurance, similar to the quality control maintenance used for radiographic intensifying screens. In addition, grids of a particular ratio and line factor are recommended for various examinations. If these recommendations are not followed, a *moiré* pattern of laser light scanning lines or data loss can occur. It must be understood that scatter radiation is detrimental to computed radiography image quality just as in conventional film-screen image quality. Grids must be used when the examination or the patient's body build warrants. Although computed radiography systems are able to correct for gross technical errors, there is a limit to the minimum dosage required for appropriate penetration and a diagnostic image. Each computed radiography operating institution must independently establish the radiation dose reduction limits. An inadequate dose will result in images demonstrating quantum mottle or areas devoid of data.

Pitfalls

In correctly produced computed radiography images, disadvantages are few and will not cause diagnostic problems, even with a relatively inexperienced computed radiography operator. The primary undesirable characteristics are edge enhancement artifacts. In certain circumstances, edge enhancement creates an appearance that may be confused with a pathologic disorder. On the edge-enhanced image, a dark band may appear at the interface between structures that differ widely in density. This effect is primarily seen in computed radiography images involving metal prostheses and barium contrast studies. The dark line of the edge-enhancement artifact is always perfectly symmetric around the dense object, which makes it relatively easy to distinguish from a lesion causing lucency. In computed radiographic images of the chest, the pulmonary vasculature is very prominent on the edge-enhanced image; however, the "standard technique" image shows the vasculature to have an appearance identical to that of standard film radiographs.

Benefits of Computed Radiography

When using a computed radiography system certain benefits are readily apparent, including the following:

IMPROVED DIAGNOSTIC ACCURACY AND EXPANDED DIAGNOSTIC SCOPE

By storing laser-scanned x-ray images on high-sensitivity imaging plates, minute differences in x-ray absorption are detected, providing highly detailed and easily readable diagnostic information. The wide exposure latitude permits diagnosis on an entire area of interest, allowing imaging from bones to soft tissue with a single exposure. Computer analysis of images can provide increased diagnostic information to assist in the medical treatment of a patient.

X-RAY DOSAGE REDUCTION

The high-speed imaging plate coupled with the efficient information read-out of the high-precision laser spot scanning device allows the patient to be exposed to a lower x-ray dose than that using a conventional film-screen system. This is especially worthwhile for pediatric examinations. Reductions vary somewhat with the type of examination performed, as shown in Table 34-3.

Table 34-3. Radiation dose for diagnostic quality image by computed radiography compared with standard radiography

Procedure	Decrease in dose relative (%)
Chest radiography	14-20
Upper GI series	5
Excretory urography	50
Pelvis radiography phantom study	12

REPEAT RATE REDUCTION

Because of the computed radiography system's wide technique latitude, technical errors are easily corrected to provide prime diagnostic information. When a film-screen combination is used, technical errors in either direction can markedly degrade the image quality. Technical errors have much less effect on the final quality of a computed radiographic image. This benefit obviously increases *throughput* and reduces the patient's discomfort, because it lessens the need to repeat the examination. The technical latitude of computed radiography is a tremendous asset in the area of portable radiography.

TELERADIOGRAPHIC TRANSMISSION

Image plate reader devices can be linked via dedicated phone lines, microwave transmission, or other teleradiographic means to centralize the review of image data. This means of image sharing could obviously benefit affiliated hospitals or clinics that are separated by large geographic distances and share professional staff. Teleradiology could also provide immediate consultation with specialists, which benefits not only the patient but also the level of efficiency of the institution.

Many radiology departments have contemplated a PACS (Picture Archive and Communication System) for the immediate or near future. Hesitation to implement PACS by many has been caused not only by fears of multimodality/multivendor interfacing, but also by the requirement that conventional projection radiography (which represents approximately 60% to 70% of a radiology department's volume) be digital format compatible. Computed radiography is the link needed for PACS. With computed radiography, all imaging modalities can be integrated and share processing, display, and archiving ventures.

Department Efficiency

The computed radiography system eliminates all darkroom work. With this factor plus the previous benefits, departmental efficiency is ultimately increased.

Summary

Computed radiography will improve both the operational and diagnostic efficiency of radiology departments. By placing conventional projection radiography in digital format, computed radiography forms the keystone for PACS. Computed radiography improves the efficiency of conventional projection radiography by providing consistent image quality, decreasing the repeat exposure rate, minimizing patient radiation exposure, and decreasing lost images. By realizing such, many departments have already found that computed radiography is proving to be a justifiable long-term investment.

Summary

Definition of Terms

analog Any information represented in continuous fashion rather than discrete units.

analog-to-digital conversion The process of converting a continuous (analog) signal to discrete (digital) units.

artifacts Observable, undesirable image features resulting from faulty image processing techniques.

bit Smallest piece of computer information.

byte 8 bits.

gigabyte (G-byte) 1000 megabytes.

megabyte (M-byte) 1000 bytes.

cathode ray tube (CRT) An electron tube (like a television tube) that makes the computer output visible; sometimes called a VDU (video display unit).

computed radiography (CR) Digital imaging process using a photostimulable chemical plate for the initial acquisition of image data; the display parameters of the image can be manipulated by a computer at a later time.

default The parameters by which the system operates; if no changes in instructions are made by the operator, the preset operating parameters or controls of the system prevail.

digital Any information represented in discrete units (see also analog).

dual energy imaging An x-ray imaging technique in which two x-ray exposures are taken of the same body part by using two different kilovoltages; the two images are processed in such a way as to remove image contrast resulting from either soft tissue or bone.

dynamic range The orders of magnitude over which the system can accurately portray information.

edge enhancement The technique of setting the spatial frequency response so that structures of a given type, usually the bones, stand out in bold relief.

gigabyte (G-byte) 1000 megabytes.

gradation processing The technique of setting the range of values over which an image is displayed, similar to the window setting in computed tomography. Gradation processing allows one to select a wide range of values to display structures with widely differing densities, or a narrow range to display structures close together in density; for example, a body part such as the mediastinum.

helium-neon laser An intense, coherent beam of light in the red wave-length.

histogram A graphic representation of the frequency distribution of gray levels, which represent the anatomy in a computed radiographic image (see Chapter 32, Fig. 32-13 for an example).

image plate reader The component of the computed radiography system that scans the image plate with a laser, converting the analog information on the image plate into an electrical signal; an analog-to-digital converter then changes the electrical signal to a digital signal.

latent image A nonobservable representation of a structure, such as the varied energy changes inherent in the crystalline structure of imaging plates.

matrix The grid-like pattern of an image, composed of a certain number of pixels, both in the horizontal and the vertical planes.

megabyte (M-byte) 1000 bytes.

moiré A fine network of wavy lines that have a watered appearance on the displayed image.

photostimulable phosphor A special luminescent material that stores x-ray energy and emits light proportional to the stored x-ray energy when stimulated by energy such as visible light from a laser.

pixels (picture elements) The small squares that form the image; pixels have depth in bits usually 8, 12, 15, etc.; the greater the pixel depth, the larger the gray scale.

region of interest (ROI) An area on the image judged of primary clinical interest.

spatial frequency response Sharpness of image that controls how prominently the "edges" are seen in one structure of one density compared with the "edges" in an adjacent structure of another density; the technique used in the computed radiography system is called "unsharp masking," in which an unsharp (blurred) image is used as the mask image to enhance the spatial frequency response.

spatial resolution How small an object can be detected by an imaging system, and how close together two similar objects can be and still be identified as separate objects. The measure usually used is line pairs per millimeter (lp/mm); for example, if the spatial resolution is 10 lp/mm, it means that 10 lines per millimeter can be distinguished as discrete lines, but if there are more than 10 lines per millimeter some lines will "run together" and appear to be a single line.

throughput The rate at which items can be processed through a system. Originally a systems analysis term, the term is now commonly used in medicine; if a radiology department can perform a maximum of 60 chest radiographs per hour, this is the maximum throughput for chest radiographs.

SELECTED BIBLIOGRAPHY

Anasuma K: Technical trends of the CR system. In Tateno Y, Iinuma T and Takano M, editors: Computed radiography, Tokyo, 1988, Springer-Verlag.

Barnes GT, Sones RA and Tesic MM: Digital chest radiography: performance evaluation of a prototype unit, Radiology 154:801-806, 1985.

Fraser RG, Breatnach E and Barnes GT: Digital radiography of the chest: clinical experience with a prototype unit, Radiology 148:1-5, 1983.

Hindel R: Review of optical storage technology for archiving digital medical images, Radiology 161:257-262, 1986.

Huebener KH: Scanned projection radiography of the chest versus standard film radiography: a comparison of 250 cases, Radiology 148:363-368, 1983.

Johnson GA and Ravin CE: A survey of digital chest radiography, Radiol Clin North Am 21(4):655-665, 1983.

Kuni CC: Introduction to computers and digital processing in medical imaging, St Louis, 1988, Mosby.

Long BW: Computed tomography: photo stimulable phosphor image plate technology, Radiol Technol 61(2):107-112, 1989.

Long BW: Image enhancement using computed radiography, Radiol Technol 61(4):276-280, 1990.

McAdams HP et al: Histogram-directed processing of digital chest images, Invest Radiol 21:253-259, 1986.

Sakuma H et al: Plain chest radiograph with computed radiography: improved sensitivity for the detection of coronary artery calcification, AJR 151:27-30, 1988.

Tateno Y: An introduction to clinical utilization of CR. In Tateno Y, Linuma T and Takeno M, editors: Computed radiography, Tokyo, 1987, Springer-Verlag.

Templeton AW et al: A digital radiology imaging system: description and clinical evaluation, AJR 149:847-851, 1987.

Tesic MM et al: Digital radiography of the chest: design features and considerations for a prototype unit, Radiology 148:259-264, 1983.

Chapter 35

DIGITAL SUBTRACTION ANGIOGRAPHY

WALTER W. PEPPLER

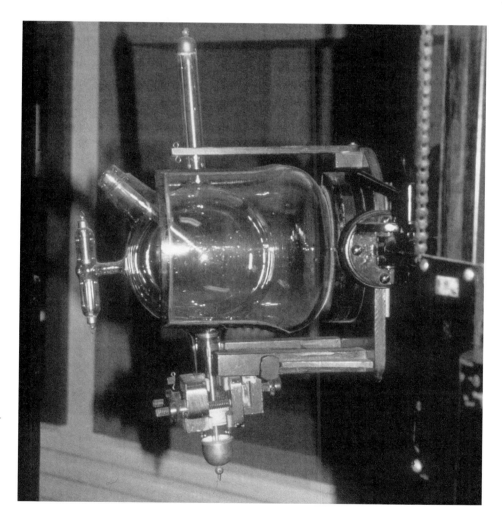

An x-ray tube surrounded by a lead glass bowl. This illustration demonstrates an early radiation safety precaution. The tube design is from approximately 1905.

Digital electronic technology has increased the speed of image processing and decreased costs to the point where totally electronic radiographic image detection, storage, and display are beginning to replace film in a number of procedures. More important, radiographic images stored in a digital memory can be manipulated in ways that are impossible with film. Such manipulation enables the radiologist to isolate image information that is too low in image contrast to be recognized on a conventional radiograph. The ability to "see" what previously had been invisible has opened new areas for radiographic study. One area that has gained widespread acceptance is *digital subtraction angiography* (DSA).

*All italicized terms are defined at the end of this chapter.
I wish to thank John C. McDermott, M.D., from the University of Wisconsin at Madison for his assistance in developing this chapter.

Historical Development

DSA was developed during the 1970s by groups at the University of Wisconsin, the University of Arizona, and the Kinderklinik at the University of Kiel. This work led to the development of commercial systems that were introduced in 1980. Within the next few years many manufacturers of x-ray equipment introduced DSA products. After several years of rapid change, the systems evolved to those available today. The primary changes since the introduction of DSA in 1980 include improved image quality, larger pixel *matrices* (up to 1024 × 1024), and fully *digital* systems. Image quality has improved for two reasons: (1) the component parts (e.g., the image intensifier, television camera) have been improved, and (2) the component parts have been more effectively integrated into the system, since the early systems were built using component parts selected "off the shelf" and they may or may not have been properly matched.

INTRAVENOUS VS. INTRAARTERIAL INJECTION

The most notable change in digital subtraction angiography was not in equipment design but in clinical practice. The initial success and promise of DSA was based on intravenous (IV) injection of contrast media. Intravenous procedures were less risky and less expensive than the intraarterial procedures used for conventional angiography and could be performed on an outpatient basis. This was advantageous, because conventional intraarterial film *angiography* usually required an overnight hospital stay. In addition, IV DSA was less painful for the patient. However, IV DSA did have serious drawbacks. Cardiac motion, diaphragmatic motion, bowel peristalsis, swallowing, or coughing all caused image *artifacts*. In patients with decreased cardiac output, the contrast bolus became seriously diluted, with resultant nondiagnostic examinations. Since large volumes of contrast were required for the IV method of DSA, contrast toxicity became a serious consideration. Finally, because all arteries in the region of interest were opacified, superimposition made the diagnosis of arterial stenosis difficult.

The standard of practice quickly evolved to performing DSA using intraarterial injection of contrast media. Since the examination was performed intraarterially, a smaller volume of more dilute contrast medium was required. With contrast being injected intraarterially near the region of interest, more *masks* could be obtained and patient motion and the attendant image degradation occurred less frequently. The evolution of smaller catheters (4 to 5 French) allowed outpatient arteriography to be performed safely. The arrival of *nonionic contrast media* has resulted in less patient discomfort (nausea and vomiting), significant reduction in the incidence of severe life-threatening reactions, with similar nephrotoxicity.

However, the main reason for the transition to intraarterial injection is the very significant increase in image quality. Intravenous injection of contrast media produces not only poorer image quality but also more variable results compared with those obtained routinely using intraarterial injections.

THE EXTINCTION OF FILM ANGIOGRAPHY?

With the widespread acceptance of DSA, and specifically intraarterial DSA, there are some proponents who believe that film arteriography may become a procedure of the past. Film arteriography still maintains an advantage in resolution with up to 10 lp/mm compared with about 2 lp/mm for DSA. Because DSA is extremely sensitive to motion artifact, the presence of bowel peristalsis and respiratory motion within the abdomen results in significant image degradation. Therefore, in visceral angiographic work, film arteriography is still considered the gold standard. This is particularly important when arteriography is performed in a patient with gastrointestinal bleeding, because resolution is critical. Cut film arteriography is still highly desirable in situations of small vessel disease (e.g., collagen vascular disease or cerebral vasculitis).

Equipment and Apparatus

An image intensifier–television system (fluoroscopy) can be used to form images with little electrical interference, provide moderate resolution, and yield diagnostic quality images when combined with a high-speed *image processor* in a DSA system as shown in Fig. 35-1.

The DSA procedure room is much like a standard angiographic suite. Both film and digital capabilities are usually present, and the fluoroscopic equipment operates in the conventional way. However, a brief review will help explain the DSA system. The input surface of the *image intensifier* is coated with an x-ray–sensitive phosphor, typically cesium iodide (CsI). The image-intensifier phosphor is contained within a vacuum and enclosed in glass. X rays that are absorbed by the CsI *input phosphor* emit visible light detected by electronics within the image intensifier. The detected light, proportional to the amount of radiation absorbed, is electronically amplified and accelerated across the image tube and is emitted at the *output phosphor* of the image intensifier by another light-emitting phosphor, approximately 1 inch in diameter. The resulting light intensity is brighter by a factor of 5000 to 10,000 times than if the CsI phosphor had been used alone.

The television camera is focused onto the image-intensifier output phosphor and converts the light intensity into an electrical signal. The television camera forms an image by electronically scanning a photosensitive *semiconductor* (called the target) on which the light has been focused. The presence of light on a small portion of the target changes the electrical properties in that target region. These changes are detected by the television camera.

The scanning of a narrow electron beam across the television target in 525 parallel lines at a rate of 525 lines per 1\30 second synthesizes an image line by line. With normal fluoroscopic operation, the video image is displayed on a television monitor. The scanning rate is so fast that the human eye does not notice the scanning process but sees a two-dimensional image on the television screen. The images are called *frames* and are presented at a rate of 30 per second.

In a DSA system, each of the television lines is further divided into segments called *pixels* (*pic*ture *el*ements). The electronic video signal corresponding to each pixel is *digitized* and stored in a digital memory. Typically each line is divided into 512 or 1024 pixels, and the digitized value (gray level) assigned to each pixel is usually in the range of zero (representing black) to 1023 (white). The image in *memory,* which is made up of a total of 512 × 512, or 1024 × 1024, pixels (the number of lines times the number of pixels per line), is also stored on a digital disk for later review, manipulation, and analysis.

The image processor consists of a computer and image processing hardware. The computer controls the various components (e.g., memories, image processing hardware, and x-ray generator), and the image processing hardware gives the system the speed to do many image processing operations in *real time*. The computer and the operator communicate via a keyboard and special function keys, or a touch-sensitive screen, to operate the DSA system.

The control room is usually separated from the procedure room and has a leaded glass window for observation (Fig. 35-2). Typically there is a video monitor on the operator's console as well as one in the procedure room next to the fluoroscopic monitor. At the operator's console there is also a computer monitor for communicating with the computer. The video monitors display the subtraction images in real time as the images are obtained during the imaging sequence. At a later time, films *(hard copy)* are produced using a multi-format camera or laser imager.

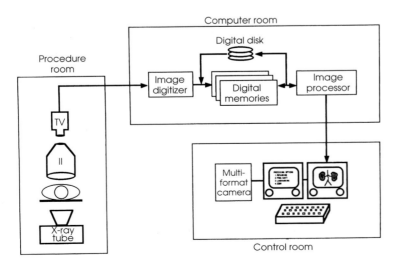

Fig. 35-1. Block diagram of a digital subtraction angiography (DSA) system.

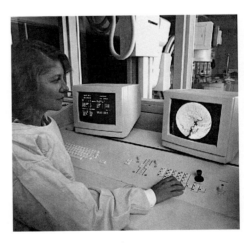

Fig. 35-2. The operator console of a digital subtraction angiography system with the procedure room in the background.

(Courtesy of Philips Medical Systems.)

Performing DSA Procedures

A DSA study begins by placing the catheter in the patient in the same manner used for conventional angiography. The injection techniques vary, but typically 40 to 50 ml of iodinated contrast medium is injected at a rate of 20 ml/sec for intravenous procedures, and 15 to 20 ml at a rate of 10 ml/sec for intraarterial procedures. An automatic pressure injector is used to ensure consistency of injection and to facilitate computer control of injection timing and image acquisition.

The intravascular catheter is positioned using conventional fluoroscopic apparatus and technique, and a suitable imaging position is selected. At this point an image that does not have a large dynamic range should be established; no part of the image should be significantly brighter than the rest of the image. This can be accomplished by proper positioning, but it often requires the use of compensating filters. The compensating filter can be either water bags or thin pieces of metal inserted in the imaging field to reduce the intensity of bright regions. Metal filters are usually affixed to the collimator, and water or saline bags are placed directly on or adjacent to the patient. If proper placement of compensating filters is not performed, significant reduction of image quality will result. The reason for this is that the DSA video camera operates most effectively with video signals that are at a fixed level. Automatic controls in the DSA system adjust the exposure factors so that the brightest part of the image is at that level. An unusually bright spot will satisfy the automatic controls and cause the rest of the image to lie at significantly reduced levels where the camera performance is worse. An alternative to proper filter placement is to adjust the automatic sensing region, which can be displayed on the image, to exclude the bright region. This solution is less desirable than using compensating filters, and for some positions of the bright spot it is not always possible.

As the imaging sequence begins, an image that will be used as a subtraction mask is digitized and stored in the digital memory. This mask image and those that follow are produced when the x-ray tube is energized and the x rays are produced, usually one exposure per second at 65 to 95 kVp, and between 5 to 150 mAs. The radiation dose received by the patient for each image is approximately the same as that used for serial film angiography. Each of these digitized images is electronically *subtracted* from the mask, and the subtraction image is amplified (contrast enhanced) and displayed in real time so that the subtraction images appear essentially instantaneously during the imaging procedure (Fig. 35-3). The images are simultaneously stored on a *digital disk* or *video tape recorder.* Video tape recorders are often used when images are acquired at a rate of 30 per second, because most digital disks cannot operate at high imaging rates. Real-time digital disks capable of recording images at a rate of 30 per second are quite expensive and are usually restricted to cardiac applications where high imaging rates are more common.

Misregistration is a major problem in DSA; it occurs when the mask and the images displaying the vessels filled with contrast medium do not exactly coincide. Misregistration is sometimes caused by voluntary movements of the patient, but it is also caused by involuntary movements, such as bowel peristalsis or the contraction of the heart. Preparing the patient by describing the sensations associated with contrast-medium injection and the importance of holding still and, of course, having the patient suspend respiration during the procedure can help eliminate volun-

tary movements. Compression bands, glucagon, and cardiac gating can be effective in reducing misregistration caused by involuntary movement. Misregistration is less of a problem in intraarterial DSA than in intravenous DSA, because there is an inherently larger signal in intraarterial DSA so the misregistration signals are less significant and also because the time is reduced between the mask and the postinjection (contrast-filled) image. In addition, because a smaller volume of contrast medium is required with intraarterial injection, the patient's discomfort and the likelihood of coughing or swallowing are reduced, so misregistration problems are also less likely.

During the imaging procedure, the subtraction images appear on the display monitor. In many cases a preliminary diagnosis can be made at this point or as the images are reviewed immediately following each exposure sequence. However, a formal reading session, typically performed from hard copy film, occurs at a later time, at which time the final diagnosis is made.

Some *post-processing* (described in the next section) is performed after each exposure sequence to improve the visualization of the anatomy of interest or to correct for misregistration. More involved post-processing, including quantitative analysis, is performed after the patient study has been completed, and then hard copies are produced using a *laser printer* or *multiformat camera.* In either case, several images appear on each film. The films are used during the formal reading session and are also kept for archival purposes.

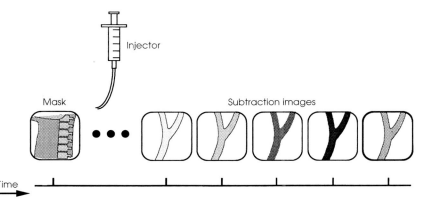

Fig. 35-3. Schematic representation of a digital subtraction angiography imaging sequence.

Image Post-Processing

After the images have been obtained and stored on a disk, there are several ways of manipulating, or post-processing, the images. The most common is to adjust the contrast and brightness to produce an optimum display of the image. The contrast and brightness adjustments are equivalent to the window and level adjustments performed on CT (Chapter 33) or MRI (Chapter 36) images. The terms "contrast" and "brightness" are often used for DSA because of the similarity to adjusting the contrast and brightness on a television set.

REMASKING

Another common post-processing task is to correct misregistered images. The most effective way to fix misregistration is simply to *remask* the image. To remask, another mask image is chosen that is properly registered with the image of interest; the procedure is usually simple. The most efficient way to remask images is as follows: Rather than choosing new masks one at a time (which may or may not work), the image containing the maximum iodine signal should be selected as the mask. Then a "live" (in this case without iodine) image that subtracts from the mask without misregistration is sought. The reversal of the role of the images reverses the polarity of the subtraction image (i.e., from white contrast to black contrast). However, the original polarity can be restored by pressing the contrast inversion button. This procedure usually produces an acceptable image with the least effort (Fig. 35-4).

PIXEL SHIFTING

In some cases an acceptable mask cannot be found. One way to salvage such runs is by *pixel shifting*. In this technique one of the images is shifted with respect to the other to compensate for the movement of the patient between the two images. Shifts of a fraction of a pixel are necessary in many cases to obtain proper registration. Most processors allow at least horizontal and vertical translation, and some permit rotation as well. Pixel shifting can be a tedious procedure that requires a great deal of patience. In addition to many possible pixel shifts, several combinations of mask and live images may have to be tried. Unfortunately, in many cases it is more expedient to simply repeat the run. A reliable automatic pixel registration routine is much more likely to be used.

EDGE ENHANCEMENT

Using *edge enhancement*, also called "unsharp masking," the edges of vessels can be accentuated (or enhanced) so that small details can be made more obvious. The procedure involves defining a *convolution matrix* that operates on the image. Predefined matrices are usually available, so an understanding of the underlying operations is not usually necessary. A real-time edge enhancement operation is available on some processors so that by simply turning a knob, various amounts of edge enhancement can be obtained.

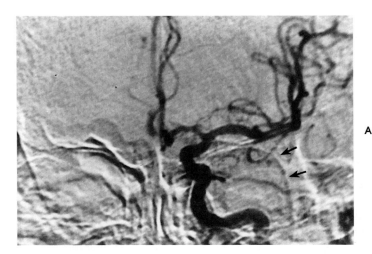

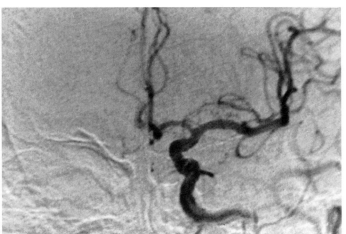

Fig. 35-4. Intraarterial DSA angiogram of the intracranial arteries, **A,** demonstrating misregistration artifacts. **B,** The same image after remasking. Notice the significant improvement in the misregistration artifacts, particularly in the region of the orbit *(arrows)*.

IMAGE ZOOM

Another post-processing option is to magnify, or *zoom*, the image. Zooming the image increases the size of a part of the image to make some subtle feature more visible. Zooming can be performed by interpolation or by pixel duplication. Interpolation produces intermediate pixels by averaging adjacent pixels and has a more pleasing appearance. However, pixel duplication is usually faster. The duplication method is often called "fast zoom," whereas the interpolation method is called "interpolative zoom." It should be noted that neither of the methods increases the resolution of the image. They simply present the same information in a more obvious way (Fig. 35-5).

LANDMARKING

In landmarking, a small amount of the original image is put back into the subtraction image. This is commonly done to give surgeons anatomic landmarks so that they can more accurately locate structures in the image. Without the landmark information it is difficult to locate the structures because the background has been so effectively eliminated. Only a fraction of the mask is added, however, so that the mask does not overwhelm the subtraction image. As an alternative to landmarking, an unsubtracted image may be printed on the same film as the subtraction images and used as a reference.

ANALYTIC TOOLS

There are a wide variety of analytic tools available on most image processors, including methods to measure distances, quantitate vessel stenoses, calculate ventricular ejection fraction, and measure blood flow. These tools are used regularly for cardiac studies. They are also used often for neuro and occasionally for vascular studies.

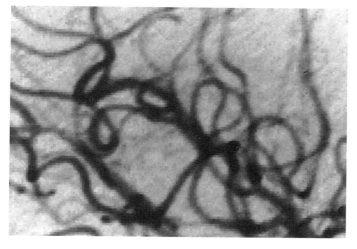

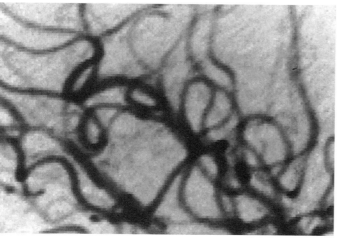

Fig. 35-5. A demonstration of the two types of image zoom on an intracranial DSA image; **A,** duplication and, **B,** interpolation. Notice the jagged appearance of the arteries when using the duplication method, **A.**

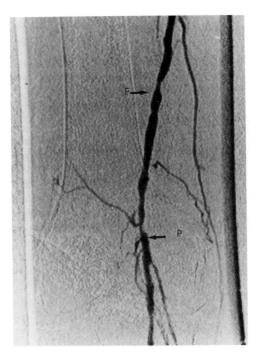

Fig. 35-6. Intraarterial DSA image of the common carotid artery demonstrating a severe stenosis of the internal carotid artery *(arrow).*

Clinical Applications

INTRAARTERIAL DSA

Nearly all peripheral and cerebrovascular arteriography is performed with intraarterial DSA (Figs. 35-6 to 35-8). Film arteriography is used whenever, in the judgment of the radiologist, the extra resolution of film is necessary or when misregistration is a problem, such as in patients with gastrointestinal bleeding where diaphragmatic motion or bowel peristalsis can cause severe image degradation.

Patients with peripheral vascular disease typically will undergo an intraarterial DSA examination of the infrarenal abdominal aorta, pelvic vessels, and runoff vessels. Because DSA has considerably greater contrast sensitivity than film, the intraarterial DSA method permits the identification of small vessels in the lower limbs of patients with severe peripheral vascular disease (Fig. 35-9). Some of these patients have been able to undergo a distal bypass procedure or angioplasty rather than amputation.

The intraarterial DSA approach can also be applied to pulmonary arteriography. To perform the examination, a catheter is placed within the main pulmonary artery, which permits the use of a small amount of contrast agent. In these situations, a rapid framing sequence (6 frames/sec to 15 frames/sec) is often used.

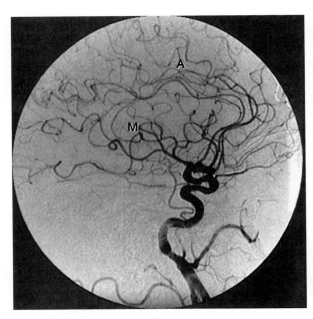

Fig. 35-7. Intraarterial DSA image of the intracranial vasculature showing patent anterior (A) and middle (M) cerebral arteries.

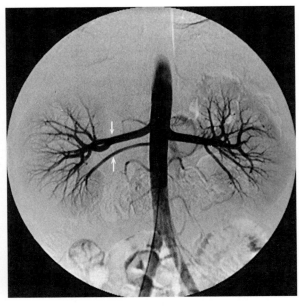

Fig. 35-8. Intraarterial DSA image of the abdominal aorta showing one renal artery on the left and two renal arteries on the right *(arrows);* all renal arteries are widely patent.

Alternatively, ECG triggering can be used with lower imaging rates. This application of the intraarterial DSA approach is particularly helpful in a patient with severe pulmonary arterial hypertension who is at significant risk from the high-rate, high-volume contrast injection used for standard pulmonary arteriography.

ROAD MAPPING

The intraarterial DSA approach has also resulted in the evolution of the road map technique. Most angiography/interventional radiologists use this technique routinely in the performance of angioplasty. The intraarterial road map technique provides the angiographer with a real-time continuous subtraction on the fluoro-scopic monitor during a procedure. An injection is made while the subtraction mask is obtained, then the fluoroscopic images are subtracted continuously from the mask. The stationary anatomy is cancelled, but the iodinated arteries remain. When the catheter is advanced it also appears on the monitor along with the iodinated arteries, which act as a road map to guide the catheter (Fig. 35-10). The road map technique is often used during the catheterization of a patient with a high-grade stenosis or an occlusion within a peripheral runoff vessel. Likewise, the intraarterial road map technique is also applied in superselective catheterization and as a monitor during the course of arterial embolization.

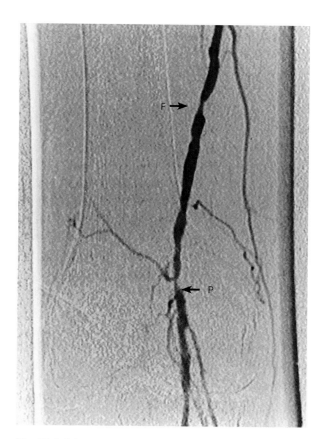

Fig. 35-9. Intraarterial DSA image of the distal superficial femoral (F), and popliteal (P) arteries showing diffuse, near occlusive disease *(arrows)*.

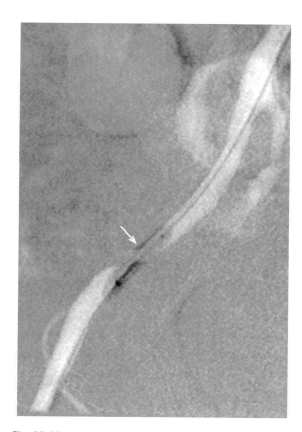

Fig. 35-10. A roadmap image of the right external iliac artery during balloon angioplasty. The roadmap image was helpful in crossing the stenosis and correctly centering the angioplasty balloon at the stenosis *(arrow)*.

INTRAVENOUS DSA

Currently, IV DSA is performed infrequently. It is occasionally employed in the evaluation of patients with malfunctioning Hickman catheters and possible superior vena cava syndrome; in such a patient, catheters are placed in each brachial vein and simultaneous contrast injections are performed to delineate the central veins (Fig. 35-11). When there is a groin hematoma or possible cellulitis, an IV DSA is helpful in excluding a pseudoaneurysm or mycotic aneurysm of the artery. When the radiologist has difficulty catheterizing the artery, and intravenous DSA examination may be helpful in determining the anatomy of the artery and in facilitating subsequent catheter placement. Rarely, IV DSA is used to determine the patency of aortobifemoral grafts.

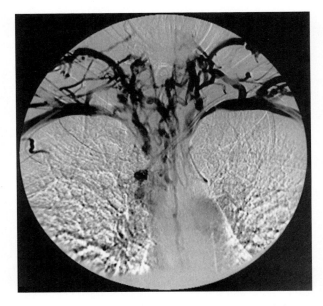

Fig. 35-11. An intravenous DSA image of the chest showing superior vena cava thrombosis.

Conclusion

Digital subtraction angiography has had a great impact on diagnostic radiology. Its advantages over film angiography are that it has much greater contrast sensitivity, lower cost, and immediate availability of results. The digital nature of the data also permits quantitative analysis of DSA images. In some cases this has proven valuable, particularly in cardiac applications. The increased contrast sensitivity has permitted the use of lower total volumes and concentrations of contrast media; decreased patient discomfort and reduced toxicity are therefore obtained.

The early interest in intravenous injection of contrast medium has yielded to the intraarterial injection technique in most cases. Intraarterial DSA has been successfully used for imaging most major arteries, but there are still procedures where film angiography is the method of choice, particularly when maximum resolution is required. A properly equipped angiography suite will have the capability for both DSA and film angiography.

Definition of Terms

angiography Producing x-ray images of the blood vessels after injection of contrast medium.

artifact Any undesirable side effect resulting from an image processing technique.

convolution matrix A two-dimensional array of values used in an operation called convolution when performing edge enhancement.

digital Information stored in discrete units, called bits. These bits are used to form a binary code for representing information.

digital disk A circular plate coated with magnetic material and used to store digital data.

digital subtraction angiography The use of digitally recorded x-ray images to produce subtraction images of vessels.

digitize The process of converting a continuous analog voltage signal into a discrete digital value.

edge enhancement Making the edges of anatomical structures more clearly visualized through intentional unsharp masking and/or computer manipulation.

frame A single image from a sequence of images.

hard copy A copy of a video image on film.

image intensifier An imaging device that converts an x-ray distribution (image) to an optical image with a large increase in brightness.

image processor A special-purpose computer designed to operate on images in a short time.

input phosphor A material that is coated on the input surface of an image intensifier tube, which emits light in response to the absorption of x rays.

ionic contrast medium A contrast agent that ionizes in solution and causes more patient discomfort than nonionic contrast medium.

laser printer A device that uses a scanning laser beam to produce a copy of images on film.

mask An image in which the arteries do not contain iodine that is subtracted from images with iodine in the arteries.

matrix A two-dimensional array of pixel values that make up an image.

memory That portion of an image processor in which the numbers that represent an image are stored.

misregistration When the two images used to form a subtraction image are slightly displaced from one another.

multiformat camera A device that produces copies of images on a single film.

nonionic contrast medium A contrast agent that does not ionize in solution and is safer, less painful, and better tolerated by the patient than ionic contrast medium.

output phosphor A material that is coated on the output surface of an image intensifier, which emits light (an image) in response to being struck by electrons.

pixel (*picture element*) One of the small cells an image breaks into when it is digitized. Each cell represents only a small fraction of an entire picture.

pixel shifting The digital image is shifted to compensate for misregistration marks caused by patient motion. It is an alternative to remasking.

post-processing Image processing operations performed when reviewing an imaging sequence.

real time Any image processing technique that can be performed within a time frame that is so short as to appear to be instantaneous.

remask Repeating the masking process by choosing a different mask image in order to correct for misregistration marks.

semiconductor Solid-state material used in the construction of electronic devices, such as transistors or integrated circuits.

subtracted When the mask image is used to remove the scout image (via electronic superimposition) from the postinjection angiogram image.

video tape recorder A device that uses magnetic tape to record video images.

zoom Magnification of the image via interpolation or pixel duplication; resolving power remains unchanged.

SELECTED BIBLIOGRAPHY

American Association of Physicists in Medicine: Performance evaluation and quality assurance in digital subtraction angiography, report no. 15, New York, 1985, American Institute of Physics Inc.

Brennecke R et al: Computerized video-image preprocessing with applications to cardio-angiographic roentgen-image series. In Nagel HH, editor: Digital image processing, Berlin, 1977, Springer-Verlag.

Carmody RF et al: Digital subtraction angiography: update 1986, Invest Radiol 21:899-905, 1986.

Christenson PC et al: Intravenous angiography using digital video subtraction: intravenous cervicocerebrovascular angiography, AJR 135:1145-1152, 1980.

Coltman JW: Fluoroscopic image brightening by electronic means, Radiology 51:359-365, 1948.

Crummy AB et al: Computerized fluoroscopy: digital subtraction for intravenous angiocardiography and arteriography, AJR 135:1131-1140, 1980.

Crummy AB: Digital subtraction angiography. In Taveras JM and Ferrucci JT: Radiology: diagnosis-imaging-intervention, Philadelphia, 1992, JB Lippincott Co.

Crummy AB et al: Digital subtraction angiography "road map" for transluminal angioplasty, Semin Intervent Radiol 1(4):247-250, 1984.

Digital subtraction angiography in clinical practice, Best, the Netherlands, 1986, Philips Medical Systems.

Fink U et al: Peripheral DSA with automated stepping, European Journal of Radiology 13:50-54, 1991.

Foley WD et al: Intravenous DSA examination of patients with suspected cerebral ischemia, Radiology 151:651-659, 1984.

Heintzen PH, Brennecke R and Bursch JH: Computer quantitation of angiocardiographic images. In Miller HA, Schmidt EV and Harrison DC, editors: Noninvasive cardiovascular measurements, vol 167, Bellingham, Wash, 1978, Society of Photooptical Industrial Engineers.

Hillman BJ: Digital radiology of the kidney, Radiol Clin North Am 23:211-226, 1985.

Kruger RA and Riederer SJ: Basic concepts of digital subtraction angiography, Boston, 1984, GK Hall Medical Publishers.

Kruger RA et al: A digital video image processor for real time subtraction imaging, Optical Engineering 17:652-657, 1978.

Kruger RA et al: Computerized fluoroscopy in real time for noninvasive visualization of the cardiovascular system, Radiology 130:49-57, 1979.

Meaney TF et al: Digital subtraction angiography of the human cardiovascular system, AJR 135:1153-1160, 1980.

Mistretta CA and Crummy AB: Digital fluoroscopy. In Coulam CM et al, editors: The physical basis of medical imaging, New York, 1981, Appleton-Century-Crofts.

Mistretta CA and Crummy AB: Diagnosis of cardiovascular disease by digital subtration angiography, Science 214:761-765, 1981.

Mistretta CA et al: Multiple image subtraction technique for enhancing low contrast periodic objects, Invest Radiol 8:43-44, 1973.

Mistretta CA et al: Digital subtraction arteriography: an application of computerized fluoroscopy, St Louis, 1982, Mosby.

Moodie DS and Yiannikas J: Digital subtraction angiography of the heart and lungs, Orlando, Fla, 1986, Grune & Stratton.

Morgan RH and Sturm RE: Johns Hopkins fluoroscopic screen intensifier, Radiology 57:556-564, 1951.

Norman D et al: Intraarterial digital subtraction imaging cost considerations, Radiology 156:33-35, 1985.

Ovitt TW et al: Intravenous angiography using digital video subtraction: x-ray imaging system, AJR 135:1141-1144, 1980.

Seeley GW et al: Computer controlled video subtraction procedures for radiology, Proc Soc Photooptical Instrumentation Engineers 206:183-189, 1979.

Strother CM et al: Clinical applications of computerized fluoroscopy: the extracranial carotid arteries, Radiology 136:781-783, 1980.

Zweibel WJ et al: Comparison of ultrasound and IVDSA for carotid evaluation, Stroke 16:633-643, 1985.

Definition of terms

Chapter 36

MAGNETIC RESONANCE IMAGING

JAMES H. ELLIS

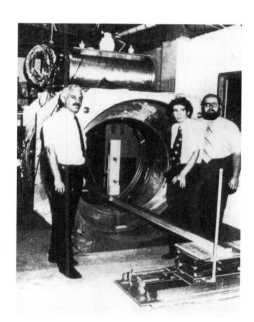

First NMR scanner for humans. Left to right, R. Damadian, L. Minkhoff, M. Goldsmith (1988).

From Eisenberg RL: Radiology: an illustrated history, ed 1, St. Louis, 1992, Mosby.

Tremendous interest among medical workers and the general public has been generated by the appearance of *magnetic resonance imaging (MRI)** as a technique for examining the human body. MRI can provide both anatomic and physiologic information noninvasively. Like computed tomography (CT), MRI is a computer-based cross-sectional imaging modality, but there the similarity to CT ends. The physical principles of MRI image production are totally different from CT and conventional radiography; no x rays, indeed no ionizing radiation of any kind, are used to generate the MRI image. MRI examines the interactions of magnetism and radio waves with tissue to obtain its images.

MRI was originally called *nuclear magnetic resonance,* or NMR. The word "nuclear" indicated that the nonradioactive atomic nucleus played an important role. The word "nuclear" has been disassociated from MR imaging because of public apprehension about nuclear energy and nuclear weapons, neither of which is associated with MRI in any way (unless by coincidence a nuclear power plant is supplying electricity to an MRI unit). In addition, there are forms of MRI that do not involve the atomic nucleus and which may, in the future, be used for imaging under the "magnetic resonance" umbrella.

---

*All italicized terms are defined at the end of this chapter.

The tireless efforts of Elaine Grech in manuscript preparation, helpful suggestions by Frank J. Londy, R.T., and photographic assistance from Robert L. Combs are greatly appreciated.

Comparison of MRI and Conventional Radiology

Since MRI provides sectional images, it serves as a useful adjunct to conventional x-ray techniques. With a radiograph, all body structures exposed by the x-ray beam are superimposed into one "flat" image. Many times, multiple projections or contrast agents are required to clearly distinguish one anatomic structure or organ from another. However, sectional imaging techniques such as ultrasound, CT, and MRI more easily separate the various organs, because there is no superimposition of structures. However, multiple *slices* (cross sections) are required to cover a single area of the body.

In addition to problems with overlapping structures, conventional radiography is relatively limited in its ability to distinguish types of tissue. In radiographic techniques, *contrast,* the ability to discriminate two different substances, depends on differences in x-ray *attenuation* within the object and the ability of the recording medium (e.g., film) to detect these differences.

Radiographs cannot detect small attenuation changes. In general, conventional radiographs can distinguish only air, fat, soft tissue, bone, and metal, where the difference in attenuation between each group is large. Most organs, for example, liver and kidneys, cannot be separated by differences in x-ray attenuation alone unless the differences are magnified through the use of contrast agents.

CT is much more sensitive than plain film radiography to small changes in x-ray attenuation. Thus CT can distinguish the liver from the kidneys on the basis of their different x-ray attenuation as well as by position.

Like CT, MRI can resolve relatively small contrast differences among tissues. It should again be emphasized, however, that these tissue differences are independent from the differences in x-ray attenuation. Contrast in MRI depends on the interaction of matter with electromagnetic forces other than x rays.

Historical Development

The basic principle (discussed more fully below) of MRI is that certain atomic nuclei, if placed in a magnetic field, can be stimulated by (absorb energy from) radio waves of the correct frequency. Following this stimulation, the nuclei release the extra absorbed energy by transmitting radio waves (the MRI signal), which can be received by an *antenna* and analyzed. *Relaxation times* represent measurements of the rates of this energy release.

These properties of magnetic resonance were first discovered in the 1940s by separate research groups headed by Bloch and Purcell. Their work led to the use of MRI *spectroscopy* for the analysis of complex molecular structure and dynamic chemical processes. Spectroscopic MRI is still in use today. The Nobel Prize in physics was shared by Bloch and Purcell in 1952 in recognition of the importance of their discoveries.

Nearly 20 years later, Damadian showed that the relaxation time of the water in a tumor differed from the relaxation time of the water in normal tissue. This indication that the relaxation times varied from tissue to tissue suggested that images of the body might be obtained by producing maps of relaxation rates. In 1973, Lauterbur published the first cross-sectional images of objects obtained with MRI techniques. These first images were crude and only large objects could be distinguished. Since then there has been an explosion in MRI technology, so that very small structures can be imaged rapidly with increased resolution and contrast.

Physical Principles
MRI SIGNAL PRODUCTION

The structure of the atom can be compared with the solar system, with the sun representing the central atomic *nucleus*. The planets orbiting the sun represent the electrons circling around the nucleus. MRI depends on the properties of the nucleus.

Many, but not all, atomic nuclei have magnetic properties; that is, they act like tiny bar magnets (Fig. 36-1). Normally the magnetic nuclei point in random directions as shown in Fig. 36-2. However, if these nuclei are placed in a strong, uniform magnetic field, they attempt to line up with the direction of the magnetic field, much as iron filings line up with the field of a toy magnet. The word "attempt" is appropriate because the nuclei do not line up precisely with the external field but at an angle to the field, and they rotate about the direction of the magnetic field similar to the wobbling of a spinning top. This wobbling motion, depicted in Fig. 36-3, is called *precession* and occurs at a specific *frequency* (rate) for a given atom's nucleus in a magnetic field of a specific strength. These precessing nuclei can absorb energy if they are exposed to *pulses* of radio waves, provided the radio waves are of the same frequency as the frequency of the nuclear precession. This absorption of energy occurs through the process of *resonance*.

After the external radio wave is turned off, the excited nuclei relax: they release their excess absorbed energy in the form of a radio wave. This radio wave transmitted by the nuclei represents the MRI *signal* and is not pulsed. The MRI signal can be picked up by a sensitive antenna, amplified, and processed by a computer to produce a sectional image of the body. This image, like the image produced by a CT scanner, represents an electronic image that can be viewed on a television monitor and adjusted to produce the most information. If desired, the image can be photographed for further study.

Most MRI currently involves the element hydrogen, the nucleus of which is a single proton. Hydrogen nuclei are the strongest nuclear magnets on a per-nucleus basis (thus giving the strongest MRI radio signal). Also, hydrogen is the most common element in the body (again giving the strongest signal). Strong signals are important to produce satisfactory im-

ages. Nevertheless, many other nuclei in the body are potential candidates for imaging. Nuclei such as phosphorus and sodium may give more useful or diagnostic information than hydrogen, particularly in efforts to understand the metabolism of normal and abnormal tissues. Changes in metabolism may prove to be more sensitive and specific in the detection of abnormalities than the more physical and structural changes recognized by

hydrogen imaging MRI or by CT. However, the MRI signal from nonhydrogen nuclei is very weak, their imaging requires more elaborate equipment, and anatomic detail is less (compared with hydrogen MRI) in sodium and phosphorus images produced to date. Nonhydrogen nuclei may be of particular importance in combined MR imaging and spectroscopy, in which small volumes of tissue may be analyzed for chemical content.

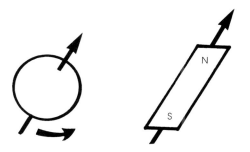

Fig. 36-1. A nucleus with magnetic properties can be compared with a tiny bar magnet. The *curved arrow* indicates that a nucleus spins on its own axis; this motion is different from that of precession.

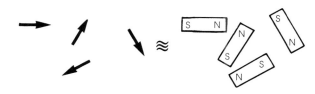

Fig. 36-2. In the absence of an external magnetic field, the nuclei *(arrows)* point in random directions and cannot be used for imaging.

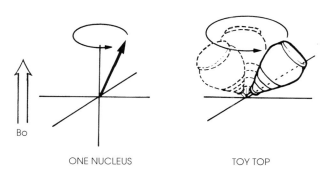

ONE NUCLEUS   TOY TOP

Fig. 36-3. Precession. Both the nucleus *(arrow)* and the toy top spin on their own axes. Both also rotate *(curved arrows)* around the direction of an external force in a wobbling motion called precession. Precessing nuclei can absorb energy through resonance. *Bo* represents the external magnetic field acting on the nucleus. The toy top precesses under the influence of gravity.

MRI SIGNAL SIGNIFICANCE

Conventional radiographic techniques, including CT, produce images based on a single property of tissue: x-ray attenuation or density. MRI images are more complex because they contain information about three properties of matter: nuclear density, relaxation rates, and flow phenomena. Each contributes to overall MRI signal strength. The computer processing converts signal strength to a shade of gray on the image. Strong signals are represented as white in the image and weak signals are black.

One determinant of signal strength is the number of precessing nuclei (spin density) in a given volume of tissue. The signal released by the excited nuclei is proportional to the number of nuclei present. Therefore signal strength depends on the nuclear concentration, or density. Since the nucleus of hydrogen is a single proton, this is often referred to as *proton density.* Most soft tissues, including fat, have a similar number of protons per unit volume, so proton density poorly separates most tissues. However, some tissues have very few hydrogen nuclei per unit of volume; examples include the cortex of bone and air in the lungs. These have a very weak signal as a result of low proton density and can be easily distinguished from other tissues.

MRI signal intensity also depends on the relaxation times of the nuclei. The process of energy release by the excited nuclei is called *relaxation,* and this can occur at different rates in different tissues. There are two processes by which excited nuclei relax. When the nuclei release their excess energy to the general environment (or lattice, the arrangement of atoms in a substance), this is called *spin-lattice relaxation.* The rate of this relaxation process is measured by *T1. Spin-spin relaxation* is the release of energy by excited nuclei through interaction among themselves. The rate of this process is measured by *T2.*

The rates of relaxation (T1 and T2) of a hydrogen nucleus depend on the chemical environment in which that nucleus is located. Chemical environment differs among tissues. For example, the chemical environment of a hydrogen nucleus in the spleen differs from that of a hydrogen nucleus in the liver. The relaxation rates of these nuclei differ, and the MRI signals given off by these nuclei differ. Liver and spleen have a different signal intensity and a different appearance on the image, enabling the viewer to discriminate between them. Similarly, fat can be separated from muscle, and many tissues can be distinguished from others, based on the rates of the relaxation of their nuclei. Indeed, the most important factor in tissue discrimination is the relaxation times.

The signals produced by MRI techniques contain a combination of proton density, T1, and T2 information. By stimulating the nuclei with certain specific radiowave *pulse sequences,* the radio signal that the nuclei release may have more information about proton density, or about T1, or about T2. Therefore one can obtain images weighted toward any one of these three parameters. In most imaging schemes, a short T1 (fast spin-lattice relaxation rate) gives a high MRI signal in T1-weighted images. Conversely, a long T2 (slow spin-spin relaxation rate) gives a high signal in T2-weighted images.

Using the data from two or more regular images, computer calculations of pure proton density, T1, or T2 images can be made. However, these calculated images have more *noise* and less resolution than regular MRI images.

The final property that influences image appearance is flow. Moving substances, for complex physical reasons, usually have weak MRI signals. (With some specialized pulse sequences, the reverse may be true. See MRI angiography later in the chapter.) With standard pulse sequences, flowing blood in vessels has a low signal, easily discriminated from surrounding stationary tissues without the need for the contrast agents required by regular radiographic techniques. Stagnant blood (such as an acute blood clot) typically has a high MRI signal in most imaging schemes, as a result of its short T1 and long T2. It may be possible to assess vessel patency or determine the rate of blood flow through vessels by employing this property of MRI (Fig. 36-4).

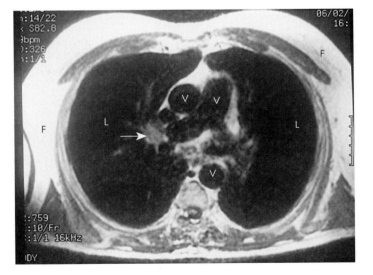

Fig. 36-4. Axial 1.5 Tesla superconductive ungated MR image through the upper chest. Lungs *(L)* have low signal as a result of low proton density. Fat *(F)* has high signal because of its short T1 relaxation rate. Moving blood in vessels *(V)* has low signal from the flow phenomenon. Hilar tumor *(arrow)* is easily identified, outlined against the low signal intensity of the lung and the vessels.

Equipment

Similar to CT, MRI requires a patient area (magnet room), a computer room, and an operator's console. A separate diagnostic viewing console is optional.

CONSOLE

The operator's console is used to control the computer. The computer then initiates the appropriate radiowave transmissions, receives the data, and analyzes it. Images are viewed on the operator's console to ensure that the proper part of the patient is being evaluated (Fig. 36-5). Images may be photographed, usually on radiographic films using a laser or multi-image camera.

The independent diagnostic viewing console may perform the same functions as the operator's console, depending on system configuration, except that usually only the operator's console can control the actual imaging process.

COMPUTER ROOM

The computer room houses the electronics necessary for transmitting the radiowave pulse sequences and receiving and analyzing the MRI signal. The *raw data* and the computer-constructed images can be stored on a computer disk temporarily and are usually transferred to magnetic tape or optical disk for permanent storage and retrieval.

MAGNET ROOM

The major component of the MRI system in the magnet room is the magnet itself. This magnet must be large enough to surround the patient and any antennas that are required for radiowave transmission and reception. Antennas are frequently wound in the shape of a coil. Most often, the patient is placed within the coil. Surface coils are placed directly on the patient and image superficial structures. However, the patient and coil must still be within the magnet to be exposed to the proper magnetic field for imaging. The patient lies on the table and is advanced into the magnetic field (Fig. 36-6).

Various magnet types and strengths may be used to provide the strong uniform magnetic field required for MR imaging.

Resistive magnets are simple, although large, electromagnets. They consist of coils of wire. A magnetic field is produced by passing an electric current through wire coils. High magnetic fields are produced by passing a large amount of current through a large number of coils. The electrical resistance of the wire produces heat and limits the maximum magnetic field strength of resistive magnets. The heat produced is conducted away from the magnet by a cooling system.

Superconductive (cryogenic) magnets are also electromagnets. However, their wire loops are cooled to very low temperatures with liquid helium and liquid nitrogen to reduce the electrical resistance. This permits higher magnetic field strengths with superconductive magnets than with resistive magnets.

Permanent magnets are a third method of producing the magnetic field. A permanent magnet has a constant field that does not require additional electricity or cooling to low temperatures. Early designs of permanent magnets were extremely heavy, even compared with the massive superconductive and resistive units, causing difficulties with placement in hospitals. With improvements in technology, permanent magnets may become more competitive with the other magnet types. Permanent magnets have the advantage that their magnetic field does not extend as far away from the magnet (*fringe field*) as do the magnetic fields of the other types. Fringe fields are a problem because of their effect on nearby electronic equipment.

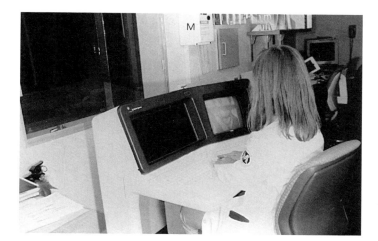

Fig. 36-5. Operator's console. This device controls the imaging process and allows visualization of images on a television monitor. The images may be manipulated to bring out the desired information. Note monitor *(M)* for magnet room oxygen concentration.

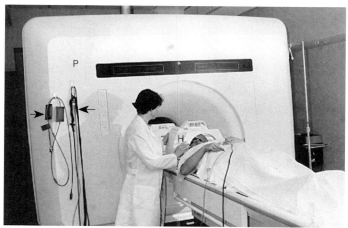

Fig. 36-6. Patient prepared for MR imaging. A protective housing *(P)* covers the magnet. The antenna coil for head *(H)* imaging is placed over the patient's head before both are advanced into the magnet. The head coil is removed when body imaging is performed. Note probes *(arrows)* for physiologic monitoring and gating.

Various MRI systems operate at different magnetic field strengths. Magnetic field strength is measured in *Tesla* or *gauss*. Most MRI has been performed with field strengths ranging from 0.1 to 1.5 Tesla, although higher strength MRI units are under development. Resistive systems generally do not exceed 0.15 Tesla, and permanent magnet systems do not exceed 0.3 Tesla. Higher field strengths require superconductive technology.

The choice of optimum field strength for imaging is controversial. Higher field strengths lead to increased MRI signal, which can be used to improve image sharpness or obtain the image data faster. However, some authorities argue that higher field strengths lead to reduced tissue contrast.

Regardless of magnet type, MRI units are relatively difficult to locate in a hospital. Current units are quite heavy, in the neighborhood of up to 10 tons for resistive and superconductive magnets and approximately 100 tons for some permanent magnets. Some hospital structures will not support this weight without reinforcement. With resistive and superconductive magnets, the fringe field extends in all directions. These fringe fields may interfere with nearby electronic or computer equipment, such as television monitors and computer tapes. In addition, metal moving through the magnetic fringe field, such as automobiles or elevators, may cause ripples in the field, similar to the ripples occurring when a pebble is thrown into a pond. These ripples can be carried into the center of the magnet where they distort the field and ruin the images. Thus MRI sites must be located far enough away from such moving metal objects to prevent this problem. Shielding of the magnetic fringe field to prevent its extension beyond the patient area continues to be developed to solve this difficulty.

The radiowaves used in MRI may be the same as those used for other nearby radio applications. These stray radiowaves from outside sources could be picked up by the MRI antenna coils and interfere with normal image production. Many MRI facilities require special room construction to shield the antenna from outside radio interference, which adds to the cost of the installation.

Safety of MRI

MRI is generally considered safe. Since MRI does not use ionizing radiation (which has known potential adverse health effects), it is often preferred over CT in imaging children, because the young and growing child's body is felt to be more susceptible to ionizing radiation's effects. Nevertheless, a number of potential safety issues concerning MRI must be raised, some related to potential direct effects on the patient from the imaging environment and others related to indirect hazards.

The question of the safety of the varying magnetic and radio frequency fields to which the patient is directly exposed remains controversial. Many studies exposing experimental animal and cell culture systems to these fields over long periods of time have reported no adverse effects, while others have reported changes in cell cultures and embryos. Some energy is deposited in the patient during imaging and is dissipated in the body as heat. These changes appear to be below the levels considered clinically significant, even in areas of the body with poor heat dissipation such as the lens of the eye. The significance of direct short-term exposure (as for imaging) or long-term exposure (as for employment) is not clear. No clear association with adverse effects in humans has been proven, but research is continuing.

A number of hazards related to MRI have been well documented. Objects containing magnetic metals (e.g., iron, nickel, and cobalt) in various combinations may be attracted to the imaging magnet with sufficient force to injure patients or personnel who may be interposed between them. Scissors, oxygen tanks, and patient gurneys are among the many items that have been drawn into the magnetic field at MRI sites. Metallic implants within patients or personnel can become dislodged within the body and cause injury if they are in delicate locations; examples include prosthetic heart valves, intracranial aneurysm clips, auditory implants, and metallic foreign bodies in the eye. On the other hand, long-standing, firmly bound surgical clips (such as from a cholecystectomy) do not pose problems. Electronic equipment can malfunction when exposed to strong magnetic fields. The most critical items in this category are cardiac pacemakers (and the similar automatic implantable cardiac defibrillators). Therefore, patients, visitors, and personnel should be screened to ensure that they do not have metallic objects on or in their bodies which might lead to adverse consequences upon exposure to strong magnetic fields.

Patients have received local burns from wires touching their skin during MRI examinations. This may result either from an electrical burn caused by currents induced in the wires or from a thermal burn caused by heating of the wires. Such burns can be prevented by checking wires for frayed insulation, avoiding wire loops within the magnetic field, and placing additional insulation between the patient and any wires exiting the MRI system.

The varying magnetic forces within an MRI unit act on the machine itself, causing motion of internal parts which results in knocking or banging sounds. These noises can be loud enough to produce temporary or permanent hearing damage. The use of earplugs or nonmagnetic headphones can be helpful in avoiding auditory complications.

Claustrophobia can be a significant impediment to MRI for up to 10% of patients (Fig. 36-7). Patient education is perhaps most important in avoiding this problem, but tranquilizers, appropriate lighting and air movement within the magnet bore, and mirrors or prisms that enable a patient to look out from inside the imager also may be helpful. Claustrophobia can also be avoided by having a family member or friend accompany the patient and be present in the room during the scan.

Rapid venting of the supercooled liquid gases (helium and/or nitrogen) used in superconductive magnet systems from the magnet or from their storage containers into the surrounding room space is a rare but potential hazard, because the relative concentration of oxygen in the air could be reduced to unsafe levels. Unconsciousness or asphyxiation could result. Oxygen monitoring devices in the magnet or cryogen storage room (Figs. 36-6 and 36-7) can signal personnel when the oxygen concentration falls too low. Personnel may then evacuate the area and activate ventilation systems to exchange the escaped gas for fresh air.

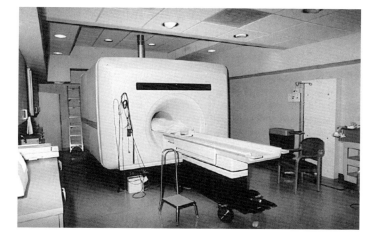

Fig. 36-7. Patient inside magnet. Some patients cannot be scanned because of claustrophobia. All items in magnet room (e.g., patient monitoring probes, foot stool, ladder to add liquid gases to the superconductive magnet) must be nonmagnetic (e.g., aluminum, plastic).

Examination Protocols

INSTRUMENT PARAMETERS

The availability of many adjustable parameters makes MRI a complex imaging technique. Knowledge of the patient's clinical condition or probable diseases is important in choosing the proper technique and imaging the correct area of the body.

A choice must be made whether to obtain a single slice image through a specific position in the body or to obtain multiple slices. Of course, a large area can be covered by making a series of single slices, just like CT. However, each standard MRI slice requires considerable time to acquire, usually 2 to 5 minutes, compared with just a few seconds or less for a CT slice. To improve throughput, MRI units can obtain multiple slices in one data acquisition. Although it may take a long time to acquire this much data, the average time per slice is reduced. As will be discussed below, some fast pulse sequences can obtain a single slice in just a few seconds.

The operator may choose to obtain MRI images in sagittal, coronal, transverse, or oblique planes. These are independently acquired images with equal resolution in any plane (Fig. 36-8). This differs from CT, in which data can be obtained only in the transverse plane. Sagittal and coronal CT images can be generated by reformatting the data from a series of transverse slices, usually with a loss of resolution.

Another MRI alternative, especially when a large number of thin slices and/or multiple imaging planes are desired, is three-dimensional (3D) imaging. In this technique, MRI data is collected simultaneously from a 3D block of tissue rather than from a series of slices. Special data collection techniques and subsequent computer analysis allow the images from the single imaging sequence to be displayed in any plane (Fig. 36-9).

Slice thickness is important in the visualization of pathology. More MRI signal is available from a thicker slice than a thinner slice, so thicker slices may provide more pleasing images that are less grainy. However, small pathologic lesions may be hidden by the surrounding tissues in the thicker slices. Therefore slice thickness may be adjusted, depending on the type of lesion under investigation.

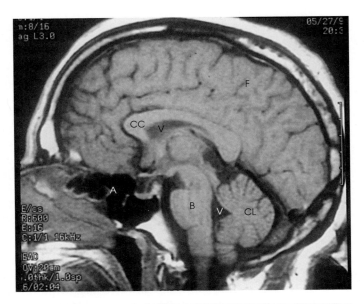

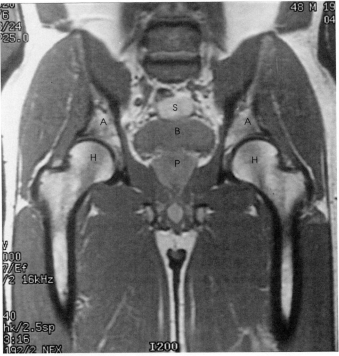

Fig. 36-8. Two images (different patients) from a 1.5 Tesla superconductive MR imager showing excellent resolution of MR images in nonaxial planes. Top image shows remarkable anatomic detail in a midline sagittal image of the head. Normal folds (*F*) on the inner surface of the brain are identified. *CC*, corpus callosum; *CL*, cerebellum; *B*, brainstem; *V*, ventricle; *A*, air in sinuses. Bottom image shows coronal image of the pelvis. Anatomic relationships of femoral heads (*H*) to acetabula (*A*) are well seen. Also excellent demonstration of the relationships of the prostate (*P*), enlarged in this case and elevating the bladder (*B*). Loop of sigmoid (*S*) on top of bladder. This degree of resolution in coronal or sagittal images would be difficult to obtain by reformatting a series of transverse CT slices.

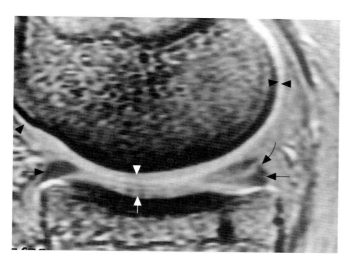

Fig. 36-9. Single slice from fast-sequence 3D acquisition of the knee on a 1.5 Tesla MR unit. Data from an entire volume within the imaging coil is obtained concurrently. It may then be reconstructed into thin slices in any plane, such as the sagittal image shown here. This imaging sequence shows hyaline cartilage *(arrowheads)* as a fairly high signal intensity rim overlying the bone. Meniscal fibrocartilage *(arrows)* has low signal intensity. High signal from joint fluid in a tear *(curved arrow)* within the posterior meniscus is visualized.

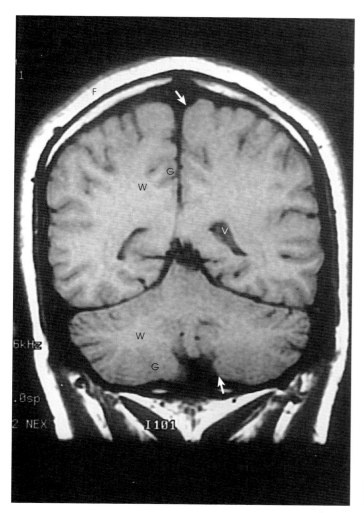

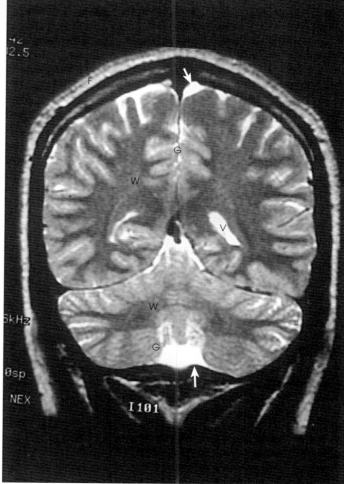

Fig. 36-10. Coronal 1.5 Tesla MR images through a normal brain. Left image is T1-weighted, showing relatively poor differentiation of gray matter *(G)* and white matter *(W)* within the brain. Right-hand image is heavily T2-weighted, showing dramatic improvement in differentiation between gray and white matter. Cerebrospinal fluid around the brain *(arrows)* and within the ventricles *(V)* also changes in appearance with change in pulse sequence (low signal on T1-weighted image and high signal on T2-weighted image). On the T1-weighted image (left-hand image), fat *(F)* shows high signal intensity, while on the T2-weighted image (right-hand image), the signal intensity of fat is less than that of cerebrospinal fluid.

Another important parameter is the overall imaging time. As imaging time (per slice) is lengthened, more MRI signal is available for analysis. Image quality thus improves with increased signal. However, fewer patients can be imaged when extended data acquisitions are performed. In addition, patient motion increases with prolonged imaging times, reducing image quality.

The radiowave pulse sequence is a crucial parameter in MRI. Depending on the choice of pulse sequence, the resulting images may be more strongly weighted toward proton density, T1, or T2 information. Normal anatomy (Fig. 36-10) or a pathologic lesion (Fig. 36-11) may be easily recognized or difficult to see depending on the relative emphasis given to these factors. It is not unusual for a lesion to stand out dramatically when one pulse sequence is used, yet be nearly invisible (same MRI signal as surrounding normal tissue) when a different pulse sequence is employed. Considerable research continues to determine the optimum pulse sequences for scanning various patient problems.

While varying the timing parameters of an individual pulse sequence can alter the relative weighting of information received, certain classes of pulse sequences tend to emphasize information about proton density, T1, T2, and even flow. *Spin echo* sequences are the classic imaging sequences, usually employed with timing parameters to yield T2-weighted images, but they can also provide proton density–weighted images and even T1-weighted images. *Inversion recovery* is a sequence which accentuates T1 information but can also provide a special result: the timing parameters can be chosen to minimize signal intensity in a particular tissue. Usually fat is the tissue chosen to have its intensity minimized, and so-called fat-suppressed images can be useful when the high signal from extensive fat overwhelms small signal intensity differences in the tissues of interest. However, techniques to suppress the signal from fat have been developed for pulse sequences other than inversion recovery, and these newer techniques have in gen-

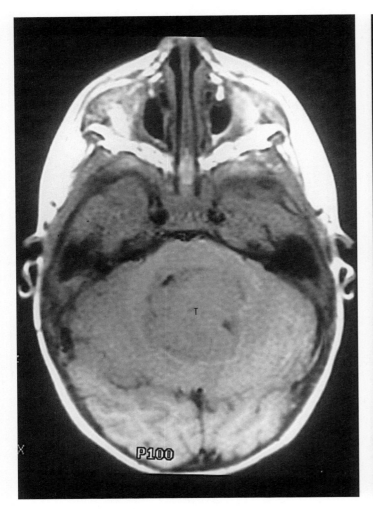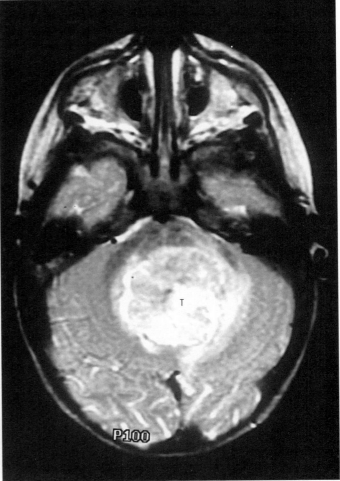

Fig. 36-11. Axial 1.5 Tesla superconductive MR images using two different radiowave pulse sequences from a child with a medulloblastoma. There is limited contrast between the tumor *(T)* and normal brain in the left image (T1-weighted); the lesion is dramatically more obvious using the pulse sequence of the right image (T2-weighted). Choice of pulse sequence is critical. These images also demonstrate the superiority of MR over CT in posterior fossa lesions due to lack of bone artifact.

eral replaced inversion recovery sequences for this purpose.

Because standard imaging sequences such as spin echo and inversion recovery are relatively time-consuming, slowing patient throughput, MRI engineers and physicists have developed faster pulse sequences to speed up examinations. Some imaging sequences are sufficiently short that imaging can be obtained during a breath hold. Many of the fast pulse sequences are sensitive to flow and may be used to provide images of blood vessels (see MR angiography later in the chapter). However, while fast pulse sequences offer scan time savings, there are prices to be paid for this advantage. Some of the faster pulse sequences tend to have less contrast among various normal and abnormal tissues, and must rely more heavily on contrast agents to provide differentiation of signal intensity between lesions and normal structures. In addition, fast MRI images may be compromised by increased noise or sensitivity to *artifacts*.

POSITIONING

Patient positioning is usually straightforward with MRI units. In general, the patient lies supine on a table that is subsequently advanced into the magnetic field. As previously discussed, it is important to check that the patient has no contraindications to MRI such as a cardiac pacemaker or intracranial aneurysm clips. Occasionally, patient positions other than the supine position are employed. For example, the patient may be turned partly to the side to obtain oblique images. Prone or decubitus positioning also may be used to shift structures under the influence of gravity or for patient comfort. As noted above, claustrophobia may be a problem for some patients, because the imaging area is tunnel-shaped in most MRI system configurations (Fig. 36-7).

COILS

The body part to be examined determines the shape of the antenna coil to be used for imaging (Fig. 36-12). Most coils are round or oval-shaped, and the body part to be examined is inserted into the coil's open center. Some coils, rather than encircling the body part, are placed directly on the patient over the area of interest. These "surface coils" are best for thin body parts, such as the limbs, or superficial portions of a larger body structure, such as the orbit within the head or the

spine within the torso. Another form of surface coil is the endocavitary coil, in which the imaging coil is designed to fit within a body cavity, such as the rectum. This enables a surface coil to be placed close to some internal organs which may be distant from surface coils applied to the exterior body. Endocavitary coils also may be used to image the wall of the cavity itself (Fig. 36-13).

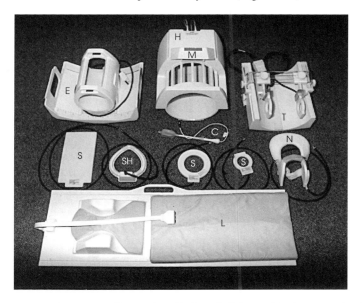

Fig. 36-12. Various coils used in MR imaging. Limb coil (*E*) is used for knee and ankles. Head coil (*H*) has open construction and mirror (*M*) allowing patient to see through coil to reduce claustrophobia. Shoulder coil (*SH*) fits over the shoulder. Neck coil (*N*) fits around neck. Surface coils in special holder (*T*) for imaging temporomandibular joints. Various shapes of general purpose surface coils (*S*) may be applied directly over the superficial part to be imaged, such as the wrist, orbit, or spine. Patient lies on larger specialized surface coil (*L*) for extensive spine imaging. Endocavitary coil (*C*) can be placed in rectum after covering balloon tip with condom. All coils shown except head and neck coils are surface coils, because the antenna does not encircle the imaged part. Any coil can act as both a radio wave transmitter and a receiver, though often an encircling coil is used as transmitter when surface coils are employed as receivers.

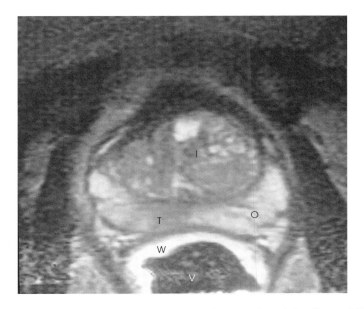

Fig. 36-13. Axial image of the prostate obtained with an endorectal coil on a 1.5 Tesla MR unit. Mixed signal intensity in the inner gland region (*I*) of the prostate due to benign prostatic hyperplasia. High intensity outer gland (*O*) is interrupted by a low intensity region representing prostatic carcinoma (*T*). Use of endorectal coil allows close proximity of coil to the area of desired imaging, improving resolution. *V*, signal void from coil within rectum (coil itself is not imaged). *W*, rectal wall.

PATIENT MONITORING

Although most MRI sites are constructed so that the operator can see the patient during imaging, often the visibility is limited and thus patients are relatively isolated within the MRI room (Fig. 36-7). Intercoms are present at most sites for verbal communication with the patient, and some units have "panic buttons" with which patients may summon assistance. However, these may be insufficient to monitor the health status of sedated, anesthetized, or unresponsive patients. MRI-compatible devices now exist to monitor multiple physiologic parameters such as heart rate, respiratory rate, blood pressure, and oxygen concentration in the blood. Typically the monitor with its display is located in the operator's room with leads extending to probes placed on the patient (Fig. 36-6). Local policy and patient condition dictate which physiologic parameters are monitored.

CONTRAST AGENTS

Contrast agents that widen the signal differences in MRI images between various normal and abnormal structures are a continuing area of research and development. The perfect agent for oral administration to identify bowel loops in MRI scans has not yet been identified. In CT scanning, high-attenuation oral contrast clearly differentiates bowel from surrounding lower attenuation structures. However, in MRI scans, the bowel may lie adjacent to normal or pathologic structures of low, medium, and high signal intensity, and these intensities may change

as images of varying T1 and T2 weighting are obtained. It is difficult to develop an agent that provides good contrast between the bowel and all other structures under these circumstances. Air, water, fatty liquids (e.g., mineral oil), solutions of dilute iron (e.g., Geritol), gadolinium compounds designed for intravenous use, barium sulfate, kaolin (a clay), and a variety of miscellaneous agents have all been employed, none with complete success.

As of this writing, the only intravenous MRI contrast agents approved in the United States for routine clinical use are gadolinium-containing compounds. Gadolinium is a metal with *paramagnetic* effects. Pharmacologically, an intravenously administered gadolinium compound acts very much like radiographic iodinated intravenous agents: it distributes through the vascular system, its major route of excretion is the urine, and it respects the blood-brain barrier (that is, it does not leak out from the blood vessels into the brain substance unless the barrier has been damaged by a pathologic process). Gadolinium compounds have lower toxicity and fewer side effects than the intravenous iodinated contrast media used in radiography and CT.

Gadolinium compounds are used most frequently in evaluation of the central nervous system. The most important clinical action of gadolinium compounds is to shorten T1. In T1-weighted images, this provides a high-signal, high-contrast focus in areas where gadolinium has accumulated by leaking through the broken blood-brain barrier into the brain substance (Fig. 36-14). Since T1-weighted

images can be obtained much faster than T2-weighted images, the use of gadolinium contrast agents can improve throughput if T2-weighted imaging sequences are eliminated. In addition, gadolinium-enhanced T1-weighted images are better at separating brain tumors or metastases from their surrounding edema than are routine T2-weighted images. Gadolinium improves the visualization of small tumors, or tumors that have signal intensity similar to normal brain, such as meningiomas. Intravenous gadolinium injections also have been used in dynamic imaging studies of body organs such as the liver and kidneys, similar to techniques using standard radiographic iodinated agents in CT.

A number of novel contrast agents for MRI are under development but, as of this writing, are not yet approved for routine clinical use. Agents specifically designed to enhance the blood may allow estimates of tissue perfusion and ischemia. Enhancement of heart muscle could assist in differentiating healthy, ischemic, or infarcted myocardial tissue. Contrast agents selectively taken up in the liver may improve detection of liver tumors or metastases. Selective enhancement of lymph nodes might enable detection of tumor involvement directly, rather than employing crude size criteria for abnormality. It may also be possible to produce contrast agents with an affinity for specific tumors; radioactive labeled antibodies against tumors are available for use in nuclear medicine, and appropriately labeled antibodies could carry paramagnetic compounds to tumor sites.

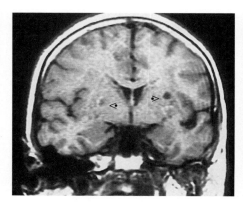
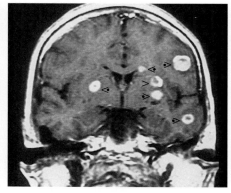
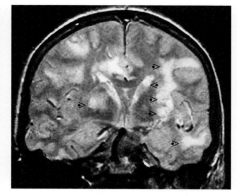

Fig. 36-14. Use of gadolinium intravenous contrast for lesion enhancement. Coronal 1.5 Tesla superconductive images of the brain. Left image shows relatively T1-weighted sequence. Two brain metastases (*arrowheads*) are identified as focal areas of low signal. Middle image employed same parameters after intravenous gadolinium contrast. Previously seen metastases are more conspicuous and additional metastases are recognized (*arrowheads*). Right image is T2-weighted. High-signal areas (*arrowheads*) represent metastases and surrounding edema; identification of focal lesion size and precise location is more difficult. In addition, scanning of entire brain took three times as long with the T2-weighted sequence as with the T1-weighted sequence. Additional high-signal intensity areas on T2-weighted image represent edema from focal lesions seen on other slices in the gadolinium-enhanced series.

GATING

Gated images are another technique for improving image quality in areas of the body where involuntary patient motion is a problem. A patient can hold his or her head still for a prolonged data acquisition but cannot stop his or her heartbeat or stop breathing for the several minutes required for standard MR imaging. Even fast pulse sequences are susceptible to motion artifact from the beating heart. This is a problem when images of the chest or upper abdomen are desired. If special techniques are not employed, part of the MRI signal may be obtained when the heart is contracted (systole) and part when the heart is relaxed (diastole). If this information is combined into one image, the image of the heart will be blurred. This is analogous to photographing a moving subject with a long shutter speed. Similar problems occur with the different phases of respiration.

To solve this problem, *gating* techniques organize the signal so that only the signal received during a specific part of the cardiac or respiratory cycle is used for image production (Fig. 36-15).

Gated images may be obtained in one of two ways. In one technique of cardiac gating, the imaging pulse sequence is initiated by the heartbeat (usually monitored by an electrocardiogram). Thus the data collection phase of the pulse sequence occurs at the same point in the cardiac cycle. Another method is to obtain data throughout the cardiac cycle, recording from what point in the cycle the data was obtained. After enough data is collected, the data is reorganized so that all data recorded within a certain portion of the cardiac cycle is collated together; for example, data collected during the first eighth of the cycle, second eighth of the cycle, etc. Each grouping of data can be combined into a single image, producing multiple images at different times in the cycle. As an analogy, consider eight children spinning on a merry-go-round. You want a high-quality picture of each child, but you have a video camera in which the image from a single frame is of insufficient quality for your purposes. If you needed an image of only one of the children, you could shoot one video frame each time that child came into the video viewfinder. Later, you could combine all the frames into one high-quality image. This is equivalent to the first gating technique. Alternately, if you wanted pictures of all the children, you could run the video camera continuously, recording which frames have which child in them. Later, you could match together all the frames showing the first child, all the frames showing the second child, and so forth, producing eight pictures, each showing one of the children. This is equivalent to the second gating technique.

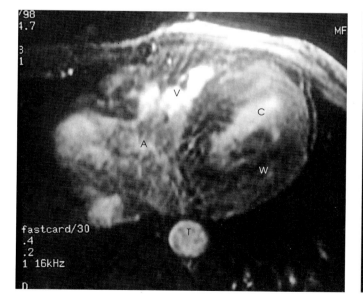
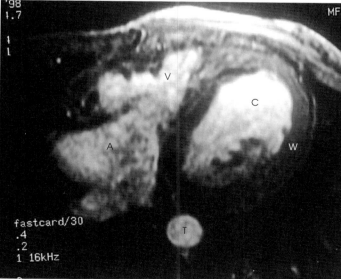

Fig. 36-15. Gated axial image of the heart in two phases of the cardiac cycle using an MR angiographic sequence on a 1.5 Tesla superconductive MR unit. Imaging was obtained continuously with incoming data subdivided into various portions of the cardiac cycle. Selected images shown were obtained in systole (left-hand image) and diastole (right-hand image). Note reduction in size of left ventricular cavity (C) and thickening of left ventricular wall (W) during systole compared with diastole. Also shown at this level are the chambers of the right atrium (A) and right ventricle (V). T, thoracic aorta. Note that moving blood has a high signal intensity on this angiographic pulse sequence.

OTHER CONSIDERATIONS

In the beginning of MRI, long imaging times were required to obtain enough information to reconstruct the sectional images, although later multiple images could be obtained during the course of one lengthy (measured in minutes) imaging run. For most routine imaging, this remains the standard. With advances in technology, however, it has become possible to quickly (within seconds) obtain enough data to reconstruct an image, using special fast-imaging pulse sequences. These fast-imaging pulse sequences are becoming more popular for specialized applications, including dynamic series of images after intravenous contrast administration. In many such sequences, fluid has very high signal intensity. This can produce a myelogram-like effect in studies of the spine or an arthrogram-like effect when joint fluid is evaluated (Fig. 36-9).

Quality assurance is important in a complex technology such as MRI. The calibration of the unit is generally performed by service personnel. However, routine scanning of phantoms can be useful to detect problems that may develop.

Clinical Applications

CENTRAL NERVOUS SYSTEM

MRI is superior to CT in imaging the posterior fossa, the portion of the brain that includes the cerebellum and brain stem. Artifact from the dense bone of the surrounding skull obscures this area with CT. There is very little MRI signal from bone, so this area is artifact-free with MRI (Fig. 36-11).

In general, the absence of bone artifact with MRI is a distinct advantage over CT. However, the inability to image calcified structures can be a disadvantage when the lesion is more easily recognized because of its calcium content. Lesions such as calcified granulomas of the lung or calcification in certain tumors are more difficult to detect with MRI than with CT.

MRI is playing an increasing role in the routine examination of the brain. Because there is more natural contrast among tissues with MRI than with CT, the differentiation of gray matter from white matter in the brain is better with MRI (Fig. 36-10). This enables MRI to be more sensitive than CT in detecting white matter disease, such as multiple sclerosis.

Primary and metastatic brain tumors, pituitary tumors, and acoustic neuromas (tumors of the eighth cranial nerve) are generally better demonstrated by MRI than by CT. The use of gadolinium-based contrast agents has improved the ability of MRI to identify meningiomas (Fig. 36-16). MRI can detect cerebral infarction earlier than can CT, but both tests provide similar information in subacute and chronic strokes.

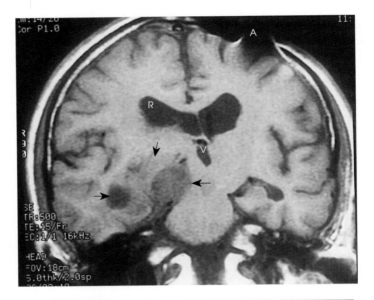

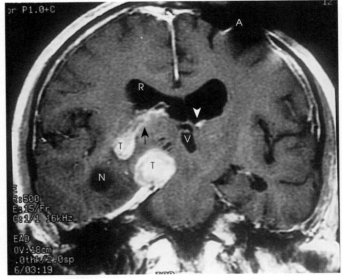

Fig. 36-16. Coronal 1.5 Tesla MR image of the brain in a patient with a meningioma arising from the tentorium cerebelli. Pre-contrast T1-weighted top image shows inhomogeneous area of abnormality (*black arrows*) with mass effect elevating the right lateral ventricle (*R*) and midline shift of the third ventricle (*V*). Bottom image shows same level after gadolinium enhancement. Active tumor (*T*) demonstrates high signal intensity. Area of necrosis (*N*) does not enhance. Additional spread of tumor towards the ventricle (*arrow*) is visualized only after contrast enhancement. Enhancement of choroid plexus (*white arrowhead*). *A*, artifact from metal in skull defect from previous surgery. Note that cerebrospinal fluid in the ventricles does not enhance (compare to CSF in Fig. 36-10).

MRI has been successfully used to image the spinal cord. The absence of bone artifact allows excellent visualization of the contents of the neural canal. In addition, the technique can separate the spinal cord from the surrounding cerebrospinal fluid (CSF) without the necessity (as is required with CT) of contrast agents injected directly into the CSF (myelogram) (Fig. 36-17). MRI is sensitive in the detection of spinal cord tumors and cystic changes of the spine (syringomyelia). MRI is also valuable in the detection of degenerated and herniated vertebral discs (Fig. 36-18).

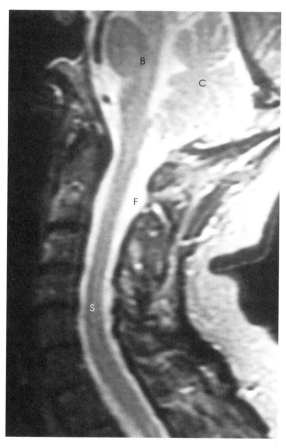

Fig. 36-17. Sagittal T2-weighted 1.5 Tesla MR image through the upper cervical spine and brainstem. The high signal from cerebrospinal fluid (F) outlines the normal brainstem (B), cerebellum (C), and spinal cord (S), giving a myelogram-like effect without contrast agents.

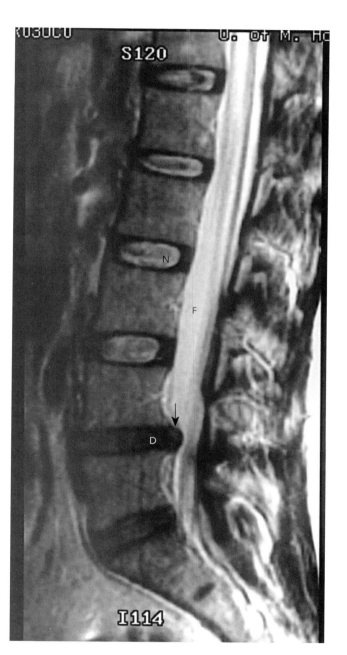

Fig. 36-18. Sagittal T2-weighted image of the lumbar spine obtained on a 1.5 Tesla MR unit. Spinal canal filled with high-signal-intensity cerebrospinal fluid (F) except for low-signal-intensity linear nerve roots running within the spinal canal. Normal vertebral discs have a high signal intensity nucleus pulposus (N). Desiccated discs (D) show low signal intensity. There is a herniated disc (arrow) at L4-L5 protruding into the spinal canal and compressing the nerve roots.

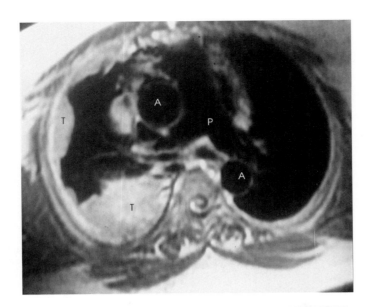

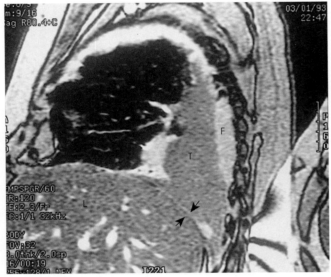

CHEST

The chest would seem to be an ideal area for MRI examination. The lungs have low signal as a result of low proton density, and the flowing blood in the great vessels of the chest also has a low MRI signal using standard pulse sequences. The heart muscle is well outlined by the lung and moving blood within the chambers. Furthermore, examination of the mediastinum is potentially fruitful since the normal structures of blood vessels and airways are of low signal. Any tumors of the mediastinum would be easily seen as areas of MRI signal standing out against the normal low signal surroundings (Fig. 36-4). The ability of MRI to image in multiple planes may be helpful in evaluating tumor spread in the thoracic inlet, chest wall, or brachial plexus region (Fig. 36-19).

However, difficulties with chest imaging remain because of cardiac and respiratory motion. Cardiac gating has markedly improved visualization of the heart with demonstration of septal defects and the cardiac valve leaflets. This is of great value in the study of congenital heart disease. Evaluation of the heart muscle for ischemia or infarction may require MRI contrast agents. Respiratory gating should also help chest images.

Fig. 36-19. Images of the chest obtained with a 1.5 Tesla MR unit in a patient with extensive mesothelioma. Top image shows axial proton-density-weighted image through the middle mediastinum. Ascending and descending aorta (A) and pulmonary artery (P) are well seen due to flow void phenomenon. Extensive rind of tumor (T) is visualized. Bottom image shows sagittal fast-sequence image obtained with breathholding. Although this is a somewhat more noisy image, the lack of motion artifact allows evaluation of the diaphragm. Thin line of diaphragm and fluid (arrows) is intact between liver (L) and tumor (T), indicating that the tumor has not invaded through the diaphragm. Some pleural fluid (F) is visualized around the tumor in the pleural space.

ABDOMEN

Respiratory and cardiac motion also detract from upper abdominal images. Again, gating should be of assistance. There is evidence that MRI is more sensitive than CT in detecting primary and metastatic tumors of the liver (Fig. 36-20). The suprarenals (adrenals), kidneys, and retroperitoneal structures such as lymph nodes are well seen, but there is limited evidence that MRI is superior to CT in this area, particularly for general screening for abnormalities. Visualization of the normal pancreas has been difficult with MRI.

MRI has some ability to predict the histologic diagnosis of certain abnormalities. For example, hepatic hemangiomas (common benign tumors of the liver) have a distinctive MRI appearance that can be helpful in ruling out other causes of hepatic masses. Patterns of enhancement with gadolinium-based contrast agents can assist in evaluating various tumors (Fig. 36-21).

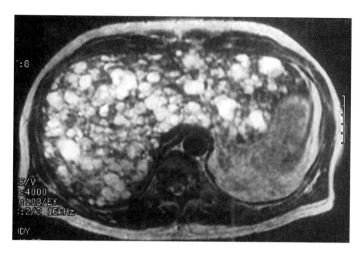

Fig. 36-20. Axial 1.5 Tesla heavily T2-weighted MR image through the liver in a patient with hemangiocarcinoma. The multiple lesions of this tumor have virtually replaced the entire liver. No contrast agents were required to demonstrate these multiple liver lesions.

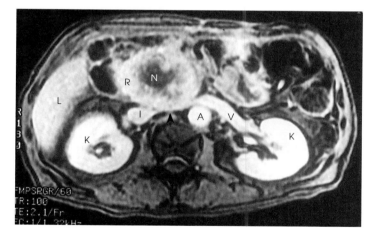

Fig. 36-21. Axial 1.5 Tesla fast-sequence MR of the central abdomen in a patient with a pancreatic islet cell tumor following gadolinium injection. Enhancement of the rim of the mass *(R)* indicates necrosis *(N)* in central portion of mass which does not enhance. Relationship of mass to vessels is also well seen, such as compression *(arrowhead)* of left renal vein *(V)*. A, aorta; I, inferior vena cava; K, kidney; L, lower tip of liver.

PELVIS

Respiratory motion has very little effect on the structures in the pelvis, leading to improved visualization compared with upper abdominal structures. The ability of MRI to image in the coronal and sagittal planes is helpful in examining the curved surfaces in the pelvis. For example, bladder tumors are well shown, including those at the dome and the base of the bladder that can be difficult to evaluate in the transverse dimension. In the prostate (Fig. 36-13) and female genital tract (Fig. 36-22), MRI is useful in detecting neoplasm and its spread.

MUSCULOSKELETAL SYSTEM

MRI produces excellent images of the limbs because they are free of involuntary motion and there is excellent MRI contrast among the soft tissues. The lack of bone artifact on MRI permits excellent visualization of the bone marrow (Fig. 36-23). Dense cortical bone frequently hides the marrow space from plain film evaluation and occasionally from CT. On the other hand, because of the lower MRI signal from calcium, calcium within tumors is better seen with CT.

Overall, the ability to image in multiple planes, along with excellent visualization of soft tissues and bone marrow, has led to a rapidly expanding role for MRI in musculoskeletal imaging. It is particularly valuable in studying joints and is replacing arthrography, and, to a lesser extent, arthroscopy, in evaluation of the injured knee (Fig. 36-9), ankle, and shoulder. Small joints also are well evaluated. Local staging of soft tissue and bone tumors is best accomplished with MRI (Fig. 36-24). Early detection of ischemic necrosis of bone is a strength of MRI (Fig. 36-25).

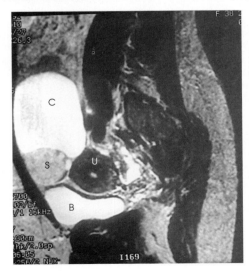

Fig. 36-22. T2-weighted images from 1.5 Tesla MR unit through the pelvis of a woman. Axial (top) and sagittal (bottom) images show solid (S) and cystic (C) components of a large ovarian tumor. Relationship to uterus (U) and bladder (B) well shown using multiple imaging planes.

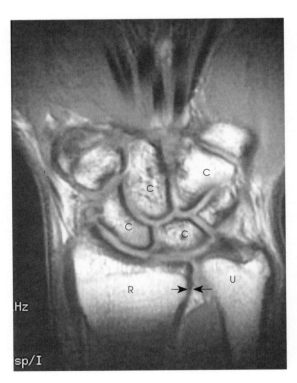

Fig. 36-23. Coronal 1.5 Tesla superconductive MR image of the wrist using a surface coil to improve visualization of superficial structures. Marrow within the carpal bones (C), radius (R), and ulna (U) has high signal as a result of its fat content. A thin black line of low-signal cortex (arrows) surrounds the marrow cavity of each bone, and trabecular bone can be seen as low signal detail interspersed within marrow.

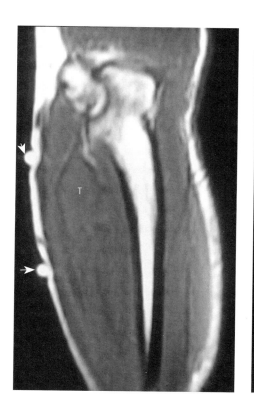

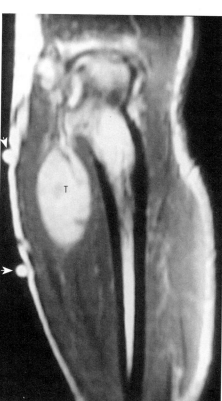

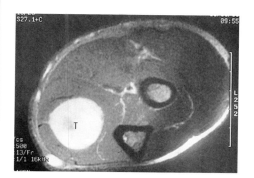

Fig. 36-24. Coronal and axial 1.5 Tesla MR images of the arm, obtained with T1-weighting, before (left-hand image) and after (middle and right-hand images) intravenous gadolinium injection. Little contrast between neurofibroma (*T*) and normal tissue prior to enhancement, but tumor is markedly enhanced after gadolinium injection. Location of tumor is evident before contrast injection only because palpable mass is marked externally with Vitamin E capsules (*arrowheads*). Relationship of tumor to other muscles and bone is evident in coronal and axial sections.

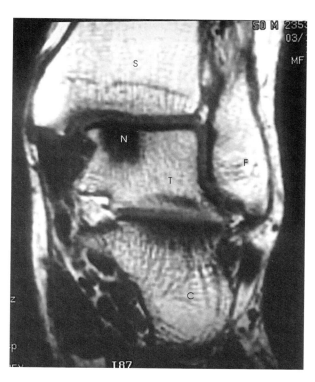

Fig. 36-25. Coronal 1.5 Tesla T1-weighted MR image of the ankle. The bone marrow demonstrates high signal intensity due to fat. A focal area (*N*) of devascularization at the dome of the talus (*T*) shows low signal intensity. However, the overlying bony cortex and cartilage are intact. *S*, tibia; *F*, fibula; *C*, calcaneus.

VESSELS

The contrast between soft tissue structures and the typical low signal of flowing blood using standard pulse sequences gives MRI the ability to visualize thrombosis within or tumor invasion of the major vessels, such as the venae cavae. Vascular anomalies, dissections, and coarctations also can be well-evaluated by MRI. Special pulse sequences allow MRI visualization of moving blood within the vascular system (Fig. 36-26). These noninvasive angiogram-like images of the vessels (MR angiograms) improve the visualization of vascular lesions.

The carotid arteries in the neck (Fig. 36-27) and their intracranial branches (Fig. 36-28) can be studied for aneurysms, arteriovenous malformations, plaques, stenoses, and occlusions, as can small arteries in the peripheral vascular system. These anatomic areas can be easily immobilized for imaging. Flow studies of the thoracic and abdominal vessels are more difficult, but specialized fast sequences do permit cardiac gated images to be obtained during a single breath hold. Typical uses include evaluation of the thoracic aorta for dissections, the abdominal aorta for aneurysms, and the renal arteries for stenoses.

Two common techniques to obtain images of flowing blood are time-of-flight and phase contrast MR angiography, either of which can be obtained in two-dimensional (obtaining a series of slices) or three-dimensional images. In time-of-flight imaging, a special pulse sequence is used which depresses the MRI signal from the anatomic area under study (Fig. 36-27). Moments later, data acquisition is performed. Only material which was outside the area when the signal-suppressing pulse occurred (e.g., blood flowing into the area from outside) will give off MRI signal. Thus incoming blood makes vessels appear bright while stationary tissue signal is suppressed. Phase contrast imaging takes advantage of the shifts in phase, or orientation, experienced by magnetic nuclei moving through the MRI field (Fig. 36-28). Special pulse sequences enhance these effects in flowing blood, producing a bright signal in vessels when the unchanging signal from stationary tissue is subtracted.

Gadolinium-based contrast agents also can be useful in MR angiography studies. Many MR angiography schemes employ fast pulse sequences to reduce overall imaging time, particularly with three-dimensional vascular imaging. To provide better contrast in images obtained with fast sequences, the T1 of blood may be shortened (to increase its signal intensity) by injection of a gadolinium-based intravascular contrast agent.

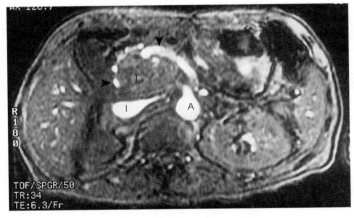

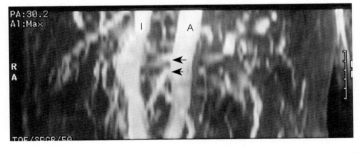

Fig. 36-26. MR angiographic sequences obtained on a 1.5 Tesla MR imager in the mid-abdomen. Time-of-flight sequence was utilized to demonstrate vessels. Blood shows high signal intensity. However, contrast of non-moving soft tissues is reduced. Top image demonstrates vessels *(arrows)* displaced around pancreatic islet cell tumor *(T)* (same patient as Fig. 36-21). Bottom image represents superimposition of multiple axial images and viewed from oblique coronal projection. Inferior vena cava *(I)*, aorta *(A)*, and their branches are demonstrated. Upper arrow marks celiac artery, and lower arrow marks superior mesenteric artery.

DIFFUSION AND PERFUSION

The sensitivity of MRI to motion can be both a handicap and a potential source of information. For example, motion artifacts interfere with upper abdominal images which are affected by heart and diaphragmatic motion, yet flow-sensitive pulse sequences can image flowing blood in blood vessels. Specialized techniques can also image the *diffusion* and *perfusion* of molecules within matter. Molecules of water undergo random motion within tissues, but the rate of this diffusion is affected by cellular membranes and macromolecules as well as by temperature. Molecules are also moving slowly through tissues through the perfusion of blood into the small capillary vessels. Tissues have structure, and this structure affects both the rate of diffusion and perfusion and its directionality; that is, diffusion and perfusion are not entirely random in a structured tissue. These microscopic motions can be detected by specialized MRI pulse sequences which can image their rate and direction. Diffusion and perfusion motion differ between tissue types. For example, diffusion patterns are different between gray matter in the brain and the more directionally-oriented fiber tracts of white matter. For technical reasons, most diffusion and perfusion imaging has focused on the central nervous system.

Diffusion and perfusion imaging can produce clinically significant images that may help in our understanding of white matter degenerative diseases such as multiple sclerosis, ischemia and infarction of the brain and possible therapies to return blood flow to underperfused brain tissue, and characterization of brain tumors. There may be similar applications in the rest of the body if technical difficulties, particularly related to patient motion such as breathing, can be overcome.

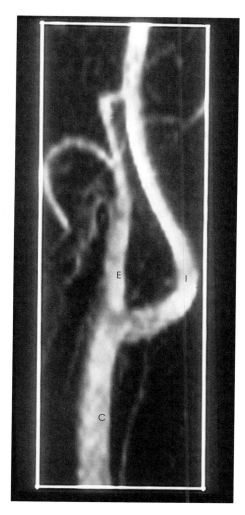

Fig. 36-27. Two-dimensional (2D) time-of-flight image of the carotid bifurcation. Normal appearance of the common (*C*), internal (*I*), and external (*E*) carotid arteries well demonstrated. Slight ribbed irregularity of edges occurs because image constructed from a series of 2D images.

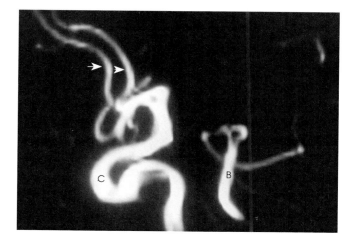

Fig. 36-28. 3D phase contrast image of the cerebral circulation obtained on a 1.5 Tesla MR unit, sagittal image. The image displays the midline and right-sided vessels. The left-sided vessels have been electronically removed for clarity. Good visualization of the carotid artery (*C*) and its major branches, including the anterior cerebral arteries (*arrows*). Basilar artery (*B*) and branches also demonstrated.

Spectroscopy

In general, for MRI we assume that each nucleus in a specific small area in space is exposed to the same magnetic field and thus precesses at and releases radiowaves of a particular frequency. If the magnetic field varies across the imaging volume in a known way, frequency can be used as one determinant of the location from which a signal is originating. There is a one-to-one relationship between frequency and location that is an integral part of creating the MRI image. In actuality, however, each nucleus in a small area in space does not see precisely the same magnetic field. The externally imposed field is the same, but the magnetic environments of the nuclei differ, depending on the magnetic effects of other nearby atoms. These differences in frequencies are very small and in general do not affect the image significantly; each signal is still placed in the correct position in the image. If we depart from imaging, however, and instead produce a detailed graph of signal strength against frequency, we are performing magnetic resonance spectroscopy and the graphs produced are called spectra.

Spectroscopy is essentially a tool for clinical analysis that can determine the relative quantity of chemical substances within a volume of tissue. Because the frequency differences are small and electronic noise is relatively high, large volumes of tissue must be studied to receive enough total signal to produce useful spectra. In addition, magnetic field strengths of 1.5 Tesla or greater are required. Nevertheless, it is possible to obtain spectra from organs (e.g., muscle and liver) or large masses to examine normal physiologic changes (e.g., with exercise), chemical alterations in persons with metabolic diseases, or differences in chemical composition between normal tissue and tumors or other pathologic processes (Fig. 36-29).

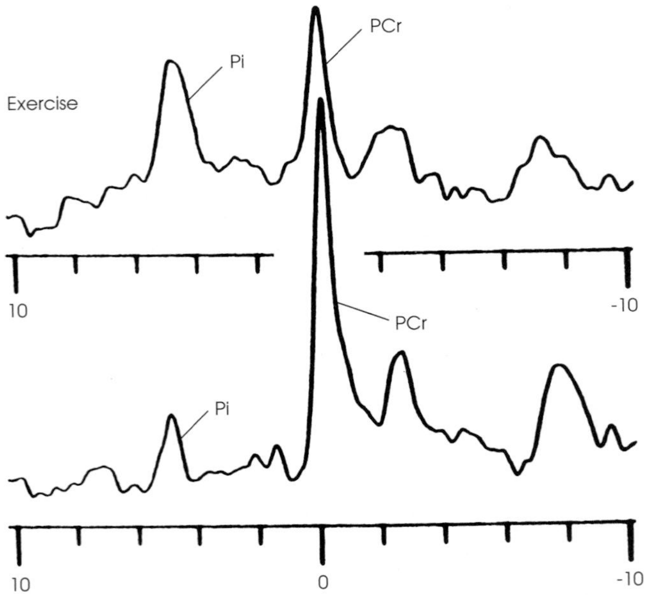

Summary

MRI is an exciting form of imaging that examines properties of tissue never before visualized. Dozens of publications have attested to MRI's efficacy in evaluating various clinical conditions. However, it is more difficult to prove that MRI is clinically superior to other imaging modalities; this analysis has been completed for some clinical situations, while for other situations, more extensive research is needed. In some cases, various modalities are complementary.

MRI is an expensive imaging technology. As a result of recent increased emphasis on cost constraints, MRI will not spread as fast as it otherwise might have. MRI also will have to compete with other modalities for an imaging "niche." Nevertheless, it is clear that MRI will be the technique of choice in many clinical situations. MRI applications continue to expand, in part because of MRI's extreme flexibility. New pulse sequences can be programmed into the computer and new contrast agents are under development; both provide new information about anatomy and pathology without requiring expensive changes in the physical structure of the imaging device. Thus, despite cost constraints, MRI continues to experience growth in the depth and breadth of its role in diagnostic imaging.

Fig. 36-29. Spectra from human muscle before (lower line) and during (upper line) exercise. Thin horizontal lines represent separate baselines for each spectrum. Each peak represents a different chemical species and the area under the peak down to the baseline indicates the amount of substance present. Inorganic phosphate (Pi) peak increases with exercise as energy-rich phosphocreatine (PCr) is used to provide energy for muscle contraction.

Definition of Terms

antenna A device for transmitting or receiving radio waves.

artifact A spurious finding in or distortion of an image.

attenuation The reduction in energy or amount of a beam of radiation when it passes through tissue or other substances.

contrast The degree of difference between two substances in some parameter. The parameter varies on the technique used; for example, attenuation in radiographic techniques or MRI signal strength in MR imaging.

cryogenic Relating to extremely low temperature. See *superconductive magnet.*

diffusion Spontaneous random motion of molecules in a medium, a natural and continuous process.

frequency The number of times that a process repeats itself in a given period of time. For example, the frequency of a radio wave is the number of complete waves per second.

fringe field That portion of the magnetic field extending away from the confines of the magnet that cannot be used for imaging but can affect nearby equipment or personnel.

gating Organizing the data so that the information used to construct the image comes from the same point in the cycle of a repeating motion, such as a heartbeat. The moving object is "frozen" at that phase of its motion, reducing image blurring.

gauss A unit of magnetic field strength. See *Tesla.*

inversion recovery A standard *pulse sequence* available on most MRI imagers, usually used for T1-weighted images. The name indicates that the direction of *precession* of the *nucleus* is reversed (inverted) before *relaxation* (recovery) occurs.

magnetic resonance (MR) The process by which certain nuclei, when placed in a magnetic field, can absorb and release energy in the form of radio waves. This technique can be used for chemical analysis or for the production of cross-sectional images of body parts. Computer analysis of the radio wave data is required.

noise Random contributions to the total signal that arise from stray external radio waves, imperfect electronic apparatus, etc. Noise cannot be eliminated, but it can be minimized. Noise tends to degrade the image by interfering with accurate measurement of the true MRI signal, similar to the difficulty in maintaining a clear conversation in a noisy room.

nuclear magnetic resonance (NMR) Another name for magnetic resonance.

nucleus The central portion of an atom composed of protons and neutrons.

paramagnetic Referring to materials that alter the magnetic field of nearby nuclei. Paramagnetic substances are not themselves directly imaged by MRI but instead change the signal intensity of the tissue where they localize, thus acting as MRI contrast agents. Paramagnetic agents shorten both the T1 and T2 of the tissues they affect, actions which tend to have opposing effects on signal intensity. In clinical practice, agents are administered in a concentration in which either T1 or T2 shortening predominates, usually the former to provide high signal on T1-weighted images.

perfusion Flow of blood through the vessels of an organ or anatomic structure. Usually refers to blood flow in the small vessels (e.g., capillary perfusion).

permanent magnet An object that produces a magnetic field without requiring an external electricity supply.

precession The rotation of an object around the direction of a force acting on that object. This should not be confused with the axis of rotation of the object itself. For example, a spinning top rotates on its own axis, but it may also precess (wobble) around the direction of the force of gravity that is acting on it.

proton density A measure of proton (i.e., hydrogen, since its nucleus is a single proton) concentration (number of nuclei per given volume). One of the major determinants of MRI signal strength in hydrogen imaging.

pulse A short burst of radio waves. If the radio waves are of the appropriate frequency, they can give energy to nuclei that are within a magnetic field by the process of *magnetic resonance.* The length of the pulse determines the amount of energy given to the nuclei.

pulse sequence A series of radio wave pulses designed to excite nuclei in such a way that their energy release has varying contribution from proton density, T1, or T2 processes.

raw data The information obtained by radio reception of the MRI signal as stored by a computer. Specific computer manipulation of this data is required to construct an image from it.

relaxation Return of excited nuclei to their normal unexcited state by the release of energy.

relaxation time A measure of the rate at which nuclei, after stimulation, release their extra energy.

resistive magnet A simple electromagnet in which electricity passing through coils of wire produces a magnetic field.

resonance The process of energy absorption by an object that is tuned to absorb energy of a specific frequency only; all other frequencies will not affect the object. For example, if one tuning fork is struck in a room full of tuning forks, only those forks tuned to that identical frequency will vibrate (resonate).

signal In MRI, the radio wave that is transmitted by nuclei upon relaxation.

slice A cross-sectional image. Can also refer to the thin section of the body from which data is acquired to produce the image.

spectroscopy Science of analyzing the components of an electromagnetic wave, usually after its interaction with some substance (to obtain information about that substance).

spin echo A standard MRI *pulse sequence* which can provide *T1-, T2-,* or *proton density*–weighted images. The name indicates that a declining MRI *signal* is refocused to gain strength (like an echo) before it is recorded as *raw data.*

spin-lattice relaxation The release of energy by excited nuclei to their general environment. One of the major determinants of MRI signal strength. T1 is a rate constant measuring spin-lattice relaxation.

spin-spin relaxation The release of energy by excited nuclei by interaction among themselves. One of the major determinants of MRI signal strength. T2 is a rate constant measuring spin-spin relaxation.

superconductive magnet An electromagnet in which the coils of wire are cooled to extremely low temperature so that the resistance to the conduction of electricity is nearly eliminated (superconductive).

T1 A rate constant measuring spin-lattice relaxation.

T2 A rate constant measuring spin-spin relaxation.

Tesla A unit of magnetic field strength. One Tesla equals 10,000 gauss or 10 kilogauss (other units of magnetic field strength). The earth's magnetic field approximates 0.5 gauss.

SELECTED BIBLIOGRAPHY

Atlas SW et al, editors: Gadolinium contrast agents in neuro-MRI, J Comput Assist Tomogr 17:S1-S48, 1993.

Axel L, editor: Glossary of MRI terms, Reston, Va, 1986, American College of Radiology.

Bellon EM et al: Magnetic resonance imaging of internal derangements of the knee, RadioGraphics 8:95-118, 1988.

Bloch F: Nuclear induction, Physiol Rev 70:460-473, 1946.

Boechat MI et al: MR imaging of the abdomen in children, AJR 152:1245-1250, 1989.

Bottomley PA: Human in vivo NMR spectroscopy in diagnostic medicine: clinical tool or research probe? Radiology 170:1-15, 1989.

Brant-Zawadzki M: MR imaging of the brain, Radiology 166:1-10, 1988.

Brasch RC: New directions in the development of MR imaging contrast media, Radiology 183:1-11, 1992.

Chenevert TL et al: Anisotropic diffusion in human white matter: demonstration with MR techniques in vivo, Radiology 177:401-405, 1990.

Chezmar JL et al: Liver and abdominal screening in patients with cancer: CT versus MR imaging, Radiology 168:43-47, 1988.

Chien D et al: Basic principles and clinical applications of magnetic resonance angiography, Semin Roentgenol 27:53-62, 1992.

Council on Scientific Affairs, American Medical Association: Magnetic resonance imaging of the abdomen and pelvis, JAMA 261:420-433, 1989.

Damadian R: Tumor detection by nuclear magnetic resonance, Science 171:1151-1153, 1971.

Ehman RL et al: MR imaging of the musculoskeletal system: a 5-year appraisal, Radiology 166:313-320, 1988.

Ellis JH et al: Resistive magnet systems: an MRI "whether" report, Diagn Imaging 6:60-62, 1984.

Ellis JH et al: NMR physics for physicians, Indiana Medicine 78:20-28, 1985.

Evens RG et al: Economic and utilization analysis of MR imaging units in the United States in 1987, Radiology 166:27-30, 1988.

Francis IR et al: Integrated imaging of adrenal disease, Radiology 184:1-13, 1992.

Glazer GM: MR imaging of the liver, kidneys, and adrenal glands, Radiology 166:303-312, 1988.

Haughton VM: MR imaging of the spine, Radiology 166:297-301, 1988.

Heiken JP et al: MR imaging of the pelvis, Radiology 166:11-16, 1988.

Hendrick RE et al: Basic physics of MR contrast agents and maximization of image contrast, JMRI 3:137-148, 1993.

Kanal E et al: Safety considerations in MR imaging, Radiology 176:593-606, 1990.

Kanal E et al: Patient monitoring during clinical MR imaging, Radiology 185:623-629, 1992.

Kanzer GK et al: Magnetic resonance imaging of diseases of the liver and biliary system, Radiol Clin North Am 29:1259-84, 1991.

Kneeland JB et al: High-resolution MR imaging with local coils, Radiology 171:1-7, 1989.

Lauterbur PC: Image formation by induced local interactions: examples employing nuclear magnetic resonance, Nature 242:190-191, 1973.

LeBihan D et al: Diffusion MR imaging: clinical applications, AJR 159:591-599, 1992.

Lee SH et al, editors: Imaging in neuroradiology, parts I and II, Radiol Clin North Am 26:701-1155, 1988.

Mitchell DG et al: The biophysical basis of tissue contrast in extracranial MR imaging, AJR 149:831-837, 1987.

Moser RP, editor: Imaging of bone and soft tissue tumors, Radiol Clin North Am 31:237-447, 1993.

Nghiem HV et al: The pelvis: T2-weighted fast spin-echo MR imaging, Radiology 185:213-217, 1992.

Owen RS et al: Symptomatic peripheral vascular disease: selection of imaging parameters and clinical evaluation with MR angiography, Radiology 187:627-635, 1993.

Potchen EJ, editor: Magnetic resonance angiography, Semin Ultrasound CT MR 13:225-310, 1992.

Purcell EM et al: Resonance absorption by nuclear magnetic moments in a solid, Physiol Rev 69:37-38, 1946.

Sartoris DJ et al: MR imaging of the musculoskeletal system: current and future status, AJR 149:457-467, 1987.

Stehling MJ et al: Whole-body echo-planar MR imaging at 0.5 T, Radiology 170:257-263, 1989.

Turner R et al: Echo-planar imaging of intravoxel incoherent motion, Radiology 177:407-411, 1990.

Webb WR et al: MR imaging of thoracic disease: clinical uses, Radiology 182:621-630, 1992.

Wehrli FW: Fast-scan magnetic resonance: principles and applications, New York, 1991, Raven Press.

Young SW: Magnetic resonance imaging: basic principles, ed 2, New York, 1988, Raven Press.

Chapter 37

DIAGNOSTIC ULTRASOUND

SANDRA L. HAGEN-ANSERT

Historical development
Physical principles
Clinical applications
Summary

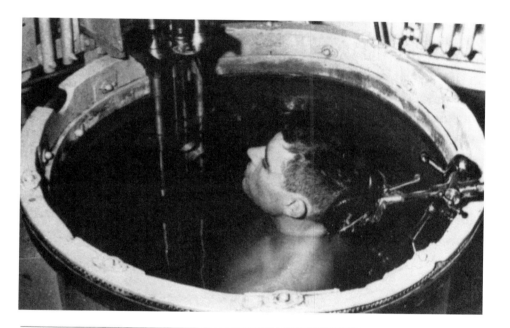

Scanning position for a patient in the fluid-filled B-29 gun turret scanner; 1954. On a transverse cross-section of the neck, the 2½-inch focus transducer is just below the water level. The transducer carriage travels around the tank on the outside track.

From Holmes JH: Diagnostic ultrasound historical perspective. In King DL (ed): Diagnostic ultrasound, St. Louis, 1974, Mosby.

Diagnostic *ultrasound,** sometimes called "diagnostic medical sonography," "sonography," or "echocardiography," has become a clinically valuable imaging technique over the past several decades. It differs from diagnostic radiology in that it uses nonionizing, high-frequency sound waves to generate an image of a particular structure. Radiography is useful in the visualization of dense bony structures and air- or contrast-filled structures, such as the lungs, stomach, colon, or small bowel. Ultrasound is employed in the visualization of soft tissue interfaces of homogeneous, fluid-filled, or "solid" organs, tumor masses, or muscles located throughout the body.

In addition, blood flow velocities may be calculated in vascular and cardiac structures with the *Doppler* technique. The *pulsed-wave, continuous wave,* or color-flow mapping techniques have proven to be very useful in determining direction of blood flow, resistance of flow, and regurgitation of flow from one structure to another.

The sonographer (an individual who performs ultrasound procedures) approaches the imaging of the body in a manner different from the conventional radiographer's. The principal difference lies in the sonographer's knowledge of detailed anatomy, physiology, and pathology. An understanding of the three-dimensional reconstruction of the image is necessary for the sonographer to produce an adequate image.

Ultrasound has many advantages over other imaging techniques in medicine. One advantage is portability of the ultrasound equipment. It may be easily moved into the operating room, special care nursery, or intensive care unit or may be manually transported by means of a mobile van service to provide ultrasound services for smaller hospitals and clinics. Ultrasound is cost-effective compared with computed tomography (CT), magnetic resonance imaging (MRI), or angiography.

The versatility of the equipment allows flexibility in hospital schedules; supplies are minimal; equipment price is low compared with other imaging modalities; and a minimal procedure time allows for a more rapid evaluation of patients. Ultrasound has generally been known as a noninvasive examination; however, recent developments in transesophageal, transrectal, and endovaginal probe designs have changed that concept. Further development in high-frequency, millimeter-size *transducers* mounted on the tip of an angiographic catheter have great potential. These miniature transducers show promise in characterizing wall thickness and plaque formation and in guiding equipment during angiographic procedures.

---

*All italicized terms are defined at the end of this chapter.

Historical Development

The development of materials, testing techniques, and sonar provided a major impetus for the development of diagnostic ultrasound. The equipment was constructed as a result of the defense effort during World War II, so the clinical development lay in the hands of various investigators who would later prove that ultrasound had a valid contribution to make to the medical community.

In 1947 Dussick was one of the earliest to apply ultrasound to medical diagnosis when he positioned two transducers on opposite sides of the head to measure ultrasound transmission profiles. He also discovered that tumors and other intracranial lesions could be detected by this technique. In the early 1950s Dussick, with Heuter, Bolt, and Ballantyne, continued to use *through-transmission* techniques and computer analysis to diagnose brain lesions through the intact skull. However, they discontinued their studies after concluding that the technique was too complicated for routine clinical use.

In the late 1940s Douglass Howry (a radiologist), John Wild (a diagnostician interested in tissue characterization), and George Ludwig (interested in reflections from gallstones) independently demonstrated that when ultrasound waves generated by a piezoelectric crystal transducer were transmitted into the human body, ultrasound waves would be returned to the transducer from tissue interfaces of different *acoustic impedances*. At this time research development in ultrasound occurred in an effort to transform naval sonar equipment into a clinically useful diagnostic tool.

In 1948 Howry developed the first ultrasound scanner, consisting of a cattle watering tank with a wooden rail anchored along the side. The transducer carriage moved along the rail in a horizontal plane, while the object to be scanned and the transducer were positioned inside the water tank. Howry also developed the *"compound"* (back and forth) double-scanning motion in an attempt to produce a more realistic anatomic image. Many of the subjects were presurgical candidates, so actual comparison of the tissue could be made with the ultrasound image.

Along with ultrasound's medical applications by physicians, veterinarians also began using it to determine the lean to fat ratio of cattle and other animals ready for slaughter.

In 1954 echocardiographic techniques were developed by Hertz and Edler in Sweden. The investigators were able to distinguish normal heart valvular motion from the thickened, calcified valve motion seen in patients with rheumatic heart disease. In 1957 the early obstetric contact-compound scanner was built by Tom Brown and Ian Donald in Scotland. The development of the contact scanner in North America came in 1962 at the University of Colorado. This equipment had a transducer that moved in a mechanical *sector scan* 30 degrees to each side of the perpendicular, while the carriage moved over the surface to be scanned.

Meanwhile, in Australia in 1959, Kossoff, Robinson, and Garrett developed diagnostic B-scanners with the use of a water bath to improve *resolution* of the image. This group was also responsible for the introduction of *gray-scale* imaging with techniques first described in 1972.

Real-time equipment is the ultrasound equipment found in hospitals, clinics, and offices today. High-frequency, high-resolution, small-diameter transducers are able to accumulate several images per second (depending on frequency and depth, as many as 30 frames per second). The flexibility of these small transducers affords the sonographer the opportunity to obtain high-quality images anywhere in the body.

Physical Principles
PROPERTIES OF SOUND WAVES

An acoustic *wave* is a propagation of energy that moves back and forth or vibrates at a steady rate. Sound waves are mechanical oscillations that are transmitted by particles in a gas, liquid, or solid medium. Generated by an external source, ultrasound is the transmission of high-frequency mechanical vibrations greater than 20 kHz through a medium.

Frequency may be explained by the following analogy. If a stick were moved in and out of a pond at a steady rate, the entire surface of the water would be covered with waves radiating from the stick. If the number of vibrations that were made in each second were counted, the frequency of vibration could be determined. In ultrasound, frequency refers to the number of oscillations per second performed by the particles of the medium in which the wave is propagating:

1 oscillation/sec = 1 cycle/second = 1 Hz
1000 oscillations/sec =
1 kilocycle/second = 1 kHz
1,000,000 oscillations/sec =
1 megacycle/second = 1 MHz

Ultrasound refers to sound waves beyond the audible range (16,000 to 20,000 cycles/second). Diagnostic applications of ultrasound use frequencies of 1 to 10 million cycles/second, or 1 to 10 MHz (Table 37-1).

Longitudinal waves

Ultrasound is a form of nonionizing radiation in which *longitudinal* pressure *waves* of high frequency are transmitted through a medium. These waves are formed by the oscillation of particles or molecules parallel to the axis of wave propagation. As illustrated in Fig. 37-1, part of the molecules are "squeezed" closer together, or *compressed*, and part undergo expansion, or *rarefaction*, by which the molecules are pulled farther apart. As sound travels through a material, alternate regions of compression and rarefaction occur.

Along with wave properties such as frequency and *intensity,* the *medium* that carries the sound is a major contributor in defining the ultrasound transmission properties. In part, the compressibility or density of a material determines the way sound is carried along with the material.

Table 37-1. Applications of sound frequency ranges

Frequency range	Manner of production	Application
Infrasound 0 to 25 Hz	Electromagnetic vibrators	Vibration analysis of structures
Audible 20 Hz to 20 kHz	Electromagnetic vibrators, musical instruments	Communications, signaling
Ultrasound 20 to 100 kHz 100 kHz to 1 MHz 1 to 20 MHz	Air whistles, electric devices Electric devices Electric devices	Biology, sonar Flaw detection, biology Diagnostic medicine

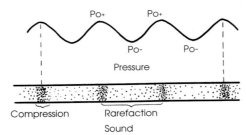

Fig. 37-1. Longitudinal wave formation occurs in pressure changes with fluctuating volume, causing compression and rarefaction.

Acoustic impedance

The ultrasound wave is similar to a light beam in that it may be *focused, refracted, reflected,* or *scattered* at interfaces between different media. At the junction of two media of different acoustic properties, an ultrasound beam may be reflected depending on the difference in acoustic impedance between the two media and the angle at which the beam hits the interface *(angle of incidence)* (Fig. 37-2). In biologic tissues, with the exception of air-tissue and bone interfaces, the differences in acoustic impedance are slight so that only a small component of the ultrasound beam is reflected at each interface. Most of the sound is passed into tissues deeper in the body and reflected at other interfaces. The acoustic impedance is the product of the *velocity of sound* in a medium and the *density* of that medium. The acoustic impedance increases if the density or propagation speed increases.

Velocity of sound

The velocity of sound in a medium is determined by the density and elastic properties of the medium. The velocity of sound differs greatly among air, bone, and soft tissue. On the other hand, the velocity of sound varies by only a few percent from one soft tissue to another. Air-filled structures, such as the lungs and stomach, or gas-filled structures, such as the bowel, impede the sound transmission. Likewise, sound is *attenuated* through most bony structures. Small differences between fat, blood, and organ tissues, as seen on an ultrasound image, may be better delineated with high-frequency transducers that improve resolution.

Measurement of sound

The *decibel* unit (dB) is often used to measure the strength or intensity of an ultrasound wave. The decibel unit allows for a quantitative statement to be made regarding the ratio of two intensities of two amplitudes. The intensity of the transmitted ultrasonic pulse on each ultrasound instrument may be varied by changing the size of excitation voltage applied to the transducer. Also, reduction of the sound beam intensity with depth or attenuation may be expressed as decibels per centimeter.

Attenuation is the sum of acoustic energy losses resulting from absorption, scattering, and reflection. If air or bone is coupled with soft tissue, more energy will be attenuated. Attenuation through a calcium interface such as a gallstone may produce an *acoustic shadow* on the B-scan image (Fig. 37-3).

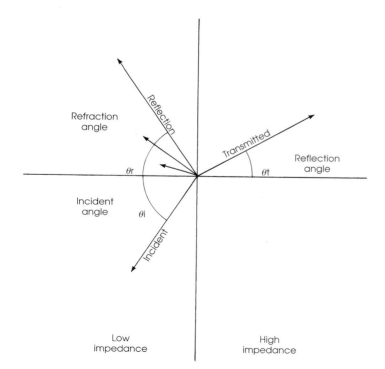

Fig. 37-2. Relationship among incident, reflected, and transmitted waves.

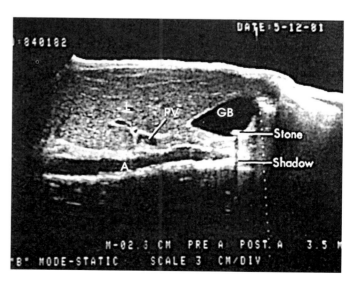

Fig. 37-3. Sagittal scan of the right upper quadrant. Anechoic gall bladder is well visualized with a solitary bright reflector along its posterior margin, representing a small gallstone. The acoustic shadow is seen posterior to the stone. GB = Gall bladder; PV = portal vein; L = Liver; A = aorta)

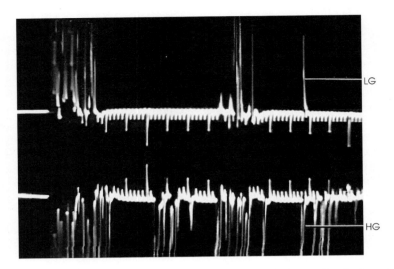

Fig. 37-4. A-mode tracing of a solid mass at low gain (upper tracing) and high gain (lower tracing). The solid mass attenuates the sound beam, giving a weak through transmission. As the gain is increased, there are multiple echoes seen within the solid mass.

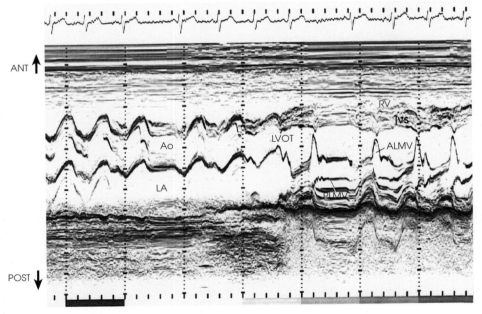

Fig. 37-5. A, M-mode tracing of a sweep from the aorta *(Ao)* and left atrium *(LA)*, to the left ventricular outflow tract *(LVOT)*, to the right ventricle *(RV)*, interventricular septum *(IVS)*, and anterior *(ALMV)* and posterior *(PLMV)* leaflets of the mitral valve. Continuity is shown between the anterior wall of the aorta and the interventricular septum; continuity is also shown between the posterior aortic wall and anterior leaflet of the mitral valve.

TRANSDUCERS

The sound beams used in diagnostic ultrasound are produced from a transducer by the *piezoelectric effect.* The transducer is a means for converting one form of energy into another (e.g., electrical energy into mechanical sound waves). The Curies first described the piezoelectric effect in 1880. They observed that when certain crystals such as quartz undergo mechanical deformation, a potential difference develops across the two surfaces of the crystals. Synthetic ceramic crystals have been developed for medical use that can be molded into various shapes and sizes and focused for ultrasonic applications. Each ceramic crystal has a *resonant frequency* that depends on the thickness of the crystal.

Most diagnostic applications use short pulsed ultrasound waves for optimum resolution. As a pulse of ultrasound is emitted, the pulse travels through tissue. When the pulse strikes an interface, part of the energy is reflected. The returning echo is a sound pressure wave that causes a slight mechanical deformation of the ceramic as it impinges on the transducer face, resulting in an electrical pulse. Each transducer has a special damping material to "silence" any continuing vibration.

DISPLAY MODES

A-mode

The *A-mode,* or amplitude modulation, display represents the time or distance it takes the beam to strike a particular interface and return its signal to the transducer. The greater the reflection at the interface, the larger the signal amplitude will appear on the A-mode screen (Fig. 37-4).

M-mode

The *M-mode,* or time-motion, trace uses the concepts of A- and B-modes (see below) as they are swept across the screen over a period of time. The M-mode is used to depict movement and is especially useful to record fetal heart motion and other cardiac functions (Fig. 37-5).

B-mode

If the tracing of the A-mode were rotated 90 degrees toward the observer, the spikes would be represented as dots. The brightness of the dots corresponds to the height, or amplitude, of the spike. *B-mode*, gray-scale, or amplitude imaging refers to the condition of varying the brightness of the dot so that brightness is proportional to the echo-signal amplitude. Thus the greater the change in acoustic impedance at the interface of a medium, the taller the spike on the A-mode tracing, which in turn presents a brighter dot on the B-mode trace. As the transducer is moved across a plane, the *echoes* are imprinted on a screen to subsequently build up a two-dimensional image. The B-mode is the basis for all real-time images in ultrasound (Fig. 37-6).

Gray-scale imaging

Gray-scale imaging allows the sonographer to selectively amplify and display the level of echoes from soft tissues at the expense of larger echoes. This signal processing is known as the compression amplication characteristic of gray-scale systems. Through digital *scan converters,* digital memory and circuitry converts echo signals into an image on a television monitor. This information then may be manipulated by the sonographer on a pre-processing or postprocessing basis, enabling the sonographer to change the presentation of the image from a softer shade of gray to a more contrasting image. This technique is useful in imaging particular tumors or small masses within the abdomen or in visualizing the lower-level "soft" echoes.

Real time

Real time or *dynamic imaging* is the presentation of multiple-image frames per second over selected areas of the body. The transducer may be composed of several elements that can be electronically focused and fired in rapid sequence to produce a real-time image. Thus structures are visible as they change position in time, such as pulsatile vascular and cardiac structures, diaphragm, and peristalsis in the bowel and stomach. The small size of the transducer allows the sonographer to easily move between intercostal spaces.

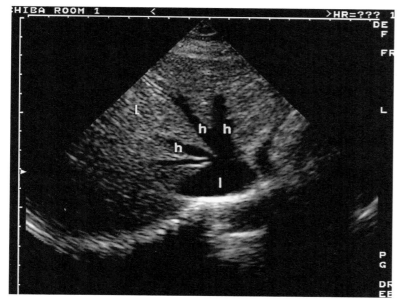

Fig. 37-6. Transverse scan over the right upper quadrant with real time ultrasound. The transducer is angled toward the diaphragm to demonstrate the homogeneous liver texture (*L*), the inferior vena cava (*l*) with the hepatic veins (*h*) draining into the cava.

Doppler principle

The *Doppler principle* refers to a change in frequency when the motion of laminar or turbulent flow is detected within a vascular structure (Fig. 37-7). In medical applications *(Doppler ultrasound)*, a sound wave is reflected from moving red blood cells (RBCs). If the cell moves along the line of the ultrasound beam, the Doppler shift is directly proportional to the velocity of the RBC. If the RBC moves away from the transducer in the plane of the ultrasound beam, the fall in frequency is directly proportional to the velocity and direction of the RBC movement. The Doppler tracing is recorded on a type of M-mode format, with a baseline serving as the "zero" point. Movement toward the transducer is recorded as a positive (above the baseline) motion, whereas movement away from the transducer is recorded as a negative (below the baseline) motion. Color-flow Doppler is a technique with the instrumentation ability to assign a "color" scale to the change in frequency or Doppler shift. Generally, red is toward the transducer, while blue is away. If the velocity of the flow is too high, the color Doppler will "alias" (wrap around the color scale). A change in the pulse repetition frequency will help to reduce this alias pattern.

Artifacts

Just as the sonographer must be able to distinguish anatomic and pathologic changes within the body, the recognition of *artifacts* is important for the production of adequate diagnostic images.

The sound beam must be perpendicular to the interface. A rarefaction artifact is produced by the bending of the beam at an interface where the beam is not perpendicular.

A *reverberation* artifact can occur when the beam strikes a reflective structure, sending the beam in multiple pathways to produce many linear reflections.

Equipment malfunction (e.g., damaged transducer), poorly adjusted time-gain compensation, incorrect sensitivity settings, or misaligned electronic calibration may have an adverse effect on the image, and the sonographer must be able to recognize these problems on a routine basis.

The sonographer must have a thorough knowledge of anatomy, physiology, pathology, and physical acoustic principles to produce a quality scan. In addition, the sonographer must be familiar with special scanning techniques, transducers, artifacts, and equipment quality control.

BIOLOGIC EFFECTS

Diagnostic ultrasound as used in clinical medicine has not been associated with any harmful biologic effects and is generally accepted as a safe modality.

Much of the work on biologic effects has come about as a result of the wide use of ultrasound in obstetrics, because it is safe and without effect on the fetus. The rationale for this conclusion is based on (1) the fact that the intensities normally used are too small to produce significant increases in temperature in exposed tissues, and (2) the tacit assumption that the pulses employed are too short to produce the selective, large-amplitude oscillation of microscopic gas bodies called *acoustic cavitation.*

Available information indicates that there are thresholds for transient *cavitation* that require peak intensities of 100m W/cm^2 in microsecond-length pulses. It should be possible to be conservative and perform all diagnostic obstetric procedures with peak intensities substantially below these levels.

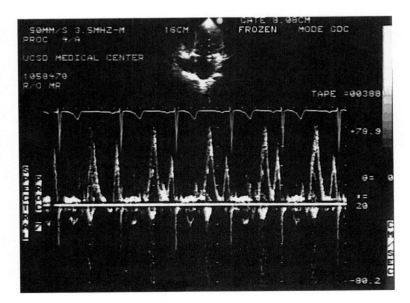

Fig. 37-7. Doppler tracing of the left atrioventricular (mitral) valve shows a positive reflective above the baseline, representing the blood as it flows toward the transducer in diastole; as the atrium begins to relax, the flow drops off. At atrial contraction, the blood flows toward the transducer with less velocity than the initial flow. The end of diastole shows the flow back to the baseline.

ANATOMIC RELATIONSHIPS AND LANDMARKS

The ability of the sonographer to understand anatomy as it relates to the *cross-sectional, coronal,* oblique, and sagittal planes is critical in performing a quality sonogram. Normal anatomy has many variations in size and position, and it is the responsibility of the sonographer to be able to demonstrate these findings on the sonogram. To complete this task the sonographer must have a thorough understanding of anatomy as it relates to the antero-posterior relationships, as well as the variations in sectional anatomy (Figs. 37-8 to 37-22). For additional information on sectional anatomy, see Volume 2, Chapter 27 of this atlas.

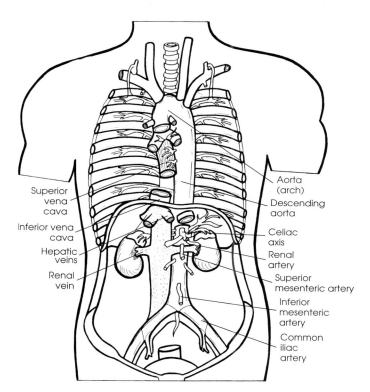

Fig. 37-8. The aorta may be visualized from its origin as it leaves the left ventricle, followed as it arches into the thoracic cavity and pierces the diaphragm to become the abdominal aorta. The major branches of the abdominal aorta (celiac trunk, superior mesenteric artery, and renal arteries) are well seen on the sonogram. The venous supply is imaged as the superior and inferior venae cavae enter the right atrium of the heart. The hepatic veins are seen to enter the inferior vena cava at the level of the diaphragm.

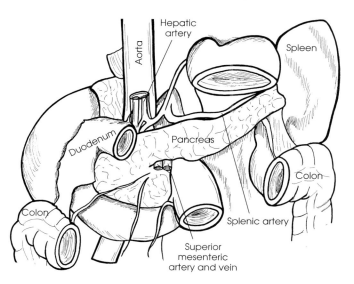

Fig. 37-9. The pancreas is a retroperitoneal structure that is recognized by locating the aorta and inferior vena cava, splenic artery, splenic vein, hepatic artery, and superior mesenteric vein. The stomach, when filled with fluid, may serve as a superior boundary of the pancreas as the fluid fills the duodenal loop that surrounds the pancreatic head.

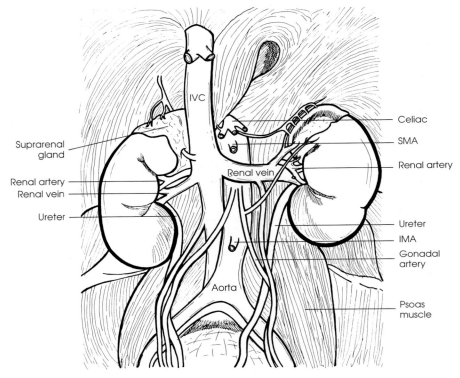

Fig. 37-10. The renal structures are best visualized by using the homogeneous liver or spleen to outline the kidneys as they lie along the psoas muscles.

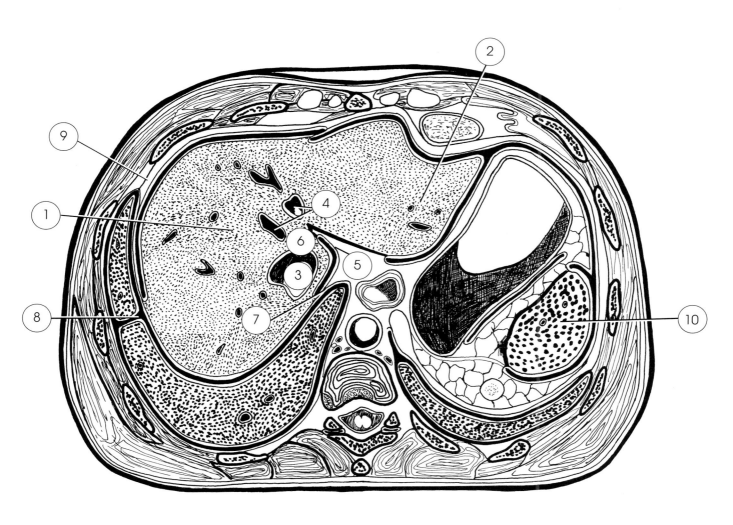

1 Right lobe of liver
2 Left lobe of liver
3 Inferior vena cava
4 Hepatic veins
5 Ligamentum venosum
6 Caudate lobe
7 Coronary hepatic
   ligament
8 Pleural cavity
9 Diaphragm
10 Spleen

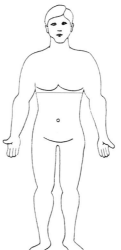

Fig. 37-11. Transverse section at the level of the xyphoid process *(blue line)*.

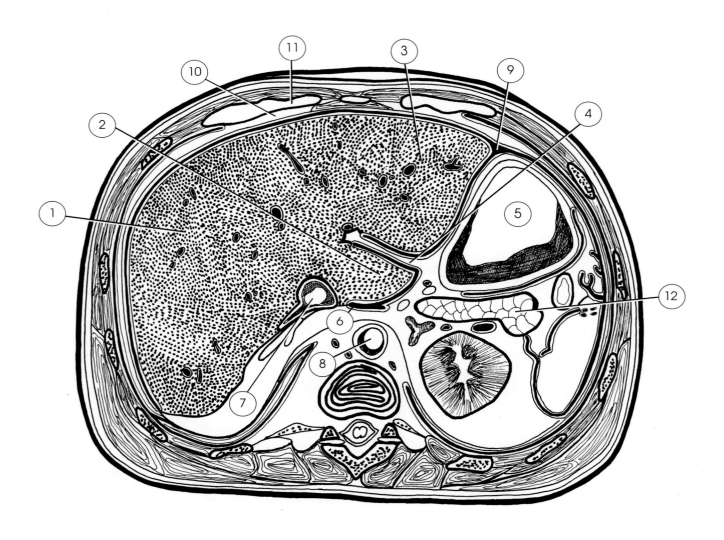

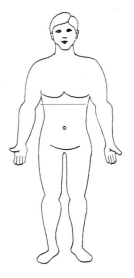

1   Right lobe of liver
2   Caudate lobe
3   Left lobe of liver
4   Hepatogastric ligament
5   Stomach
6   Omental bursa
7   Inferior vena cava
8   Aorta
9   Peritoneal cavity
10 Diaphragm
11 Rectus abdominis
    muscle
12 Tail of pancreas

Fig. 37-12. Transverse section 2 cm below the xyphoid process *(blue line).*

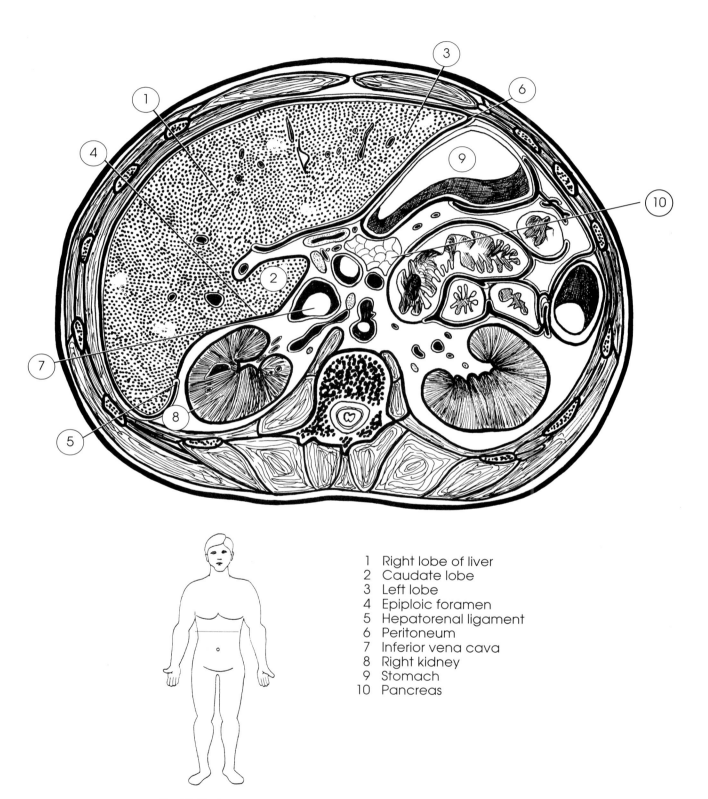

1 Right lobe of liver
2 Caudate lobe
3 Left lobe
4 Epiploic foramen
5 Hepatorenal ligament
6 Peritoneum
7 Inferior vena cava
8 Right kidney
9 Stomach
10 Pancreas

Fig. 37-13. Transverse section 4 cm below the xyphoid process *(blue line).*

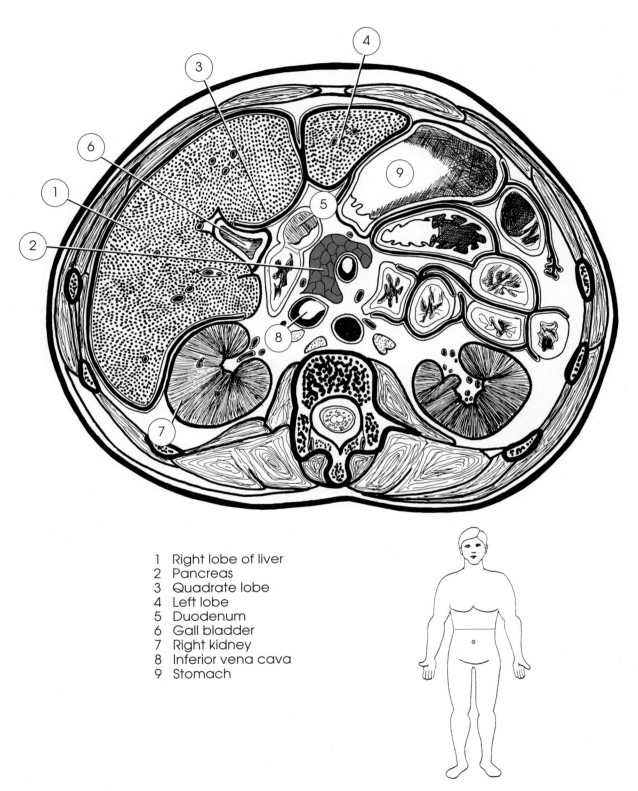

1 Right lobe of liver
2 Pancreas
3 Quadrate lobe
4 Left lobe
5 Duodenum
6 Gall bladder
7 Right kidney
8 Inferior vena cava
9 Stomach

Fig. 37-14. Transverse section 6 cm below the xyphoid process *(blue line)*.

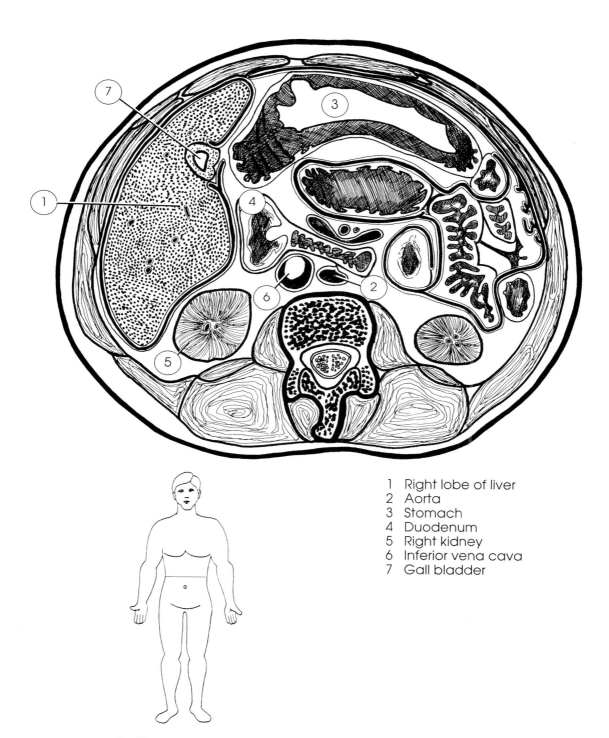

1 Right lobe of liver
2 Aorta
3 Stomach
4 Duodenum
5 Right kidney
6 Inferior vena cava
7 Gall bladder

Fig. 37-15. Transverse section 8 cm below the xyphoid process *(blue line)*.

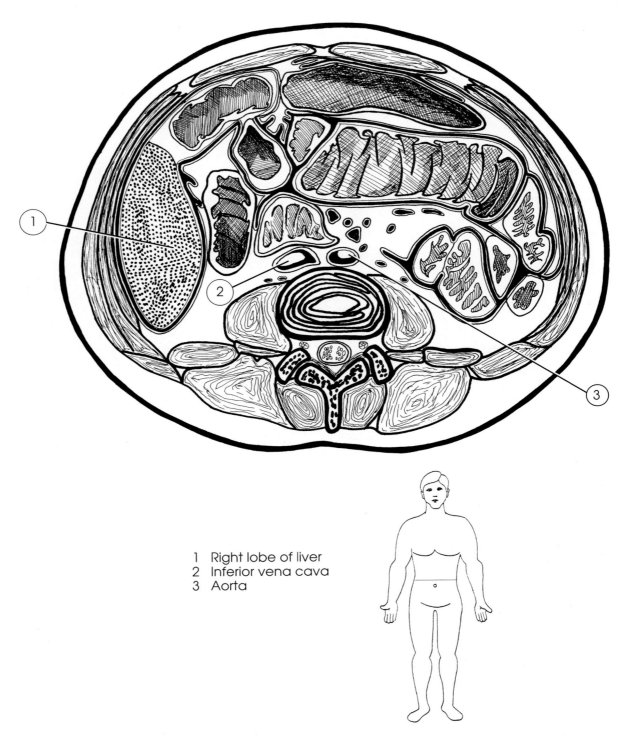

1 Right lobe of liver
2 Inferior vena cava
3 Aorta

Fig. 37-16. Transverse section 10 cm below the xyphoid process *(blue line)*.

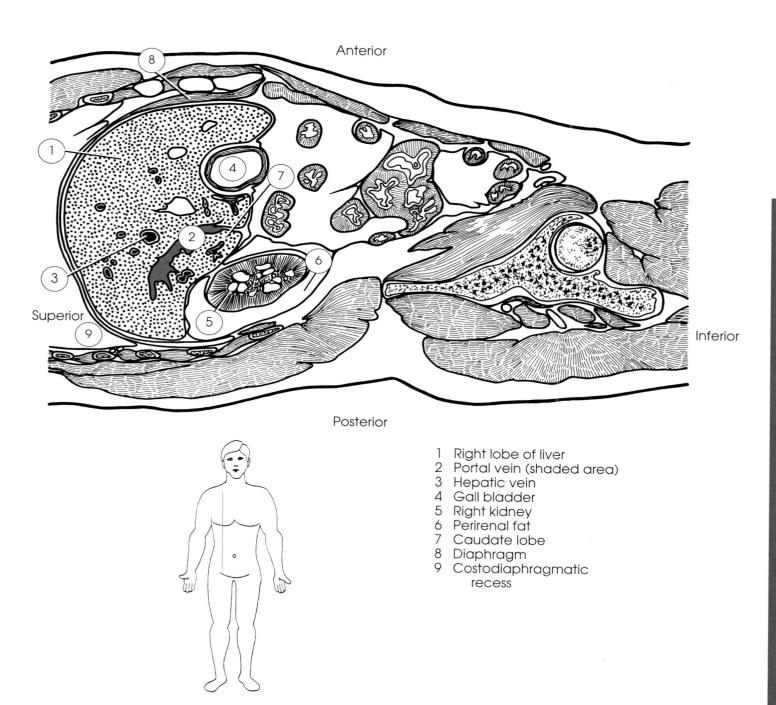

Anterior

Superior

Inferior

Posterior

Fig. 37-17. Longitudinal section 8 cm to the right of midline *(blue line)*.

1 Right lobe of liver
2 Portal vein (shaded area)
3 Hepatic vein
4 Gall bladder
5 Right kidney
6 Perirenal fat
7 Caudate lobe
8 Diaphragm
9 Costodiaphragmatic
   recess

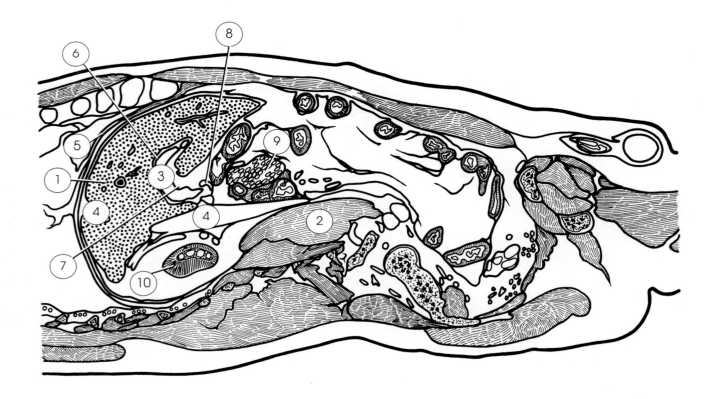

1 Right lobe of liver
2 Psoas muscle
3 Left portal vein
4 Inferior vena cava
5 Diaphragm
6 Fissure for the
   ligamentum teres
7 Hepatic artery
8 Common bile duct
9 Head of the pancreas
10 Right kidney

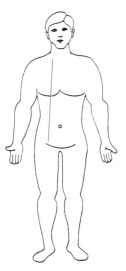

Fig. 37-18. Longitudinal section 6 cm to the right of midline (*blue line*).

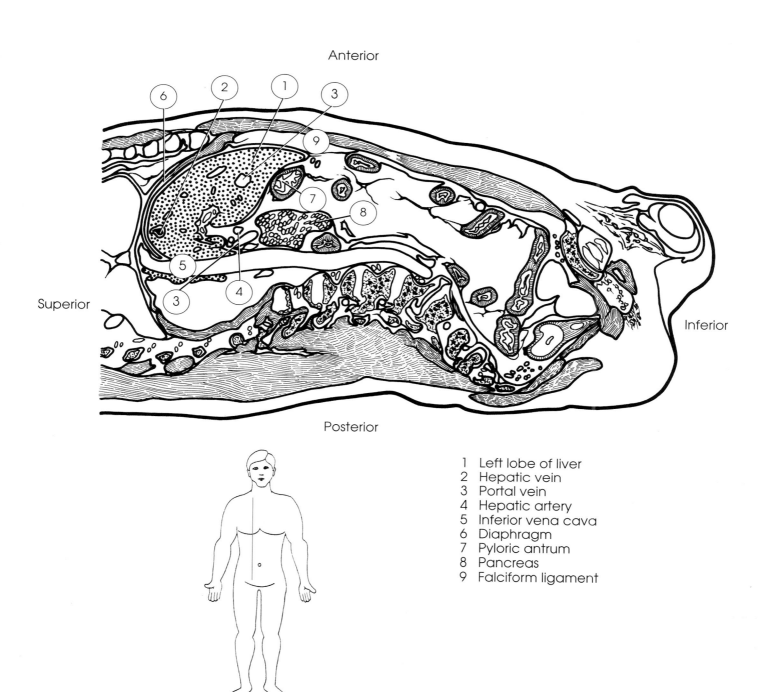

Anterior

Superior

Inferior

Posterior

1 Left lobe of liver
2 Hepatic vein
3 Portal vein
4 Hepatic artery
5 Inferior vena cava
6 Diaphragm
7 Pyloric antrum
8 Pancreas
9 Falciform ligament

Fig. 37-19. Longitudinal section 4 cm to the right of midline *(blue line)*.

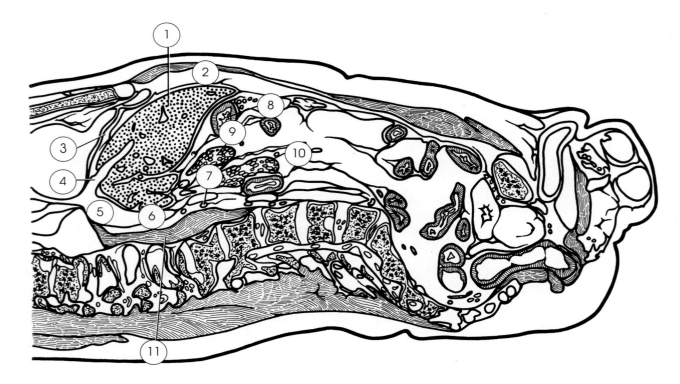

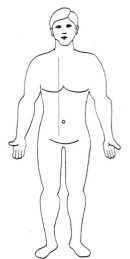

1 Left lobe of liver
2 Omentum
3 Diaphragm
4 Hepatic vein
5 Inferior vena cava
6 Hepatic artery
7 Right renal artery
8 Pyloric antrum
9 Pancreatic head
10 Uncinate process
11 Crus of the diaphragm

Fig. 37-20. Longitudinal section 2 cm to the right of midline *(blue line)*.

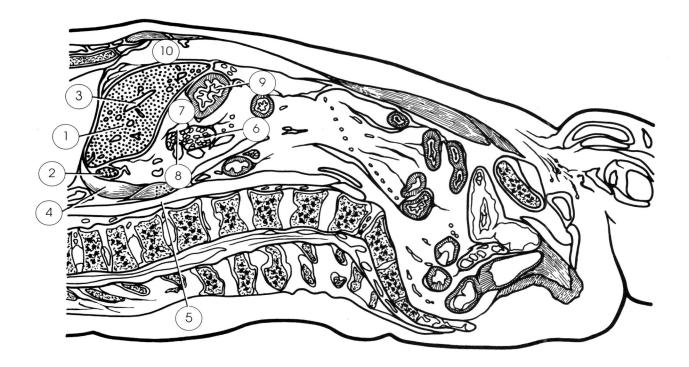

1   Left lobe of liver
2   Caudate lobe
3   Portal vein
4   Crus of the diaphragm
5   Aorta
6   Pancreas
7   Lesser omentum
8   Lesser sac
9   Stomach
10 Omentum

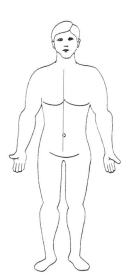

Fig. 37-21. Longitudinal section in the midline *(blue line).*

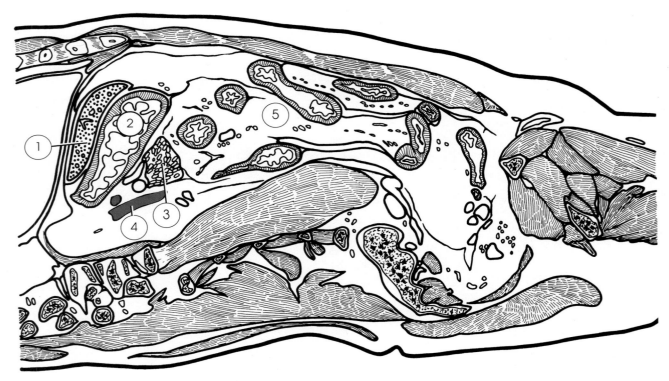

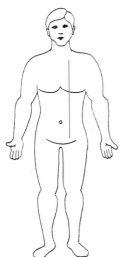

1 Left lobe of liver
2 Body of stomach
3 Pancreas
4 Left suprarenal gland
5 Mesentery

Fig. 37-22. Longitudinal section 4 cm to the left of midline *(blue line)*.

Clinical Applications
ABDOMEN AND RETROPERITONEUM

The upper abdominal ultrasound examination includes visualization of the liver, portal system, biliary system, prevertebral vessels, pancreas, spleen, kidneys, diaphragm, spine, and muscles. The patient is examined in the supine, decubitus, upright, or prone position. Generally a high-frequency, 3.5 MHz, sector or curved array transducer is used for optimal resolution. In obese patients, a 2.25 MHz transducer may be used. In pediatric patients, a 5.0 MHz transducer is used for improved resolution (Figs. 37-23 to 37-32).

For an upper abdominal scan, the patient does not eat or drink anything for 6 hours prior to the examination so that an adequate image of the biliary system may be obtained. Scanning may consist of transverse and sagittal planes, with additional scans made in the subcostal, coronal, and oblique planes.

If the left upper quadrant is not adequately visualized secondary to overlying bowel gas or air in the stomach, a liquid such as water or tomato juice may be given to dilate the stomach and fill the duodenum to serve as a landmark for the visualization of the pancreas.

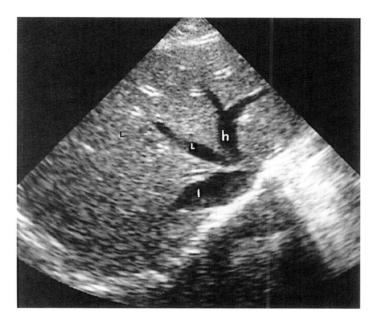

Fig. 37-23. Transverse scan of the right upper quadrant demonstrates the liver (L), the hepatic veins (h) as they drain into the inferior vena cava (I) at the level of the diaphragm.

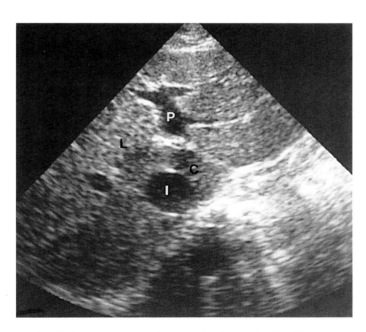

Fig. 37-24. Transverse scan 2 cm below the xyphoid of the right upper quadrant shows the liver (L), portal vein (p), caudate lobe (C) of the liver, and inferior vena cava (I).

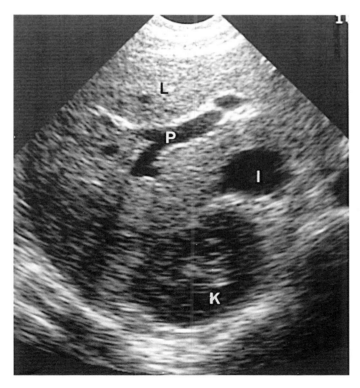

Fig. 37-25. Transverse scan 4 cm below the xyphoid of the right upper quadrant shows the homogeneous liver (L), right portal vein (p), inferior vena cava (I), and midpole of the right kidney (K).

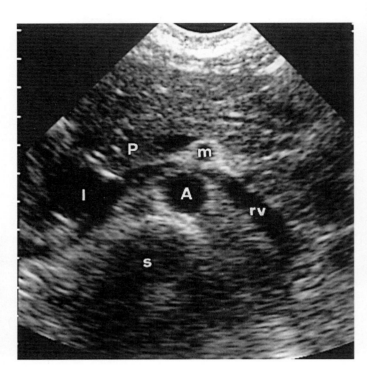

Fig. 37-26. Transverse scan of the pancreatic area 5 cm below the xyphoid shows the spine (s), the aorta (A) and inferior vena cava (l), the superior mesenteric artery (m), the left renal vein (rv) as it crosses anterior to the aorta and posterior to the superior mesenteric artery, and the pancreas (p) anterior to the prevertebral vessels.

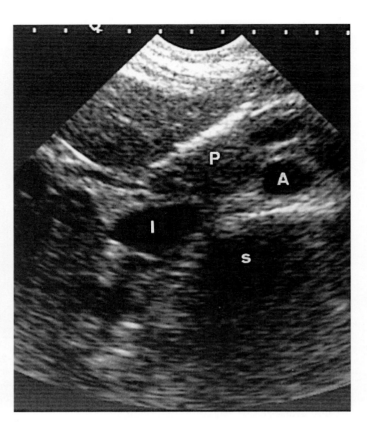

Fig. 37-27. Transverse scan of the pancreatic area 6 cm below the xyphoid shows the spine (s), aorta (A), and inferior vena cava (l) with the head of the pancreas anterior (p).

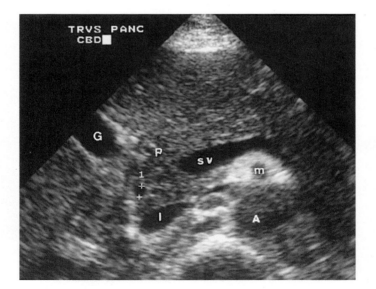

Fig. 37-28. Transverse scan 6 cm below the xyphoid shows the gall bladder (G), the head and body of the pancreas (p), the common bile duct (between the + markers), the splenic vein (sv) as it drapes anterior to the superior mesenteric artery (m), the aorta (A) and the inferior vena cava (l).

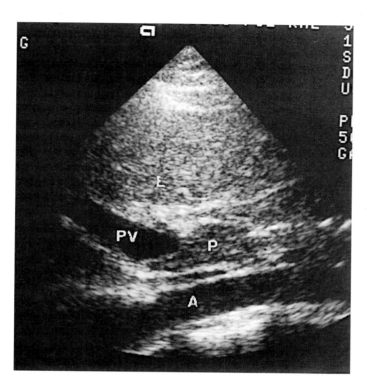

Fig. 37-29. Longitudinal scan slightly to the left of midline shows the aorta (A), the body of the pancreas (p) as it lies anterior to the aorta and inferior to the portal vein (PV) under the left lobe of the liver (L).

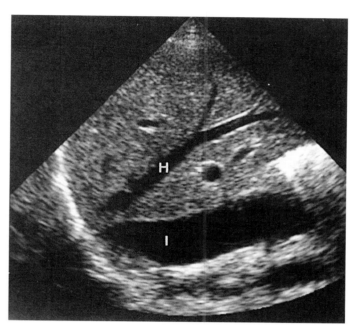

Fig. 37-30. Longitudinal scan slightly to the right of midline shows the dilated inferior vena cava (I) with the hepatic vein (H) draining into its anterior border at the level of the diaphragm.

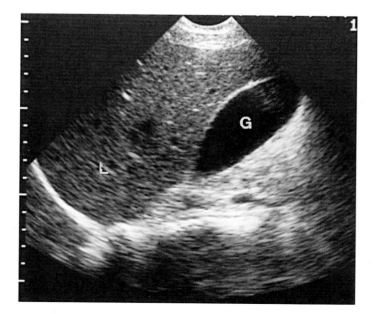

Fig. 37-31. Longitudinal scan 4 cm to the right of midline shows the homogeneous liver texture with the gall bladder (G) near the right inferior border.

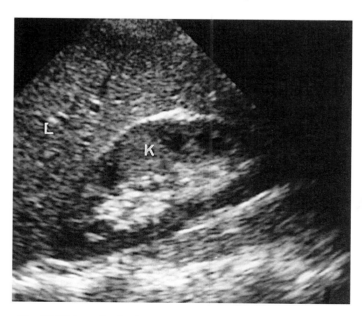

Fig. 37-32. Longitudinal scan 8 cm to the right of midline shows the liver (L) and right kidney (K).

Clinical applications

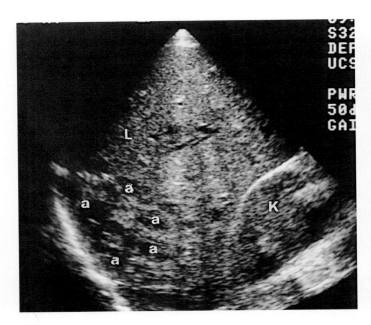

Fig. 37-33. Longitudinal scan 8 cm to the right of midline shows the inhomogeneity of the liver texture due to multiple abscess pockets (a) throughout the right lobe of the liver (L, liver; K, kidney).

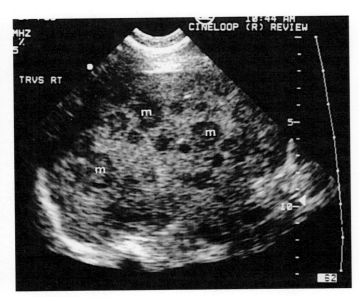

Fig. 37-34. Transverse scan of the right upper quadrant shows the hepatomegaly with multiple hypoechoic lesions throughout the liver. These represent metastatic (m) involvement of the liver secondary to colon cancer.

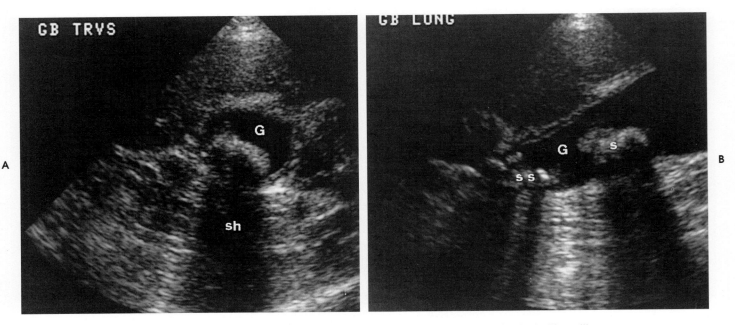

Fig. 37-35. A, Transverse and **B,** longitudinal scans of the gall bladder (G) filled with multiple large echogenic stones (s) causing shadowing posterior to the stones (sh).

The sonographer must have an understanding of the patient's clinical history and symptoms to produce an adequate scan. The normal sonographic patterns of abdominal and pelvic organs and vascular structures must be adequately imaged to detect any pathologic condition that might require further investigation. Although ultrasound cannot diagnose a lesion, the clinical picture may lead to a more specific difficult diagnosis to rule out infection, diffuse disease, mass, hematoma, or other infiltrative process. The liver, spleen, and pancreas are evaluated to assess size and homogeneity of tissue, or the presence of dilated vessels is assessed to determine flow patterns, thrombus, or collateral circulation (Figs. 37-33 and 37-34). The gall bladder and biliary system are evaluated to assess size, wall thickness, and the presence of sludge, stones, polyps, or other masses (Fig. 37-35). The kidneys are assessed for size, dilatation of the clinical structures, obstruction, cyst, tumor, abscess, infarct, hematoma, or infiltrative process and for localization for renal biopsy (Fig. 37-36). Renal transplanted kidneys may be evaluated for size, presence of hydronephrosis, texture pattern (to rule out rejection), extrarenal fluid collections, and ureter size. The retroperitoneal space is evaluated for the presence of mass lesions, increased fluid or ascites, hematoma, or other abnormal omental or mesentary echo patterns.

Once a mass is suspected, the sonographer must evaluate its acoustic properties to determine if it is heterogeneous, homogeneous, *hypo-* or *hyperechoic,* isoechoic, or *anechoic.* A hypoechoic lesion is fluid-filled, homogeneous, or necrotic tissue. A hyperechoic mass may be a tumor, thrombus, or calcification. A mixed pattern would show characteristics of both solid and cystic patterns as seen in an abscess, a necrotic tumor with hemorrhage, a decomposing thrombus, a complex tumor, or a septated mass. An isoechoic mass would show the same *echogenicity* as the surrounding organs. An anechoic lesion would show no internal echoes, smooth walls, and increased through transmission.

The sonographer must be able to analyze the borders of a mass to determine whether they are smooth, irregular, ill-defined, thin, or thick to further define its characteristics. A hyperechoic attenuated mass would show decreased through transmission, whereas a hypoechoic mass would show increased through transmission posterior to the borders.

A small calculus within a structure, such as a renal stone or gallstone, may produce a sharp, well-defined acoustic shadow posterior to its border. This shadow depends on the transducer's being perpendicular to the calculus. A thrombus within a vessel may produce a low-level echo pattern within the dilated structure. Color-flow Doppler may be used to outline the patency of the vascular structure. Reduced flow would indicate obstruction of flow.

Once a mass has been localized, ultrasound can aid the clinician in the aspiration or biopsy procedure. The sonographer may locate the site of the lesion, calculate its depth, and determine the direction and angulation of needle placement for the procedure.

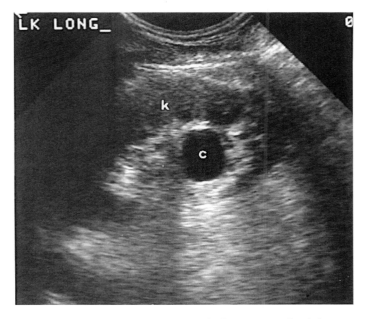

Fig. 37-36. Longitudinal scan over the left upper quadrant shows the left kidney *(k)* with an anechoic cystic lesion *(c)* near its midpole. There is good through transmission of the sound through the simple cyst.

PELVIS AND OBSTETRICS

Anatomic features of the pelvis

The pelvis is divided into the greater and lesser pelvic cavity with the pelvic brim being the circumference of a plane dividing these two portions. The greater, or false, pelvis is superior to the pelvic brim and is bounded on each side by the ilium. The lesser, or true, pelvis is situated caudal to the pelvic brim. The walls of the pelvic cavity are formed by muscles collectively called the pelvic diaphragm.

The female peritoneal cavity extends inferiorly into the lesser pelvis and is bounded by the peritoneum, which covers the rectum, bladder, and uterus (Fig. 37-37). In the female, the peritoneum descends from the anterior abdominal wall to the level of the pubic bone onto the superior surface of the bladder. It then passes from the bladder to the uterus to form the vesicouterine pouch. The peritoneum covers the fundus and body of the uterus and extends over the posterior fornix and the wall of the vagina. Between the uterus and the rectum the peritoneum forms the deep rectouterine pouch.

Pelvis

Gynecologic examination Examination of the female pelvis includes ultrasonic visualization of the distended urinary bladder, uterus, cervix, vagina, ovaries, and supporting pelvic musculature (Figs. 37-38 and 37-39). The rectum and other bowel structures are often visualized and, if necessary, filled by way of a water enema to separate normal structures from extra fluid or masses that may lie close to these structures. The uterine (fallopian) tubes and broad ligament may be imaged, especially if the patient has excessive free fluid in the pelvic cavity.

Ultrasonic examination of the pelvis has been useful in imaging normal pelvic anatomy and musculature, identifying the size of ovarian follicles, measuring endometrial thickness, evaluating the texture of the myometrium, localizing intrauterine or extrauterine pregnancies, detecting masses or abscess collections, or localizing an intrauterine contraceptive device in the transabdominal approach. Evaluation of the pelvis may be performed with transabdominal or endovaginal techniques.

To adequately visualize the pelvic anatomy, the patient must have a very full bladder. This allows the small bowel to be pushed superiorly out of the pelvic cavity, elevates the uterus, and serves as a *sonic window* to image the pelvic structures.

Distinct echo patterns of an enlarged uterus allow the sonographer to distinguish a leiomyoma from endometriosis or from an early gestational sac. The sonographer is able to identify a cystic, solid, or complex mass within the ovaries or pelvic cavity. The sonographer must be able to distinguish the mass from bowel by observing peristalsis in the bowel or change in the shape of the bowel over time. The ultrasound interpretation, correlated with the patient's history and clinical symptoms, often allows for differential diagnosis.

Ultrasound also has been applied to women receiving fertility medication to monitor the serial growth of follicular cysts within the ovaries. A large follicular cyst may be an indication that the egg is ready for stimulation with subsequent fertilization.

Endovaginal ultrasound is another technique that allows the transducer to be inserted into the vagina to image the pelvic cavity in coronal and sagittal planes (the bladder must be completely empty for this procedure). A higher frequency transducer (6 to 7.5 MHz) is employed for very high–resolution images. This technique has become a clinical aid in the visualization of the ovaries, follicles, uterus, endometrium, and cervix.

In postoperative patients who have developed a fever of unknown origin, ultrasound may play a role in excluding abscess formation in the cul-de-sac of the pelvis (Douglas' pouch), the peripheral margins, or "gutters," of the abdomen, or the perirenal space.

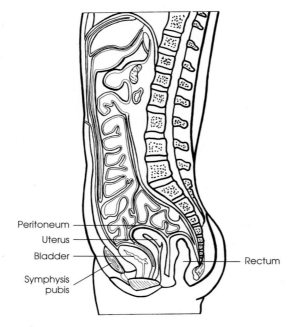

Fig. 37-37. Sagittal line drawing of the abdominal and pelvic cavity. The reflections of the peritoneal cavity are shown as it drapes over the rectum, uterus, and bladder.

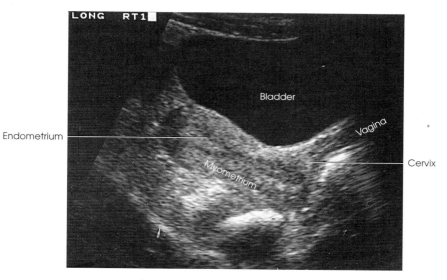

Fig. 37-38. Normal sagittal sonogram of the midline of the pelvic cavity. The distended urinary bladder is shown anterior to the uterus. The endometrium is shown as the bright linear echo within the uterus. The myometrium is the homogeneous smooth echo tissue surrounding the endometrium of the uterus. The cervix and vagina are well seen.

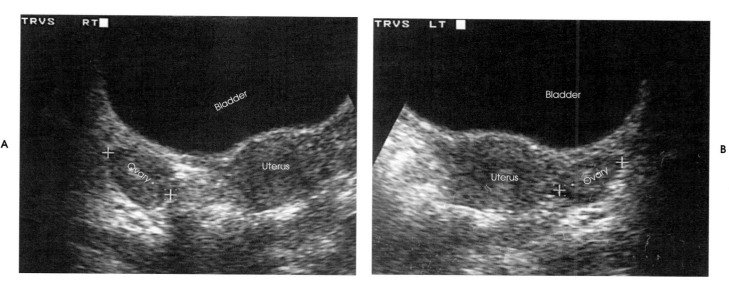

Fig. 37-39. A and **B,** Normal transverse scans over the lower pelvic segment show the distended bladder, uterus, and respective ovaries. If the ovaries are not visualized on transabdominal scans, the endovaginal technique is used.

Obstetrics

Obstetric examination The pregnant woman is the ideal candidate for an ultrasound examination. The amniotic fluid enhances sound penetration to differentiate fetal echo patterns from those of the placenta.

Endovaginal ultrasound is successfully used during the first trimester of gestation to define specific fetal anatomy. The fetal skeleton is not calcified during the first trimester to allow for adequate visualization of fetal structures. A gestational sac can be visualized as early as 4 weeks from the date of conception, and the embryo, heart, and placenta site can be seen at the sixth week of gestation. Heart motion and fetal size, position, and anomalies can be assessed in the second trimester of pregnancy. Serial examinations provide information relevant to the normal or abnormal (intrauterine growth retardation) growth of the fetus. The location and homogeneity of the placenta can be accurately defined in a patient who, presenting with pain and bleeding, may be diagnosed with placenta previa or abruptio placentae. Ultrasound is an aid to the perinatologist in localization techniques for amniocentesis, chorionic villus sampling, fetal blood sampling, or cord transfusion. Color flow Doppler has been helpful in defining the vascularity of the placenta in difficult cases such as placenta previa or placenta accreta.

In a pregnant patient whose uterus is too large for the calculated elapsed time, ultrasound allows the sonographer to assess for problems such as multiple gestation, hydatidiform mole development, a developing fibroid or other extrauterine mass, or simply a fetus that is more developed than the patient or physician suspected.

The fetal *biparietal diameter* may be visualized around the twelfth week of gestation and, along with the fetal abdomen, femur, and chest, is useful in monitoring fetal growth by measurement calculations and serial evaluation (Fig. 37-40).

Many developmental complications of pregnancy such as neural tube defects, skeletal anomalies, cardiac defects, gastrointestinal and genitourinary defects, and head anomalies may also be assessed by ultrasound (Figs. 37-41 to 37-45).

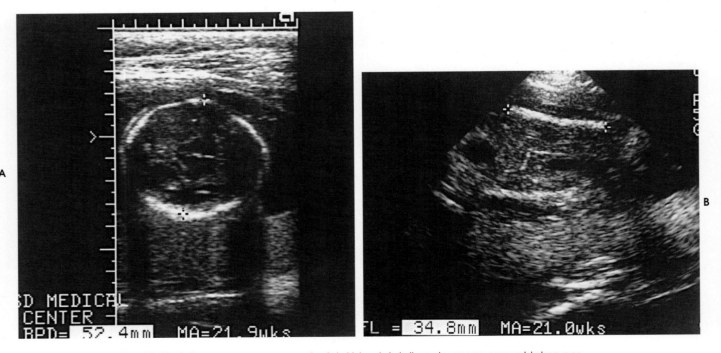

Fig. 37-40. A, Transverse sonogram of a fetal biparietal diameter measurement taken perpendicular to the falx of the midline. This particular measurement (marked on image) correlates with a gestational age of 21.9 weeks. **B,** Further correlation of the gestational age is made by taking measurements of the abdominal circumference and femur length as shown in this sagittal scan.

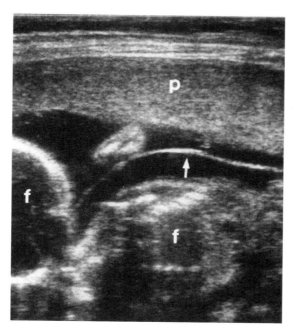

Fig. 37-41. Twin pregnancy with membrane *(arrow)* separating the two sacs *(p,* placenta; *f,* fetus).

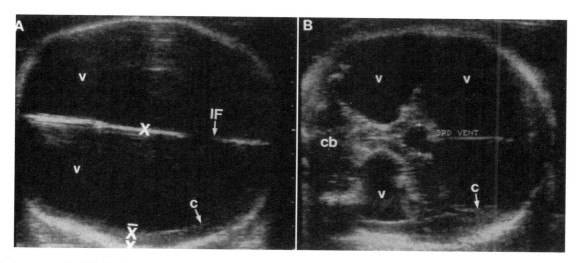

Fig. 37-42. A and **B,** Transverse section through cranium at the level of the temporal ventricular horns in a fetus with ventriculomegaly. Ventrical dilation *(v)* is apparent in both hemispheres. Cortical tissue *(c)* is noted. The interhemispheric fissure *(IF)* is noted dividing the cranial hemispheres.

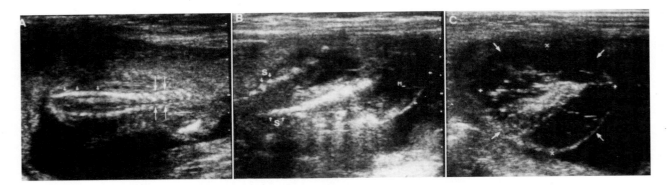

Fig. 37-43. A, Sagittal scan denoting the splaying of the thoracic, lumbar, and sacral spine in a fetus with a large spinal defect (small *arrows*). Long *arrows*, upper thoracic spine. **B,** Magnified view of spinal defect demonstrating marked widening of the spine (*s*) and protruding meningomyelocele sac (*m*). **C,** Tangential view of meningomyelocele (*arrows*) with multiple neural components.

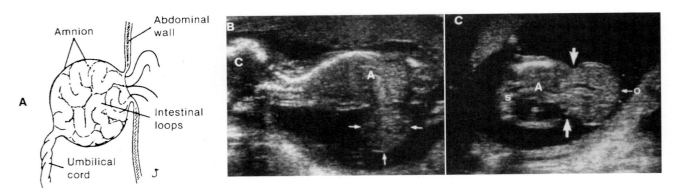

Fig. 37-44. A, Schema of omphalocele—failure of the intestinal loops and/or liver to return to the abdominal cavity. The herniated loops are surrounded by a membranous sac formed by the amnion. **B,** Sagittal scan of 18-week fetus in a spine-up position with evidence of a contained mass projecting from the anterior abdominal wall representing an omphalocele (*arrows*). (*C,* cranium; *A,* abdomen). **C,** Transverse plane, in same patient, localizing herniation of liver in the omphalocele (*o*). Note the portal vessel within the herniated liver. (*s,* spine; large *arrows*, first border of omphalocele; *A,* abdomen).

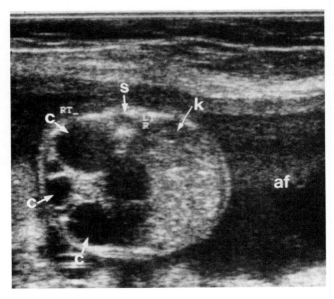

Fig. 37-45. Unilateral right multicystic kidney (*arrows*) at 21.5 weeks of gestation. Note the varying sizes of the cysts (*c*) and the normal contralateral kidney (*k*). (*af,* amniotic fluid).

Superficial structures

High-frequency (6 to 10 MHz) transducers have tremendously aided quality visualization of superficial structures such as the thyroid, breast, scrotum, and penis.

The visualization of minute structures such as the lactiferous ducts within the breast and spermatic cord within the testes are imaged in a routine ultrasound examination. Pathologic hypoechoic and hyperechoic areas (e.g., cyst, adenoma, carcinoma, or hydrocele) may be demonstrated.

Another development, used for imaging pelvic structures, is *endorectal* transducers. This very high–resolution transducer is inserted into the rectum to visualize the anatomy of the prostate gland or uterus. If an abnormality is detected, guidance for the biopsy may be given with this ultrasound study.

Neonatal neurosonography

The neonatal skull is evaluated with a high-frequency small sector or linear array transducer. A series of scans are produced through the coronal suture. The transducer is angled from the frontal lobe of the cerebrum to the occipital lobe (Fig. 37-46). Subsequent scans are made in the sagittal plane to outline the ventricular system, septum pellucidum, corpus collosum, and choroid plexus (Fig. 37-47). Axial scans may be made to image the posterior fossa, vermis, and fourth ventricle (Fig. 37-48).

Abnormalities may be evaluated in meningomyelocele (Chiari II malformation), intracranial cystic abnormalities (e.g., hydrocephalus and Dandy-Walker syndrome), and other congenital malformations such as agenesis of the corpus callosum, holoprosencephaly, and arteriovenous malformations.

Ultrasound is useful in evaluating the infant for an intracranial infection, hemorrhage, or tumor or for following ventricular shunt function.

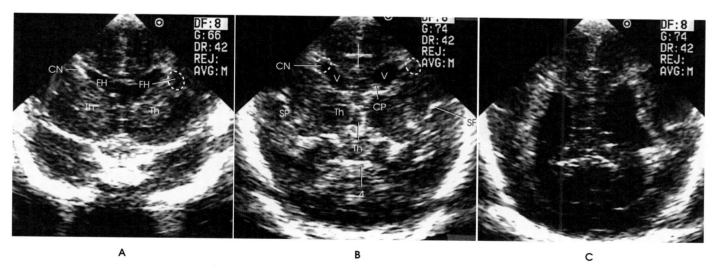

Fig. 37-46. Multiple coronal images of the neonatal skull; the coronal image is taken along the axis of the coronal suture. **A,** The transducer is angled toward the anterior skull (face); the small semilunar slits are anterior to the frontal horns *(FH)* of the lateral ventricle; the caudate nucleus *(CN)* is adjacent to the frontal horns, with the thalamus *(Th)* posterior. **B,** The transducer is perpendicular to the skull; the body of the ventricle *(V)* is seen, along with the third *(3)* and fourth *(4)* ventricles; the choroid plexus *(CP)* is the dense echogenic material found along the floor of the ventricle; the sylvian fissure *(SF)* is easily seen on the lateral aspect of the brain. **C,** The transducer is angled toward the posterior skull; the body of the lateral ventricles *(V)* is easily seen.

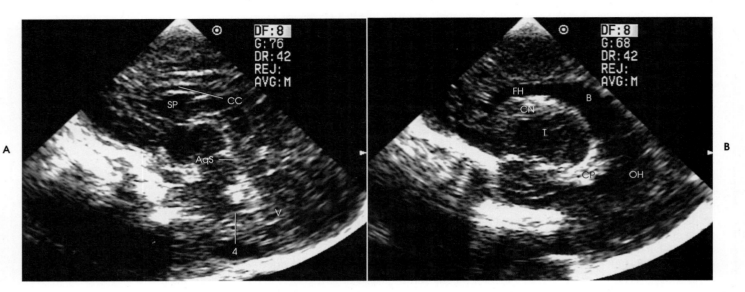

Fig. 37-47. Sagittal images of the neonatal skull. **A,** Midline sagittal view shows the cavum septi pellucidi *(SP)*, the corpus callosum *(CC)*, the cerebral aqueduct *(aqS)*, the fourth ventricle *(4)*, and the vermis of the cerebellum *(V)*. **B,** Sagittal scan shows the lateral ventricle (frontal horn *(FH)*, body *(B)*, occipital horn *(OH)*; the caudate nucleus *(CN)* and choroid plexus *(CP)* are shown as echodense structures; the thalamus *(T)* is also seen.

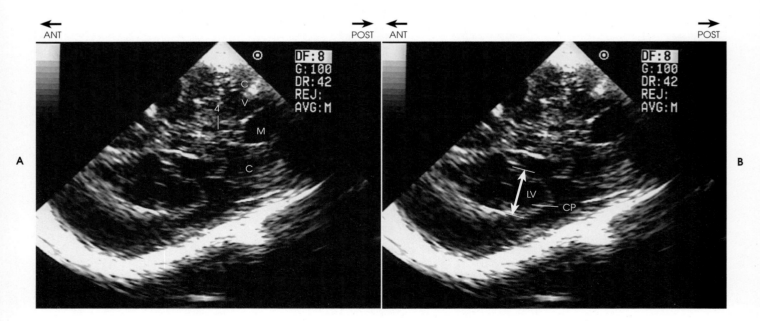

Fig. 37-48. Axial views of the neonatal skull obtained by placing the transducer on the lateral aspect of the neonatal head: anterior is to the left; posterior to the right. **A,** Axial view showing the area of the fourth ventricle *(4)*, cerebellum *(C)*, and medulla oblongata *(M)*. **B,** Axial view with a slight superior angulation shows the lateral ventricles *(LV)* with the choroid plexus lying along the far lateral edge; this is a good view to measure the size of the lateral ventricles.

PERIPHERAL VASCULAR ULTRASOUND

The use of ultrasound, Doppler, and color-flow Doppler has enhanced the ability to image the peripheral vascular structures in the body. Visualization of the common carotid artery and its branches is routine with ultrasound imaging. Ultrasound can be used to detect the presence of plaque, thrombosis, obstruction, or stenosis.

In addition, the femoral artery and vein, as it extends into the lower limb, can be imaged by high-frequency ultrasound transducers. The visualization of thrombus is made through the inability of the venous structure to be fully compressed by the sonographer performing the study. Careful mapping of the arterial and venous structures may be reliably made with the ultrasound vascular mapping technique.

Ultrasound is also useful to image the patency of other vascular structures, such as the subclavian artery and vein, the brachial artery and vein, and radial grafts.

CARDIOLOGY APPLICATIONS

The echocardiographic examination includes visualization of the four chambers of the heart (right and left ventricles, right and left atria), the four valvular structures (left and right atrioventricular [mitral, tricuspid], aortic, and pulmonic valves), the interatrial and interventricular septa, the delineation of cardiac musculature (endocardium, myocardium, epicardium), the papillary muscles and chorda tendineae cordis, and the pericardium (Fig. 37-49). The application of real-time two-dimensional ultrasound in the adult, pediatric, neonatal, and fetal patient has proven to be a tremendous diagnostic aid for the echocardiographer.

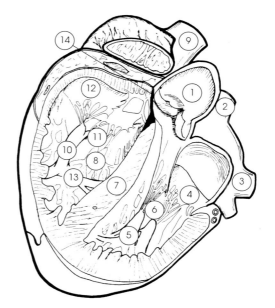

1 Ascending aorta
2 Right pulmonary vein
3 Left pulmonary vein
4 Left atrioventricular (mitral) valve
5 Posterior papillary muscle
6 Left ventricle
7 Muscular interventricular septum
8 Right posterior papillary muscle
9 Superior vena cava
10 Septal band
11 Right ventricle
12 Right atrioventricular (tricuspid) valve
13 Moderator band
14 Membranous interventricular septum

Fig. 37-49. Schematic drawing of the right and left ventricles of the heart. The left ventricle is slightly larger than the right. Its wall is thicker because of increased pressure on the left. The interventricular septum separates the two chambers.

Procedure for echocardiography. The examination usually begins with the patient in a slightly left lateral, semidecubitus position, to move the heart away from the sternum and closer to the chest wall, thus producing a better cardiac window. The transducer should be placed slightly to the left of the sternum in the third, fourth, or fifth intercostal space.

The real-time procedure includes the following views:

1. Long-axis views: from the base of the heart to its apex (Fig. 37-50)
2. Multiple short-axis views (Fig. 37-51)
3. Apical or subxiphoid views: to image the four chambers and valves simultaneously
4. Suprasternal view: to image the aortic arch and its branches, right pulmonary artery, left atrium, and left main bronchus

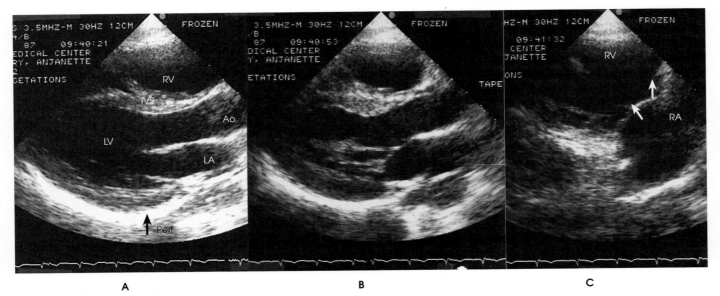

A   B   C

Fig. 37-50. A, Diastolic frame of the parasternal long-axis view in the heart as the (mitral) valve opens in diastole to allow blood to fill the ventricular cavity as it flows through the orifice from the left atrium. **B,** When the (mitral) valve closes, the ventricle pumps blood through the aortic cusps into the ascending aorta. **C,** Parasternal long-axis view with the transducer angled medially and to the right shows the right ventricle *(RV)* right atrioventricular (tricuspid) valve *(arrows)*, and right atrium *(RA)*.

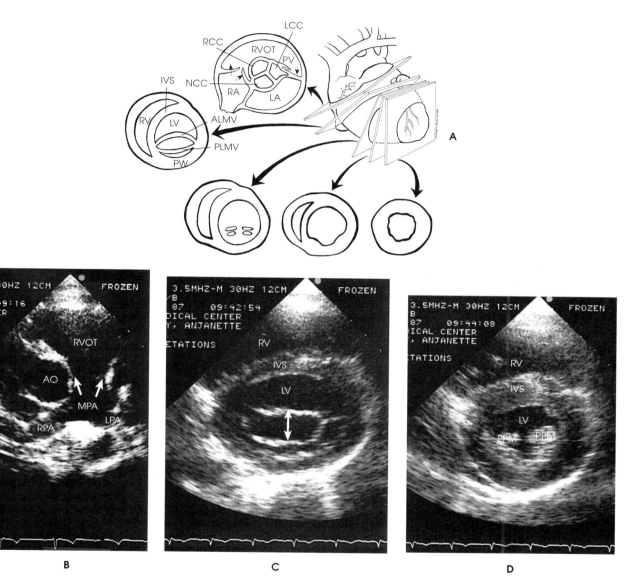

Fig. 37-51. A, Schematic drawings of multiple parasternal short-axis views of the heart. The transducer has been rotated 90 degrees from the long-axis plane. Right ventricle *(RV),* interventricular septum *(IVS),* left ventricle *(LV),* anterior leaflet mitral valve *(ALMV),* posterior leaflet mitral valve *(PLMV),* and posterior wall of left ventricle *(PW),* right ventricular outflow tract *(RVOT),* right atrium *(RA),* left atrium *(LA),* aortic cusps *(RCC, LCC, NCC),* pulmonary valve *(PV).* **B,** High-parasternal short-axis view of the heart shows the right ventricular outflow tract wrapped anterior to the aorta. The main pulmonary artery *(MPA)* shows the pulmonary valve *(arrows)* before it bifurcates into right and left pulmonary arteries. **C,** Mid-parasternal short-axis view over the right ventricle, septum, and left atrioventricular (mitral) valve within the left ventricle. **D,** Low-parasternal short-axis views of the heart show the right ventricle wrapped anterior to the septum and left ventricular cavity. The two prominent projections into the left ventricle represent the posterior papillary muscles *(PPM).*

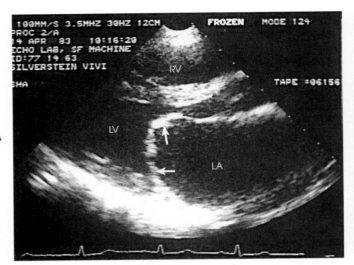

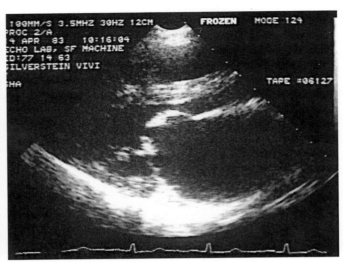

Fig. 37-52. A, Systolic and, **B,** diastolic frames taken in the parasternal long-axis view in a patient with severe mitral stenosis. The anterior leaflet *(arrows)* is thickened and does not open to its full excursion. The left atrium is dilated because of the calcified mitral valve, causing mitral regurgitation.

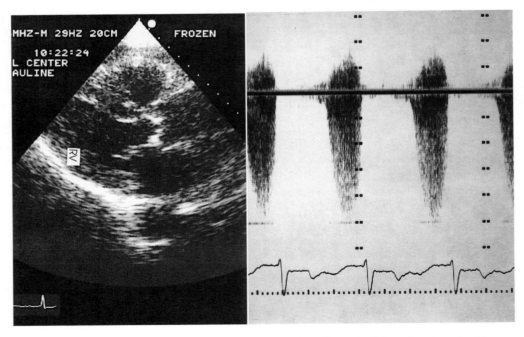

Fig. 37-53. Two-dimensional and Doppler tracings (from the apical five-chamber view) in a patient with significant aortic stenosis. The leaflets are thickened with restrictive opening. There is a 4.5 m/sec of aortic stenosis.

Cardiac pathology The echocardiographic evaluation of cardiac pathology may be used to evaluate calcification, thickening of the valve leaflets, or thrombus formation in the atrial cavities secondary to rheumatic heart disease. This process may lead to significant stenosis and regurgitation of the leaflet with subsequent chamber enlargement (Figs. 37-52 and 37-53). An infectious process such as bacterial endocarditis may lead to the formation of vegetations, rupture, or tear of the valve leaflet with regurgitation into the atrial cavity. Congestive cardiomyopathy would show generalized cardiac enlargement, valve leakage, and thrombus formation (Fig. 37-54). Cardiac cysts and tumors may be seen with subsequent valve damage if the tumor is adjacent to the valvular structures (Fig. 37-55). The presence of pericardial or pleural effusion may be readily assessed with echocardiography (Fig. 37-56).

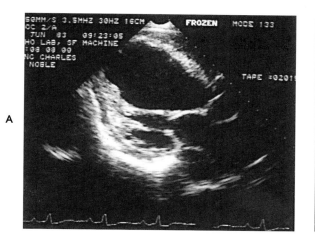
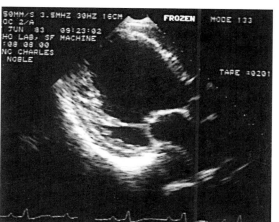
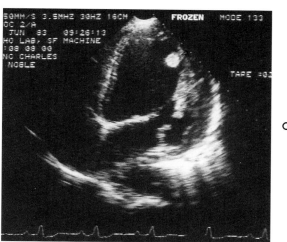

Fig. 37-54. A, Systolic and, **B,** diastolic long-axis views of a very dilated heart in a patient with congestive cardiomyopathy. **C** shows a four-chamber view of the cardiac dilation with a bright echo from a thrombus formation near the apex of the heart.

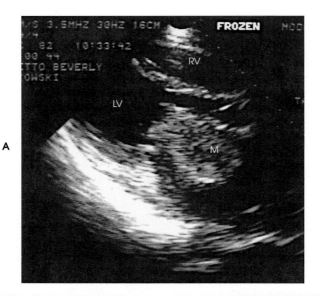

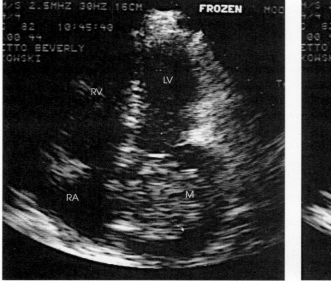

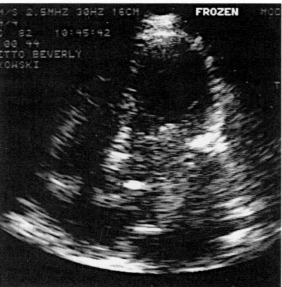

Fig. 37-55. A, Parasternal long-axis view and, **B** and **C,** apical four-chamber views of a patient with a large left atrial myxoma. The tumor mass is seen throughout the cardiac cycle as it flops behind the mitral valve and falls into the left atrial cavity.

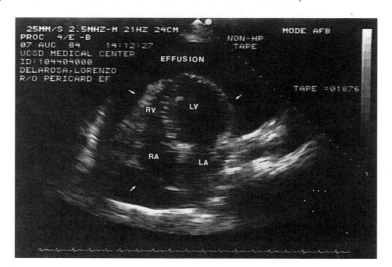

Fig. 37-56. In this apical four-chamber echocardiographic view, the four chambers of the heart are completely surrounded by the huge effusion *(arrows)* from the atrioventricular junction to the basal segment of the right atrium.

The analysis of left ventricular function and the serial evaluation of patients after myocardial infarction are investigated with computer analysis to measure changes in the intraventricular and posterior left ventricular wall thickness and contractility (Fig. 37-57). The gray-scale reflections of normal myocardial tissue, scar tissue, and newly infarcted tissues are being evaluated with myocardial contrast studies.

Simple and complex congenital lesions of the heart have been diagnosed with the use of echocardiography. With careful evaluation, the sonographer can determine the location, number, and size of the valves (e.g., agenesis, atresia, stenosis, deformed, domed, redundant); the number, size, thickness, and continuity among the cardiac chambers with the interventricular and interatrial septa; and the orientation of the great vessels and their relationship to the ventricles.

The critically ill neonate has a much better chance for survival if the correct diagnosis is made early. Thus, with the aid of sonography, the condition of the cyanotic infant can be diagnosed as congenital heart disease or severe respiratory distress. Critical heart disease in a cyanotic infant would include a hypoplastic left heart, transposition of the great vessels, truncus arteriosus, or pulmonary atresia with tetralogy of Fallot (Fig. 37-58).

The Doppler technique with color flow has added a new dimension to understanding flow patterns within the heart. Shunt flow across a ventricular or atrial septal defect is well defined with this technique. In addition, multiple defects may be detected with color mapping. Areas of narrowing, or stenosis, cause a specific turbulent pattern within the vessel. Areas that leak or regurgitate cause a smooth back flow from the valve into the chamber below.

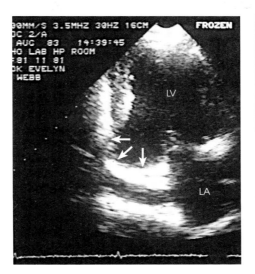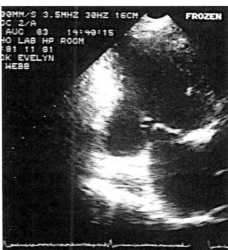

Fig. 37-57. Parasternal long-axis views of the left ventricle with an aneurysmal formation in the posterior basal segment *(arrows)*. This condition may occur secondary to a myocardial infarction as the tissue becomes scarred and weakened.

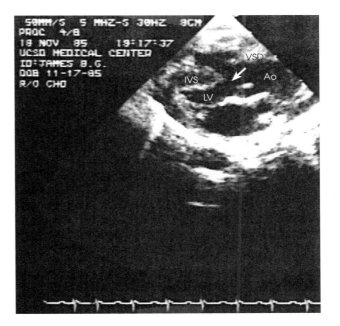

Fig. 37-58. A common congenital heart lesion in infants is tetralogy of Fallot. This syndrome is characterized by the presence of a ventricular septal defect *(VSD)*, overriding of the aorta *(Ao)*, pulmonary stenosis, and right ventricular hypertrophy.

Summary

Diagnostic ultrasound has made significant progress during the last decade in the management and differential diagnosis of the patient. The development of high-frequency transducers with endoscopic visualization (transvaginal, transrectal, and transesophageal) has aided the visualization of previously difficult areas. Better equipment design enables the sonographer to obtain more information and to process more data points to obtain a comprehensive report from the ultrasound or echocardiographic study. Color-flow mapping enables the sonographer to distinguish the direction and velocity of arterial and venous blood flow from other structures in the body. It can differentiate to determine areas of obstruction from areas of regurgitation.

Improvements in resolution and transducer design has allowed for progress in resolving small structures within the abdomen, pelvis, heart, and neonatal head. Obstetric patients benefit from these improvements because of the increased ability to detect neural tube defects, cleft palates, shortened extremities, and gastrointestinal and genitourinary abnormalities, in addition to other fetal anomalies. The examination of the fetal heart has become routine in high-risk obstetric patients and in patients with an increased risk for cardiac disease.

Continued research and development of computer analysis and tissue characterization of echo reflections should further contribute to the total diagnostic approach for the patient. Research into contrast agents for ultrasound is also being conducted in efforts to tag vascular molecules to improve visualization in order to separate normal organ structures from pathologic tumor growth patterns.

Ultrasound has rapidly emerged into a useful, noninvasive, high-yield clinical diagnostic examination for various applications in medicine. The field will continue to grow in importance with further development in transducer design, image resolution, tissue characterization applications, color flow increased sensitivity, and three-dimensional reconstruction.

Definition of Terms*

acoustic cavitation Formation of partial vacuums in a liquid by high-frequency sound waves.

acoustic impedance The ratio of acoustic pressure to particle velocity at any point in the acoustic field.

acoustic shadow The loss of acoustic power of structures lying behind an attenuating or reflecting target.

A-mode (amplitude) A method of acoustic echo display in which time is represented along the horizontal axis and echo amplitude is displayed along the vertical axis.

anechoic The property of being free of echoes or without echoes.

angle of incidence The angle at which the ultrasound beam strikes an interface with respect to normal (perpendicular) incidence.

array A spatial arrangement of two or more transducers.

artifact An echo that does not correspond in distance or direction to a real target.

attenuation Reduction of acoustic amplitude along the propagation pathway as a result of diffraction, absorption, scattering, reflections, or any other process that redirects the signal away from the receiver.

attenuation compensation The compensation for attenuation of acoustic signals along the propagation pathway as a result of losses and geometric divergence. When accomplished electronically this is called *time-gain compensation* (TGC).

backscatter The part of the acoustic energy reflected from a small (compared with the wavelength) target back toward the source.

biparietal diameter (BPD) The largest dimension of the fetal head perpendicular to the median sagittal plane. Measured by ultrasonic visualization; used to measure fetal development.

B-mode (brightness) A method of acoustic display on an oscilloscope in which the intensity of the echo is represented by modulation of the brightness of the spot and in which the position of the echo is determined from the position of the transducer and the transit time of the acoustic pulse; displayed in the x-y plane.

cavitation Acoustic cavitation is an activity produced by sound in liquids or any medium with liquid content, involving bubbles or cavities containing gas or vapor.

characteristic acoustic impedance The impedance determined by the product of the undisturbed density and velocity (pc), which occurs in equations, describing plane progressive propagation in homogeneous media; hence, often regarded as "characteristic" of the medium.

compound scan A method of scanning that combines at least two basic scanning motions.

compression Process of decreasing the difference between the smallest and largest amplitudes.

continuous wave (CW) ultrasound A waveform in which the amplitude modulation factor is less than or equal to a small value.

coronal image plane An anatomic term used to describe a plane perpendicular to both the sagittal and transverse planes of the body.

cross-sectional display A display that presents ultrasound interaction echo data from a single plane within a tissue. It is produced by sweeping the ultrasound beam through a given angle, by translating it along a line, or by some combination of linear and angular motions. The depth in the tissue is represented along one coordinate and the position in the scan is represented by the second coordinate. The intensity of the echoes produced in echo ranging is displayed by modulation of the brightness of the image produced. The plane of the section may be sagittal, coronal, or transverse. The lateral resolution is determined by the beam width of the transducers.

decibel A unit used for expressing the ratio of two quantities of electrical signal or sound energy.

density Mass divided by volume.

Doppler effect A shift in frequency or wavelength, depending on the conditions of observation, caused by relative motions among sources, receivers, and the medium.

Doppler ultrasound Application of the Doppler effect to ultrasound to detect movement of a reflecting boundary relative to the source, resulting in a change of the wavelength of the reflected wave.

dynamic imaging Imaging of an object in motion at a frame rate sufficient to cause no significant blurring of any one image and at a repetition rate sufficient to adequately represent the movement pattern. This is frequently referred to as imaging at a real-time (frame) rate.

echo Reflection of acoustic energy received from scattering elements or a specular reflector.

echogenic A medium that contains echo-producing structures.

endorectal High-frequency transducer that can be inserted into the rectum to visualize the bladder and prostate gland.

endovaginal High-frequency transducer (and decreased penetration) that can be in-

*Interim AIUM Standard Nomenclature, November, 1978. M Central Office, Washington, D.C.
Kremkau, Frederick W, PhD: Diagnostic ultrasound. In Physical principles and exercises, 1980, Grune & Stratton. By permission.

serted into the vagina to obtain high-resolution images of the pelvic structures.

focal zone The distance along the beam axis of a focused transducer assembly, from the point where the beam area first becomes equal to four times the focal area to the point beyond the focal surface where the beam area again becomes equal to four times the focal area.

focus To concentrate the sound beam into a smaller beam area than would exist without focusing.

frequency Number of cycles per unit of time, usually expressed in Hertz (Hz), or megahertz (MHz—million cycles per second).

gray scale A property of the display in which intensity information is recorded as changes in the brightness of the display.

hard copy A method of image recording in which the data is stored on paper, film, or other recording material.

hyperechoic Producing more echoes than normal.

hypoechoic Producing fewer echoes than normal.

intensity Power divided by beam area.

linear scan The motion of the transducer at a constant speed along a straight line at right angles to the beam.

longitudinal wave Wave in which the particle motion is parallel to the direction of wave travel.

matching layer Material placed in front of the face of a transducer element to reduce the reflection at the transducer surface.

medium Material through which a wave travels.

M-mode (motion) A method of display in which tissue depth is displayed along one axis and time is displayed along the second axis.

piezoelectric effect Conversion of pressure to electrical voltage or conversion of an electrical voltage to a mechanical pressure.

power Rate at which work is done; rate at which energy is transferred.

pulsed-wave ultrasound Sound waves produced in pulse form by applying electrical pulses to the transducer.

rarefaction The state of minimum pressure in a medium transversed by compression waves.

real time imaging Imaging with a real-time display whose output keeps pace with changes in input.

reflection Acoustic energy is reflected from a structure where there is a discontinuity in the characteristic acoustic impedance along the propagation path.

refraction The phenomenon of bending wave fronts as the acoustic energy propagates from the medium of one acoustic velocity to a second medium of differing acoustic velocity.

resolution A measure of the ability to display two closely spaced structures as discrete targets.

resonant frequency Operating frequency.

reverberation The phenomenon of multiple reflections within a closed system.

scan A technique for moving an acoustic beam to produce an image for which both the transducer and the display movements are synchronized.

scan converter Device that stores a grayscale image and allows it to be displayed on a television monitor.

scattering Diffusion or redirection of sound in several directions on encountering a particle suspension or a rough surface.

sector scan A system of scanning in which the transducer or transmitted beam is rotated through an angle, the center of rotation being near or behind the surface of the transducer.

sonic window The sonographer's ability to visualize a particular area. For example, the full urinary bladder is a good sonic window to image the uterus and ovaries in a transabdominal scan. The intercostal margins may be a good sonic window to image the liver parenchyma.

speed of sound The product of the frequency and the wavelength of the generated wave for a plane, longitudinal wave.

through transmission The process of imaging by transmitting the sound field through the specimen and picking up the transmitted energy on a far surface or a receiving transducer.

time gain compensation (tgc) An electronic amplification of increasing or decreasing returning amplitude information as the pulse travels in distance.

transducer Device that converts energy from one form to another.

transonic A region of material, such as a cyst, or a tissue that is relatively unattenuating.

ultrasound Sound of frequency greater than 20 kHz.

velocity Speed with direction of motion specified.

velocity of sound Speed with direction of motion specified.

watt per square centimeter (W/cm²) A unit of power density or intensity.

wave An acoustic wave is a mechanical disturbance that propagates through a medium.

SELECTED BIBLIOGRAPHY

Babcock DS and Han BK: Cranial ultrasonography of infants, Baltimore, 1981, Williams & Wilkins.

Callen PW: Ultrasonography in obstetrics and gynecology, Philadelphia, 1991, WB Saunders.

Cooperberg P et al: Advances in ultrasonography of the gallbladder and biliary tract, Radiol Clin North Am 20(4):611-633, 1982.

Hagen AD et al: Two-dimensional echocardiography: clinical-pathological correlations in adult and congenital heart disease, Boston, 1991, Little, Brown & Co.

Hagen-Ansert SL: Textbook of diagnostic ultrasonography, ed 4, St Louis, 1994, Mosby.

Hatle L and Angelsen B: Doppler ultrasound in cardiology: physical principles and clinical applications, Philadelphia, 1982, Lea & Febiger.

Holmes JH: Perspectives in ultrasonography: early diagnostic ultrasonography, J Ultrasound Med 2:33-43, 1983.

Lerski RA: Ultrasonic tissue characterization, Diagn Imaging 51(5):238-248, 1982.

McDicken WN: Diagnostic ultrasonics: principles and use of instruments, London, 1976, Granada Publishing.

Powis RL: Ultrasound physics for the fun of it, Denver, 1978, Unirad Corp.

Sanders RC and James AE: The principles and practice of ultrasonography in obstetrics and gynecology, New York, 1990, Appleton-Century-Crofts.

Sickles EA et al: Breast cancer detection with sonography and mammography: comparison using state-of-the-art equipment, AJR 140(5):843-845, 1983.

Zweibel WJ, editor: Introduction to vascular ultrasonography, New York, 1993, Grune & Stratton.

Definition of terms

Chapter 38

NUCLEAR MEDICINE

MEL ALLEN

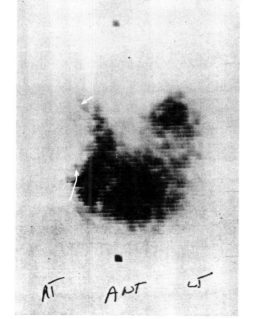

Abnormal thyroid rectilinear scanner image showing the medial border of a "cold spot" lesion *(arrows)*; early 1970s.

Introduction

The clinical application of *radioactive** materials used to diagnose and treat disease is known as nuclear medicine. Modern day nuclear medicine technology utilizes chemistry, physics, physiology, and computer science information to provide diagnostic images and radionuclide therapy for a variety of organ systems in the human body. Nuclear medicine began as a medical specialty area for diagnosis and treatment of disease in the late 1950s and early 1960s. However, long before that, in the early 1800s scientists such as John Dalton and Amedeo Avogadro were proposing theories on atomic and molecular structure that would serve as the basis for later research and eventually the discovery of radioactivity by A.H. Becquerel in 1896. This discovery lead to more research, and 2 years later a Nobel prize was awarded to Marie Curie, who identified the radioactive elements of polonium and radium.

Radioactive compounds were first used for medical application in the 1930s in the treatment of cancers in laboratory animals and humans. Through a slow evolution other radioactive compounds were eventually discovered and used to diagnose, as well as treat disease. Along with these new radioactive elements *(radionuclides)* came new devices capable of imaging these radionuclides and demonstrating their distribution inside the body. Through the use of chemistry these radioactive elements were attached, or tagged, to a variety of compounds which allowed them to be selectively taken up by a particular organ system in the human body. This lead to the rapid development of a large number of radionuclides targeted at different functions within the human body.

*Italicized terms are defined at the end of this chapter.

Today very complex imaging and computer systems are used with these different radioactive components, not only to image and treat diseases but also to provide functional and quantitative analysis of many body systems. Nuclear medicine has found a unique niche in the medical imaging field by virtue of its functional imaging capacity.

Other imaging modalities such as diagnostic x-ray, computed tomography (CT), interventional procedures, sonography, and magnetic resonance imaging (MRI) provide images of anatomy based primarily on structure, whereas nuclear medicine looks at anatomy based on physiology. This is accomplished by administering *radiopharmaceuticals* which are distributed in the body based on the physiology or function of the particular organ of interest. Nuclear medicine imaging makes it possible to look at function as well as structure inside the body.

Nuclear medicine is used to identify or diagnose and treat a wide range of abnormalities or disease processes including infections, inflammations, tumors, and infarctions, as well as a wide variety of functional/physiological changes within the human body including cardiac, renal, lung, and GI functions as well as blood flow and distribution in almost any organ system (see Appendix A at end of this chapter). These images and their quantitative results provide physicians with detailed information regarding the function of a particular organ. Although nuclear medicine images can be very specific regarding function, they may not provide the resolution seen in conventional radiography. Therefore, these two modalities are often used to complement each other to provide a complete picture of the patient's condition.

Physical Principles of Nuclear Medicine

To grasp the principles of nuclear medicine and how images are created using radioactive compounds, one must first understand "radioactivity." The term "radiation" is taken from the Latin word *radii,* referring to the spokes of a wheel leading out from a central point. The term "radioactivity" is used to describe the radiation of energy (in the form of particles or waves) from the nucleus of an atom.

BASIC NUCLEAR PHYSICS

The basic components of an atom include a *nucleus,* composed of varying numbers of *protons* and *neutrons,* and orbiting *electrons,* which revolve around the nucleus in discrete energy levels. Protons have a positive electric charge, electrons have a negative charge, and neutrons are electrically neutral. Both protons and neutrons have masses approximately 2000 times that of the electron. Therefore the nucleus composes most of the mass of an atom. This configuration can be described by the Bohr atomic model (Fig. 38-1). The total number of protons, neutrons, and electrons in an atom determine its characteristics.

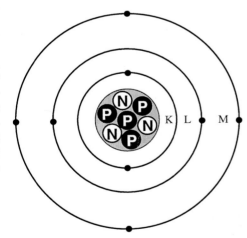

Fig. 38-1. Diagram of Bohr atom containing a single nucleus of protons and neutrons with surrounding orbital electrons of varying energy levels (K, L, M . . .).

The term *nuclide* is used to describe an atomic species with a particular arrangement of protons and neutrons in the nucleus. Elements with the same number of protons but a different number of neutrons are referred to as *isotopes*. Isotopes have the same chemical properties as one another since the total number of protons and electrons is the same. They simply differ in the total number of neutrons contained in the nucleus. The neutron-proton ratio in the nucleus determines if that atom is stable. When these ratios vary, atoms may become unstable, and a process known as spontaneous *decay* can occur as the atom attempts to regain stability. The nucleus of an atom has energy levels similar to those of orbital electrons. Energy is liberated in a variety of ways during this decay or return to ground state. Radionuclides decay by giving off emissions of alpha, beta, and gamma radiation. Most of these radionuclides reach ground state through a variety of decay processes including *alpha, beta, positron,* and electron capture, as well as several other methods. These decay methods are dependent on the type of particles or *gamma rays* used and given off in the decay process. To better explain this process, decay schemes have been created to show the details of how a "parent" nuclide decays to the *daughter* and/or ground state (Fig. 38-2, *A*). These decay schemes are unique for each radionuclide and identify the type of decay, the energy associated with each process, the probability of a particular decay process, and the *half-life* of each radionuclide.

Radioactive decay is considered to be a purely random and spontaneous process that can be mathematically defined by complex equations and represented by average decay rates. The term "half-life" ($T_{1/2}$) is used to describe the time it takes for a particular radionuclide to decay to one-half its original activity. This radioactive decay is a measure of the physical time it takes to reach one-half the original number of atoms in a given radionuclide through disintegration. The rate of decay has an exponential function, as demonstrated when plotted on a linear scale (Fig. 38-2, *B*). If plotted on a logarithmic scale, the decay rate would be represented as a straight line. Half-lives of radionuclides range from milliseconds to years. Most of the radionuclides used in nuclear medicine have half-lives that range from several hours to several days.

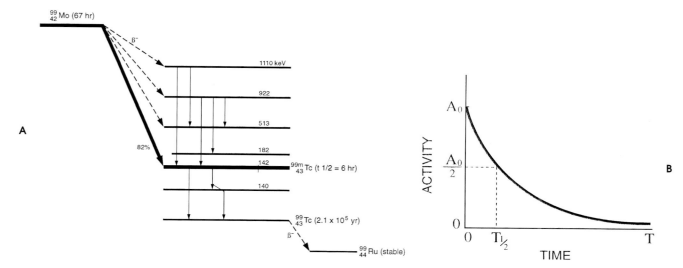

Fig. 38-2. A, Decay scheme illustrating the method by which radioactive molybdenum (Mo-99) decays to technetium (Tc^{99m}), one of the most commonly used radiopharmaceuticals in nuclear medicine. **B,** Graphic representation showing the rate of physical decay of a radionuclide. The y (vertical axis) represents the amount of radioactivity and the x (horizontal axis) represents time. The half-life ($T_{1/2}$) is referred to as the time at which a specific amount of acitivity has decreased to one half its initial value. Every radionuclide has an associated half-life which is representative of its rate of decay.

Nuclear Pharmacy

The radionuclides used in nuclear medicine are produced in *nuclear reactors* or particle accelerators *(cyclotrons)*. Naturally occurring radionuclides have very long half-lives, making them unsuitable for nuclear medicine imaging because of the high absorbed dose the patient would receive. To produce radionuclides in a cyclotron, nuclear reactions are created between a specific target chemical and high-speed charged particles. The number of protons in the target nuclei is changed when bombarded by the high-speed charged particles, and a new radiochemical is produced. Radionuclides can be produced in nuclear reactors by either inserting a target chemical into the reactor core or using spent fuel from the nuclear reactor.

The most commonly used radiopharmaceutical in nuclear medicine today is technetium (Tc^{99m}), which is produced from a radionuclide *generator* system. This generator system uses molybdenum-99 as the "parent." Molybdenum-99 can be the product of either U-235 fission in a nuclear reactor or neutron radiation of Mo-98 in a reactor. Molybdenum-99 has a half-life of 66.7 hours and decays (82%) to a daughter product known as metastable technetium (Tc^{99m}). Since technetium and molybdenum are chemically different, they can be easily separated through a radionuclide generator system. Technetium exhibits near ideal characteristics for use in nuclear medicine examinations, including a relatively short physical half-life of 6.04 hours and a high-yield (98.6%) 140 KeV gamma photon (Fig. 38-2, *A*).

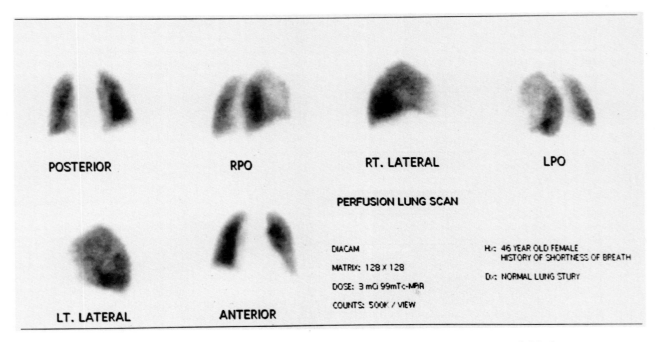

Fig. 38-3. Normal perfusion lung scan using 3 millicuries of Tc^{99m} – MAA on a large field of view gamma camera approximately five minutes post-injection.

(Courtesy Siemens Medical Systems).

Technetium can be bound to biologically active compounds or drugs to create a radiopharmaceutical which will localize in a particular organ system or structure when administered intravenously or orally. A commonly used radiopharmaceutical is technetium tagged or labeled with macro-aggregated albumin (MAA), which is distributed and trapped throughout the small capillaries in the lungs based on blood flow to the lungs (Fig. 38-3). Blood clots in the lungs will prevent this radiopharmaceutical from concentrating in the area beyond the clot, therefore showing a void or clear area when imaged. There are over 30 different radiopharmaceuticals used in nuclear medicine (Table 38-1).

Radiopharmaceutical doses vary, depending on the radionuclide used, the examination being performed, and the size of the patient. The measure of radioactivity can be stated as either the *becquerel (Bq)*, which corresponds to the decay rate of one disintegration per second, or the *curie (Ci)*, which equals 3.7×10^{10} disintegrations per second.

Table 38-1.

Radionuclide	Symbol	Physical half-life	Chemical form	Diagnostic use
Chromium	^{51}Cr	27.8 days	Sodium chromate	Red blood cell volume and survival
			Albumin	Gastrointestinal protein loss
Cobalt	^{57}Co	270 days	Cyanocobalamin (vitamin B_{12})	Vitamin B_{12} absorption
	^{58}Co	72 days	Cyanocobalamin	Vitamin B_{12} absorption
Gallium	^{67}Ga	77 days	Gallium citrate	Inflammatory process and tumor imaging
Indium	^{111}In	67.4 hours	Diethylenetriamine penta-acetic acid (DTPA)	Cerebrospinal fluid imaging
			Oxine	White blood cell/abscess imaging
Iodine	^{123}I	13.3 hours	Sodium iodide	Thyroid function and imaging
	^{125}I	60 days	Triiodothronine	Thyroid hormone assay
			Thyroxine	Thyroid hormone assay
			Other hormones or drugs	Radioassays
			Human serum albumin	Plasma volume
			Sodium iodide	Thyroid function, imaging, and therapy
			Hippurate	Renal function
Technetium	^{99m}Tc	6 hours	Sodium pertechnetate	Imaging of brain, thyroid, scrotum, salivary glands, renal perfusion, and pericardial effusion; evaluation of left-to-right cardiac shunts
			Sulfar colloid	Imaging of liver and spleen and renal transplants
			Human albumin microspheres	Lung imaging
			Isonitriles	Cardiovascular imaging, myocardial perfusion
			DTPA	Brain and renal imaging
			Dimethylsuccinic acid (DMSA)	Renal imaging
			Mercaptoacetylglycylglycylglycine(MAG3)	
			Diphosphonate	Bone imaging
			Pyrophosphate	Bone and myocardial imaging
			Red blood cells	Cardiac function imaging
			Hexamethylpropylene (HMPAO)	Functional brain imaging
			Iminodiacetic (IDA derivations)	Liver function imaging
Thallium	^{201}Tl	73.5 hours	Thallous chloride	Myocardiac imaging
Xenon	^{133}Xe	5.3 days	Xenon gas	Lung ventilation imaging

Radiation Safety in Nuclear Medicine

The radiation protection requirements in nuclear medicine are unique and different from general radiation safety measures used for diagnostic x-ray. Most of the radionuclides used in nuclear medicine are in either liquid or gaseous form. Because of the nature of radioactive decay, these liquids or gases continually emit radiation (unlike diagnostic x-rays which can be turned on and off mechanically) and therefore require special precautions.

When dealing with high concentrations or activities of radionuclides such as those used in a nuclear pharmacy to prepare doses, a designated preparation area must be utilized, including isolated ventilation, protective lead glass, protective lead shielding that includes vial and syringe shields, absorbent material, and gloves. For handling and administering diagnostic doses to patients, lead *syringe shields* and gloves should be utilized at all times (Fig. 38-4). Any radioactive material that is spilled will continue to emit radioactivity and therefore must be immediately contained and cleaned up. Radioactive contamination on the skin can be absorbed and may not be easily washed off. This is why it is very important to wear gloves when handling radiopharmaceuticals. Technologists and nuclear pharmacists should also wear appropriate radiation monitoring (dosimetry) devices such as *film badges* and *thermoluminescent dosimetry (TLD)* rings to monitor radiation exposure to the body and hands. If radiopharmaceuticals are handled inappropriately and an accident occurs, fingers and hands are likely to become contaminated.

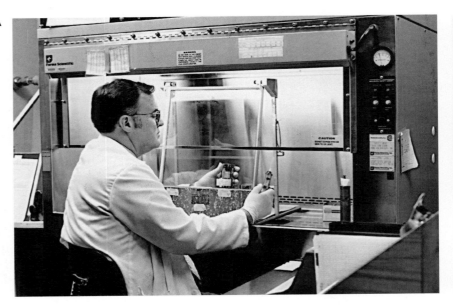
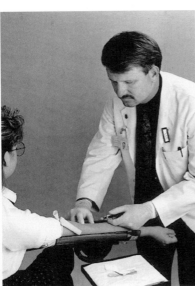

Fig. 38-4. A, Radiopharmacy dose area where radiopharmaceuticals are prepared in a clean and protected environment. **B,** Nuclear medicine technologist administering a radiopharmaceutical intravenously utilizing appropriate radiation safety precautions including gloves and a syringe shield.

Instrumentation

RADIOACTIVE DETECTORS
Gas-Filled Detectors

In order for radioactivity to be detected, it must first interact with matter. When radioactivity strikes matter, as with gas molecules inside a gas-filled detector, the gas ionizes and creates a voltage potential between two electrodes. This voltage potential is then used as a measure of the radioactivity present.

Two common gas-filled detectors used in nuclear medicine are:

1. *Geiger-Mueller Survey Meter* (Geiger Counter)
2. *Dose Calibrator:* an ionization chamber used to measure the amount of radioactivity in a sample (syringe, vial, test tube, etc.)

These devices are used to detect and estimate the amount of radioactivity present (Fig. 38-5).

Scintillation Detectors

The term "scintillate" means to emit light photons. A.H. Becquerel discovered that ionizing radiation caused certain materials to scintillate. *Scintillation* is a product of excitation produced by radiation interacting with a molecule or crystal rather than ionization as seen in *gas detectors*. Devices have been created to capture, detect, and count/display these scintillations.

Scintillation detectors were used in the development of the first-generation nuclear medicine scanner—the *rectilinear scanner* built in 1950. This was a moving detector and image-producing system that traveled in a horizontal manner across the area of interest, incremented vertically, and repeated the process. This system was able not only to detect radioactivity but also to create an image based on the distribution of the radioactive tracer in the structure of interest.

A

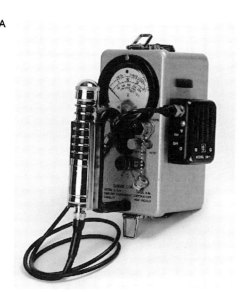

B

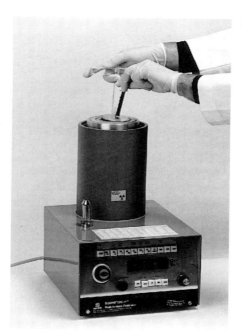

Fig. 38-5. A, GM-Survey Meter used to detect and determine the relative amount of radioactivity present. **B,** Dose calibrator used to determine the amount of radioactivity in syringes or vials.

The Modern-Day Gamma Camera

Rectilinear scanners have evolved into very complex imaging systems known today as gamma cameras (because they detect gamma rays). These cameras are still scintillation detectors that use a very large sodium iodide crystal (NaI) to detect and transform specific radioactive emissions into light photons. Through a very complex process these light photons are amplified and their location electronically recorded to produce an image.

Gamma cameras may be either stationary or mobile. Mobile gamma cameras are used to perform bedside studies on critically ill patients who cannot be transported to the nuclear medicine department. Mobile gamma cameras typically have limitations, including a smaller field of view and less detector shielding, limiting the types of examinations that can be performed.

Basic Components and Structure of a Gamma Camera: The gamma camera is made up of many components that work together to produce an image (Fig. 38-6). Located at the face of the detector where radioactive photons first enter the camera is what is referred to as a *collimator.* Collimators are used to limit the field of view in order to increase resolution and vary sensitivity by limiting the number and direction of photons entering the detector. These "exchangeable" collimators are usually made of material with a high atomic number, such as lead. Different collimators are used for different types of examinations in order to gain the best combination of sensitivity and resolution.

Crystal: Scintillation crystals commonly used in gamma cameras are made of sodium iodide (NaI) with trace quantities of thallium (Tl) added. This crystal configuration is effective in stopping most common gamma rays emitted from the radiopharmaceuticals used in nuclear medicine. The thickness of the crystal may vary from 1/4 to 1/2 inch. Thicker crystals are better for imaging radiopharmaceuticals with higher energies (over 180 KeV) but have decreased resolution, whereas thinner crystals provide improved resolution but cannot efficiently image higher KeV photons. A light pipe may also be used to attach the crystal to the *photomultiplier tubes (PMT)*. This light pipe helps direct photons.

Detector Electronics: Attached to the crystal or light pipe inside the detector are photomultiplier tubes. These devices are used to detect and convert light photons emitted from the crystal. Once the PMTs have detected the light emission from the crystal, they convert this light into an electronic signal and multiply or amplify the electronic signal by a factor of as much as 10^7. A typical gamma camera detector head may contain as many as 80 to 100 PMTs.

The PMTs then send the detected signal through a series of processing steps. These steps include determining location (x, y) and amplitude or energy (z). The x and y values are determined by where the photon strikes the crystal. Electronic circuitry known as *pulse height analysis* is used to discriminate those z signals that are not within a desired preset energy range for a particular radionuclide. This helps eliminate scatter and other unwanted photons that would generally degrade resolution.

Once this information is processed, these signals are transmitted to the display system, which includes a *cathode ray tube (CRT)* and a film imaging system or computer to record the image.

Multihead Gamma Camera Systems

Gamma camera systems may include as many as three detectors (heads). The standard gamma camera is a single detector that can be moved in a variety of positions around the patient. There are also dual-head gamma camera systems which allow for the simultaneous imaging of anterior and posterior views. Dual-head systems may be used for whole body bone or tumor imaging.

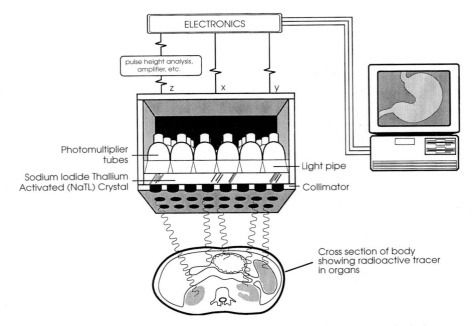

ELECTRONICS

pulse height analysis, amplifier, etc.

z   x   y

Photomultiplier tubes

Sodium Iodide Thallium Activated (NaTL) Crystal

Light pipe

Collimator

Cross section of body showing radioactive tracer in organs

Fig. 38-6. Basic schematic of a typical gamma camera system. This system includes complex computers and electronic mechanical components for acquiring, processing, displaying, and analyzing nuclear medicine images.

SPECT

Single photon emission computed tomography (SPECT) may utilize from one to three gamma camera detectors to produce tomographic or sectional images of a structure (Fig. 38-7). These systems are designed to allow the detector heads to rotate around the body while collecting data. The detector(s) may rotate as much as 360 degrees around the patient. This tomographic data is reconstructed in a computer in any number of formats including transaxial, sagittal, coronal, planar, or 3-D representations. These computer-generated images allow for the display of thin slices through different planes of an organ or structure. This display helps identify small abnormalities in different planes.

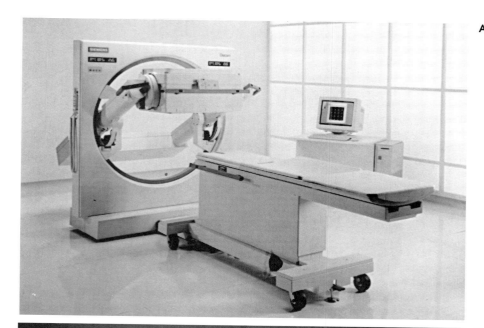

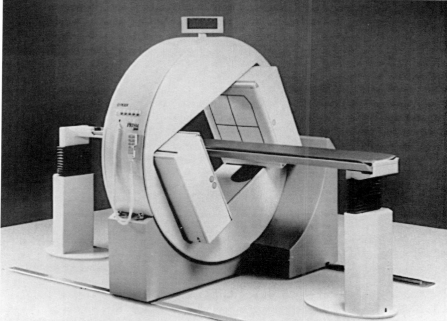

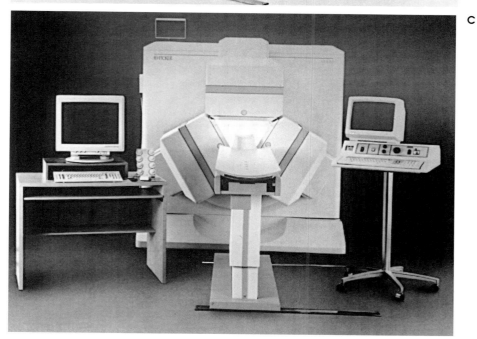

Fig. 38-7. Example of single photon emission computed tomography (SPECT) camera systems ranging from **(A)** single- to **(B)** dual- to **(C)** triple-headed systems.

(Courtesy Picker and Siemens Medical Systems.)

A common example of a SPECT study is the myocardial perfusion study used to identify perfusion defects in the left ventricular wall. The patient is injected intravenously with a radiopharmaceutical while exercising, usually on a treadmill. The radiopharmaceutical will distribute in the heart muscle in the same fashion as blood flows to heart muscle. An initial set of images is made after injection of the radiopharmaceutical toward the end of exercise. A second set of images is taken several hours later when the patient is rested to determine if any blood perfusion defects seen on the initial images have resolved. By comparing these images the physician may be able to tell if the patient has damaged heart tissue due to a myocardial infarction or myocardial ischemia (Fig. 38-8).

COMPUTERS

Computers have become an integral part of the nuclear medicine imaging system. Computer systems are used to acquire and process data from gamma cameras. They allow for the collection of data over a specific time frame; the data can then be analyzed to determine functional change over time (Fig. 38-9, *A* and *B*). A common example of this is the functional renal study where the radiopharmaceutical administered is cleared by normal functioning kidneys in about 20 minutes. The computer can collect images of the kidney over a 40-minute time frame and analyze these images to determine how quickly the kidneys clear the radiopharmaceutical (Fig. 38-9, *C*). The computer also allows the user to interactively manipulate the image to enhance a particular structure by adjusting the contrast and brightness of the image.

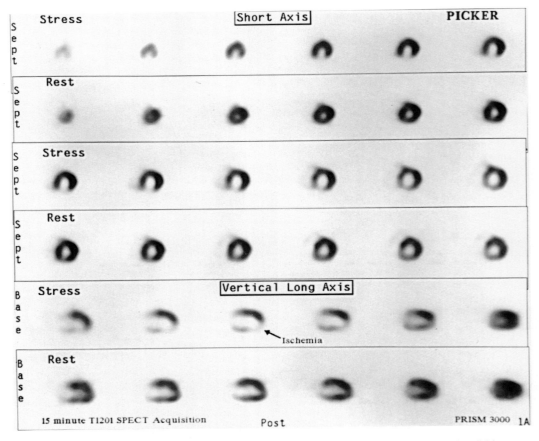

Fig. 38-8. Myocardial perfusion study using thallium 201. Comparison of stress and redistribution (resting) images in various planes of the heart (short axis and long axis). A perfusion defect is identified in the stress images but not seen on the redistribution (rest) images, indicating an ischemia.

(Courtesy Siemens Medical Systems.)

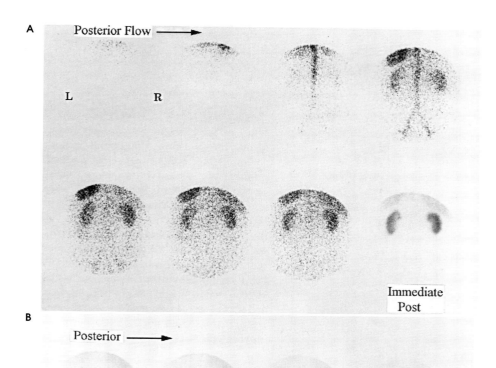

A

Posterior Flow ⟶

L   R

Immediate
Post

B

Posterior ⟶

L   R

Fig. 38-9. A, Posterior renal blood flow in an adult patient using 10 millicuries of Tc^{99m} – DTPA imaged at 3 seconds per frame. The image in the lower right corner is a blood pool image taken immediately following the initial flow sequence. These images demonstrate normal renal blood flow to both kidneys. **B,** The same patient undergoing a renal function study utilizing 5 millicuries of Tc^{99m} – mag 3. These images are taken for 5 minutes each for a total of 40 minutes. These images demonstrate delayed clearance by the left kidney. **C,** Graphical representation of the right and left kidney function taken from the mag 3 study. These curves show a normal functioning right kidney and delayed uptake and clearance in the left kidney.

C

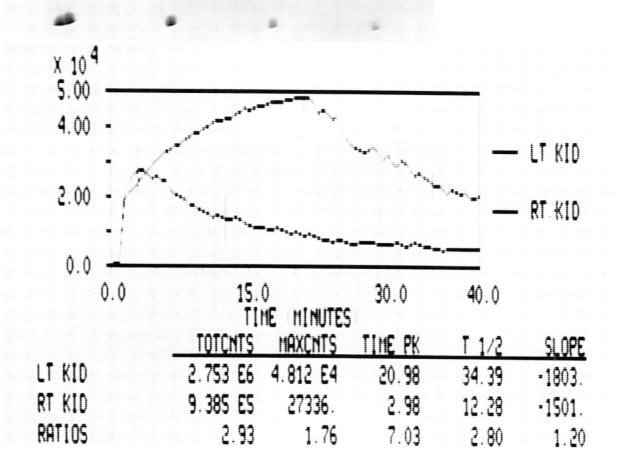

X 10^4

5.00

4.00

2.00

0.0

0.0   15.0   30.0   40.0

TIME (MINUTES)

— LT KID

— RT KID

	TOTCNTS	MAXCNTS	TIME PK	T 1/2	SLOPE
LT KID	2.753 E6	4.812 E4	20.98	34.39	-1803.
RT KID	9.385 E5	27336.	2.98	12.28	-1501.
RATIOS	2.93	1.76	7.03	2.80	1.20

Computers are necessary to acquire and process SPECT images. SPECT studies are complex, requiring a great deal of computer processing to create images in a transaxial, sagittal, or coronal plane similar to that of CT and MRI. Three-dimensional images can also be generated from SPECT data (Fig. 38-10).

QUANTITATIVE ANALYSIS

Many of the procedures being performed in nuclear medicine departments require some form of quantitative analysis, which provides physicians with numeric results based on function. Specialized software allows nuclear medicine computers to collect, process, and analyze functional information obtained from nuclear medicine imaging systems. Cardiac ejection fractions are one of the more common quantitative results provided from nuclear medicine procedures (Fig. 38-11). This study is a dynamic acquisition of the heart contracting and expanding in which the computer quantitatively determines the "ejection fraction" or amount of blood pumped out of the left ventricle with each contraction.

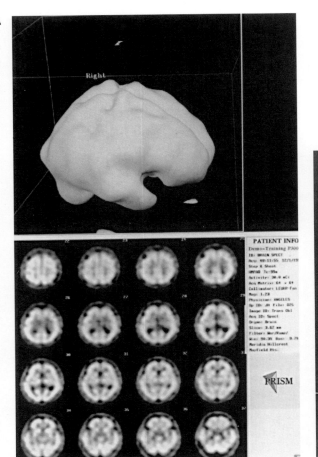

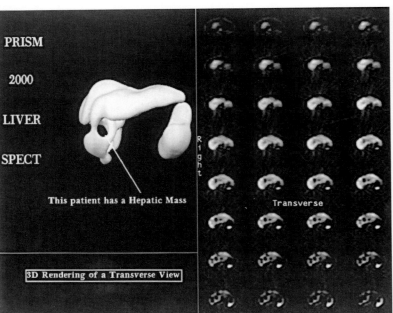

Fig. 38-10. A, Three-dimensional SPECT brain study using 30 mCi of Tc^{99m} HMPAO. Three-dimensional representation of a normal brain with transaxial slices shown below. **B,** Three-dimensional SPECT liver study using 8 mCi of Tc^{99m} Sulfar Colloid. Hepatic mass is seen on both the 3D and transaxial images.

(Courtesy Picker International.)

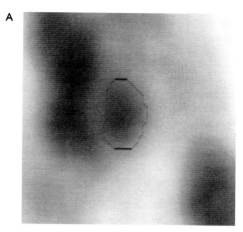

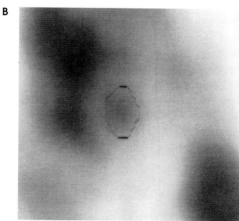

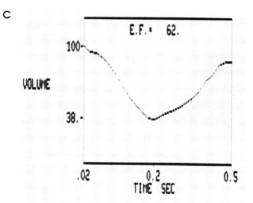

Clinical Nuclear Medicine

Nuclear medicine procedures are generally divided into three basic categories: *in vivo, in vitro/radioimmunoassay (RIA),* and radionuclide therapy procedures.

IN VIVO PROCEDURES

The term *in vivo* is defined as "within the living body." This category includes all diagnostic nuclear medicine imaging procedures. Since diagnostic imaging procedures are based on the distribution of radiopharmaceuticals "within the body," they are classified as in vivo examinations.

There are a wide variety of in vivo/diagnostic imaging examinations performed in nuclear medicine. These examinations can be described based on the imaging method used: *static,* whole body *dynamic,* SPECT, and positron emission tomography (PET) (see Chapter 39).

Static Imaging

Static nuclear medicine images are obtained by acquiring a single image of a particular structure. This could be thought of as a "snapshot" of the radiopharmaceutical distribution within the body. Examples of this include lung scans, "spot" bone scan images, and thyroid images. Static images are usually obtained in a variety of orientations, or "views," around a particular structure in order to demonstrate all aspects of that structure. Anterior, posterior, and oblique views are often obtained. In order to minimize the radiation exposure to patients, low radiopharmaceutical activity levels are used. Because of these low activity levels, images must be acquired for a preset time or number of counts or radioactive emissions. This may vary from a few seconds to several minutes or from 100,000 counts to over 1 million counts. Generally, static images require from 30 seconds to 5 minutes in order to obtain a sufficient number of emissions to produce a satisfactory image.

Fig. 38-11. A, Cardiac-gated study showing heart wall motion as well as quantitative results including cardiac ejection fraction. This is a left anterior oblique (LAO) image of the left ventricle at end-diastole (relaxed phase) with a region of interest drawn around the left ventricle. **B,** Same LAO image showing end-systole (contracted phase). **C,** A curve representing the volume change in the left ventricle of the heart prior to, during, and after contraction. This volume change is referred to as the ejection fraction (EF), with a normal value being approximately 64% ± 10%.

Whole Body Imaging

Whole body imaging utilizes a specially designed gamma camera system to produce an image of the entire body or a large section of the body. This imaging is performed by having the gamma camera collect data while it moves over the body. Over the past several years the detector width for whole body systems has been increased to allow for a single pass from head to foot or from foot to head encompassing the entire body from side to side. These systems may also include dual heads for simultaneous anterior and posterior imaging. Previous detector systems were smaller and required as many as two or three incremental passes over the body in order to encompass the entire width of the body. Whole body imaging systems are utilized primarily for whole body bone scans, whole body tumor or abscess imaging, and many other clinical and research applications (Fig. 38-12).

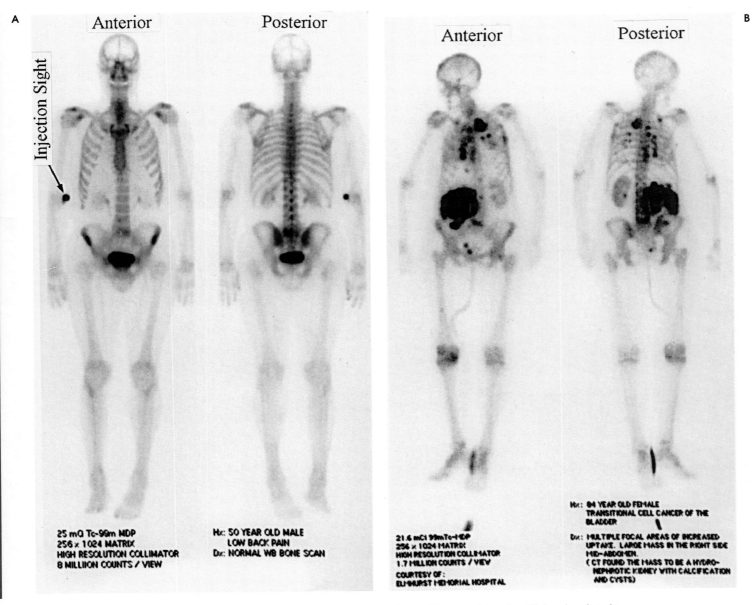

A

Anterior   Posterior

Injection Sight

25 mQ Tc-99m MDP
256 x 1024 MATRIX
HIGH RESOLUTION COLLIMATOR
8 MILLIION COUNTS / VIEW

Hx: 50 YEAR OLD MALE
LOW BACK PAIN
Dx: NORMAL WB BONE SCAN

B

Anterior   Posterior

21.6 mCi 99mTc-MDP
256 x 1024 MATRIX
HIGH RESOLUTION COLLIMATOR
1.7 MILLION COUNTS / VIEW
COURTESY OF:
ELMHURST MEMORIAL HOSPITAL

Hx: 84 YEAR OLD FEMALE
TRANSITIONAL CELL CANCER OF THE
BLADDER
Dx: MULTIPLE FOCAL AREAS OF INCREASED
UPTAKE. LARGE MASS IN THE RIGHT SIDE
MID-ABDOMEN.
(CT FOUND THE MASS TO BE A HYDRO-
NEPHROTIC KIDNEY WITH CALCIFICATION
AND CYSTS)

Fig. 38-12. A, Whole body bone scan perfomed on a 50-year-old male with low back pain using 25 millicuries of Tc⁹⁹ᵐMDP. The study was normal; however, note the injection site in the right antecubital fossa. **B,** Bone scan on an 84-year-old female with cancer of the bladder showing multiple focal areas of increased uptake, which represent abnormalities.

(Courtesy Siemens Medical Systems.)

Dynamic Imaging

Dynamic images represent the distribution of a particular radiopharmaceutical over a specific time period. A dynamic or "flow" study of a particular structure is generally used to evaluate the blood flow to that structure. This can be thought of as a sequential or time-lapse image. Images may be acquired and displayed in time sequences as short as one tenth of a second to longer than 10 minutes in each image. Two common examples of dynamic imaging are brain flow studies (Fig. 38-13) and renal flow studies (see Fig. 38-9).

Single Photon Emission Computed Tomography Imaging

Single photon emission computed tomography (SPECT) imaging produces images similar to CT or MR images in that thin slices through a particular organ are created by a computer and displayed as transaxial, sagittal, or coronal slices. This imaging technique has proven very beneficial in delineating small lesions within a structure and can be used on virtually any structure or organ. The most common SPECT studies include cardiac perfusion, brain imaging, liver imaging (see Fig. 38-10, B), and bone imaging.

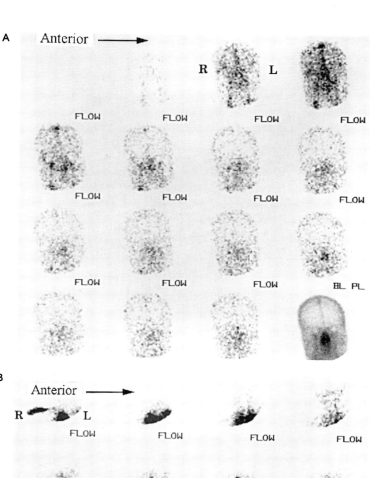

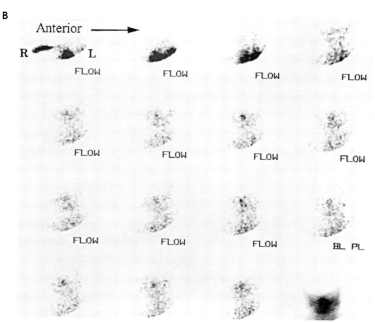

Fig. 38-13. A, Normal portable cerebral brain flow study performed using 30 millicuries of Tc^{99m} – DTPA injected as a bolus. **B,** Abnormal portable brain flow study in a patient demonstrating little or no blood flow activity in the brain, indicating brain death.

Positron Emission Tomography Imaging

Positron emission tomography (PET) imaging utilizes positron emissions from selected radionuclides to produce very detailed functional images within the body. A positron emitter releases two identical photons at 180 degrees (opposite directions), which can be detected and imaged by two opposing detectors. These photons are extremely high energy (511 KeV) and require special imaging detectors. The positron radiopharmaceuticals generally have a very short half-life of anywhere from a few seconds to a few minutes. Therefore these radiopharmaceuticals must be produced in a cyclotron convenient to the imaging facility or through a specially designed generator system. One of the more common PET procedures is the use of fluorodexyglucose (FDG) to measure glucose metabolism in the brain (Fig. 38-14).

IN VIVO NONIMAGING

In vivo procedures usually involve the labeling of a particular target substance, such as red blood cells, with a radioactive tracer. These labeled biological products are readministered to the patient, allowing them to be normally distributed or metabolized. A representative sample is then taken for analysis. Sodium iodide counters are used to determine the amount of radioactivity present in these samples. No diagnostic images are produced from these examinations, only quantitative results. Examples of these would include blood volume determination by radioactive labeling, B_{12} absorption, and red blood cell survival time.

IN VITRO PROCEDURES

In vitro is defined as "within a glass; observable in a test tube; in an artificial environment." This category is used to describe those nuclear medicine examinations that require an evaluation or analysis of radioactive samples taken from the human body. Results from these examinations are usually a specific quantitative value rather than a diagnostic image.

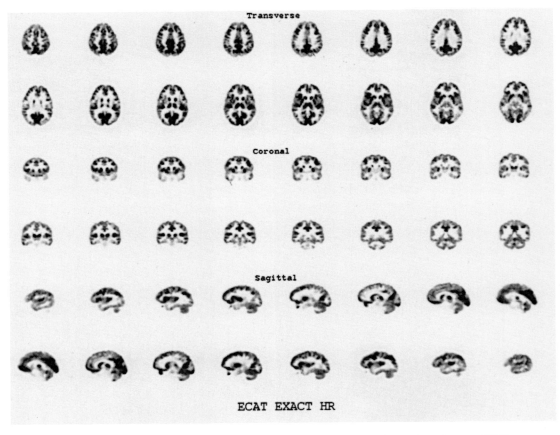

Fig. 38-14. Positron emission tomography (PET) brain study using fluorodexyglucose (FDG) to measure metabolic changes in the brain.

Radioimmunoassay

Radioimmunoassay (RIA) procedures are performed on body samples such as whole blood, serum, spinal fluid, and urine. Specific target structures or *ligands,* such as antibodies or metabolically active drugs, are labeled with a radioactive tracer to determine their levels. Examples of radioimmunoassays include thyroid hormone values (T3—Triiodothyronine, T4—thyroxine, or TSH—thyroid stimulating hormone), drug levels (digoxin, digitoxin, methyltrexate, theophylline, aminophylin, cyclosporin), and vitamins (vitamin B_{12}, folic acid). Levels of these particular hormones, drugs, and vitamins are determined by counting these labeled samples in a specialized scintillation counter. These assays are very sensitive and specific and are used to determine minute levels ($\mu G/dl$) of a wide range of ligands.

THERAPEUTIC NUCLEAR MEDICINE

Radionuclides are also utilized to treat specific diseases and cancers in the body. These radioactive compounds are administered, taken up, and distributed within a particular tumor, thereby providing continuous radiation to that structure. Radionuclide therapy includes treatment of thyroid diseases and cancers with radioactive iodine-131; in addition, radioactive phosphorus, including chromic phosphate and sodium phosphate (P32), is used to treat ovarian carcinoma and polycythemia vera. Radiopharmaceuticals such as Strontium-89 (Sr^{89}) are also being used to provide palliative therapy for patients with widespread bone cancer.

Summary

The field of nuclear medicine provides a diagnostic and therapeutic tool that continues to expand into new areas with the help of new radiopharmaceuticals and advancements in imaging technology. New areas of development for nuclear medicine include *monoclonal-antibody imaging,* which involves the attachment of radionuclides to specific monoclonal-antibodies in order to demonstrate or identify particular tumors within the body. This particular technique offers great potential in pinpointing specific tumors such as colon and ovarian forms. Also continuing to expand is the area of functional analysis, which utilizes computer information to produce quantitative results. This would include results from functional analyses of the heart, brain, and GI/biliary system, to name a few.

Developments in imaging and computer equipment utilized in nuclear medicine continue to improve the resolution of images and decrease the imaging time needed. Multihead camera systems can collect and analyze data two to three times faster than the previous single-head camera systems. These imaging systems allow for greater flexibility of image acquisition and processing, including the generation of three-dimensional images of a particular structure.

The future of nuclear medicine may lie in its unique ability to identify functional or physiological abnormalities. Other modalities are just beginning to develop techniques for assessing physiology or function. With continued development in new radiopharmaceuticals and imaging technology, nuclear medicine will continue to be a unique and valuable tool for diagnosing and treating disease.

Summary

The following is a summary of the major nuclear medicine procedures. The physiological principle of each study as well as the most common radiopharmaceutical(s) and standard adult dose are given for each procedure, followed by the procedure's indications and limitations. Finally, some complementary procedures are listed. The word "tracer" will be used in reference to the specific radiopharmaceutical by which the physiological or pathophysiological localization process occurs.

Endocrine System

THYROID UPTAKE

Principle. Thyroid function is proportional to its uptake of iodine, which is a substrate for thyroid hormones.

Radiopharmaceutical. Oral sodium iodide; ^{131}I (0.01 mCi).

Indications. Assessment of overall function of the thyroid, primarily hyperthyroidism; useful in metabolic errors of the thyroid, thyroiditis, and some cases of hypothyroidism; necessary for ^{131}I therapy.

Limitations. Inaccurate if body iodide pool is expanded (often due to radiographic contrast media) or if thyroid function is pharmacologically blocked, except to determine the effectiveness of the block.

Complementary procedures. Thyroid hormonal serum assays should be used to determine thyroid functional status.

Examination time. Two visits required 24 hours apart; first day, 30 minutes; second day, 1 hour.

THYROID IMAGING

Principle. See thyroid uptake; if part of the gland is functioning abnormally, the amount of tracer will be different in this part of the gland. Pertechnetate is concentrated but not fixed in the thyroid.

Radiopharmaceutical. ^{99m}TcO$_4$—(pertechnetate) (10.0 mCi) IV.

Indications. Assessment of the functional status of nodules, the size of the thyroid gland, or the presence and location of aberrant functioning thyroid tissue (metastatic thyroid carcinoma).

Limitations. Cannot distinguish between cyst, nonfunctioning tumor, etc.

Complementary procedures. Ultrasound will determine if nodule is solid or cystic.

Examination time. 1 hour.

THYROID METASTATIC IMAGING

Principle. Metastatic thyroid lesions will concentrate orally administered Iodine (I-131) just as normally functioning thyroid tissue will.

Radiopharmaceutical. Orally administered ^{131}I (10 mCi) or post-therapy.

Indications. Assessment and follow-up of patients with known thyroid cancer; useful in determining extent or recovery of metastatic thyroid disease.

Limitations. See thyroid uptake; usually not effective for functioning metastatic thyroid carcinoma when nonmetastatic thyroid tissue (thyroid gland) is present.

Complementary procedures. None.

Examination time. Examination begins 48 hours post-administration or approximately 1 week post-therapy and requires about 1.5 hours to scan.

SUPRARENAL (ADRENAL) CORTICAL IMAGING

Principle. Suprarenal (adrenal) cortical function is proportional to its uptake of cholesterol, which is its hormonal substrate.

Radiopharmaceutical. ^{131}I labeled 6-iodomethyl 19-norcholesterol (2 mCi) IV.

Indications. Localization of hyperplasia or tumor of the suprarenal (adrenal) cortex.

Limitations. Not particularly useful for diagnosis of hyperfunctioning suprarenal (adrenal) cortex; usually used in conjunction with suprarenal (adrenal) cortical suppression; need to block thyroid with iodide.

Complementary procedures. CT, MRI, ultrasound or arteriography, and venography for assessing enlargement or tumor of the suprarenal (adrenal) cortex.

Examination time. Examination begins 48 hours after administration of radiopharmaceutical and continues daily for 5 to 6 days.

Examination time. 1 hour.

PARATHYROID IMAGING

Principle. Active glandular tissue in the neck (parathyroid and thyroid) is imaged with ^{201}Tl, an intracellular tracer. The competing and interfering thyroid image is removed by subtracting a pertechnetate image.

Radiopharmaceutical. ^{201}TlCl (1.0 mCi) and later ^{99m}Tc4—(1.0 mCi) IV.

Indications. Preoperative localization of a parathyroid adenoma; should be used only when the diagnosis is reasonably established by other means.

Limitations. Will not image normal parathyroids or adenomas less than 0.5 g; cannot be used after contrast procedures or in the presence of iodide suppression of thyroid uptake.

Complementary procedures. Ultrasound, CT, arteriography of the neck, and direct neck vein parathyroid hormone sampling.

Examination time. 1 hour.

Nuclear medicine

Central Nervous System

CAROTID AND CEREBRAL BLOOD FLOW

Principle. An intravenous bolus of tracer will follow the flow of blood in major arteries.

Radiopharmaceutical. ^{99m}Tc compounds, usually ^{99m}Tc DTPA (30.0 mCi) or ^{99m}Tc Glucoheptonate (30.0 mCi) IV.

Indications. Internal carotid artery insufficiency, middle cerebral artery vascular accident, intracranial A-V malformation, early subdural hematoma or cerebral death, "stroke syndrome," suspected encephalitis (herpes simplex), or brain abscess.

Limitations. Not usually useful for TIA; may be false negative for cerebral death but no known false positives.

Complementary procedures. Arteriography, MRI, or CT may show results of vascular disease; Doppler ultrasound may be useful for carotid flow and subdural hematoma; EEG for cerebral death.

Examination time. 45 minutes.

BRAIN IMAGING

Principle. An intact blood brain barrier excludes tracer from diffusing into cerebral tissue. Ischemia, tumor, etc., destroys the integrity of the blood brain barrier, so tracer can diffuse into area and will appear as a "hot" area on delayed static images.

Radiopharmaceutical. ^{99m}Tc compounds, usually ^{99m}Tc DTPA (30.0 mCi) or ^{99m}Tc HMPAO (20.0 mCi) IV.

Indications. Cerebral vascular accident, primary or metastatic tumor, cerebral infection and inflammation (H.S.V.), or subdural hematoma; sometimes will show abnormality when CT does not.

Limitations. In general, not as sensitive or specific as CT; may not distinguish between tumor, infarction, abscess, etc.; not useful for acute subdural hematomas (7 to 10 days post-trauma).

Complementary procedures. CT or MRI usually has better sensitivity and specificity and better anatomical definition.

Examination time. Examination begins 1.5 hours after injection and requires 1 hour.

CEREBRAL SPINAL FLUID IMAGING

Principle. The tracer will follow the flow of the CSF.

Radiopharmaceutical. ^{111}In DTPA. Administered via lumbar puncture.

Indications. Low pressure hydrocephalus, CSF leak, or shunt malfunction.

Limitations. Tracer must be introduced by experienced person, since multiple or poor dural puncture will result in extravasation of tracer at site of puncture and the tracer will not follow the CSF flow.

Complementary procedures. CT or MRI will show size of ventricles but not flow and rate of absorption of CSF.

Examination time. Examination begins 24 to 48 hours post-injection and requires 1 hour to scan.

Respiratory System

LUNG PERFUSION

Principle. A particulate tracer, if injected into the venous circulation, will be stopped by the precapillary arterioles and capillaries in the lung. The particles will be well mixed with the blood before reaching the lungs and will therefore be distributed in the lungs in proportion to the regional blood flow.

Radiopharmaceutical. ^{99m}Tc macro aggregated albumin (MAA) (3.0 mCi) IV.

Indications. Suspected pulmonary embolism or thrombosis or evaluation of regional pulmonary function and regional pulmonary blood flow.

Limitations. Will not distinguish between perfusion defect due to pulmonary embolism and that due to poor ventilation (see lung ventilation below) or other vascular disease. Severe COPD or pulmonary vascular disease generally limits diagnostic specificity.

Complementary procedures. Lung ventilation and pulmonary angiography.

Examination time. 30 to 45 minutes.

LUNG VENTILATION

Principle. A tracer gas or aerosol will be distributed in the lungs in proportion to the regional ventilation.

Radiopharmaceutical. ^{133}Xe (10 mCi) or ^{127}Xe (3 mCi) (gas); Aerosolized ^{99m}Tc DTPA (40 mCi); ^{81}Kr (10 to 20 mCi).

Indications. Evaluation of ventilation in region(s) of decreased perfusion for lung perfusion is better for evaluating overall regional pulmonary function.

Limitations. Small areas of ventilation/perfusion (V/Q) match or mismatch usually cannot be detected, especially in the presence of marked COPD.

Complementary procedures. None.

Examination time. 30 to 45 minutes.

Respiratory system

Cardiovascular System
MYOCARDIAL PERFUSION

Principle. The tracer (thallium) is a potassium analog and thus concentrates intracellularly in metabolically active myocardium in proportion to the blood flow to the muscle. ^{99m}Tc Isonitrile derivatives are also used and function similar to thallium. Usually performed in conjunction with a stress treadmill study.

Radiopharmaceutical. ^{201}Tl (4.0 mCi) IV or ^{99m}Tc Isonitrile (30 mCi) IV.

Indications. To assess extent of ischemic or infarcted myocardial tissue and differentiate between the two processes.

Limitations. Adequate stress is required of the patient in order to differentiate between ischemia and infarction.

Complementary procedures. Coronary arteriography (much more invasive).

Examination time. There is a 3-hour delay between the stress and redistribution scans, each requiring 1 hour.

ACUTE MYOCARDIAL INFARCT

Principle. Tracer is a calcium analog and concentrates in areas of acute infarction.

Radiopharmaceutical. ^{99m}Tc pyrophosphate (20 mCi) IV.

Indications. Most tissue infarctions including but not limited to myocardial, cerebral, and muscle.

Limitations. Accurate only 1 to 10 days post-infarction.

Complementary procedures. EKG and real-time sonography.

Examination time. Examination begins 3 to 4 hours post-injection and requires 1 hour.

GATED CARDIAC BLOOD POOL

Principle. The tracer is labeled to red blood cells and equilibrates with the blood pool. As the RBC-labeled tracer is pumped in and out of the cardiac chambers, computerized images are recorded of the cardiac cycle.

Radiopharmaceutical. ^{99m}Tc-labeled RBCs (30.0 mCi) 1 ml PYP (cold) IV.

Indications. General overall assessment of cardiac function (ejection fraction and wall motion); useful in following patients receiving cardiotoxic drugs (chemotherapeutic).

Limitations. Cardiac arrhythmias such as uncontrolled atrial fibrillation may compromise the results.

Complementary procedures. Exercise cardiac gated blood pool. First pass study to assess right ventricle function, left ventricle cine angiography.

Examination time. 1 to 1.5 hours.

ARTERIAL/VENOUS IMAGING

Principle. Intravascular blood pool tracer will show patency and distribution of major arteries and veins.

Radiopharmaceutical. ^{99m}Tc labeled homologous red cells or ^{99m}Tc human serum albumin (30 mCi) IV.

Indications. Major vascular occlusion.

Limitations. Useful only for major central or peripheral vessels.

Complementary procedures. Ultrasound, digital subtraction angiography, MRI, and CT.

Examination time. 1 hour.

Gastrointestinal System
SALIVARY GLAND FUNCTION

Principle. Tracer is concentrated by salivary glands and secreted following administration of a secretagogue.

Radiopharmaceutical. ^{99m}TcO$_4$- (5.0 mCi) IV.

Indications. Salivary gland malfunction (Sjogren's syndrome, radiation obstruction); Warthin's tumor (concentrates tracer; other masses show as a cold defect in the gland).

Limitations. None.

Complementary procedures. Sialography.

Examination time. 1 hour.

ESOPHAGEAL REFLUX

Principle. Tracer put into stomach can be detected in esophagus during reflux or in lung if aspirated.

Radiopharmaceutical. ^{99m}Tc Sulfur Colloid (0.5 mCi) orally.

Indications. Suspected esophageal reflux; nocturnal reflux and aspiration (tracer detected in lungs).

Limitations. None.

Complementary procedures. X-ray barium contrast study and prolonged esophageal pH probe monitoring.

Examination time. 1 hour.

GASTRIC EMPTYING

Principle. Retention of tracer put into stomach can be quantitated.

Radiopharmaceutical. ^{99m}Tc Sulfur Colloid (0.3 mCi) with semisolid test analog orally.

Indications. Gastric obstruction or decreased stomach motility.

Limitations. Not valid if vomiting occurs.

Complementary procedures. Upper GI.

Examination time. 1 hour.

MECKEL'S DIVERTICULUM

Principle. Bleeding Meckel's contains gastric mucosa which can be detected by tracer that concentrates in gastric mucosa.

Radiopharmaceutical. $^{99m}TcO_4-$ (10 mCi) IV.

Indications. Unexplained GI bleeding, particularly in a child.

Limitations. Meckel's may be missed if diverticulum is adjacent to bladder, ureteral diverticulum may be false positive.

Complementary procedures. Small bowel barium studies less sensitive.

Examination time. 1 hour with possible delay images.

GASTROINTESTINAL BLEEDING

Principle. Nondiffusible tracer injected into blood pool will localize at site of extravasation.

Radiopharmaceutical. ^{99m}Tc red blood cells (30 mCi) IV.

Indications. Acute GI bleeding after excluding sites in or above duodenum and in or below sigmoid.

Limitations. Must be actively bleeding (0.1 ml/minute) during study; anatomical bleeding site only approximated. Poor tracer label may invalidate procedure.

Complementary procedures. Upper and/or lower endoscopic examination when possible.

Examination time. 1 hour with possible delay images.

LIVER/SPLEEN IMAGING

Principle. Reticuloendothelial cells in liver and spleen remove tracer colloid from circulation.

Radiopharmaceutical. ^{99m}Tc Sulfur Colloid (8 mCi) IV.

Indications. Space occupying lesions of the liver or spleen, cirrhosis, liver or spleen size, accessory splenic tissue and trauma.

Limitations. Lesions less than 1 cm in diameter may not be detected; may not distinguish between tumor, cyst, abscess, etc; accessory spleen may not be detected if adjacent to the liver; mild cirrhosis may show no changes.

Complementary procedures. CT, MRI, or ultrasound will distinguish cystic versus solid lesions; Gallium imaging will indicate abscess and hepatoma. Heat damaged, labeled RBCs can be used to identify accessory splenic tissue.

Examination time. 1 hour.

HEPATOBILIARY FUNCTION

Principle. Hepatic polygonal cells concentrate tracer and excrete it through the biliary system, similar to bilirubin.

Radiopharmaceutical. ^{99m}Tc aminodiaceticacid (IDA derivatives) (2 to 5 mCi) IV.

Indications. Acute and chronic cholecystitis, biliary obstruction, bile leak, biliary atresia, or decreased hepatocyte function.

Limitations. Serum bilirubin over 20 to 30 may interfere with uptake of tracer by liver, delayed images needed to distinguish acute from chronic cholecystitis.

Complementary procedures. Ultrasound for bile duct dilatation, stones in ducts, or gall bladder.

Examination time. 1 hour with possible delay images.

SCHILLING'S TEST

Principle. The absorption of vitamin B_{12}, with and without Intrinsic Factor, from the terminal ilium is estimated by measuring the urinary excretion of an orally administered dose of radioactive vitamin B_{12}.

Radiopharmaceutical. ^{57}Co vitamin B_{12} (.0005 mCi) or ^{58}Co vitamin B_{12} (.008 mCi) orally.

Indications. Pernicious anemia or malabsorption (especially distal ilium).

Limitations. Incomplete or inaccurate 24-hour urine collection will invalidate results; radioactivity in urine from recent nuclear medicine study may cause problems; loading dose of 1 mg of "cold" vitamin B_{12} IM is needed as part of procedure.

Complementary procedures. Vitamin B_{12} serum levels.

Examination time. Two-day visit with 24-hour urine collection; first day, approximately 45 minutes; second day, 10 minutes.

Genitourinary System

RENAL BLOOD FLOW

Principle. Initial bolus flow of the tracer to the kidneys will reveal gross changes in blood flow.

Radiopharmaceutical. Any ^{99m}Tc renal radiopharmaceutical (10 mCi) IV.

Indications. Renal artery thrombosis or major obstruction.

Limitations. Decreases such as 70% renal artery stenosis not detected.

Complementary procedures. Digital angiography may show smaller lesions and anatomy.

Examination time. 30 minutes.

RENAL MORPHOLOGIC IMAGING

Principle. Renal tubular concentration of tracer.

Radiopharmaceutical. ^{99m}Tc DMSA (dimethylsuccinic acid) (10 mCi) IV.

Indications. Mass lesion of kidney, renal infarction, relative function of right and left kidneys, trauma, or acute pyelonephritis; differentiate normal versus abnormal renal morphology.

Limitations. May not distinguish between cyst, tumor, abscess, etc.

Complementary procedures. CT, ultrasound, or MRI will distinguish cysts and solid lesions; IVP less sensitive for suspected tumor or relative renal function.

Examination time. 1 hour.

RENAL GLOMERULAR FUNCTION

Principle. Tracer is primarily and rapidly excreted through the kidneys by glomerular filtration.

Radiopharmaceutical. ^{99m}Tc DTPA (10 mCi) IV.

Indications. Right and left kidney glomerular filtration rates (GFRs); renal excretory function; differentiate ureteropelvic and ureterovesical (UPJ and UVJ) obstruction from dilated, non-obstructed system using Lasix.

Limitations. Not particularly effective for mass lesions of the kidney; detailed anatomy of obstruction not seen.

Complementary procedures. Abdominal radiograph, CT, or ultrasound may show renal stone; IVP may show ureteral anatomy and cause of obstruction; creatinine clearance provides total GFR; Hippuran Sequential Function study better for acute tubular necrosis.

Examination time. 1 hour.

RENAL FUNCTIONAL IMAGING

Principle. Tracer is primarily and rapidly excreted through the kidneys by tubular concentration and excretion.

Radiopharmaceutical. ^{131}I Hippuran (0.3 mCi) IV or ^{99m}Tc MAG-3 (5 mCi) IV.

Indications. Acute tubular necrosis, right and left renal function (equivalent to PAH clearance), or possible ureteral obstruction.

Limitations. Anatomy seen even less than with renal glomerular filtration study.

Complementary procedures. Abdominal radiograph, CT, or ultrasound may show renal stone; IVP may show ureteral anatomy and cause of obstruction; renal glomerular filtration study generally better for evaluating obstruction unless obstructed kidney function is severely decreased.

Examination time. 1 hour.

URETERAL OBSTRUCTION

See renal glomerular filtration and renal function imaging above.

Examination time. 1 hour.

SCROTAL IMAGING

Principle. Initial flow through the testes shows flow or lack of flow on affected side.

Radiopharmaceutical. ^{99m}TcO$_4-$ (20 mCi) IV.

Indications. Testicular torsion (decreased flow) versus epididymitis (increased flow).

Limitations. Cyst or hydrocele in scrotum may cause false positive for torsion.

Complementary procedures. Ultrasound.

Examination time. 1 hour.

Musculoskeletal System

SKELETAL IMAGING

Principle. Labeled phosphate localizes normally in bone and in region of osteoblastic activity which is the repair reaction of the bone.

Radiopharmaceutical. ^{99m}Tc phosphonate (20 mCi) IV.

Indications. Skeletal primary or secondary tumor, infection (osteomyelitis), injury (stress fractures), or aseptic necrosis.

Limitations. May not distinguish between etiological factors of bone injury.

Complementary procedures. Bone radiographs are less sensitive in detecting disease but more specific as to etiological factor; CT and MRI.

Examination time. 15 to 30 minutes for injection, then scan begins 2.5 hours later.

BONE MARROW IMAGING

Principle. Reticuloendothelial cells in bone marrow concentrate particular tracer.

Radiopharmaceutical. ^{99m}Tc Sulfur Colloid (10 mCi) IV.

Indications. Bone marrow replacement or expansion.

Limitations. Subtle degrees of expansion or replacement not detected; of no value in aplastic anemia; imaging of the reticuloendothelial system usually, but not always, correlates with bone marrow disease.

Complementary procedures. MRI.

Examination time. Imaging begins 30 minutes after injection and requires about 1 hour to scan.

Hematologic System

RED CELL VOLUME

Principle. Dilution of labeled red cells in the body.

Radiopharmaceutical. ^{51}Cr-labeled red cells (.02 to 0.1 mCi) IV.

Indications. Polycythemia or anemia.

Limitations. Must have good IV injection.

Complementary procedures. Plasma volume determination.

Examination time. 1.5 hours.

PLASMA VOLUME

Principle. Dilution of labeled albumin in the vascular space.

Radiopharmaceutical. ^{125}I human serum albumin (0.005 mCi) IV.

Indications. Hypovolemia or hypoalbuminemia.

Limitations. Plasma volume alone cannot be used to evaluate total blood volume, must have good IV injection.

Complementary procedures. Red cell volume.

Examination time. 1 hour.

RED CELL SURVIVAL

Principle. Labeled red cells follow the same fate as other red cells.

Radiopharmaceutical. ^{51}Cr labeled red cells (0.1 mCi) IV.

Indications. Anemia.

Limitations. Procedure may take several days; transfusions during procedure may alter results.

Complementary procedures. Splenic sequestration.

Examination time. 1 hour a day for several days (4 to 7).

SPLENIC SEQUESTRATION

Principle. Splenic accumulation of labeled red cells.

Radiopharmaceutical. ^{51}Cr labeled red cells (0.1 mCi) IV.

Indications. Hemolytic anemia or hypersplenism.

Limitations. Only indirectly useful for splenic sequestration of other formed elements of the blood and hypersplenism of any cause.

Complementary procedures. Red cell survival.

Examination time. Same as red cell survival.

Miscellaneous

INFLAMMATION/INFECTION: GALLIUM/INDIUM

Principle. Tracer follows white cells and localizes in region of infection or inflammation.

Radiopharmaceutical. ^{67}Ga Citrate (6 to 10 mCi) or ^{111}In labeled WBCs (0.5 mCi) IV or ^{99m}Tc HMPAO WBC (15 mCi) IV.

Indications. Fever of unknown origin, osteomyelitis, possible abscess, or evaluation of extent of inflammation/infection. Indium better for acute infections and in abdomen; Gallium better for chronic infections.

Limitations. Procedure takes hours or days; localization in osteomyelitis may be obscured by overlying acute cellulitis; Gallium uptake in the abdomen may be obscured by uptake in the gut and liver, Indium by uptake in liver; Gallium uptake in tumor may be confusing.

Complementary procedures. Gallium and Indium complement each other; CT, MRI, and ultrasound.

Examination time. 1-hour scan may be required 24, 48, and even 72 hours post-injection.

TUMOR IMAGING

Principle. Gallium binds to the proteins present in certain tumors.

Radiopharmaceutical. ^{67}Ga Citrate (10mCi) IV or ^{111}In Satumomab Pendetide (4 mCi) IV.

Indications. Lymphomas or multiple solid malignancies (especially lung and head/neck cancer or melanoma).

Limitations. Uptake by tumor is variable even within metastatic sites in the same patient; infected sites may cause false positive; not useful for GI adenocarcinoma.

Complementary procedures. CT, MRI, and ultrasound.

Examination time. 1-hour scan may be required 24, 48, and even 72 hours post-injection.

RADIOIMMUNOASSAY (RIA) LIGAND ASSAY

Principle. An in vitro procedure in which tracer-labeled ligand, such as a hormone, is displaced from a binding agent (such as a specific antibody) in proportion to the amount of nonlabeled (native) ligand present in the test tube.

Radiopharmaceutical. ^{125}I labeled ligands.

Indications. Quantitation of amount of ligands.

Limitations. May be subject to cross reactions or interfering substances in serum.

Complementary procedures. Other laboratory procedures.

Examination time. Requires one blood sample (15 to 60 minutes).

Therapy

HYPERTHYROIDISM

Principle. Overactive thyroid cells concentrate radioactive iodine and the beta radiation from the decay kills the cells, thus reducing the production of thyroid hormone.

Radiopharmaceutical. ^{131}I as sodium iodide (2 to 30 mCi) orally.

Indications. Thyrotoxicosis secondary to overactive thyroid, either diffuse toxic goiter (Grave's disease) or toxic nodule. There is no evidence that thyroid carcinoma is induced by this treatment, even in children.

Limitations. Should not be used if patient is pregnant or nursing; should not be used in neonatal thyrotoxicosis; patient cannot be treated if there is an expanded body iodide pool or if thyroid is blocked by drug therapy.

Complementary procedures. Surgery or propylthiouracil (PTU) drug therapy may be used but generally is not as safe or effective; drug therapy (particularly propanolol and sometimes PTU) should be used adjunctively since ^{131}I may take several weeks for full effect.

Examination time. About .5 to 1 hour.

THYROID CARCINOMA

Principle: Many well-differentiated papillary and follicular thyroid carcinomas will concentrate iodide, although usually less well than normal thyroid tissue; thus administration of radioactive iodide will result in intense beta irradiation of those cells which concentrate the tracer.

Radiopharmaceutical. ^{131}I as sodium iodide (50 to 200 mCi) orally.

Indications. Demonstrated uptake of ^{131}I by foci of thyroid carcinoma on a whole body iodide scan.

Limitations. Thyroid carcinomas which do not take up iodide cannot be treated by this method (e.g., medullary or anaplastic); patient must not have any substantial amount of normal thyroid remaining and must be off any replacement thyroid for several weeks or the carcinoma will not take up enough ^{131}I.

Complementary procedures. Other chemotherapy or external radiation may be used but they are not as effective; they should not be used just prior to ^{131}I therapy because they will decrease uptake.

Examination time. May require hospital stay of 3 to 5 days.

POLYCYTHEMIA

Principle. Radioactive phosphorus will concentrate in the precursor cells of the formed blood elements and will therefore irradiate them with beta irradiation.

Radiopharmaceutical. ^{32}P as sodium phosphate (2 to 5 mCi) IV.

Indications. Treatment of choice for polycythemia rubra vera that is not controlled by one phlebotomy every 3 months; thrombocytosis; some leukemias.

Limitations. Not as effective as chemotherapy for most leukemias.

Complementary procedures. Chemotherapy and phlebotomy.

Examination time. 1 hour.

SKELETAL METASTASES

Principle. The tracer, Strontium, is a calcium analog which concentrates in areas of osteoblastic activity.

Radiopharmaceutical. ^{89}Sr Strontium Chloride IV.

Indications. Bone pain secondary to metastases, especially from breast and prostate cancers.

Limitations. Palliative not curative. Ninety percent pain response in breast cancer patients; 80% in prostate cancer patients.

Complementary procedures. Chemotherapy, beam therapy, and pain medication.

Examination time. 1 hour.

Definition of Terms

alpha particle A particle that is identical to the helium nucleus, consisting of two protons and two neutrons. It carries a positive charge of 2.

becquerel (Bq) Measure of radioactive decay stated as the decay rate of 1 disintegration per second.

beta decay The radioactive disintegration of a nucleus resulting in the emission of an electron (beta particle).

beta particle An electron, either positive or negative. Positive beta particles are called positrons (B^+). Negative beta particles are sometimes called negatrons (B^-). The term "beta particle" and the symbol "B" are reserved for electrons originating in a nucleus.

cathode ray tube (CRT) Device used to record an event by exciting its phosphor.

collimator An apparatus, often consisting of a pair of slits, used to confine radiation to a narrow beam.

curie (Ci) Measure of radioactive decay equaling 3.7×10^{10} disintegrations per second.

cyclotron A device used to produce neutron-poor radionuclides.

daughter The decay product produced by a radioactive nuclide. When the parent nuclide undergoes decay, a daughter nuclide is produced.

decay The radioactive disintegration of a nucleus.

dose calibrator Especially designed gas-filled ionization chamber used to measure the amount of radioactivity in a sample such as a syringe, vial, or test tube.

dynamic image A nuclear medicine image representing the distribution of a radiopharmaceutical over a specific time period. Also called a "flow study," which refers to the blood flow being imaged in a particular area. This is a sequential or time-lapse sequence in which images are collected every few seconds for a preset time.

electron An elementary particle of nature having a charge of 1 and a mass of 9.1×10^{-28} grams.

film badge A piece of photographic film contained in a lightproof holder and worn by an individual to measure the amount of radiation to which he or she is exposed.

gamma rays Electromagnetic radiation having its origin in an atomic nucleus.

gas detector A device employing a gas plus a high-voltage power supply for detection of radiation.

Geiger-Mueller Survey Meter A small ionization chamber operated by gas amplication and used to detect small quantities of radioactivity.

generator A method of producing radioactivity in a nuclear medicine department.

half-life The time required for one half of a given number of radioactive atoms to undergo decay; symbol $T_{1/2}$.

in vivo Within the living body. This term is used to describe many of the routine nuclear medicine imaging studies.

in vitro Within a glass; observable in a test tube; or in an artificial environment. This term is used to describe the nonimaging laboratory studies performed in nuclear medicine.

isotope One of a group of nuclides of the same element (same Z) having the same number or protons in the nucleus but differing in the number of neutrons, resulting in different values of A.

ligand A molecule that binds to another molecule; this term is used especially to refer to a small molecule that binds specifically to a larger molecule (e.g., an antigen binding to an antibody, a hormone binding to a receptor).

microcurie (μCi) One millionth of a curie.

millicurie (mCi) One thousandth of a curie.

monoclonal-antibody imaging Technique utilizing antibodies produced from a single strain and cloned to create identical copies which are tagged to a particular isotope in order to image a specific antibody structure such as a tumor site (e.g., colorectal or ovarian cancer).

neutron A neutral elementary particle having a mass number of 1. In the free state (outside the nucleus), it is unstable, having a half-life of about 12 minutes. It decays by the process $n = p + e + v$.

nuclear reactor A device for supporting a self-sustained nuclear chain reaction under controlled conditions.

nucleus The positively charged core of an atom in which almost all the mass is concentrated.

nuclide Any one of the more than 1000 species of atoms characterized by the number of protons and number of neutrons in the nucleus.

photocathode Photosensitive layer (cathode) of a photomultiplier tube.

photomultiplier tube (PMT) A phototube of exceptionally high sensitivity; the electron or electrons released at the photocathode initiate a cascade from one dynode to another with a resultant electron amplication as high as 10.

positron A positive electron.

positron emission tomography (PET) Imaging technology that utilizes high-energy positron-emitting radiopharmaceuticals. These high-energy positrons are emitted from the nucleus and rapidly lose energy and interact with an electron to release two 511-KeV photons, which are emitted at an angle of approximately 180 degrees. The detector and computer systems allow for the coincidence counting (i.e., the detection of these two photons by opposing detectors within a given time window [typically 5 to 20 nanoseconds]), compensating for attenuation and electronically collimating field of view to permit precise location of the emission. Primary radiopharmaceuticals used for PET imaging have extremely short physical half-lives and therefore usually require an on-site cyclotron to produce these isotopes.

proton A positively charged elementary particle having a mass number of 1; the nucleus of a hydrogen atom of mass 1.

pulse height analysis Electronic circuitry used to select some pulses and reject others that are not within a desired preset range.

radioactive Giving off radiant energy in the form of alpha, beta, or gamma rays by the breaking up of atoms.

radioimmunoassay (RIA) A highly sensitive and specific assay method that uses the competition between radiolabeled and unlabeled substances in an antigen-antibody reaction to determine the concentration of the unlabeled substance.

radioisotope Any isotope that is unstable, thus undergoing decay with the emission of a characteristic radiation. Synonym for radioactive isotope.

radionuclide A nuclide that disintegrates with the emission of corpuscular or electromagnetic radiations. Synonym for radioactive nuclide.

radiopharmaceutical A radioactive substance used especially for diagnostic purposes or treatment of disease.

rectilinear scanner A device that generates an image of an organ by detecting radioactivity within that organ and recording it on film.

scintillation The flash of light produced in a phosphor by radiation.

scintillation camera An imaging device using all of the components of a scintillation counter.

scintillation counter A counter employing a phosphor, photomultiplier tube, and associated circuits for the detection of radiation.

scintillation detector Sensitive device used to detect ionizing radiation by electronically measuring the light (scintillation) produced.

single photon emission computed tomography (SPECT) An imaging technique in which the gamma camera rotates around the patient to collect and reconstruct data in various planes including transaxial, sagittal, and coronal orientations.

static image A single stationary nuclear medicine image of a particular structure.

syringe shield Device used to house syringes containing radioactive material. These shields are made of lead and include leaded glass, with the primary purpose of decreasing radiation exposure from the radioactive material within the syringe.

thermoluminescent dosimetry (TLD) A method of measuring radiation exposure.

BIBLIOGRAPHY

Bernier DR, Langan JK, and Christian PE: Nuclear medicine technology and techniques, ed 3, St Louis, 1994, Mosby.

Bogardus CR, Jr: Clinical applications of physics of radiology and nuclear medicine, St Louis, 1969, Warren H. Green.

Casarett AP: Radiation biology, Englewood Cliffs, NJ, 1968, Prentice-Hall.

Chandra R: Introductory physics of nuclear medicine, ed 3, Philadelphia, 1987, Lea & Febiger.

Data FL, Patch GG, Arias JM, and Morton KA: Nuclear medicine a teaching file, St Louis, 1992, Mosby.

Dillman LT and von der Lage FC: Radionuclide decay schemes and nuclear parameters for use in radiation-dose estimation, MIRD Pamphlet No. 10, New York, 1975, Society of Nuclear Medicine.

Early PJ and Sodee BD: Principles and practice of nuclear medicine, St Louis, 1985, Mosby.

Gerson MC: Cardiac nuclear medicine, ed 2, 1991 New.

Goodwin PN and Rao DV: The physics of nuclear medicine, Springfield, Ill, 1977, Charles C. Thomas, Publisher.

Gottschalk A and Potchen EJ: Diagnostic Nuclear Medicine, ed 2, 2 volumes, Baltimore, 1988, Williams & Wilkins.

Harness B, Christian P, and Rowell K: Clinical computers in nuclear medicine, New York, 1992, Society of Nuclear Medicine.

Hendee WR: Medical radiation physics, ed 2, St Louis, 1979, Mosby.

Johns HE: The physics of radiology, ed 4, Springfield, Ill, 1983, Charles C. Thomas, Publisher.

King ER and Mitchell TG: A manual for nuclear medicine, Springfield, Ill, 1961, Charles C. Thomas, Publisher.

Kowalsky RJ and Perry JR: Radiopharmaceuticals in nuclear medicine practice, East Norwalk, 1987, Appleton & Lange.

Metler FA and Guiberteau MJ: Essentials of nuclear medicine imaging, ed 3, Philadelphia, 1991, WB Saunders.

Quimby EH and Feitelberg S: Radioactive nuclides in medicine and biology, ed 3, Philadelphia, Lea & Febiger.

Rocha AFG and Harbert JE: Textbook of nuclear medicine: basic science, ed 2, Philadelphia, 1984, Lea & Febiger.

Rollo FD: Nuclear medicine physics, instrumentation, and agents, St Louis, 1977, Mosby.

Saha GB: Fundamentals of nuclear pharmacy, ed 3, New York, 1992, Springer-Verlag.

Shapiro J: Radiation protection, ed 3, Cambridge, Mass, 1990, Harvard University Press.

Shilling CW: Atomic energy encyclopedia in the life sciences, Philadelphia, 1964, WB Saunders.

Sorenson JA and Phelps ME: Physics in nuclear medicine, ed 2, New York, 1987, WB Saunders.

Wagner HN: Principles of nuclear medicine, Philadelphia, 1968, WB Saunders.

Wahner H: Nuclear medicine: quantitative procedures, Boston, 1983, Little, Brown & Co.

Definition of terms

Chapter 39

POSITRON EMISSION TOMOGRAPHY

RICHARD D. HICHWA

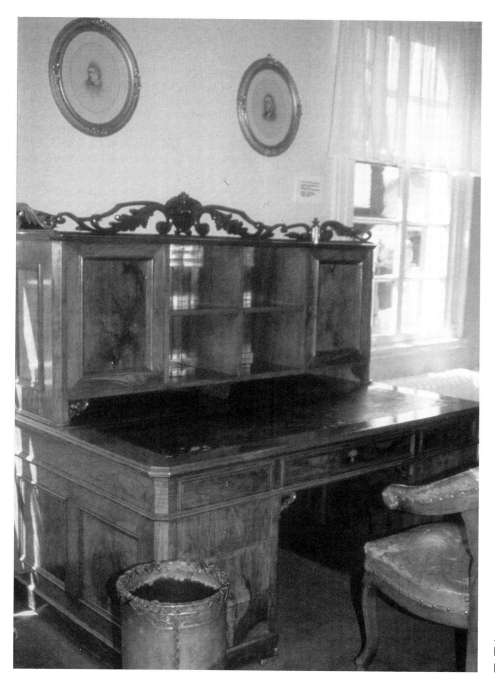

Dr. Roentgen's desk on display at his birthplace.

*Positron emission tomography** (PET) is a noninvasive nuclear imaging technique that involves the administration of a *radiopharmaceutical* and subsequent imaging of the distribution and *kinetics* of the radioactive material. PET imaging of the heart, brain, lungs, or other organs is possible if an appropriate radiopharmaceutical, also called a *radiotracer,* can be synthesized and administered to the patient.

Three important factors distinguish PET from all radiologic procedures and from other nuclear imaging procedures. The first factor is that the results of the data acquisition and analysis techniques yield an image related to a particular physiologic parameter, such as blood flow or metabolism. The ensuing image is aptly called a functional or *parametric image.*

Secondly, the images are created by the simultaneous detection of a pair of *annihilation* radiations that result from a *positron* annihilation occurrence as illustrated in Fig. 39-1.

*All italicized terms are defined at the end of this chapter.

The third feature distinguishing PET is the actual chemical and biologic form of the radiopharmaceutical. The radiopharmaceutical is specifically chosen for its similarity to naturally occurring biochemical constituents of the human body. Because very small amounts of the radiopharmaceutical are administered, equilibrium conditions within the body are not altered. If, for instance, the radiopharmaceutical is a form of sugar, it will behave very much like the natural sugar in the body. The kinetics of uptake and distribution of the radioactive sugar within the body are followed by measuring the distribution of the *radioactivity concentration* with the PET scanner as a function of time. From this, the distribution of metabolism of the sugar may be deduced by converting the many images that demonstrate the tracer kinetics into a single parametric image that indicates tissue function.

In this chapter, the basic concepts of PET are discussed and examples of PET imaging studies are presented.

Comparison with Other Modalities

PET is predominantly used to measure human cellular, organ, or system function. That is, a parameter that characterizes a particular aspect of human physiology is determined from the measurement of the radioactivity emitted from a radiopharmaceutical in a given volume of tissue. In contrast, conventional radiography measures the structure of organs or human anatomy by determining x-ray transmission through a given volume of tissue. X-ray attenuation by structures interposed between the x-ray source and the radiographic film provides the contrast necessary to visualize an organ. Computed tomography (CT) creates cross-sectional tomographic images by computer reconstruction of multiple x-ray transmissions. A comparison of various modalities is given in Table 39-1.

Radionuclides used for conventional nuclear medicine include ^{99m}Tc, ^{123}I, ^{131}I, ^{111}In, ^{201}Tl, and ^{67}Ga. Labeled compounds with these high atomic weight radionuclides often do not mimic the physiologic properties of natural substances because of their size, mass, and distinctly different chemical properties—unlike hydrogen, carbon, nitrogen, and oxygen, which are the predominant constituents of natural compounds. Thus compounds labeled with conventional nuclear medicine radionuclides are poor radioactive *analogs* for natural substances. Imaging studies with these agents are qualitative and emphasize nonbiochemical properties. Nature has provided ^{11}C (carbon), ^{13}N (nitrogen), ^{15}O (oxygen), and ^{18}F (fluorine). These positron-emitting radionuclides can directly replace their stable counterparts in substrates, metabolites, drugs, and other biologically active compounds without disrupting normal biochemical properties.

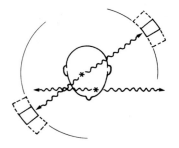 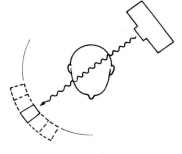

Fig. 39-1. Positron emission tomography relies on the simultaneous detection of a pair of annihilation radiations emitted from the body (left), unlike computed tomography (CT), which depends on the detection of x-rays transmitted through the body (right).

Table 39-1. Comparison of imaging modalities*

	PET	SPECT	MRI	CT
Measures	Physiology	Physiology	Anatomy (Physiology)*	Anatomy
Resolution	4.5-5 mm	8-10 mm	0.5-1 mm	1-1.5 mm
Technique	Positron annihilation	Gamma emission	Nuclear magnetic resonance	Absorption of x-ray transmissions
Harmful effects	Radiation exposure	Radiation exposure	None known	Radiation exposure
Use	Research (Clinical)	Clinical	Clinical (Research)*	Clinical
Number of examinations per day	3-6	4-8	10-15	15-20

(Secondary use of modality.)

Single photon emission computed tomography *(SPECT)* (also discussed in Chapter 38) employs nuclear imaging techniques to determine tissue function. Use of collimators and lower-energy photons offer reduced sensitivity by 10^1 to 10^5 and accuracy when compared with PET. In general, resolution with SPECT is decreased in comparison. PET easily accounts for photon loss through attenuation by performing a *transmission scan.* This is difficult to achieve and not routinely done with SPECT imaging.

To emphasize the differences between the various modalities, consider a study of the blood flow within the brain. Without an intact circulatory system, an IV injection of the radiopharmaceutical could not make its way into the brain and be distributed throughout the capillary network within the brain. Therefore, a PET scan would not be possible. For radiographic procedures such as CT, structures within the brain may well be intact but there may be no blood flow to and through the brain tissues. A CT scan (see Chapter 33) under these circumstances may appear almost normal. The use of contrast materials for brain studies requires a working circulatory system for transport to the brain. Their use, however, is to help define structures of interest by providing increased x-ray absorption, and this does not help to visualize underlying tissue function.

The contrast agents used in many of the radiographic studies to enhance image contrast are toxic. The x-ray dose to the patient from these radiographic studies is greater than in nuclear imaging studies. Radiopharmaceuticals used in PET studies are similar to the body's own biochemical constituents and are administered in very small amounts. Biochemical compatibility of the tracers with the body minimizes the risks to the patient because the tracers are not toxic. Trace amounts minimize the alteration of the body's *homeostasis.*

An imaging technique that augments both CT and PET is *magnetic resonance imaging (MRI)* (see Chapter 36). Images of each modality are shown in Fig. 39-2. MRI is used primarily to measure anatomy or morphology. Unlike CT, which derives its greatest image contrast from varying tissue densities (bone from soft tissue), MRI better differentiates tissue by its proton content and the degree to which these protons are bound in lattice structures. The

tightly bound protons of bone make it virtually transparent to MRI. Advances in spectroscopic imaging of fluorine, phosphorus, and other elements now permit to some degree the determination of organ and cellular function of relatively large tissue volumes. The image *resolution* obtained from spectroscopic techniques is poorer than conventional proton MRI imaging. Measurement of large-vessel blood flow is already achieved and new capabilities make possible capillary flow measurements. Development of paramagnetic contrast agents, improved MRI imaging instrumentation, absolute quantification, and spectroscopy remain the major areas of MRI research.

It is important to note that CT, MRI, and other anatomic imaging modalities provide complementary information to PET. PET benefits from *image coregistration* with CT and MRI by pinpointing physiologic function from precise anatomic locations. PET remains unique in its ability to measure in vivo physiology.

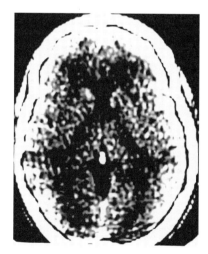
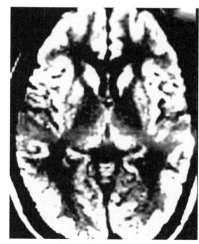
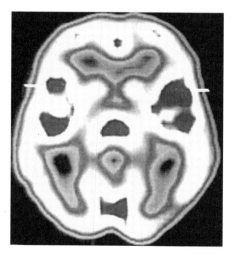

Fig. 39-2. Brain images of the same patient in the same position with CT (left), MRI (center), and PET (right).

Historical Development

The use of positron-emitting radio-pharmaceuticals for medical purposes was first conceived by the inventor of the *cyclotron*, E.O. Lawrence, in the early 1930s. Simple compounds with positron-emitting radionuclides were synthesized, and Geiger counters were used to qualitatively measure the relative uptake in various parts of the body.

It was not until more suitable *scintillators* such as sodium iodide (NaI) and more sophisticated nuclear counting electronics became available that positron coincidence localization was possible. F.W. Wrenn demonstrated the use of positron-emitting radioisotopes for the localization of brain tumors in 1951. G.L. Brownell further developed instrumentation for similar studies in 1953.

The next major advance came in 1967 when G. Hounsfield demonstrated the clinical use of CT. The mathematics of PET image reconstruction are very similar to CT reconstruction techniques. Instead of x-rays from a point source traversing the body and being detected by a single detector, PET imaging counts the resulting pairs of 0.511 MeV photons from the positron-electron annihilation by using two opposing detectors.

During the next 8 years, significant developments were made in computer technology, scintillator design, and *photomultiplier tube (PMT)* speed for the detection of high-energy photons. In 1975, the first closed-ring transverse positron tomograph was built for PET imaging by M.M. Ter-Pogossian and M.E. Phelps.

Since 1975, developments on two fronts have accelerated the use of PET. First, with vastly improved imaging instrumentation, scientists are nearing the theoretical limits (1 to 2 mm) of PET tomograph resolution by employing smaller, more efficient scintillators and photomultiplier tubes. Microprocessors now tune and adjust the entire ring of *detectors* that surround the patient, which may number as many as 500 to 800 detectors per ring. The second major area of development is in the design of new radiopharmaceuticals. Agents are being developed to measure blood flow, metabolism, protein synthesis, lipid content, receptor binding, and many other physiologic parameters. During the mid-1980s, PET was predominantly used as a research tool; but by the early 1990s clinical PET centers had been established, and PET was routinely used for diagnostic procedures on the brain, heart, and tumors.

Principles and Facilities

In this section, the major concepts and facilities for the use of PET are discussed. To better understand the multidisciplinary nature of PET, four major functions are presented. These are radionuclide production, radiopharmaceutical production, data acquisition, and image reconstruction and image processing. A short discussion of the particles called positrons is also presented.

POSITRONS

Living organisms are composed primarily of compounds containing the elements hydrogen, carbon, nitrogen, and oxygen. In PET, radiotracers are made by synthesizing compounds with radioactive isotopes of these elements. Chemically, the radioactive isotope is indistinguishable from its equivalent stable isotope. Neutron-rich (more neutrons than protons) radionuclides emit electrons or beta particles. The effective range or distance traveled for a 1 MeV beta particle (β^-) in human tissue is only 4 mm. These radionuclides typically do not emit other types of radiation that can be easily measured externally with counters or scintillation detectors. The only radioisotopes of these elements that can be detected outside the body are positron-emitting nuclides. Fig. 39-3 (from a portion of the Chart of the Nuclides) depicts the stable and radioactive nuclides of several elements.

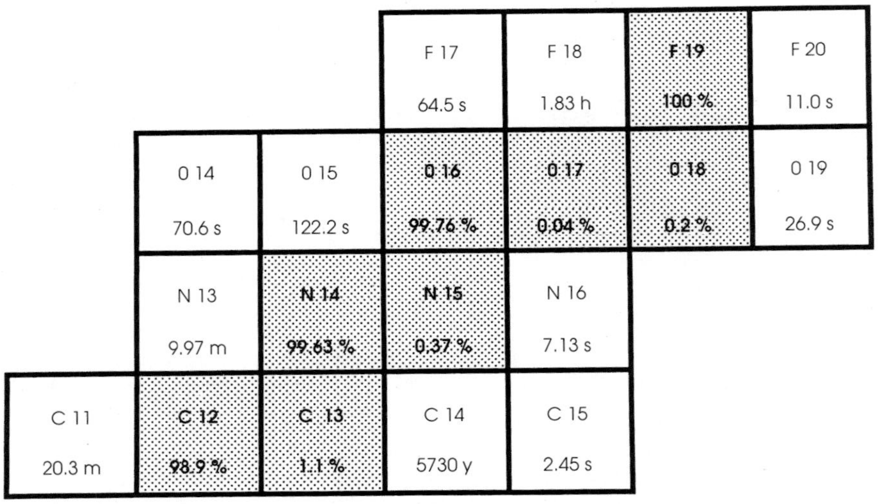

F 17	F 18	F 19	F 20
64.5 s	1.83 h	100 %	11.0 s

O 14	O 15	O 16	O 17	O 18	O 19
70.6 s	122.2 s	99.76 %	0.04 %	0.2 %	26.9 s

N 13	N 14	N 15	N 16
9.97 m	99.63 %	0.37 %	7.13 s

C 11	C 12	C 13	C 14	C 15
20.3 m	98.9 %	1.1 %	5730 y	2.45 s

Fig. 39-3. Excerpt from the Chart of the Nuclides showing the stable elements (shaded boxes), positron emitters (to the left of stable elements), and beta emitters (to the right of stable elements). Isotopes farther from their stable counterparts have very short half-lives.

Positron-emitting radionuclides have a neutron-deficient nucleus (more protons than neutrons or proton-rich). Positrons (β+) are identical in mass to electrons, but they possess positive instead of negative charge. The characteristics of positrons are given in Table 39-2. Positron decay occurs in unstable *radioisotopes* only if the nucleus possesses excess energy greater than the energy equivalent of two electron rest masses or a total of 1.022 MeV. After a positron is emitted from the nucleus, it is rapidly slowed by interactions in the surrounding tissues until all of its kinetic energy is lost. At this point, the positron combines momentarily with an electron. The combination of particles totally annihilates or disintegrates, and the combined positron-electron mass of 1.022 MeV is transformed into two equal energy photons of 0.511 MeV, which are emitted at 180 degrees from each other (Fig. 39-4). These annihilation photons behave like *gamma rays,* have sufficient energy to traverse the body tissues, and can be detected externally. Because two identical, or isoenergetic, photons are emitted at exactly 180 degrees from each other, the near simultaneous detection of both photons defines a line passing through the body, and the line is located precisely between the two scintillators that detected the photons. A simplified block diagram for a single coincidence circuit is shown in Fig. 39-5. Creation of images from coincidence detection is discussed in the section on data acquisition. The important point to note is that the positron annihilation photons can be used for external detection from the positron-emitting radionuclides of carbon, nitrogen, and oxygen. Table 39-3 depicts the positron ranges for three positron energies in tissue, air, and lead. Hydrogen has no positron-emitting radioisotope; however, fluorine-18 (^{18}F) is a positron (β+) emitter that is used as a hydrogen substitute in many compounds. This is successfully accomplished because of its small size and strong bond with carbon.

Table 39-2. Positron characteristics

Definition	Positively charged electron
Origin	Neutron-deficient nuclei
Production	Accelerators
Nuclide decay	p = n + β+ + neutrino
Positron decay	Annihilation to two 0.511 MeV photons
Number	~240 known
Range	Proportional to kinetic energy of β+
Routine PET nuclides	^{11}C, ^{13}N, ^{15}O, ^{18}F, ^{68}Ga, ^{82}Rb

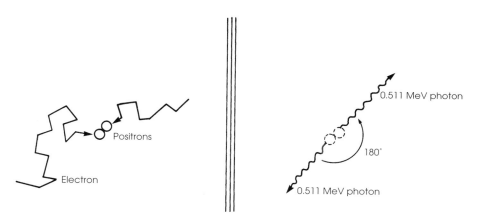

Fig. 39-4. Neutron-deficient nuclei decay by positron emission. A positron is ejected from the nucleus and loses kinetic energy by scattering (erratic line on left) until it comes to rest and interacts with a free electron. Two photons of 0.511 MeV ($E = m_0c^2$) result from the positron and electron annihilation (right).

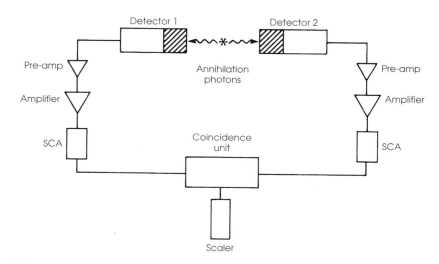

Fig. 39-5. Simplified coincidence electronics for one pair of detectors in a PET tomograph.

Table 39-3. Range (R) of positrons in centimeters

β+ Ē (MeV)	R_{tissue}	R_{air}	R_{lead}
0.5	0.15	127	0.01
1.0	0.38	279	0.03
1.5	0.64	508	0.05

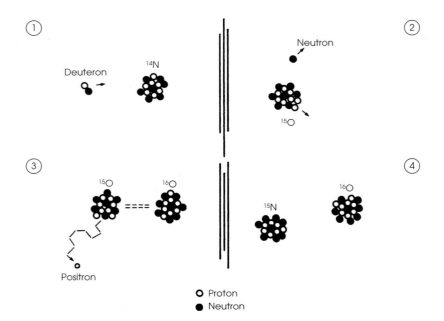

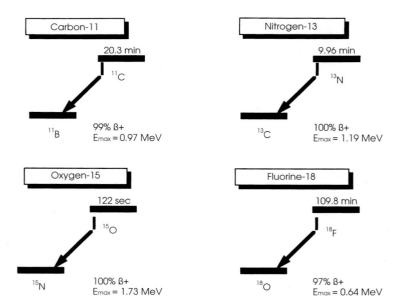

Fig. 39-6. Typical radionuclide production sequence. The $^{14}N(d,n)^{15}O$ reaction is used for making ^{15}O-^{16}O molecules. A deuteron ion is accelerated to high energy (10-17 MeV) by a cyclotron and impinges on a stable ^{14}N nucleus *(1)*. As a result of the nuclear reaction, a neutron is emitted, leaving a radioactive nucleus of ^{15}O *(2)*. The ^{15}O atom quickly associates with an ^{16}O atom to form an O_2 molecule. Sometime later the unstable ^{15}O atom emits a positron *(3)*. As a result of positron decay (positron exits nucleus), the ^{15}O atom is transformed into a stable ^{15}N atom and the O_2 molecule breaks apart *(4)*.

Fig. 39-7. Decay schemes for ^{11}C, ^{13}N, ^{15}O, and ^{18}F. Each positron emitter decays to a stable nuclide by ejecting a positron from the nucleus.

RADIONUCLIDE PRODUCTION

To produce positron-emitting radionuclides, a *nuclear particle accelerator* is used to bombard appropriate nonradioactive *target* atoms with nuclei accelerated to high energies. The high energies are necessary to overcome the electrostatic and nuclear forces of the target nuclei so that a nuclear reaction can take place. An example is the production of oxygen-15 (^{15}O). Deuterons (a deuteron is an atom stripped of its electrons, leaving a nucleus with one proton and one neutron) or heavy hydrogen ions are accelerated to approximately 10 MeV. The target material is stable nitrogen-14 (^{14}N) gas in the form of an N_2 molecule. The resultant nuclear reaction yields a neutron and an ^{15}O atom which can be written for this sequence in the following form: $^{14}N(d,n)^{15}O$. The ^{15}O atom quickly associates with a stable ^{16}O atom that has been intentionally added to the target gas in order to produce a radioactive ^{15}O-^{16}O molecule in the form of O_2. The unstable or radioactive ^{15}O atom emits a positron. This radioactive decay transforms a proton into a neutron. Hence, the ^{15}O atom becomes a stable ^{15}N atom and the O_2 molecule breaks apart. This process is shown in Fig. 39-6. Fig. 39-7 shows the decay schemes for the four routinely produced PET radionuclides.

The common reactions used for production of positron-emitting forms of carbon (C), nitrogen (N), oxygen (O), and fluorine (F) are given in Table 39-4.

The very short half-lives of routinely used positron-emitting nuclides require nearby access to a nuclear particle accelerator to produce sufficient quantities of these radioactive materials. The most common device to achieve nuclide production within reasonable space (250 ft²) and energy (150 kW) constraints is a compact medical cyclotron, which is specifically designed to accomplish the following: (1) simple operation by the technologic staff, (2) reliable and routine operation with minimal downtime, and (3) computer-controlled automatic operation to reduce overall staffing needs. A cyclotron consists of four major parts: the ion source, the magnet, the radio-frequency high-voltage acceleration system, and the extraction system (Fig. 39-8).

The ion source, as the name suggests, is used to create ions for acceleration from simple stable gases (protons from ionized hydrogen gas or deuterons from ionized deuterium gas). These ions, which are positive ions if their electrons have been stripped away or negative ions if an extra electron has been added, are extracted from the ion source and accelerated toward the outer rim of the cyclotron magnet. The cyclotron magnet is used to constrain the charged particles or ions to move in circular orbits. As one might expect, higher energy particles move with greater velocity and therefore travel in orbits of greater radii than lower energy particles. Fig. 39-9 shows a typical cyclotron used for radionuclide production. The cyclotron must either be located in a thick concrete vault (a room with 5- to 6-foot-thick walls and ceiling) or have shielding material located directly on all machine exterior surfaces (self-shielded cyclotron) in order to reduce the radiation levels to safe values when the cyclotron is in operation (<2 mR/hr).

Ions are accelerated by traversing the electric field gradient between the copper "dee" electrodes; these structures somewhat resemble the capital letter D. This gradient is created by charging the dees to a high voltage (30 to 50 kV), much like charging a large capacitor. As an ion is repelled by the polarity of the charge on one dee and attracted toward the opposite polarity of the charge on the other dee, it gains kinetic energy and its velocity increases. Once an ion is inside the conducting dee structure, it no longer experiences electrostatic forces and is constrained to move in a circular orbit toward the opposite dee by the magnetic field (1.4 to 1.8 Tesla). During this time, the polarity of the dees is automatically reversed. The alternating voltage cycle occurs at radio frequencies (RF) of 10 to 30 MHz. Therefore each time the ion traverses the gap between the two dees, it is accelerated by the respective attractive and repulsive electrostatic forces. It gains approximately twice the voltage difference between the two dees for every orbit or complete circular path. If the dee-to-dee voltage is 30 kV, then a proton gains 60 keV per orbit and undergoes approximately 280 to 300 orbits to achieve the maximum output energy, which is 17 MeV for the cyclotron shown in Fig. 39-9. During this time, the ion increases its orbital radius from the center of the cyclotron to near the outer edge of the main magnetic field in an increasingly larger spiral path.

Table 39-4. Production of the most useful PET nuclides

Nuclide	Half-life	Reaction(s)		Target material
		Proton	Deuteron	
^{11}C	20.4 min	$^{14}N(p,\alpha)^{11}C$		N_2 (gas)
^{13}N	9.97 min	$^{16}O(p,\alpha)^{13}N$		H_2O (liquid)
^{15}O	2.03 min	$^{15}N(p,n)^{15}O$	$^{14}N(d,n)^{15}O$	$N_2 + 1\% O_2$ (gas)
^{18}F	109.8 min	$^{18}O(p,n)^{18}F$		95% $^{18}O - H_2O$ (liquid)
			$^{20}Ne(d,\alpha)^{18}F$	Ne + 0.1% F_2 (gas)

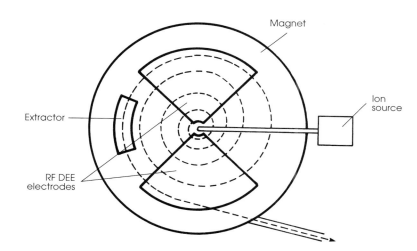

Fig. 39-8. Cyclotron schematic. The dashed line indicates the path of accelerated particles for a positive ion cyclotron. Ions originate at the ion source, are constrained to circular paths by the magnetic field, are accelerated to higher energy and thus larger orbits by the *RF* applied to the dee electrodes, and are finally directed toward the target by the extractor.

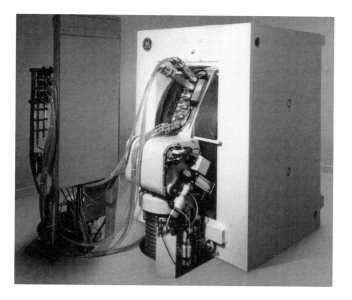

Fig. 39-9. Small cyclotron used for routine production of PET isotopes. The cyclotron can either be located in a concrete vault or be self-shielded. Particles are accelerated in vertical orbits and impinge on targets located near the top of the machine near the center. This is an example of a negative ion.

(Courtesy of GE Medical Systems)

A high-voltage electrostatic deflector operating at 20 to 50 kV is used to nudge positive ions from the edge of the magnetic field to a point where they can be extracted from the cyclotron. Negative ions are extracted by removing the added electrons by passing the ions through an extremely thin carbon foil (0.0001 in. thick). Because these ions were once negative (H$^-$) and are now positive (H$^+$), they rotate in the opposite direction under the influence of the constant magnetic field produced by the large electromagnet of the cyclotron. Hence, negative ions are easily extracted from the cyclotron.

The ion source emits ions with every cycle (1/RF frequency of the cyclotron) of the RF voltage applied to the dees regardless of ion polarity. Therefore ions arrive at the extraction system in packets synchronized with the RF frequency. These packets, or beam of particles (10 to 50 μA of protons or deuterons), are focused and directed toward the targets for production of positron-emitting radioisotopes. The radioisotopes produced in the target may be solid, liquid, or gaseous and may be created either continuously or in batches.

Proton-only cyclotrons produce nuclides by reactions shown under the proton column of Table 39-4. For cyclotrons that can produce both protons and deuterons, all reactions in Table 39-4 are possible, but the $^{14}N(d,n)^{15}O$ deuteron reaction is used primarily to produce ^{15}O while all other nuclides are typically produced with protons.

RADIOPHARMACEUTICAL PRODUCTION

Radiopharmaceuticals are synthesized from radionuclides derived from the target material. These agents may be very simple, as are the ^{15}O-^{16}O molecules described earlier, or they may be very complex. However, regardless of the chemical complexity of the radioactive molecule, each must be synthesized very rapidly. This entails specialized techniques not only to create the labeled substance but also to verify the purity (chemical, radiochemical, and radionuclidic) of the radiopharmaceutical.

There are two important radiopharmaceuticals presently used in many PET studies. The first is ^{15}O water (^{15}O-H_2O), which is produced continuously or in batches from the $^{14}N(d,n)^{15}O$ or $^{15}N(p,n)^{15}O$ nuclear reaction. As discussed earlier, the radioactive oxygen quickly combines with a stable ^{16}O atom, which has been added to the stable N_2 target gas, to form an oxygen molecule (O_2). The ^{15}O-^{16}O molecule is combusted over a platinum catalyst with small amounts of stable H_2 and N_2 gas. Radioactive water vapor is produced and collected in sterile saline for injection. A typical bolus injection of ^{15}O-H_2O is approximately 30 to 50 mCi in a volume of 1 to 2 ml of saline. A dose of radioactive water can be prepared every few minutes (2 to 5 minutes). Radioactive ^{15}O-H_2O is used primarily for determination of *local cerebral blood flow (LCBF)*. A PET LCBF image and MRI image of the same slice of brain from the same subject are shown in Fig. 39-10.

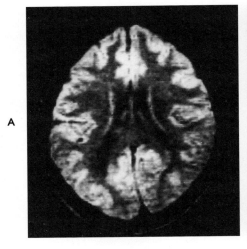 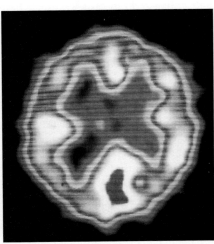

Fig. 39-10. MRI image (left) and PET LCBF image (right) of the same normal, awake 30-year-old male subject. Both transverse images have the same slice thickness and are seen from the vantage point of one standing at the patient's head.

The second major radiopharmaceutical used routinely in PET employs ^{18}F labeled fluoride ions (F⁻) to form a sugar analog called [^{18}F]-2-fluoro-2-deoxy-D-glucose, or *[18]F-FDG*. This agent is used to determine the *local metabolic rate of glucose utilization (LMRG)* in brain, heart, tumor, or other tissues that utilize glucose as a metabolic substrate. For example, glucose, obtained from food, is metabolized by the brain to provide the adenosine triphosphate (ATP) necessary for maintaining the membrane potential of the neurons within the brain. The metabolism of glucose is proportional to the neural activity of the brain and thus brain metabolism. Radioactive ^{18}F-FDG and glucose enter the same biochemical pathways in the brain. However, ^{18}F-FDG cannot be completely metabolized in the brain, as can glucose, because its metabolism is blocked at the level of fluoro-deoxyglucose-6-phosphate ([^{18}F] FDG-6-PO$_4$). However, since ^{18}F-FDG follows the glucose pathway into the brain, the concentration of [^{18}F]-FDG-6-PO$_4$ within the brain cells is proportional to brain tissue metabolism. These pathways for glucose and ^{18}F-FDG are schematically drawn in Fig. 39-11.

^{18}F-FDG is synthesized by displacing the triflate-leaving group of 1,3,4,6-tetra-O-acetyl-2-O-trifluoromethanesulfonyl-E1-D-mannopyranose with anhydrous ^{18}F-fluoride, obtained from drying ^{18}F-fluoride ions generated by proton bombardment of stable ^{18}O-water (see Table 39-4). The intermediate is deacetylated by acid hydrolysis and purified chromatographically to give [^{18}F]-2-fluoro-2-deoxy-D-glucose, or ^{18}F-FDG. A standard dose of 5 to 10 mCi in a few ml of isotonic saline is administered intravenously. The total time for target irradiation (1 hour), radiochemical synthesis (1.3 hour), and purity certification (0.2 hour) is approximately 2.5 hours.

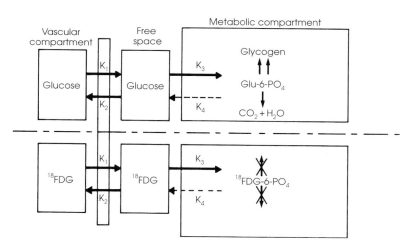

Fig. 39-11. Glucose compartmental model (above dashed line) versus ^{18}F-FDG model (below dashed line). Note that ^{18}F-FDG does not go to complete storage (glycogen) or metabolism ($CO_2 + H_2O$) as does glucose.

Principles and facilities

DATA ACQUISITION

The positron-electron annihilation photons are detected and counted with a PET scanner or tomograph (Fig. 39-12). In general, for neurologic PET scanners the distance between detector faces is 70 cm. This is increased to 90 cm for whole body scanners. The radial field of view (FOV) for these scanners is approximately 24 and 55 cm respectively, as shown in Fig. 39-13. Typical scanners have between 500 and 800 detectors per ring. A detector module consists of *BGO scintillators* organized into a matrix (6 × 6, 7 × 8, or 8 × 8) of small BGO cubes (3 to 6 mm long, 6 mm wide, and 20 to 30 mm deep) which are coupled to photomultiplier tubes. Individual tubes are no longer mated to single scintillator crystals, as in the first PET scanners, but are arranged in an overlapping fashion similar to NaI crystals and PMTs in conventional gamma cameras. Early scanners had only a single ring of detectors. Current tomographs are constructed of 18 to 24 rings. Not only are coincidence counts collected for detector pairs within each ring (direct-plane information), but data are also collected between adjacent rings (cross-plane information) as shown in Fig. 39-14. Therefore, 35 to 47 tomographic slices (2 × number of rings - 1) can be acquired simultaneously for 18- to 24-ring tomographs which have a total of 10,000 to 20,000 detectors (BGO crystals). Fig. 39-14 schematically shows the organization of rings.

The concept of PET scanner resolution can be explained using a bicycle wheel as an example. The highest density of spokes is located at the hub. In the case of PET, *rays* between detectors correspond to the bicycle spokes. At the rim of the wheel, the density of spokes is reduced, and the number of detector rays is also reduced. That is why the imaging field of view for these scanners is approximately one-third the distance from one detector face to the opposite detector face. Adequate ray density for the best resolution for image reconstruction is achieved only within this field of view.

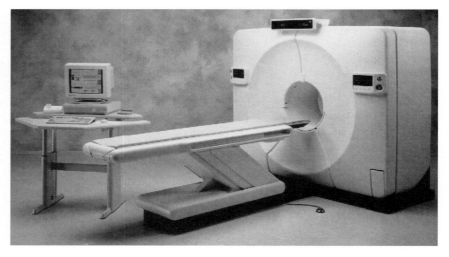

Fig. 39-12. Typical whole-body PET scanner. The bed is capable of moving in and out of the scanner to measure the distribution of PET radiopharmaceuticals throughout the body and adjusts to a very low position for easy patient access. Sophisticated computer workstations are required to view and analyze data.

(Courtesy of GE Medical Systems.)

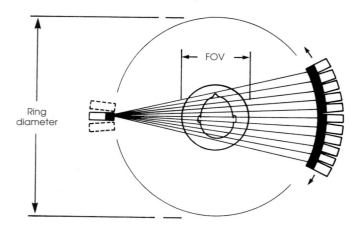

Fig. 39-13. Detector arrangement in neurologic PET ring (head-only scanner). Coincidences from opposed detector pairs at the edge of the ring are measured for each ray shown (lines between detectors). The useful FOV is delineated by the central circle.

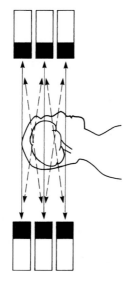

Fig. 39-14. A side view schematic of a multi-ring PET tomograph. Solid black squares indicate the scintillator matrix. Photomultiplier tubes are attached to the rear of the scintillators. Solid lines indicate the direct planes and dashed lines depict the cross-planes. The X formed by the pair of cross-planes forms a data-plane located between direct-planes.

The resolution within the image plane for PET scanners is between 4 and 6 mm FWHM (full width at half maximum). Thus an image of a point source of radioactivity appears to be 4 to 6 mm wide at one-half the maximum intensity of the source image. The theoretical limit of resolution for PET tomographs is 1 to 2 mm FWHM and depends on the finite range of the positron in tissue for the particular radionuclide used. The resolution between tomographic planes or slices, that is, along the z axis (axis parallel to the PET scanner couch), is between 5 and 6 mm FWHM.

Further improvements in image resolution require that the number of rays between detectors be increased. This implies that the number of detectors in the tomograph must be increased. On some devices now being constructed, well over 1,000 detectors are being installed per ring. Of course, as the number of detectors in the tomograph increases, so does the complexity of acquiring and cataloging each annihilation event. The electronics systems, wiring, and heat loads generated from the associated electronics also increase. Previously, methods for improving resolution employed rotation of the detector array with respect to the patient.

This achieved an increase in the number of rays used for image reconstruction. However, the complexity of detector rotation and the additional costs to engineer these systems limited the usefulness of this technique. Therefore, increasing the number of detectors in the ring is the most effective way to improve image resolution, and it does so without detector motion.

Not all photons emitted from the patient can be detected. Some of the pairs of 0.511 MeV photons from the positron annihilation impinge on detectors in the tomograph ring and are detected; most do not. Recall that the photon pairs are emitted 180 degrees from each other. The emission process is isotropic, which means that the gamma rays are emitted with equal probability in all directions so that only a small fraction (10%) of the total number of photons emitted from the patient actually strike the tomograph detectors (Fig. 39-15).

Originally, PET scanners used ray information only from the nearest adjacent planes (cross-plane on either side of direct-plane or ring). However, with improvements in software reconstruction techniques, the second, third, fourth, and even fifth adjacent plane can be used to produce three-dimensional PET images. PET scanner *sensitivity* is greatly increased by this technique. Hence, the injected dose of radiopharmaceutical can be significantly reduced (50 to 90% less radioactivity given) to yield equivalent quality PET images compared with images obtained from the original dose levels. If the dose is only moderately reduced (50%), then the total imaging time can be decreased and the overall patient throughput improved.

When pairs of photons are detected, they are counted as valid events, i.e., true positron annihilation, if and only if they appear at the detectors within the resolving time for the coincidence electronics. For many PET tomographs, this is typically 8 to 12 nanoseconds. If one photon is detected and no other photon is observed during that time window, the original event is discarded. This is essentially electronic collimation; hence, no conventional lead collimators are used in PET scanners. These detector systems must also be able to handle very high count rates with minimal deadtime losses.

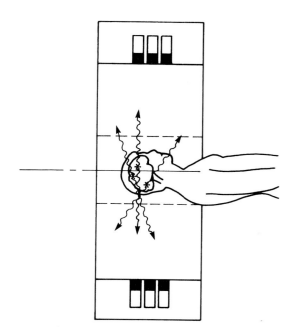

Fig. 39-15. Only 10% of the total number of emitted photons from the patient are capable of being detected in a whole body tomograph (ring diameter = 100 cm). This is increased to 17% for a head tomograph (ring diameter = 60 cm). In both cases, the z-axis coverage is 10 cm. The actual number of detected coincidences is reduced, since the detector efficiency is less than 100% (typically 30%).

For PET procedures, data acquisition is not limited to just the tomographic count rates. To create *quantitative* parametric images of glucose metabolism, for example, the blood concentrations of the radiopharmaceutical must be measured. This is accomplished in one of the following ways: (1) by discrete or continuous arterial sampling, (2) by discrete or continuous venous sampling, or (3) by *region of interest (ROI)* analysis of major arterial vessels observed in reconstructed tomographic images. For arterial sampling, an indwelling catheter is placed in the radial artery. Arterial blood pressure forces blood out of the catheter when needed for collection and radioactivity measurement. For venous sampling, blood is withdrawn through an indwelling venous catheter. However, to obtain *arterialized venous blood,* the hand must be heated to between 40 and 42°F (8°C). In this situation arterial blood is shunted directly to the venous system. If plasma radioactivity is required while collecting discrete samples, the red blood cells are separated from whole blood by centrifugation and the radioactivity concentration within plasma is determined by discrete sample counting in a gamma well counter. Continuous counting is performed on whole blood by directing blood through a radiation detector via small bore tubing and a peristaltic pump. In ROI analysis, the arterial blood curve is generated directly from each image of a multiple frame time series PET scan. An ROI is placed around an arterial vessel visualized in the PET images. The average number of counts for the ROI from each frame is plotted against time. Actual blood sampling is not usually required for ROI analysis.

A typical set of curves is given in Fig. 39-16. Curves created from plasma data, as well as other information (e.g., nonradioactive plasma glucose level), is supplied to a mathematical model that appropriately describes the physiological process being measured. Parametric or functional images are created by applying the model to the original PET data.

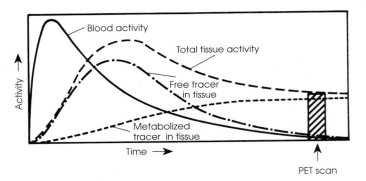

Fig. 39-16. Decay-corrected radioactivity curves for ^{18}F-FDG in brain tissue and blood (plasma). Injection occurs at the origin. The blood activity rapidly peaks after the injection. The metabolized tracer ((^{18}F)-FDG-6-PO$_4$) slowly accumulates in tissue. Typical static PET scanning occurs after an incorporation time of 40 to 60 minutes in which the uptake of ^{18}F-FDG is balanced with the slow washout of the labeled metabolite.

IMAGE RECONSTRUCTION AND IMAGE PROCESSING

Images are created from raw data collected as rays corresponding to each detected annihilation event. A typical image (one slice) has 128×128 or 256×256 picture elements, or pixels. Each pixel represents 2 bytes of information. The image storage requirement of a PET study can be computed by the following: (image size)$^2 \times$ (2 bytes) $\times$ (number of slices) $\times$ (number of frames in a dynamic scan). For a LCBF study, the calculated storage is (128 pixels)$^2 \times$ (2 bytes) $\times$ (47 slices) $\times$ (10 frames) = 15 MB (megabytes). When multiple injections are contemplated for test/retest studies, the image storage requirements increase further.

An FOV of 15 to 20 cm (axial direction) is required to adequately encompass the entire volume of the brain from the top of the cerebral cortex to the base of the cerebellum. Array processors are used to perform the filtered backprojection reconstruction that converts the raw sinogram data into PET images. This technique is similar to that employed for CT image reconstruction.

The disintegration of radionuclides follows Poisson statistics. As a result of this random process, photons from the different annihilation events may strike the tomograph detectors simultaneously. This is registered as a true event because it occurs within the coincidence time window. A simple approximation allows for the subtraction of the random events after image acquisition and is based on the individual count rates for each detector and the coincidence resolving time (8 to 12 nanoseconds) of the tomograph electronics.

Photons traversing biologic tissues undergo absorption and scatter. An attenuation correction is applied to account for those photons that should have been detected but were not, as shown in Fig. 39-17. The correction is based on a transmission scan acquired with a radioactive rod or pin source of ^{68}Ge (271 day half-life) that circumscribes under computer control the portion of the patient's body within the PET scanner. For brain studies, another attenuation correction technique is used, but it is less accurate. It approximates the outline of the skull with an ellipse and calculates the attenuation of photons based on the dimensions of the ellipse. A transmission scan measures the actual attenuation of photons based on the true cross-sectional area of head. The *attenuation coefficient* for 0.511 MeV photons in tissue is 0.096 cm^2/gm. In either case, the coincidence data for each image plane are multiplied by a matrix of numerical values within the boundaries of the skull to correct the observed count rates to the true count rates for losses that result from attenuation.

Count rates from the detectors are also corrected for deadtime losses. At high-count rates the detector electronics cannot process every event; therefore some of these events are lost. By measuring the tomograph response to known input count rates, empirical formulations for the losses are determined and applied to the image data.

Not every detector in the system responds exactly the same way to a uniform distribution of radioactivity. A calibration scan is performed to measure the count rate for each detector in the system from a homogenous source. A correction mask is created from this calibration scan and the raw data are multiplied by this mask to yield a uniform count-rate image from the homogenous (flood) source. This correction is then applied to all PET images.

Finally, the corrected images and the blood data are used as input to the physiologic model to create a parametric image. Each pixel in the parametric image represents a physiologic value for that volume of brain tissue. As an example, recall that a ^{18}F-FDG image represents local glucose metabolism of the brain (LCMRG). The pixel will contain a number between 0.0 and approximately 6 in units of mg of glucose utilization per minute per 100 gm of brain tissue. For LCBF, each pixel represents blood flow in that particular volume of brain and possesses a value between 0.0 and 150 in units of ml of blood flow per minute per 100 grams of brain tissue.

Once the raw data are converted to functional images, regions of interest (ROI) are drawn on the images. Average values of counts/area or counts/pixel are determined for each ROI. The data analysis task then is to correlate the physiologic value obtained from the PET image data of the patient to normative data. Intrinsically, biologic parameters have approximately a 15% standard deviation. To observe a true intersubject difference, variations in LCBF and LCMRG values must be greater than 15%. Intrasubject variability from PET studies has been shown to be about 7%. Therefore if a research or clinical protocol can be designed so that the patient serves as his or her own control, greater reliability and reduced errors are achieved.

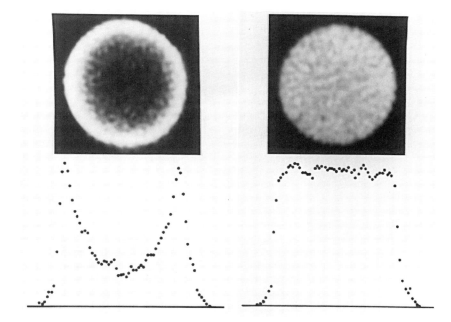

Fig. 39-17. Uncorrected image of a phantom homogeneously filled with a water-soluble PET nuclide of ^{68}Ga or ^{18}F − (left) versus an attenuation-corrected image (right). Cross-sectional cuts through the center of each image are shown in the lower panels. The attenuation correction for the 20-cm-diameter phantom shown can be as large as 70% in the center of the object.

Clinical Studies

PET imaging is relatively costly. It is best used for answering complex questions that involve tissue function (Figs. 39-18 and 39-19). It is unlikely that PET will be used as a broad-based clinical screening tool since the actual imaging time for PET studies is long (1 to 3 hours) compared with other imaging procedures.

It is important, then, that patients and normal volunteers be selected according to very stringent protocols. Before each imaging procedure, subjects typically receive a brief physical examination and laboratory blood tests. External landmarks (specifically, for brain imaging the head diameter and distance from the top of the head to an imaginary line passing from the lateral canthus of the eye to the meatus of the ear, or *CM line*) are measured. For quantitative studies, a radial artery is catheterized to obtain arterial blood samples, or heated hand techniques are used to obtain arterialized venous blood. Blood curves are collected and used as input functions for the physiologic models. Patients are oriented in the scanner in the supine position, either head or feet first.

Injection of the appropriate radiopharmaceutical by intravenous bolus, infusion, or a combination of these two techniques is performed. For dynamic studies, the injection is synchronized with the start of imaging. For quantitative studies, blood samples are collected according to established protocols. For ^{18}F-FDG studies, a decay-corrected plasma activity curve is constructed from blood samples (approximately 20×1 ml samples) acquired over the entire imaging procedure (1 to 1.5 hours) using discrete blood sampling techniques. For ^{15}O-H$_2$O studies, arterial samples are continuously withdrawn at a rate of 5 to 7 ml/minute for 2 minutes using a peristaltic pump. Radioactivity detectors measure whole blood ^{15}O-H$_2$O concentration while the blood is being withdrawn. As much as 200 to 300 ml of blood may be drawn over a long study (5 to 8 injections of ^{15}O-H$_2$O).

^{18}F-FDG studies require a 40- to 60-minute incorporation period of the radiopharmaceutical after which 5- to 25-minute static scans for each bed position are acquired to measure the almost static distribution of ^{18}F-FDG glucose metabolism in tissue. The scanning procedure including incorporation period takes about 1.5 to 2.5 hours for a single injection of ^{18}F-FDG. The long half-life of ^{18}F (109.8 minutes) precludes multiple injections on the same day in most cases. Whole-body images are created by piecing together PET data acquired from several scans as the bed automatically moves out of the PET scanner. For safety reasons, bed operation is outward from the scanner when controlled by the computer in order to avoid contact between the PET scanner opening and the patient's body (head, arms, or shoulders).

For ^{15}O-H$_2$O LCBF studies, a separate injection is necessary for each axial FOV (35 to 47 slices). Often for research studies, several injections are administered and data are collected which show the differences in brain blood flow between each injection. The scanning procedure takes only 40 seconds to 6 minutes for blood flow studies. From one injection to the next, a total of 10 to 15 minutes is required for the ^{15}O radioactivity to reach low enough levels to repeat the study.

After the scanning procedures, the catheters are removed and the patient is permitted to leave the facility. There is little residual radioactivity remaining in the patient after ^{18}F-FDG imaging, especially after voiding, and practically none after ^{15}O-H$_2$O studies. Patients may immediately resume normal activities.

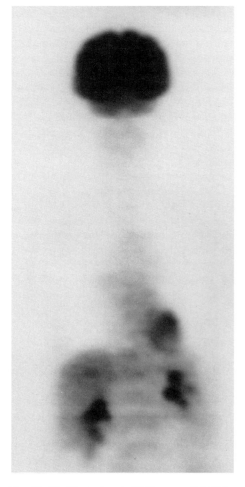

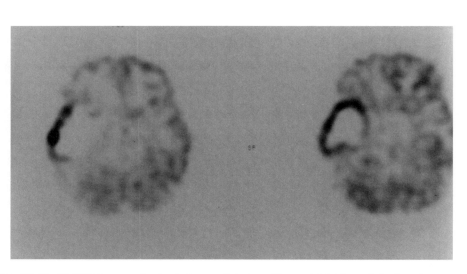

Fig. 39-18. ^{18}F-FDG image of a brain tumor. Exterior of tumor is highly metabolic, whereas the interior is necrotic.

Fig. 39-19. Whole-body PET image. ^{18}F-FDG image of tumor metastases. Normal uptake of ^{18}F-FDG is observed in brain, heart, and bladder.

Table 39-5. LCMRG* and LCBF† rates in normal subjects

	Cerebellum	Temporal cortex	Visual cortex	Left hemisphere	Right hemisphere	Whole brain
LCMRG	4.7	5.1	6.6	4.6	4.5	4.6
LCBF	60.8	65.3	82.7	54.5	55.3	54.8

*mg glucose utilization per minute per 100 gm tissue.
†ml flow per minute per 100 gm tissue.

NORMAL SUBJECTS

Normal volunteers studied using PET provide a database of normal values for comparison with patient data. Table 39-5 depicts local cerebral glucose metabolic rates and local cerebral blood flow rates for normal subjects. Three primary areas of brain LCMRG and LCBF are presented. The first area is associated with control and coordination of voluntary muscle movements (cerebellum), the second reflects the intact gray matter cortical regions (temporal cortex), which may be related to such functions as memory and fine motor movements, and the last region is responsible for decoding visual images (primary visual cortex). In virtually all cases the visual cortex depicts the highest glucose utilization rates and the cerebellum the lowest metabolic rates. The hemispheric averages do not differ significantly from each other nor do they differ from the cerebellar values.

Future Studies

Considerable research has been conducted to study brain function with radiopharmaceuticals to measure metabolism, flow, and receptor density. PET scanners have been specifically designed to optimally acquire data from the brain, heart, lung, organ transplants, and tumors. As the technology matures, even greater emphasis will be placed on expanding clinical and research investigation of these tissues and organ systems.

Summary

PET is a very complex diagnostic imaging procedure. Consequently, it is both a clinical tool and a research tool. It involves the multidisciplinary support of the physician, physicist, physiologist, chemist, engineer, and radiographer. PET permits the investigator to peer into the working human body to examine numerous biologic parameters without disturbing the normal equilibrium physiology. It measures regional function that cannot be determined by any other means including CT and MRI imaging.

Current PET studies involve PET imaging of patients with epilepsy, Huntington's disease, stroke, schizophrenia, brain tumors, Alzheimer's disease, and other disorders of the brain. PET studies of the heart are providing routine diagnostic information on patients with coronary artery disease by identifying viable myocardium for revascularization. Other areas of PET scanning include determination of organ transplant function, tumor imaging, effects of therapeutic drug regimens, and differentiation of necrosis from viable tumor. Our understanding of physiology will increase as the technology advances, yielding higher resolution instruments, new radiopharmaceuticals, and improved analysis of PET data.

Definition of Terms

analog PET radiopharmaceutical biochemically equivalent to a naturally occurring compound in the body.

annihilation Total transformation of matter into energy. Occurs after the antimatter positron collides with an electron. Two photons are created; each equals the rest mass of the individual particles.

arterialized venous blood Arterial blood passed directly to the venous system by shunts in the capillary system by heating surface veins to between 40 and 42°F (8°C). Blood gases from the vein under these conditions reflect near arterial levels of pO_2, pCO_2, and pH.

attenuation coefficient A number that represents the statistical reduction in photons that exit a material (N) from the value that entered (N_o) the material. The reduced flux is the result of scatter and absorption, which can be expressed in the following equation: $N = N_o e^{-\mu \chi}$ where μ is the attenuation coefficient and χ is the distance traversed by the photons.

BGO scintillator Bismuth Germanate scintillator with an efficiency twice that of NaI. BGO is used in nearly all commercially produced PET scanners.

CM line Canthomeatal line defined by an imaginary line drawn between the lateral canthus of the eye and meatus of the ear.

cyclotron Cyclic particle accelerator used to increase the kinetic energy of nuclei such as protons and deuterons so that radioactive materials may be produced from the resultant nuclear reactions of the ions on stable materials.

detector Device that is a combination of a scintillator and photomultiplier tube. It is used to detect x rays and gamma rays.

^{18}F-FDG Radioactive analog of naturally available glucose. It follows the same biochemical pathways as glucose but is not totally metabolized to CO_2 and H_2O as is glucose.

gamma ray Electromagnetic radiation or photon emitted from the decay of a radioactive nucleus. Its energy is expressed in the equivalent energy of the photon in units of electron volts (eV) or millions of electron volts (MeV).

homeostasis State of equilibrium of the body's internal environment.

image coregistration Computer technique that permits realignment of images acquired from different modalities, which have different orientations and magnifications, so that each possesses the same orientation and size. The images can then be overlaid one on the other in order to demonstrate similarities and differences between the images.

Definition of terms

289

kinetics Movement of materials into, out of, and through biological spaces. A mathematical expression is often used to describe and quantify how substances traverse membranes or participate in biochemical reactions.

local cerebral blood flow (LCBF) Description of the parametric image of blood flow through the brain. It is expressed in units of ml blood flow per minute per 100 gm brain tissue.

local metabolic rate of glucose utilization (LMRG) Units of mg glucose utilization per minute per 100 gm tissue. Used in conjunction with parametric images of tissues such as brain, heart, or tumor. LCMRG is specific to brain and corresponds to the local cerebral metabolic rate of glucose utilization.

magnetic resonance imaging (MRI) Technique of nuclear magnetic resonance (NMR) as it is applied to medical imaging. Also abbreviated MR.

nuclear particle accelerator Device to produce radioactive material by accelerating ions (electrons, protons, deuterons, etc.) to high energies and projecting them towards stable materials. The list of accelerators includes linac, cyclotron, synchrotron, Van de Graaff accelerator, and betatron.

parametric image Image that relates anatomic position (the x and y position on an image) to a physiological parameter such as blood flow (image intensity or color). It may also be referred to as a "functional image." Parametric images contrast anatomical or structural images.

photomultiplier tube (PMT) Vacuum tube that transforms visible light photons into minute electron currents that are subsequently amplified by a factor of approximately 10^6. Typically the output current is proportional to the energy of the incident photon.

positron Positively charged particle emitted from neutron-deficient radioactive nuclei.

positron emission tomography (PET) Imaging technique that creates transaxial images of organ physiology from the simultaneous detection of positron annihilation photons.

quantitative Type of PET study in which the final images are not simply distributions of radioactivity, but rather correspond to units of capillary blood flow, glucose metabolism, receptor density, etc. Studies between individuals and repeat studies in the same individual permit comparison of pixel values on an absolute scale.

radioactivity concentration Amount of radioactivity per unit volume. It can be expressed in units of mCi/ml.

radioisotope Synonym for radioactive isotope. Any isotope that is unstable undergoes decay with the emission of characteristic radiation.

radiopharmaceutical Radioactive material that is inhaled, ingested, or injected into humans or animals. Synonymous with radiotracer.

radiotracer Synonym of radiopharmaceutical.

ray The imaginary line drawn between a pair of detectors in the PET scanner or between the x-ray source and detector in a CT scanner.

region of interest (ROI) Area that circumscribes a desired anatomic location on a PET image. Image processing systems permit drawing of ROIs on images. The average parametric value is computed for all pixels within the ROI and returned to the radiographer.

resolution Smallest separation of two point sources of radioactivity that can be distinguished for PET or SPECT imaging. Highly attenuating materials are used for CT measurements and $CuSO_4$ for MRI measurements of resolution instead of radioactivity.

scintillator Material either organic or inorganic that transforms high-energy photons such as x rays or gamma rays into visible or near visible light (UV) photons for easy measurement.

sensitivity Ability to measure the total number of photons incident on a detector. In this case, the term is synonymous with efficiency. PET scanner sensitivity is often reported in units of counts/sec/μCi/cc in a 20-cm-diameter phantom homogeneously filled with ^{18}F, ^{68}Ge, or ^{68}Ga.

SPECT Single photon emission computed tomography. A nuclear medicine scanning procedure that measures conventional single photon gamma emissions (^{99m}Tc) with a specially designed rotating gamma camera.

target Device used to contain stable materials and subsequent radioactive materials during bombardment by high-energy nuclei from a cyclotron or other particle accelerator. The term is also applied to the material inside the device, which may be solid, liquid, or gaseous.

transmission scan Type of PET scan that is equivalent to a low-resolution CT scan. Attenuation is determined by rotating a rod of radioactive ^{68}Ge around the subject. Photons that traverse the subject either impinge on a detector and are registered as valid counts or are attenuated (absorbed or scattered). The ratio of counts with and without the attenuating tissue in place provides the factors to correct PET scans for the loss of counts from attenuation of the 0.511 MeV photons.

SELECTED BIBLIOGRAPHY

Barnes WE, editor: Basic physics of radiotracers, vols I and II, Boca Raton, Fla, 1983, CRC Press.

Bergmann SR and Sobel BE, editors: Positron emission tomography of the heart, Mount Kisco, New York, 1992, Futura Publishing Company.

Bergstrom M et al: Correction for scattered radiation in a ring detector positron camera by integral transformation of the projections, J Comput Assist Tomogr 7:42-50, 1983.

Burns HD et al: (3-N-[^{11}C] Methyl) Spiperone, a ligand binding to dopamine receptors: radiochemical synthesis and biodistribution studies in mice, J Nucl Med 25:1222-1227, 1984.

Clark JC et al: Short-lived radioactive gases for clinical use, Boston, 1975, Butterworth Publishers.

Frackowiak RSJ et al: Quantitative measurement of cerebral blood flow and oxygen metabolism in man using ^{15}O and positron emission tomography: theory, procedure and normal values, J Comput Assist Tomogr 4:727-736, 1980.

Freedman GS, editor: Tomographic imaging in nuclear medicine, New York, 1973, The Society of Nuclear Medicine.

Heiss WD et al: Regional kinetic constants and cerebral metabolic rate for glucose in normal human volunteers determined by dynamic positron emission tomography of [^{18}F]-2-fluoro-2-deoxy-D-glucose, J Cereb Blood Flow Metab 4:212-223, 1984.

Helus F, editor: Radionuclides production, vols I and II, Boca Raton, Fla, 1983, CRC Press.

Hendee WR: The physical principles of computed tomography, Boston, 1983, Little, Brown & Co.

Herman TG, editor: Image reconstruction from projections—implementation and applications, New York, 1979, Springer-Verlag New York.

Hoffman EJ et al: Quantitation in positron emission computed tomography: 1. Effect of object size, J Comput Assist Tomogr 3:299-308, 1979.

Hubner KF et al: Clinical positron emission tomography, St Louis, 1992, Mosby.

Livingood JJ: Principles of cyclic particle accelerators, Princeton, NJ, 1961, D Van Nostrand Company.

Mazziotta JC et al: Tomographic mapping of human cerebral metabolism: normal unstimulated state, Neurology 31:503-516, 1981.

Minton MA et al: Brain oxygen utilization measured with 0-15 radiotracers and positron emission tomography, J Nucl Med 25:177-187, 1984.

Phelps ME et al: Tomographic measurements of local cerebral glucose metabolic rate in humans with (F-18)-2-fluoro-2-deoxy-D-glucose: validation of method, Ann Neurol 6:371-388, 1979.

Reivich M et al: The [^{18}F]Fluorodeoxyglucose method for the measurement of local cerebral glucose utilization in man, Circ Res 44:127-137, 1979.

Riggs DS: The mathematical approach to physiological problems, Cambridge, Mass, 1963, Williams & Wilkins.

Robertson JS, editor: Compartmental distribution of radiotracers, Boca Raton, Fla, 1983, CRC Press.

Schelbert HR et al: Regional myocardial perfusion assessed with N-13 labeled ammonia and positron emission computerized axial tomography, Am J Cardiol 43:209-218, 1979.

Sokoloff L et al: The ^{14}C-deoxyglucose method for the measurement of local cerebral glucose utilization: theory, procedure and normal values in conscious and anesthetized albino rats, J Neurochem 28:897-916, 1977.

Chapter 40

RADIATION ONCOLOGY

CHARLES H. MARSCHKE

Historical development
Theory
Clinical applications
Future trends
Summary

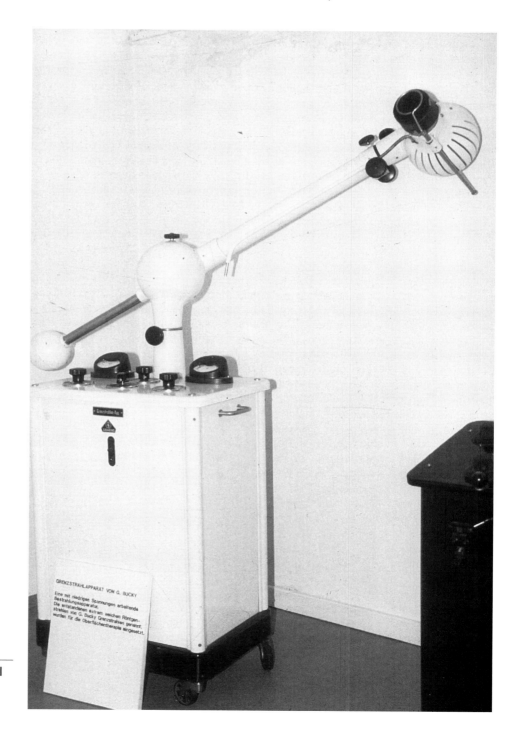

A Grenz x-ray device for superficial therapy treatments from approximately 1940.

Radiation oncology,* radiation therapy, or radiotherapy involves the treatment of cancerous tumors or lesions by the precise application of ionizing radiation. The radiation is administered by a *radiation therapist* under the supervision of a *radiation oncologist,* a physician skilled in the art of applying radiation in the treatment of malignant disease.

Different specialists are routinely consulted in virtually all cases involving selection of a best plan of treatment for the patient. The individuals often consulted are specialists in tumor growth, spread, and response to treatment. Other specialists are usually the surgical and medical *oncologists.* As the name implies, the surgical oncologist is a surgeon who deals primarily with cancer patients. The medical oncologist is usually a physician certified in internal medicine who has gained additional expertise in the application of chemical agents in the treatment of cancer.

This coordinated "team approach" to the diagnosis, care, and treatment of cancer patients is essential to ensure the best possible therapeutic results.

Although radiation oncology may be used as the only method of treatment for malignant disease, a more common approach is to use radiation oncology in conjunction with surgery, chemotherapy, or a combination of the two. Some patients may be treated by only surgery or chemotherapy; however, approximately 70% of all diagnosed cancer patients are treated with radiation. The choice of treatment involves consideration of a number of patient variables such as the patient's overall physical and emotional condition, the histologic type of the disease, and the extent and anatomic position of the tumor. If a tumor is small and its margins are well defined, a surgical approach alone may be prescribed. On the other hand, if the disease is systemic, a chemotherapeutic approach may be chosen. Most tumors, however, exhibit degrees of size, invasion, and spread and require variations in the treatment approach that in all likelihood will include radiation oncology as an adjunct to or in conjunction with surgery or chemotherapy. These limitations determine the goal of treatment—definitive, palliation, or as an adjunct to surgery.

*All italicized terms are defined at the end of this chapter.

Once the patient has been fully evaluated and radiation oncology chosen as the form of treatment, the optimum therapeutic approach must be determined. Options include *teletherapy* versus *brachytherapy,* single-field versus multifield irradiation, temporary or permanent implant, particulate versus nonparticulate irradiation, and *fractionated* versus *protracted* dose application. Whatever treatment approach or regimen is chosen, a number of variables must be considered, and the opportunities for error are many. The radiation therapist participates in this planning process and is responsible for administering and keeping accurate records of the dose and monitoring the patient's physical and emotional well-being once the patient has begun the treatment schedule. The therapist should have an understanding of *oncology,* radiobiology, radiation physics, anatomy, mathematics, pathology, communication skills, *dosimetry,* and methods of patient care.

This chapter provides an overview of some of the aforementioned subject areas to enable the reader to have a greater understanding of the therapeutic approach. A complete and effective treatment plan is dependent on precise patient evaluation and diagnosis, excellent patient care, and meticulous attention to the patient setup throughout the course of treatment. The bibliography includes a list of references for further study.

Historical Development

Historically, ionizing radiation was applied to obtain a radiographic image of an individual's internal anatomy for diagnostic purposes. The resulting image depended on many variables, including the energy of the beam, processing techniques, the material on which the image was recorded, and most importantly, the amount of energy absorbed by the various organs of the body. This transfer of energy from the beam of radiation to the biologic system and the observation of the effects of this interaction became the foundation of radiation oncology.

Two of the most obvious, and sometimes immediate, biologic effects observed during the early diagnostic procedures were loss of hair (epilation) and a reddening of the patient's skin (erythema). Epilation and erythema resulted primarily from the great amount of energy absorbed by the skin of the patient during the radiographic procedure. These short-term radiation-induced effects afforded radiographic practitioners an opportunity to expand the use of radiation to treat conditions ranging from relatively benign maladies such as hypertrichosis (excessive hair), acne, and boils to grotesque and malignant diseases such as lupus vulgaris and skin cancer.

The first reported application of ionizing radiation to a patient for the treatment of a more in-depth lesion was begun on January 29, 1896, by Dr. Émile H. Grubbé (Table 40-1). Dr. Grubbé is reported to

Table 40-1. Time line of development of radiation therapy

Dates	Persons	Events
1895	W.C. Roentgen	Discovery of x-rays
1896	Ē. Grubbé	First use of ionizing radiation in treatment of cancer
	A.H. Becquerel	Discovery of radioactive emissions by uranium compounds
1898	M. and P. Curie	Discovery of radium
1902	C.E. Skinner	First documented case of cancer "cure" using ionizing radiation
1906	J. Bergonié and L. Tribondeau	Postulation of first law of radiosensitivity
1932	E.O. Lawrence	Invention of cyclotron
1934	F. Joliot and I. Joliot-Curie	Production of artificial radioactivity
1939	E.O. Lawrence and R.S. Stone	Treatment of cancer patient with neutron beam from cyclotron
1940	D.W. Kerst	Construction of betatron
1951		Installation of first cobalt 60 teletherapy units
1952		Installation of first linear accelerator (Hammersmith Hospital, London)

have irradiated for therapeutic purposes a woman with carcinoma of the left breast. This event occurred only 3 months after the discovery of x rays in November 1895 by Dr. W.C. Roentgen. Although Dr. Grubbé neither expected nor observed any dramatic results from irradiation of the patient, the event is significant simply because it occurred.

The first reported case of a patient being treated with ionizing radiation and considered to have been *cured* was performed by Dr. Clarence E. Skinner of New Haven, Connecticut, in January 1902. Dr. Skinner treated a woman who had a diagnosed malignant fibrosarcoma. During the next 2 years and 3 months the woman received a total of 136 applications of the x rays. In April 1909, 7 years after the initial application of the radiation, the woman was free of disease and considered cured.

As more and more data were collected, the interest in radiation therapy grew. More sophisticated equipment, a greater understanding of the effects of ionizing radiation, an appreciation for time-dose relationships, and a number of other related medical breakthroughs gave impetus to the interest in radiation therapy that led to the evolution of a distinct medical specialty.

Theory

The biologic effectiveness of ionizing radiation in living tissue is dependent partially on the amount of energy that is deposited within the tissue and partially on the condition of the biologic system. The terms used to describe this relationship are "linear energy transfer" (LET) and "relative biologic effectiveness" (RBE).

LET values are expressed in thousands of electron volts deposited per micron of tissue (keV/μm) and will vary, of course, depending on the type of radiation being considered. Particles, because of their mass and possible charge, tend to interact more readily with the material through which they are passing and therefore have a greater LET value. As an example, a 5-meV alpha particle has an LET value of 100 keV/μm in tissue. Nonparticulate radiations such as 250-kVp x rays and 1.2-meV gamma rays have much lower LET values: 1.5 and 0.3 respectively.

RBE values are determined by calculating the ratio of the dose from a standard beam of radiation to the dose required of the radiation beam in question to produce a similar biologic effect. The standard beam of radiation is 250-kV x rays, and the ratio is set up as follows:

$$RBE = \frac{\text{Standard beam dose to obtain effect}}{\substack{\text{Similar effect using beam} \\ \text{in question}}}$$

Table 40-2. RBE and LET values for certain forms of radiation

Radiation	RBE	LET
250-keV x-rays	1.0	1.5
^{60}Co gamma rays	0.85	0.3
14-meV neutrons	12.0	75.0
5-meV alpha particles	20.0	100.0

It is now accepted that, as the LET increases, so too will the RBE. Some RBE and LET values are listed in Table 40-2.

The effectiveness of ionizing radiation on a biologic system depends not only on the amount of radiation deposited but also on the state of the biologic system. One of the first laws of radiation biology, postulated by Bergonié and Tribondeau, stated in essence that the *radiosensitivity* of a tissue is dependent on the number of *undifferentiated* cells in the tissue, the degree of mitotic activity of the tissue, and the length of time that cells of the tissue remain in active proliferation. Although exceptions exist, the preceding is true in most tissues. The primary target of ionizing radiation is the DNA molecule, and the human cell is most radiosensitive during mitosis. Current research tends to indicate that all cells are equally radio-"sensitive," however the manifestation of the radiation injury occurs at different time frames (i.e., acute versus late effects).

Because tissue cells are comprised primarily of water, most of the ionizing interactions occur with water molecules. These events are called indirect effects and result in the formation of free radicals such as OH, H, and HO$_2$. These highly reactive free radicals may recombine, resulting in no biologic effect whatsoever, or they may combine with other atoms and molecules to produce biochemical changes that may be deleterious to the cell. The possibility also exists that the radiation may interact with an organic molecule or atom, which may result in the inactivation of the cell; this reaction is called the "direct effect." Because ionizing radiation is nonspecific—i.e., it will interact with normal cells as readily as with tumor cells—it is obvious that cellular damage will occur in both normal and abnormal tissue. The deleterious effects, however, will be greater in the abnormal cells because a greater percentage of the abnormal cells are undergoing mitosis; they also tend to be more poorly differentiated. In addition, normal cells have a greater capability for repairing sublethal damage than do tumor cells. Because of these reasons, greater cell damage will occur to abnormal than to normal cells for any given increment of dose. The effects of the interactions in either normal or tumor cells may be expressed in a number of ways:

1. Loss of reproductive ability
2. Metabolic changes
3. Cell transformation
4. Acceleration of the aging process
5. Cell mutation

Certainly the greater the number of interactions that occur, the greater the possibility of cell death.

The preceding information leads to a categorization of tumors according to their radiosensitivity:

1. Very radiosensitive
   a. Gonadal germ cell tumors (seminoma of testis, dysgerminoma of ovary)
   b. Lymphoproliferative tumors (Hodgkin's disease, lymphoma)
   c. Embryonal tumors (Wilms' tumor of kidney, retinoblastoma)
2. Moderately radiosensitive
   a. Epithelial tumors (squamous and basal cell carcinomas of skin)
   b. Glandular tumors (adenocarcinoma of prostate)
3. Relatively radioresistant
   a. Mesenchymal tumors (sarcomas of bone, connective tissue, and muscle)
   b. Nerve tumors (glioma, melanoma)

Although many of the concepts originating in the laboratory have little practical application, they are beginning to influence the selection of treatment modalities and techniques of radiation oncology. The physician's understanding of cellular function and the effects of radiation on the cell have initiated research and interest in using drugs, or simply oxygen, to enhance the effectiveness of the radiation.

CANCER

Cancer has yet to be precisely defined; however, a number of attempts, such as the following, have been made:

1. Cells in which the normal growth-controlling mechanism is altered, permitting progressive growth
2. A group of diseases of unknown causes that occur in all human and animal populations and arise in all tissues that are composed of potentially dividing cells
3. A disease of tissue organization
4. A genetic disease of somatic cells resulting from a mutation of a previously normal cell into a new cell of enduring malignancy
5. So-called spontaneous autoaggressive disease of a tissue initiated by random gene mutation in a stem cell

Although the number of definitions may indicate confusion, some basic facts are known about cancer:

1. Cancers can arise from cells that have the ability to proliferate.
2. Tumor cells may mature inadequately and may be spoken of as *"anaplastic"* or "dedifferentiated."
3. Cancers may arise after a variety of stimuli (chemical, physical, or viral) but usually only after a prolonged latent period.
4. Cancer cells may lie dormant for prolonged periods.
5. No distinctive ultrastructural or biochemical difference between a cancer and a normal cell has been positively identified.
6. A few cancers regress spontaneously.

More than 300 types of cancers have been recognized and defined histologically, and the degrees of variation within a single tumor type can be infinite. Finally, the physiologic, immunologic, and indeed the entire physical condition of the host will play an important part in the prevention or development of a cancer.

Malignant tumors, or cancers, are cells that have been influenced by a *carcinogen* to produce abnormal and uncontrolled growth. If the tumor is allowed to progress untreated, it will most likely result in the death of the host. The growth or spread *(metastasis)* of a malignant tumor is accomplished by invasion of the tumor into adjacent tissue and permeation of cancer cells into the blood or lymph vessels. The size of the tumor, its depth of penetration, whether it has invaded the lumina of the blood of lymph vessels, and whether it has metastasized determine the curability of the cancer.

Although cancers may arise in any human tissue, they are usually categorized under six general headings according to their tissue or origin, as in the following examples:

Tissue of origin	Type of tumor
Epithelium	
Surface epithelium	Carcinoma
Glandular epithelium	Adenocarcinoma
Connective tissue	
Bone	Osteosarcoma
Fat	Liposarcoma
Lymphoreticular-	
Hematopoietic tissue	
Lymph nodes	Lymphoma
Plasma cells	Multiple myeloma
Erythrocytic tissue	Erythroleukemia
Nerve tissue	
Glial tissue	Glioma
Neuroectoderm	Neuroblastoma
Tumors of more than	
one tissue	
Embryonic kidney	Nephroblastoma
Tumors that do not fit	
into above catego-	
ries	
Testis	Seminoma
Thymus	Thymoma

To facilitate the exchange of patient information from one physician to another, a system of classifying tumors based on anatomic and histologic considerations was designed by the International Union Against Cancer (UICC) and the American Joint Committee for the Cancer Staging and End Results Reporting (AJC). The system designed was the "TNM" classification (Table 40-3), which describes a tumor according to (1) the size of the primary lesion, (2) the involvement of the regional lymph nodes, and (3) occurrence of metastasis.

Table 40-3. Application of the TNM classification system*

Classification	Description of tumor
$T_0N_0M_0$	Occult lesion; no evidence clinically
$T_1N_0M_0$	Small lesion confined to organ of origin with no evidence of vascular and lymphatic spread or metastasis
$T_2N_1M_0$	Tumor of less than 5 cm invading surrounding tissue and first-station lymph nodes but no evidence of metastasis
$T_3N_2M_0$	Extensive lesion greater than 5 cm with fixation to deeper structure and with bone and lymph invasion but no evidence of metastasis
$T_4N_3M_+$	More extensive lesion than above with distant metastasis

*Although variations of the TNM classification system exist, the general description of the tumor does not change, that is, a T_1 lesion is confined to the organ of origin regardless of whether it is 0.5 or 1.5 cm in diameter.

Because of the various types of tumors, their sizes, the degree of spread, and symptoms exhibited by the patient, a number of classification and staging techniques are available. All have been designed to assist in describing the extent of the tumor for the purpose of treatment and prognosis.

Effective treatment of a malignant tumor with ionizing radiation depends on (1) the extent of the disease at diagnosis, (2) the histologic type of the tumor, (3) the general well-being of the patient, (4) the location of the tumor, and (5) whether the tumor is *radiocurable*. The first three concerns have been dealt with briefly in this chapter; the last two, however, will be expanded before discussion of treatment planning.

To treat a tumor definitively requires that the tumor be located in a tissue that is more radioresistant than the tumor itself. The therapeutic ratio (TR) was designed to assist in the determination of whether a tumor could be treated for cure, taking into account the normal tissue tolerance dose and the tumor lethal dose:

$$TR = \frac{\text{Normal tissue tolerance dose}}{\text{Tumor tissue lethal dose}}$$

If the TR is less than 1, the chances of cure are much less likely than if the TR is greater than 1.

A tumor must have some degree of radiosensitivity to be considered for radiation treatment; however, radiosensitivity does not necessarily imply radiocurability. The characteristics that make a tumor radiosensitive, for example, fast growth and vascularity, also cause it to spread more rapidly, giving rise to a more extensive lesion (e.g., lymphosarcoma). This situation tends to compromise the treatment approach. Conversely, some tumors that have been classified as radioresistant, for instance, carcinoma of the tongue, may be considered radiocurable.

BASIC PHYSICS

As stated earlier, the effectiveness of radiation oncology is partially dependent on the amount of energy that is deposited within the *tumor volume* while at the same time minimizing the amount of energy deposited in the normal surrounding tissue. If available, a beam of radiation with high LET and resulting RBE values, as well as the ability to deliver a cancercidal dose to only the lesion no matter what its anatomic depth, would be appropriate to use. Although beams of this nature are not available at present, research is being conducted in this area of radiation physics. Until the ideal beam can be produced and supplied for therapeutic purposes, currently available beams must be applied so that a cancercidal dose can be deposited to the lesion with a limited amount of damage to the surrounding normal tissue.

Most radiation oncology departments have available some or all of the following units, the dose depositions of which are compared in Fig. 40-1:

1. 120 keV superficial x-ray unit for treating lesions on or very near the surface of the patient
2. 250 keV orthovoltage x-ray unit for moderately superficial tissues.
3. 4 to 35 meV linear *accelerator* or *betatron* to serve as a source of high-energy, or megavoltage, electrons and x rays
4. Cobalt 60 *gamma ray* source with an average energy of 1.25 meV

Nonparticulate irradiations

The penetrability, or energy, of an x ray or gamma ray is totally dependent on its wavelength: the shorter the wavelength, the more penetrating the photon, and conversely the longer the wavelength, the less penetrating the photon. A low-energy beam (120 keV or less) of radiation tends to deposit all or most of its energy on or near the surface of the patient and thus is suitable for lesions on or near the skin surface. In addition, with the low-energy beam a greater amount of absorption or dose deposition takes place in bone than in soft tissue.

A high-energy beam of radiation (1 meV or greater) tends to deposit its energy throughout the entire volume of tissue irradiated, with a greater amount of dose deposition occurring at or near the entry port than at the exit port. In this energy range the dose is deposited about equally in soft tissue and bone. The high-energy, or megavoltage, beam is most suitable for in-depth tumors.

The *skin-sparing* effect, a phenomenon that occurs as the energy of a beam of radiation is increased, is of value from a therapeutic standpoint. In the superficial and orthovoltage energy range the maximum dose occurs on the surface of the patient, with decreasing deposition of dose as the beam traverses the patient. As the energy of the beam increases into the megavoltage range, the maximum dose absorbed by the patient occurs at some point below the skin surface. The skin-

sparing effect is of importance clinically because the skin is a radiosensitive organ and excessive dose deposition to the skin may compromise the treatment dose to a tumor that is at some depth within the patient. The greater the energy of the beam, the more in-depth the maximum dose will occur (Fig. 40-2).

Particulate irradiations

Particles in motion have kinetic energy; the greater their speed, the more kinetic energy they have, resulting in increased penetrability of the material irradiated. Once the particles have expended their kinetic energy and are no longer capable of *ionization,* they essentially cease to exist from a therapeutic standpoint.

Alpha particles (+2 charge and relatively large mass), when set in motion, have a large LET value but are virtually nonpenetrating and are essentially useless as a therapeutic tool. Moreover, they are a nuisance from a radiation protection standpoint.

Electron beam therapy, on the other hand, has become commonplace in most radiation oncology departments. Obtaining a beam of high-energy electrons involves removal of the transmission target from the path of the accelerated electrons, which are used for the production of x rays in the linear accelerators and betatrons. The usefulness of high-energy electrons is their deposition of energy within a given depth of tissue dependent on their kinetic energy (in million electron volts) and not any deeper. The general rule for determining the depth of tumor placement and depth of penetration in centimeters of a given beam of electrons is to divide the number of million electron volts of the beam by 3 and 2 respectively. For example, an 18 meV beam would be chosen for a tumor located 6 cm in depth (18 ÷ 3), and the resulting total depth of penetration of the beam would be 9 cm (18 ÷ 2). This phenomenon of the electrons depositing their energy within a given depth of tissue and no deeper allows the therapist to irradiate a tumor that may be in close proximity to a vital organ (Fig. 40-3). The LET values of electrons are dependent on their energy, but in the therapeutic ranges the value is similar to that of *cobalt 60* (^{60}Co).

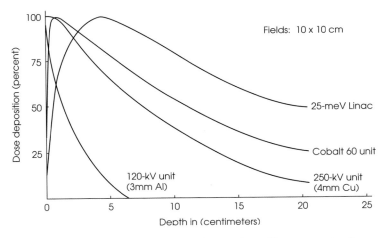

Fig. 40-1. Plot of percent depth of dose deposition versus depth in centimeters of tissue for various energies of photon beams.

Neutrons are of interest therapeutically for a variety of reasons, including the following:

1. The LET value for 20 meV neutrons is 7.
2. The biologic effectiveness of neutrons is not significantly altered by a lack of oxygen within the tumor cell.

However, only a few neutron therapy facilities are currently available, and research is still being conducted in this area.

Two other charged particles deserve mention: the proton and the pion. Although these particle beams are not available to most cancer centers in the United States, they are being investigated for their therapeutic use in a number of medical research facilities.

Most cancer patients are treated by teletherapy units; however, some may also be treated with an implant technique called brachytherapy. The theory behind brachytherapy is to deliver low-intensity radiation over an extended period of time to a relatively small volume of tissue. Brachytherapy may be accomplished in a number of ways:

1. Mould technique: placement of a *radioactive* source or sources on or in close proximity to the lesion.
2. Intracavitary implant technique: placement of a radioactive source or sources in a body cavity.
3. Interstitial implant technique: placement of a radioactive source or sources directly into the tumor site and adjacent tissue.

The majority of brachytherapy applications tend to be temporary; the sources are left in the patient until a designated tumor dose has been attained, possibly 3 to 4 days. A radioactive nuclide frequently used for intracavitary implants is cesium 137. For interstitial implants Iridium 192 is used. The nuclides may be reused after being sterilized or disinfected.

Permanent implant therapy may also be accomplished. An example of permanent implant nuclide is iodine 125 seeds. Permanent implant nuclides have *half-lives* of hours or days and are left in the patient essentially forever. The amount and distribution of the radionuclide implanted in this manner are dependent on the total dose that the radiation oncologist is trying to deliver. In most if not all cases of brachytherapy implantation, the implant is applied as part of the patient's overall treatment plan and may be followed by more external beam radiation therapy or possibly a surgical approach.

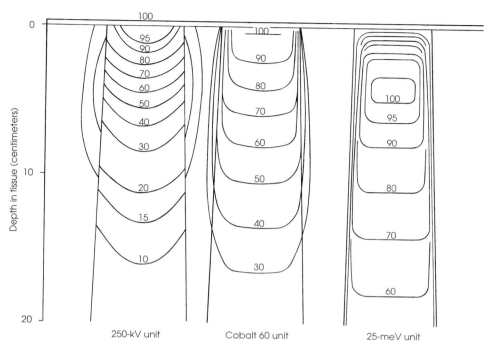

Fig. 40-2. Three isodose curves showing comparison of percent dose deposition from three x-ray units of different energies. As energy of beam is increased, percentage of dose deposited on surface of patient decreases.

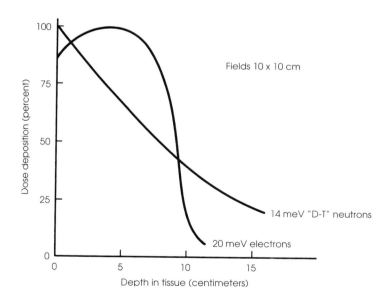

Fig. 40-3. Plot of percent dose deposition versus depth in centimeters of tissue for high-energy neutrons and electrons.

297

Clinical Applications

TREATMENT PLAN

If a patient has been diagnosed as having a particular histologic type of cancer and the extensiveness of the tumor has been determined to include possible nodal involvement, extension into any adjacent tissues, and possible metastasis, the decision is made as to what part, if any, radiation oncology will play.

If radiation oncology is considered of value in offering the patient the best possible prognosis, a treatment plan must be outlined and implemented for the patient. The following variables must be determined:

1. Type and extent of tumor
2. Emotional and physical well-being of the patient
3. Time-dose fractions (size of dose over period of time)
4. Radiation oncology unit capabilities
5. Goal of treatment (cure or palliation)

Each member of the radiation oncology department (e.g., radiation oncologist, radiation therapist, oncology nurse, physicist, dosimetrist) plays an active and integral part in the planning and implementation of the optimum treatment plan.

DOSIMETRY

Dosimetry is the design and monitoring of a technique for the precise application of a dose of ionizing radiation to the tumor without irreparably damaging the surrounding normal tissue. Many approaches may be used to accomplish this purpose; following are some examples of teletherapy.

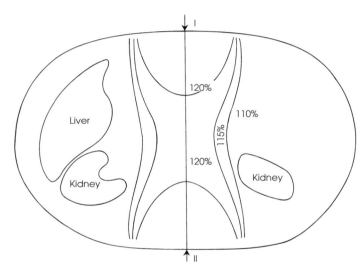

Fig. 40-4. Opposing ports teletherapy. Summated isodose lines represent equal dose contributions from fields **I** and **II**.

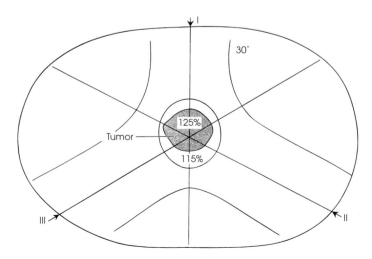

Fig. 40-5. Multifield teletherapy. Summated isodose lines represent equal dose contributions from fields **I** to **III**.

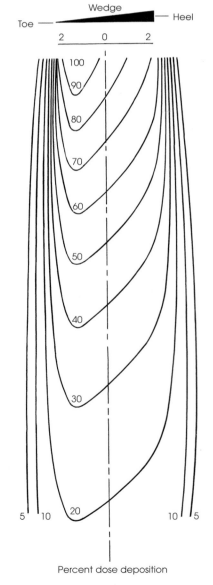

Percent dose deposition

Fig. 40-6. Isodose curve obtained from cobalt 60 unit with wedge placed between source and absorbing material.

Single field

In some cases the entire tumor dose is delivered through only one treatment port or *field*. An example of this approach is the treatment of skin cancer, although skin cancer is now being treated surgically.

Opposing ports

In this approach the tumor dose is the result of contributions from fields I and II (Fig. 40-4). If the tumor dose is to be 200 rads per treatment day, 100 rads can be delivered through each of the treatment ports or can be weighted more to one side than the other to protect a non-involved structure.

Multifield

This technique is basically an expansion of the opposing ports approach but employs the use of three or more fields to deliver the tumor dose (Fig. 40-5). Again, in most cases, the tumor dose can be delivered by equal contributions or outweighted contributions from the involved fields.

Rotational field

In this case the patient is positioned so that the tumor is located at the axis of rotation of the treatment unit. When the unit is turned on, the source of radiation rotates around the patient until the dose has been delivered. This treatment technique is usually applied to centrally located lesions such as cancer of the prostate. The advantage of this technique is that the maximum dose deposition is at the axis of rotation with minimal dose buildup to other parts of the anatomy.

Wedge field

Occasionally, the primary beam must be altered to accomplish the treatment goal; one way is to apply a wedge field technique. To obtain the desired isodose distribution, a wedge-shaped device, usually made of lead, is placed in the beam approximately halfway between the source of radiation and the patient. When the wedge is correctly placed within the beam of radiation, an *isodose curve* similar to that illustrated is obtained (Fig. 40-6). The wedges, as well as the wedge fields they produce, are usually oriented in a heel-to-heel manner with extreme care given to the daily setups. A combination of two wedge fields may be used to obtain the desired treatment plan. Although wedge fields may be used for tumors located at any anatomic site, they are often employed in head and neck tumors and intact breast set-ups (Fig. 40-7).

Shaped field

Most radiation oncology units have field-defining *collimators* that are rectangular in nature. Often irradiation of the entire rectangular area is not necessary to deliver the tumor dose. To reduce the radiation exposure to only portions of the field, shaper blocks, such as those illustrated in Fig. 40-8, are placed at some point between the source and patient. The shaper blocks are generally a lead alloy or an equivalent material and reduce the intensity of the beam to 5% or less of the original intensity.

To assist in the treatment planning and dosimetry of many treatment setups, computers, ultrasonography, magnetic resonance imaging (MRI), and computed tomography (CT) are used not only to locate the tumor but also to localize the boundaries of noninvolved organs, to indicate doses outside the tumor volume, or possibly to evaluate the effectiveness of the treatment plan by recording tumor regression. In addition, new techniques are being investigated which, it is hoped, will enhance the effectiveness of cancer therapy. Specific areas of interest include intraoperative irradiation of selected tumors, the treatment of patients twice a day instead of the usual once-a-day regimen, and the use of radiosensitizing agents, hyperthermia, and high-energy particulate irradiation.

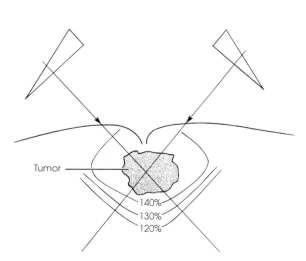

Fig. 40-7. Summated isodose curves obtained when pair of wedge fields are applied for therapeutic purposes. Wedges are oriented "heel to heel."

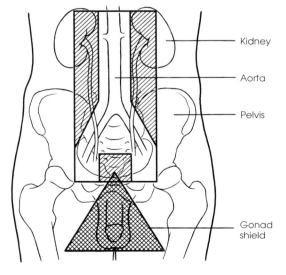

Fig. 40-8. "Inverted Y" radiation field frequently used to treat lymphatic disease below diaphragm. Darker area over gonads represents double thickness of lead shaper blocks.

CLINICAL ENTITIES

Because the ability of the oncologist to treat any tumor for cure depends on early diagnosis of the disease, the following discussions assume that the disease process is in a beginning stage.

Larynx cancer

Lesions of this nature are best treated with megavoltage radiation. Tumors that are confined to the true vocal cord, with normal cord mobility, have a 90% 5-year cure rate; in addition, the voice remains useful. The method of treatment is usually accomplished by using opposing lateral wedged fields of 4 × 5 cm or 5 × 5 cm and delivering a dose of 6500 rads in a 6-week period.

Skin cancer

Carcinomas of the skin are usually squamous cell or basal cell lesions and are best treated with superficial radiation. Cure rates tend to run between 80% and 90%, and basal cell lesions less than 1 cm in diameter have a cure rate of almost 100%. The method of treatment is usually a single-field approach with attention given to shielding the uninvolved skin and delivering 5000 rads in a 4-week period.

Medulloblastoma

Children with this disease are usually referred to the radiation oncology department after a biopsy and shunt procedure. The tumor is radiosensitive, and patients who have had treatment of the entire cerebrospinal axis have a 5-year cure rate of 40% to 50%. The therapeutic approach tends to be complicated because the entire brain is irradiated with 4500 rads, the spinal cord receives a dose of between 3500 and 4500 rads, and the cerebellum receives an additional 1000 rads (Fig. 40-9). This irradiation is usually accomplished with parallel opposed fields to the cranial vault with an extended single field to the spinal cord. A megavoltage unit is often used with extreme care given to any areas of abutting fields.

Retinoblastoma

Retinoblastoma is a disease which usually manifests itself before the individual is 3 years of age. If the tumor is diagnosed early and occurs in only one eye, the chances of controlling the disease are about 50%. The tumor dose of 4500 to 5500 rads in 4½ to 5½ weeks may be accomplished with either high-energy electrons or a megavoltage unit. Lateral ports are generally used with care given to dosimetry. Two important complications that often occur are radiation-induced cataracts and facial asymmetry caused by growth-retarding effects of radiation on bone.

Radiation oncology may be the only therapeutic approach used in the treatment of some cancers, or it may be used in conjunction with chemotherapy or surgery. The decision of how a patient is treated is determined by weighing many factors and options and then integrating them with the capabilities of the medical facility. Following are some generally agreed-upon treatment factors (which may vary from institution to institution) for a number of frequently treated cancers.

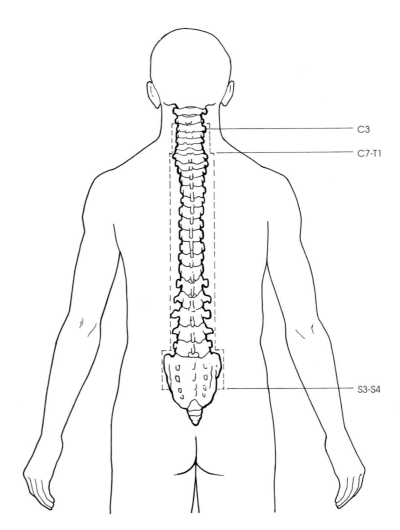

Fig. 40-9. Spinal treatment portal for medulloblastoma.

Cancers treated primarily by radiation therapy

Larynx cancer Irradiation from opposing lateral ports with small field sizes and possibly wedges is employed. A megavoltage unit delivers a total dose of 6500 rads in 6 weeks.

Skin cancer This treatment involves a single field large enough to cover the lesion and any possible extension. The uninvolved tissue should be well protected. For lesions 2 to 3 cm in size, 5000 rads in 4 weeks are delivered by a superficial unit.

Oral cavity cancer A number of approaches may be used depending on the size and the extent of the tumor. An intraoral cone may be used to deliver 6000 rads in 4 weeks, with an orthovoltage beam for small lesions. Larger lesions may be treated with irradiation through opposing lateral ports from a megavoltage unit possibly followed by brachytherapy.

Cervical cancer Early diagnosed lesions can be treated with either surgery or therapy. A four-field technique using AP, PA, and R and L lateral ports using a megavoltage unit, preferably 10 meV or greater, deliver 4500 to 5000 rads in 5 weeks to an area of the primary and regional lymph nodes (Fig. 40-10). An intracavitary implant may also be indicated.

Hodgkin's disease and malignant lymphoma The age of the patient and extent of the disease may determine the prognosis. Extended field therapy includes the lymphatic chain above and/or below the diaphragm and is applied by a megavoltage unit that delivers 4500 rads through AP-PA ports. Chemotherapy may also be indicated for more advanced cases.

Nasopharynx cancer Shaped lateral opposing ports are used to deliver 7000 rads in 6 to 8 weeks with the possibility of an intracavitary application (Fig. 40-11). The tumor dose is delivered by a megavoltage unit.

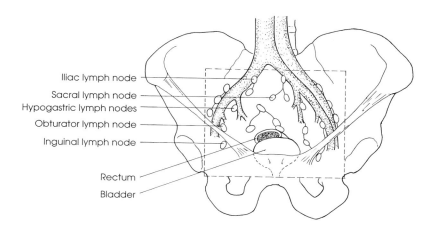

Iliac lymph node
Sacral lymph node
Hypogastric lymph nodes
Obturator lymph node
Inguinal lymph node
Rectum
Bladder

Fig. 40-10. Field employed for irradiation of primary tumor and adjacent lymph nodes.

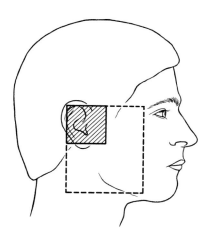

Fig. 40-11. Opposing ports for treatment of nasopharyngeal cancer. Shaded area represents the use of lead shaper blocks.

Cancers treated with radiation and surgery and/or chemotherapy

Breast cancer Using two tangential fields to the chest wall or intact breast, megavoltage radiation delivers 5000 rads in 5 weeks (Fig. 40-12). Chemotherapy may also be indicated.

Uterine cancer External megavoltage irradiation may be used preoperatively or postoperatively using the four-field technique. After total hysterectomy an intracavitary implant may be indicated.

Lung cancer Treatment for some small lesions involves surgical resection followed by postoperative irradiation by a megavoltage unit that delivers 6000 to 7000 rads through opposing ports (Fig. 40-13). The total dose depends on the radiosensitivity of the surrounding tissue. Chemotherapy may also be indicated in some types of lung cancer.

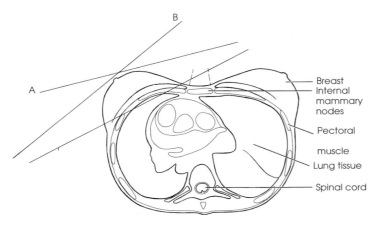

Fig. 40-12. Cross section of thorax. *A* and *B,* Field arrangements to tangentially irradiate intact breast.

Breast
Internal mammary nodes
Pectoral muscle
Lung tissue
Spinal cord

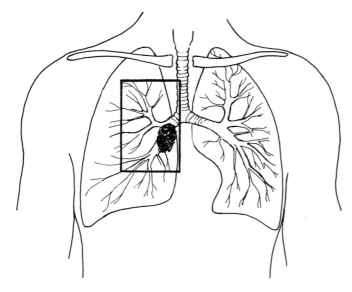

Fig. 40-13. Typical field for irradiation of carcinoma of the lung.

Future Trends

Because of the nature of cancer, it is wishful thinking to expect dramatic breakthroughs in research that will result in a cure for all cancers. A more realistic expectation is that research will continue to supply important bits of information that, when added to the present body of information, will afford a greater understanding of the disease and how to treat it effectively. The continued application of ionizing radiation as a treatment modality will not require the discovery of new radiation or the design of larger, more costly radiation-producing units. The future will more likely revolve around three specific questions: (1) when to irradiate, (2) under what altered biologic conditions to irradiate, and (3) how much radiation to use over what period of time. It is not the usefulness of radiation that is the question—we know it works and we have a basic understanding of how it works. Instead, efforts will be directed toward effectively controlling and/or manipulating the biologic and physical environment to maximize the desired positive effects.

WHEN TO IRRADIATE

Evidence supports the argument that the earlier a tumor is diagnosed and treated, the better the patient's prognosis will be. This truism will not change; however, it is hoped that, with increased public education efforts coupled with available screening programs, patients will be seen even earlier than at present. Additionally, increased diagnostic capabilities, such as those available with MRI, CT scans, and newly devised medical laboratory examinations, will allow for determinations of the extent and histologic type of a tumor far beyond the present capabilities.

ALTERING THE BIOLOGIC ENVIRONMENT

The effort to alter the biologic environment will be two-pronged: (1) involving the immunotherapist approach, in which physicians will be able to trigger the body's own immune mechanism to recognize and destroy abnormal growth, and (2) incorporating the oncology effort to alter the biologic and/or physical environment to increase the radiosensitivity of the malignancy. Radiation oncology will be concerned with the latter effort.

Altering the biologic and physical environment will have much impact on therapists because it will require them to accommodate and become more knowledgeable in such diverse areas as hyperthermia, fractionated brachytherapy procedures, monoclonal antibodies, and possibly hyperbaric treatment techniques. These adaptations, coupled with a plethora of chemotherapeutic agents, will not only alter the tumor environment but also greatly increase the day-to-day patient care and treatment responsibilities of the radiation therapist.

HOW MUCH RADIATION AND IN WHAT TIME PERIOD

Finally, the appropriateness of delivering an established number of rads for a given type of tumor over a certain time frame is being questioned. For example, delivering 180 rads per day for 5 weeks for a total dose of 4500 rads (45 Gy) may no longer be the method of choice to obtain the desired biologic response. Radiation oncologists are investigating various therapeutic procedures that will enhance the biologic effects of radiation to tumors, while at the same time diminishing the harmful effects to normal tissue. Techniques might include treating the patent twice a day, or using three-dimensional treatment planning approaches.

There is little doubt that currently accepted radiation oncology treatment techniques will change. However, the changes will not take place overnight; rather, the changes will be subtle and well thought out. They will include some or all of the above three subject areas and, it is hoped, will result in increased patient survival statistics.

The twenty-first century will present innovations and challenges in radiation oncology and should be entered with enthusiasm and a certain degree of cautious optimism.

Summary

From a somewhat questionable beginning, radiation therapy has emerged as one of the primary modalities employed in the treatment of malignant disease. Radiation therapy departments are currently examining and treating approximately 75% of all newly diagnosed cancer patients. The radiation oncologists and therapists are integral members of the health team that discusses and selects the appropriate treatment regimens for all cancer patients.

As our understanding of those factors that initiate cellular change, growth, and spread increases, our ability to treat patients more effectively will also increase. The irradiation techniques presently used may change dramatically based on this new information. Additionally, new, more sophisticated radiation-producing equipment is being designed that may cause us to reevaluate the presently accepted therapeutic techniques and dose levels. Finally, new chemotherapeutic agents are being produced that, when used by themselves or in combination with other drugs, may enhance tumor sensitivity when used in conjunction with radiation.

The positive role of radiation oncology in the treatment of cancer has been established. Certainly changes will occur, and if the present trend continues, it appears that radiation therapy will play an ever-increasing role in cancer treatment.

Definition of Terms

absorbed dose Amount of ionizing radiation absorbed per unit of mass of irradiated material.

accelerator (particle) Device that accelerates charged subatomic particles to great energies. These particles or rays may be used for direct medical irradiation and basic physical research. Medical units include linear accelerators, betatrons, and cyclotrons.

air dose Dose of radiation measured in roentgens in free air, uncorrected for absorption or backscatter.

anaplasia Alteration of cell to more embryonic primitive state; may be used to describe particular type of tumor.

attenuation Removal of energy from beam of ionizing radiation when it traverses matter, by disposition of energy in matter and by deflection of energy out of beam.

betatron Electron accelerator that uses magnetic induction to accelerate electrons in circular path; also capable of producing photons.

bolus Tissue-equivalent material (e.g., rice, beeswax, petroleum gauze, Silly Putty) placed around curved, irregularly shaped anatomic areas to obtain more uniform dosage distribution.

brachytherapy Placement of radioactive nuclide(s) in or on neoplasm to deliver cancercidal dose.

cancer Term frequently applied to malignant disease: neoplasm (new growth) or oma (tumor).

carcinogen Any cancer-producing substance or material such as nicotine, radiation, or ingested uranium.

chemical dosimeter Detector for indirect measurement of radiation by indicating extent to which radiation causes measurable chemical change to take place.

cobalt 60 (^{60}Co) Radioisotope with half-life of 5.26 years, average gamma-ray energy of 1.25 meV (1.17 and 1.33), and ability to spare skin with buildup depth in tissue of 0.5 cm.

collimator Diaphragm or system of diaphragms made of radiation-absorbing material that define dimension and direction of beam.

compensating filter Filter designed to modify dose distribution within patient. Filters may be designed to account for patient shape, size, or position (e.g., wedge filter).

contamination Radioactivity in inappropriate places such as radiographer's hands.

cure Usually, 5-year period after completion of treatment during which time patient exhibits no evidence of disease.

decay or disintegration Transformation of radioactive nucleus, resulting in emission of radiation.

differentiation Acquisition of cellular function/structure that differ from function/structure of original cell type.

dose rate Radiation dose delivered per unit of time, usually rads per minute.

dosimeter Device (e.g., film badge, ionization chamber, Geiger counter) that measures radiation exposure.

dosimetrist Person responsible for the calculation of the proper radiation treatment dose who assists the oncologist in designing individual treatment plans.

etiology Study of causes of diseases.

field Geometric area defined by collimator or radiotherapy unit at skin surface.

filter Attenuator inserted in beam near source to modify beam quality in desired way. Materials used most often are copper, aluminum, and lead.

fission Breaking apart of uranium 235 nucleus, liberating energy and neutrons, which are used in producing radioactive isotopes in reactor (^{60}Co).

fractionation Dividing of total planned dose into number of smaller doses to be given over longer period. Consideration must be given to biologic effectiveness of smaller doses.

gamma ray Electromagnetic radiation that originates from radioactive nucleus and causes ionization in matter; identical in properties to x ray.

grenz rays X rays generated at 20 kVp or less.

half-life Time (specific for each radioactive substance) required for radioactive material to decay to half its initial activity. Types are biologic and physical.

half-value layer Thickness of attenuating material inserted in beam to reduce beam intensity to half of the original intensity.

ionization Process in which one or more electrons are added to or removed from atoms, creating ions. Can be caused by high temperatures, electrical discharges, or nuclear radiations.

isodose curve Curve or line drawn to connect points of identical amounts of radiation in given field.

metastasis Transmission of cells or groups of cells from primary tumor to site(s) elsewhere in body.

oncologist Doctor of medicine specializing in study of tumors.

oncology Study of tumors.

protraction Delivery of tumor dose over an extended time period.

radiation oncologist Doctor of medicine specializing in use of ionizing radiation in treatment of disease.

radiation oncology Medical specialty involving the treatment of cancerous lesions using ionizing radiation.

radiation therapy Older term used to define medical specialty of treatment with ionizing radiations.

radiation therapist Person trained to assist and take directions from radiation oncologist in use of ionizing radiations in treatment of disease.

radioactive Pertaining to atoms of elements that undergo spontaneous transformation, resulting in emission of radiation.

radiocurable Susceptibility of neoplastic cells to cure (destruction) by ionizing radiation.

radiosensitivity Responsiveness of cells to radiation.

radium (Ra) Radionuclide (atomic number, 88; atomic weight, 226; half-life, 1622 years) used clinically for radiation therapy. In conjunction with its subsequent transformations, radium emits alpha and beta particles and gamma rays. In encapsulated form it is used for various intracavitary radiation therapy applications such as that for cancer of cervix.

reactor Cubicle in which isotopes are artificially produced.

roentgen (R) Unit of exposure dose, based on extent of ionization in air and defined as $2.58 \times 10\text{-}4$ coulombs/kg of dry air, which is equivalent to 1 electrostatic unit of charge/cc or 0.001293 gm of dry air; 1.16×1012 ion pairs/gm of air; 2.08×109 ion pairs/gm of air; or absorption of 87 ergs of energy/gm of air.

scattering Process in which trajectory of particle or photon is changed; caused by collision with atoms, nuclei, and other particles.

sequelae Reaction or side effects of ionizing radiation on tissue.

skin sparing In megavoltage beam therapy, reduced skin injury per rad exposure when electron equilibrium is not present at advance portal but occurs below skin. Occurs from 0.5 to 5 cm deep depending on energy.

teletherapy Radiation therapy technique for which source of radiation is at some distance from patient.

tumor volume Portion of anatomy that includes tumor and adjacent areas of invasion.

undifferentiation Lack of resemblance of cells to cells of origin.

unstable nuclide In excited, active state; with nucleus possessing excess energy.

Van de Graff generator Electrostatic machine in which electronically charged particles are sprayed on moving belt and carried by it to build up high potential on insulated terminal. Charged particles are then accelerated along discharge path through vacuum tube by potential difference between insulated terminal and opposite end of machine. Often used to inject particles into larger accelerators.

SELECTED BIBLIOGRAPHY

Bentel GC et al: Treatment planning and dose calculation in radiation oncology, ed 3, New York, 1982, Pergamon Press.

Blake SW: Advances in treatment planning dosimetry for a high energy neutron beam, Br J Radiol 64:341, 1991

Brenner DJ: Dose, volume, and tumor-control predictions in radiotherapy, J Radiat Oncol Biol Phys 26:171, 1993.

Cooper JS et al: Concepts in cancer care, Philadelphia, 1983, Lea & Febiger.

Dische S: Radiotherapy in the nineties: increase in cure, decrease in morbidity, Acta Oncol 31:501, 1992.

Grabowski CM, Unger JA, Potish RA: Factors predictive of completion of treatment and survival after palliative radiation therapy, Radiology 184:329, 1992.

Hall EJ: Radiobiology for the radiologist, New York, 1973, Harper & Row Publishers.

Johns HE and Cunningham JR: The physics of radiology, ed 4, Springfield, Ill, 1983, Charles C Thomas, Publisher.

Marks JE, Armbruster JS: Accreditation of radiation oncology in the U.S., Int J Radiat Oncol Biol Phys 24:863, 1992.

Meredith WJ et al: Fundamental physics of radiology, ed 3, Bristol, 1977, Wright & Sons.

Morgan HM: Quality assurance of computer controlled radiotherapy treatments, Br J Radiol 65:409, 1992.

Moss WT et al: Radiation oncology rationale, technique, and results, ed 5, St Louis, 1979, Mosby.

Mould RF: Radiotherapy treatment planning, Bristol, 1981, Hilger.

Order SE: Training in systemic radiation therapy, Int J Radiat Oncol Biol Phys 24:895, 1992.

Perez CA: Quest for excellence: ultimate goal of the radiation oncologist: astro gold medal address 1992, Perez, CA, Int J Radiat Oncol Biol Phys 26:567, 1993.

Pizzarello DJ et al: Medical radiation biology, ed 2, Philadelphia, 1982, Lea & Febiger.

Rafla S et al: Introduction to radiotherapy, St Louis, 1974, Mosby.

Rubin P et al: Clinical oncology for medical students and physicians, ed 6, 1983, American Cancer Society.

Selman J: The basic physics of radiation therapy, ed 2, Springfield, Ill, 1976, Charles C Thomas Publisher.

Wagner LK: Absorbed dose in imaging: why measure it? Radiology, 178:622, 1991.

Walter J et al: A short textbook of radiotherapy for technicians and students, ed 3, Boston, 1969, Little, Brown & Co.

Chapter 41

INTRODUCTION TO RADIOGRAPHIC QUALITY ASSURANCE

WILLIAM F. FINNEY III

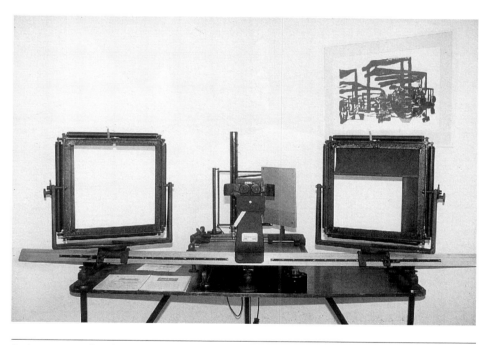

A stereoscopic viewer used to show depth of field within the human body. Two radiographs were placed on each screen (left and right), and the viewer observed them through the eyepiece in the center viewing device.

In a medical diagnostic radiographic imaging system there are numerous sources of variability. These sources can produce subquality images if they are not controlled. Most subquality radiographs often require repeat examinations, resulting in additional radiation exposure to the patient and an increased cost to the department. A systematic and structured mechanism to control these variables is the foundation upon which radiographic *quality assurance (QA)* is built.

The intent of this chapter is to acquaint the reader with radiographic quality assurance. It is not designed to be a procedures manual for the various quality control tests but is written as an overview of the radiographic quality assurance concept. For additional information on any topic discussed in this chapter, please refer to the bibliography at the end of this chapter.

The information in this chapter draws heavily from the quality assurance series developed and published by the National Center for Devices and Radiological Health *(NCDRH*)* and from material by Radiation Measurements Incorporated (RMI). These organizations have been active in promoting quality assurance and instrumental in creating a practical approach to quality assurance, allowing its concepts to be realized by *diagnostic radiology facilities* regardless of their size (Figs. 41-1 and 41-2).

---

*All italicized terms are defined at the end of this chapter.

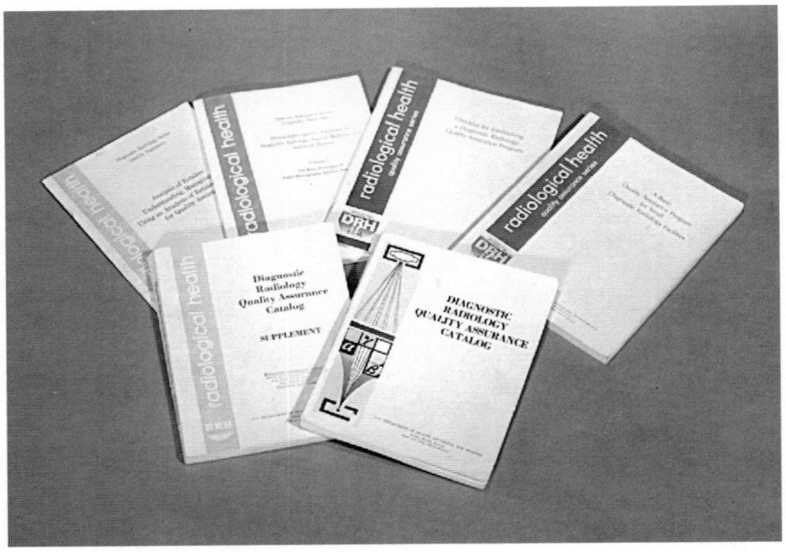

Fig. 41-1. NCDRH quality assurance publications.

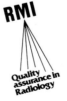

Quality Assurance Handbook

RADIATION MEASUREMENTS, INC.
P.O. BOX 44, 7617 DONNA DR.
MIDDLETON, WI 53562
608/831-1188

Fig. 41-2. RMI specializes in quality control test tools for radiology.

Quality Assurance Versus Quality Control

"Radiographic quality assurance" and "radiographic quality control" are terms that are often used synonymously. Both terms refer to concepts that define a mechanism used to enhance the quality of the services and products rendered. Their main difference is the scope of their intent.

One concept of radiographic quality assurance encompasses the total picture of radiographic care delivery with its primary objective being the enhancement of patient care. Patient selection parameters, management techniques, departmental polices and procedures, technical effectiveness and efficiency, and inservice education are examples of some of the elements that are included. The Joint Commission for Accreditation of Healthcare Organizations (JCAHO) uses this quality assurance concept in their hospital accreditation process.

The NCDRH's concept of radiographic quality assurance focuses primarily on the enhancement of radiographic image quality and on the reduction of unnecessary patient exposure by using *quality administrative procedures* and quality control techniques.

Quality control (QC) as defined by the NCDRH deals with the techniques used in the monitoring and maintenance of the technical elements of the system that affect the quality of the image. Although the idea of control is basic to this concept, the goal of optimizing the performance and ensuring the accuracy of these elements must not be forgotten. This chapter uses the terms "radiographic quality assurance" and "radiographic quality control" in the context as defined by the NCDRH.

Historical Development

Quality assurance in diagnostic radiology is not new. Many radiography departments have been systematically monitoring their equipment since long before "quality assurance/control" became a buzzword. This interest in radiographic quality assurance can be traced to actions taken by the federal government.

In 1968 the Radiation Control for Health and Safety Act was passed. This act required the U.S. Department of Health, Education and Welfare, now designated Health and Human Services (HHS), to conduct a radiation control program through the development and administration of standards to reduce human exposure to radiation from electronic products. The Bureau of Radiological Health (BRH), now designated The National Center for Devices and Radiological Health (NCDRH), was given the responsibility of carrying out this act.

In 1974 the BRH set forth regulatory action to control the manufacture and installation of medical/dental diagnostic x-ray equipment to reduce the production of useless radiation. This action, known as the X-ray Equipment Standard, was designed to regulate the performance of *x-ray systems,* not the use of such systems.

Another approach to help realize the goal of reducing the patient's exposure to unnecessary radiation was the development of facility-based *quality assurance programs.* Support for this concept came from numerous studies, which pointed out that many diagnostic radiology facilities produce subquality images and deliver unnecessary amounts of radiation while examining patients. It was believed that the best way to discourage such practices was to educate the radiologic community about the concept of radiographic quality assurance. The professional community was made aware of the BRH's intent to develop recommendations concerning quality assurance programs in 1976. The professional community was solicited for input in the development of quality assurance recommendations, and in 1978 the proposed Recommendation for Quality Assurance Programs in Diagnostic Radiology Facilities was published. Comments on the proposal were solicited, and in 1979 the recommendation was published in its final form in the Federal Register.

The Consumer-Patient Radiation Health and Safety Act of 1981 established guidelines for further reducing unnecessary patient exposure. This act addressed issues such as unnecessary repeat examinations, quality assurance techniques, radiation exposure, referral criteria, and unnecessary mass screening programs. In addition, the act established minimum standards for accreditation of educational programs in the radiologic sciences and for the certification of radiographic equipment operators.

Benefits

The benefits of having a well-administered radiographic quality assurance program are numerous. The use of such a program in diagnostic radiology facilities is one of the methods that can minimize unnecessary radiation to patient consumers. Studies have demonstrated that the number of repeated radiographs, which result in additional radiation to the patient, can be reduced with the implementation of quality assurance procedures. Although the reduction in unnecessary patient exposure is significant, the potential to improve the overall efficiency of the radiologic service delivery can also be realized. These advantages result in satisfied patient consumers.

The radiology facility is also the beneficiary of quality assurance. Improvement of radiographic image quality is achievable, as is increased consistency of image production. Quality control procedures can increase the reliability, efficiency, and cost effectiveness of the equipment used by the facility. These are important gains, considering the current emphasis on cost containment in health care delivery. Although increased overall departmental efficiency in itself is a major advantage, the betterment of personnel morale resulting from such improvements may be the most important benefit in the long run.

Not all facilities engaged in quality assurance gain from all the benefits possible; the goal is to provide a more effective and efficient delivery of radiologic services along with a reduction in unnecessary radiation to the patient consumer. With the proper planning, design, and management of a quality assurance program, these benefits are easily achievable.

National Center for Devices and Radiological Health Quality Assurance Program Recommendation

The National Center for Devices and Radiological Health's (NCDRH) recommendation for establishing quality assurance programs in diagnostic radiology facilities was developed from research, empirical data, and feedback from the professional community. Although the recommendation is not mandatory, the NCDRH strongly believes that the establishment of quality assurance programs helps to achieve the goals of reducing unproductive patient radiation, minimizing unnecessary costs, and improving the consistency of quality images.

The NCDRH's recommendation includes 10 elements that are considered essential for a viable program. All facilities would not require an approach to quality assurance as comprehensive as that recommended; the NCDRH suggests that the size, objectives, and available resources of a facility should determine the extent to which each element should be implemented. The recommendation provides some valuable insight into the concepts of quality assurance. A brief description of each of the 10 elements follows.

RESPONSIBILITY

Although quality assurance is the responsibility of the entire staff of the diagnostic radiographic facility, an efficient and effective quality assurance program requires accountability. Distinct and documented assignments of responsibility for the program and its components are essential for success. The size of the facility, scope of the program, and available resources are some of the factors that dictate the levels to which these responsibilities are assigned (e.g., physicist, field or in-house service engineer, chief radiographer, supervisory personnel, staff radiographer, and consultant). Regardless of facility size, the primary responsibility for quality assurance is that of the owner or practitioner in charge.

EVALUATION

The element of evaluation within a quality assurance program should be addressed at different levels. First, the performance of the facility should be evaluated. This information can be used to determine the scope and design of a quality assurance program for the facility and/or to provide data that can be used for comparison with data generated at future points in time. These comparison evaluations demonstrate the effectiveness of the quality assurance program. The most popular procedure used to evaluate facility performance is the analysis of rejected radiographs, commonly known as *reject analysis*. On another level, equipment monitoring results should be evaluated to assess the need for corrective action or to determine trends that may indicate that preventive maintenance is required.

PURCHASE SPECIFICATIONS

When new equipment is purchased, the facility should determine the desired performance criteria for the equipment. These performance criteria are then reflected in the purchase specifications. Before final acceptance of the equipment, it should be tested to ensure that the actual performance meets the criteria requested in the purchase specifications. The future monitoring and testing of the equipment can be compared with the equipment performance criteria to determine if the equipment is continuing to perform at the acceptable level.

STANDARDS FOR IMAGE QUALITY

Standards for image quality should be established for the performance parameters of the x-ray system that are of interest to the facility. The creation of these standards should, when possible, *objectively* indicate the amount of performance variation that can be accepted before the quality of the image is affected. A *subjective* determination of the standards is often used when objective standards cannot be defined. If the equipment monitoring results show that the equipment does not meet the acceptance limits of the standard, then corrective actions should be taken.

MONITORING AND MAINTENANCE

This element is sometimes referred to as the quality control portion of the program. Equipment monitoring and maintenance is the center of a quality assurance program. The NCDRH suggests that every facility should consider monitoring the following system components:

1. Film processing
2. Performance of radiographic/fluoroscopic units
3. Cassettes and grids
4. Illuminators
5. Darkroom

The system component parameters that should be monitored vary from facility to facility, depending on such factors as program goals, available resources, and cost. The NCDRH includes a listing of parameters for all system components in its recommendation (Table 41-1). A maintenance program including both the preventative and corrective aspects of equipment maintenance is an important aspect of any quality assurance program.

TRAINING

A plan for the training of personnel with quality assurance responsibilities is recommended. A mechanism for the continuing education of these individuals should also be included. A subtle but important aspect of this element is educating the facility's staff to the importance, design, and goals of the quality assurance program. The real strength of a quality assurance program is based on the support and commitment of the entire staff.

Table 41-1. X-ray system component parameters

I. Film processing
   a. An index of speed
   b. An index of contrast
   c. Base plug fog
   d. Solution temperatures
   e. Film artifact identification
II. Fluoroscopic x-ray units
   a. Tabletop exposure rates
   b. Centering alignment
   c. Collimation
   d. kVp accuracy and reproducibility
   e. mA accuracy and reproducibility
   f. Exposure time accuracy and reproducibility
   g. Reproducibility of x-ray output
   h. Focal spot size consistency
   i. Half-value layer
   j. Representative entrance skin exposures
III. Image intensified systems
   a. Resolution
   b. Focusing
   c. Distortion
   d. Glare
   e. Low-contrast performance
   f. Physical alignment of camera and collimating lens

IV. Radiographic x-ray units
   a. Reproducibility of x-ray output
   b. Linearity and reproducibility of mA stations
   c. Reproducibility and accuracy of timer stations
   d. Reproducibility and accuracy of kVp stations
   e. Accuracy of source-to-image receptor distance indicators
   f. Light/x-ray field congruence
   g. Half-value layer
   h. Focal spot size consistency
   i. Representative entrance skin exposures
V. Automatic exposure control (AEC) devices
   a. Reproducibility
   b. kVp compensation
   c. Field sensitivity matching
   d. Minimum response time
   e. Back-up timer verification
VI. Cassettes and grids
   a. Cassettes
      1. Film-screen contact
      2. Screen condition
      3. Light leaks
      4. Artifact identification
      5. Uniformity of screen speed
   b. Grids
      1. Alignment and focal distance
      2. Artifact identification

VII. Illuminators
   a. Consistency of light output with time
   b. Consistency of light output from one illuminator to another
   c. Illuminator surface conditions
VIII. Darkrooms
   a. Darkroom integrity
   b. Safelight conditions
IX. Tomographic systems
   a. Accuracy of depth and cut indicator
   b. Thickness of cut plane
   c. Exposure angle
   d. Completeness of tomographic motion
   e. Flatness of tomographic field
   f. Resolution
   g. Continuity of exposure
   h. Flatness of cassette
   i. Representative entrance skin exposures
X. Computed tomography
   a. Precision (noise)
   b. Contrast scale
   c. High- and low-contrast resolution
   d. Alignment
   e. Representative entrance skin exposures

COMMITTEE

This element might better be described as communication. Large facilities may require a quality assurance committee structure for planning, review, and evaluation purposes. Smaller facilities may not require a formal committee but instead rely on input directly from the staff. The intent of this element is to emphasize the importance of maintaining open communication among all participants in the quality assurance program.

RECORDS

The documentation of equipment monitoring results, maintenance actions, and other such activities should be included in a quality assurance program. A regular and systematic method of collecting and recording data is the foundation on which the review and evaluation elements of the program are based.

MANUAL

A quality assurance program should develop and maintain a complete, comprehensive, and up-to-date manual. The manual should serve as a source document or guide for all elements of the program. The manual should include items such as quality assurance personnel, monitoring procedures, monitoring schedules, monitoring evaluations, corrective actions, and service records.

REVIEW

Periodic review is necessary to determine the status of the quality assurance program. A look at the entire program will determine if it is operating at its maximum effectiveness or if changes must be made. Inspection of the important program elements will reveal their currentness, appropriateness, consistency, regularity, and effectiveness in achieving the goals of the program.

Quality Assurance Program Design

Every radiographic facility is a unique entity. Although their missions may be the same, the process and environment of each are different. With this in mind, a facility must custom-fit quality assurance to its own situation. A review of the quality assurance literature provides valuable guidance for the design of a program. A systematic approach to fitting a quality assurance program to the needs of a facility makes such a seemingly large task manageable. Begin by planning an assessment of the facility's performance. This information may reveal areas that should be attended to first, along with providing documentation for supporting the program plan. One method of assessing the facility's performance is by the use of reject analysis. A reject analysis is a planned, systematic procedure in which rejected subquality radiographs are collected, analyzed, and categorized according to cause, which may be related to the competence of technical personnel, equipment problems, specific difficulties associated with the examination, or some combination of these elements. The analysis of rejected radiographs is an effective method of identifying equipment performance problems. A reject analysis program as a routine part of the quality assurance program acts as a link between a department's quality assurance efforts and the consistency of its image quality. It may be used to evaluate problems leading to poor image quality, as a self-improvement tool for the staff, as a management database, or as an excellent method of evaluating the impact of the quality assurance program on the quality of the radiographic images. Organizing the program plan is the next step. Training personnel, establishing image quality standards, developing and documenting monitoring procedures, and procuring the necessary monitoring equipment are some of the aspects of the organization phase. Implementation of the plan is next, followed by an evaluation of the program's impact, which can be assessed by repair records, monitoring results, reject analysis results, or subjective methods. The feedback from the evaluation phase provides input to the original planning steps and should be used to make any necessary adjustments to make the program more effective and efficient.

BASIC QUALITY CONTROL TESTS

The quality control tests used to monitor x-ray system components usually require some type of device to measure the parameter being evaluated. Quality control tools range from simple homemade devices to sophisticated microprocessors (Fig. 41-3). Radiation Measurements Incorporated (RMI) manufactures a comprehensive line of quality control test tools that are relatively inexpensive and easy to use. These tools can be purchased as a complete quality control kit (Fig. 41-4) or individually. The multiple test cassette, which tests several x-ray unit parameters with a single exposure, is especially popular in smaller facilities (Fig. 41-5). Multiple-function digital meters are also available which will display digital readouts of the measurements for the tested parameters (e.g., exposure time, kVp, and mR output). The decision of what quality control tools to use depends on such factors as cost, ease of use, accuracy, and dependability. Most vendors of x-ray supplies carry a wide variety of quality control test tools. To familiarize the reader with some examples of quality control test tools, the following section briefly reviews some of the basic tests for quality control.

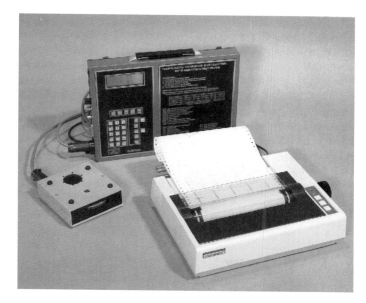

Fig. 41-3. NERO is a microprocessor that can be programmed to acquire and analyze exposure data, providing quality control test results for numerous parameters.

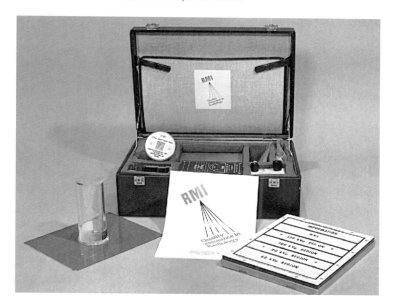

Fig. 41-4. RMI radiographic/fluoroscopic quality control kit.

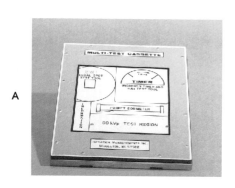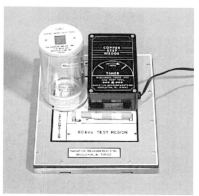

Fig. 41-5. RMI multitest cassette. **A,** Cassette only. **B,** Cassette with quality control tools in place.

Film processing

Film processors are one of the biggest contributors of variability to an x-ray system. Most authorities suggest in-house sensitometric monitoring of the film processor. This approach provides a quantitative means of recording processor variability. Sensitometric monitoring requires the use of a *sensitometer* and a *densitometer* (Fig. 41-6). In addition, a dependable thermometer should be considered to accurately measure developer temperature, and one specific box of radiographic film should be reserved for use as control film in the testing procedure. The sensito-

meter is used to deliver a graduated series of controlled light intensities to a piece of radiographic control film. The exposed control film is then processed, producing a series of graduated or stepped densities known as a sensitometric *control strip* (Fig. 41-7). A densitometer is used to quantitatively measure the densities of the developed sensitometric control strip. Normally only three measurements are needed. A midrange step, which is close to having an optical density of 1, is known as the speed step. The optical density of the second step above the speed step is measured. The difference between this

step and the speed step is known as the density difference, or contrast. The gross, or *base plus fog*, should also be measured. It is good practice to also measure the developer temperature at the time the sensitometric control strip is processed using an accurate thermometer. The data generated are then plotted on a processor control chart (Fig. 41-8). This procedure should be performed at least daily. By charting these processing characteristics, one can interpret the processor's operating condition on a daily basis and also detect any trends in the data that may lead to problems. The measurements should fall within the facility's film processing standard for image quality (speed, contrast, base plus fog), which are established when the processor is considered to be operating in an optimum fashion. If the measurements fall outside the standards, the situation should be analyzed and immediately corrected. The NCDRH recommends the following processing standards of quality: base plus fog ± 0.05 optical density units; contrast ± 0.10 optical density units; speed ± 0.10 optical density units. The integrity and condition of the darkroom should also be tested periodically. This is usually accomplished by visually inspecting the darkroom for light leaks and testing the safelights to determine the level of fog they contribute to the radiographic film.

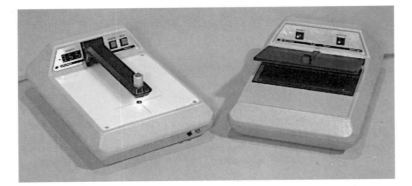

Fig. 41-6. Processor quality control program requires a sensitometer (right) and a densitometer (left).

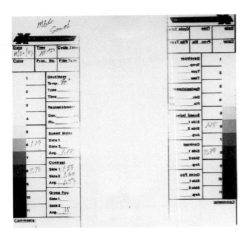

Fig. 41-7. Sensitometric control strip. Both sides of the control film emulsion are sensitometrically exposed. The densitometer measurements of both sides are averaged and recorded on the control strip.

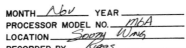

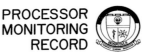

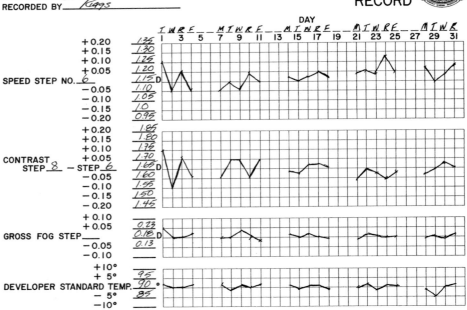

Fig. 41-8. Typical processor control chart.

Radiographic x-ray units

Numerous radiographic x-ray unit parameters can be monitored. A few of the more basic tests are described here.

Beam alignment and beam/light field congruence. This test is designed to check the centering and perpendicularity of the beam, as well as the *congruence* or the *alignment* of the collimator light field and the x-ray beam field. This is an important test since a great deal of unproductive radiation can be delivered to the patient if the system is misaligned. Radiographing straightened paper clips aligned with the edges of the collimator light field is a quick, simple method to evaluate beam/light field alignment accuracy. A tool specifically designed to test these parameters is shown in Fig. 41-9. Light field/x-ray beam alignment is measured by exposing the collimator template. Beam alignment and perpendicularity is assessed by the plastic cylinder, which has a small metallic bead enclosed in each end. The cylinder is centered to the template and exposed. These tests are usually performed on the tabletop and can be used to test both the manual and automatic collimator modes. Beam/light field alignment should be within ± 2% of the SID. Beam perpendicularity is acceptable if both beads are projected within the center ring (Fig. 41-10).

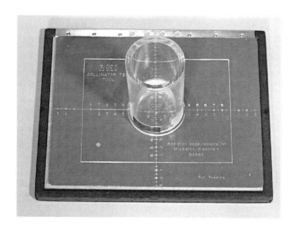

Fig. 41-9. Beam perpendicularity and beam/light field alignment test tools.

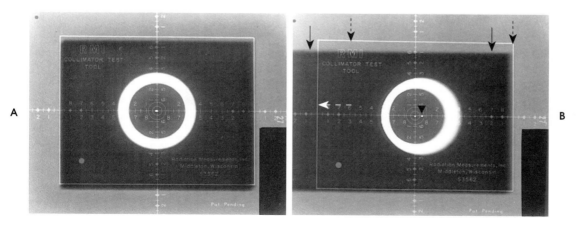

Fig. 41-10. A, Acceptable beam perpendicularity and beam/light field alignment. **B,** Unacceptable beam perpendicularity and beam/light field alignment. Radiation beam *(arrows)* does not agree with collimator light field *(broken arrows)*. Perpendicularity is out of alignment. Note top bead is shifted to the right *(arrowhead)*.

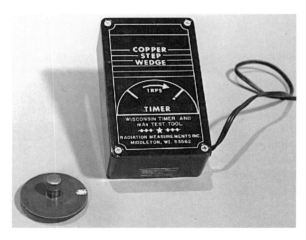

Fig. 41-11. Spinning top (left) and RMI motorized synchronous top (right).

Exposure time. This test determines if the x-ray unit is delivering the same time of exposure as indicated by the control panel's radiographic exposure time. A manually operated spinning top is appropriate for single-phase generators, but three-phase, and high frequency, generators require a motorized synchronous top (Fig. 41-11). The radiopaque face of the synchronous motor device contains a radius slit aperture. An exposure is made of the rotating top. As the slit rotates, it allows radiation to pass, producing an arc of density on the radiograph. By measuring the angle of arc, the time of exposure can be calculated and compared with the time selected on the control panel. This calculation is simplified by using a template to determine the actual exposure time, as shown in Fig. 41-12. Digital x-ray exposure timer test tools are also available that can be used to test both single and three-phase generators. When exposed, these meters measure the x-ray exposure time and display it as a direct digital readout on the face of the meter.

A

B

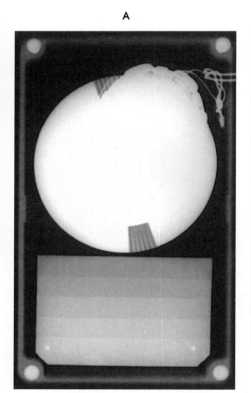

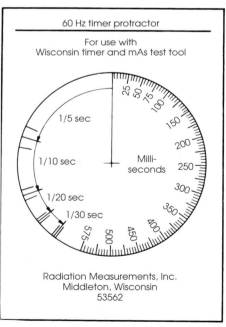

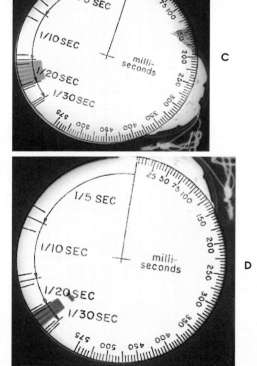

C

D

Fig. 41-12. A, Radiograph produced at 200 mA and 1/20-second exposure. **B,** RMI protractor template. **C,** Radiograph A with template showing acceptable results for a 1/20-second exposure. **D,** Radiograph produced at 300 mA and 1/30-second showing unacceptable results.

Beam quality. The quality of the primary x-ray beam refers to the energy of the x-ray photons that comprise it and is generally described by the *half-value layer (HVL)*. The HVL is a measurement of the x-ray beam quality or average energy. It is an indication of the total equivalent filtration in the path of the x-ray beam (it is not a direct measure of the total filtration). Total equivalent filtration includes the filtration properties of the x-ray glass envelope, the mirror and plastic underside of the collimator, and any added filtration at the port of the x-ray tube. Added filtration is used to increase the *beam hardness,* or average beam energy, by removing more low- than high-energy photons from the beam. This is an important radiation protection consideration, since low-energy x-ray photons are absorbed more readily by the patient. The *beam quality* test verifies that the beam's HVL is sufficient to reduce the patient's exposure to low-energy radiation. The HVL is determined by plotting the thickness of aluminum *attenua-tors* (Fig. 41-13, *A*) that are added to the beam versus the resultant exposures that are measured with a dosimeter (Fig. 41-13, *B*). The acceptable HVL for a single phase generator 80 kVp beam is 2.3 mm of aluminum. An HVL less than this indicates that the total filtration of the beam must be increased (Fig. 41-13, *C*), assuming that the kVp is accurate. Inaccurate HVL values may also indicate inaccurate kVp calibration or tube problems.

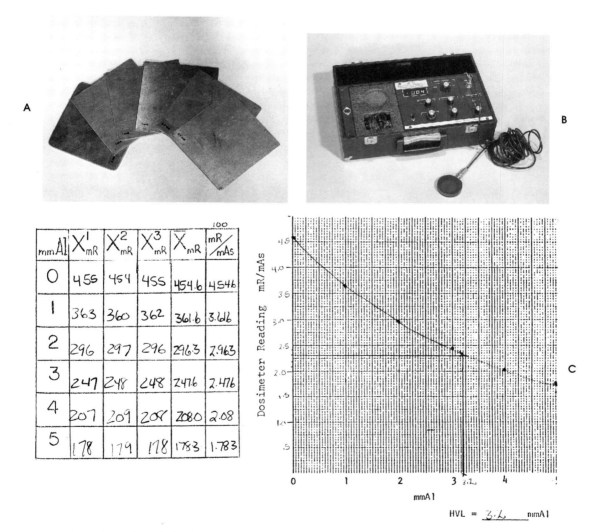

mmAl	X^1_{mR}	X^2_{mR}	X^3_{mR}	$\overline{X}_{mR}$	mR/mAs
0	455	454	455	454.6	4.546
1	363	360	362	361.6	3.616
2	296	297	296	296.3	2.963
3	247	248	248	247.6	2.476
4	207	209	208	208.0	2.08
5	178	179	178	178.3	1.783

HVL = 3.2 mmAl

Fig. 41-13. A, Set of aluminum attenuators of various thicknesses. **B,** Digital dosimeter used to measure exposure output. **C,** HVL layer is calculated by plotting the average output of exposure in mR/mAs versus thickness of added Al attenuator. Graph shows acceptable results.

kVp. The maximum or peak electrical potential (kVp) across the x-ray tube affects the radiation intensity reaching the image receptor and the subject contrast of the final image. Radiographic density and contrast can be adversely affected by inaccurate kVp calibration. Noninvasive electronic digital kVp meters are available that will accurately measure kVp and provide a digital readout of the measured kVp in a fast and convenient manner. Another device used to test the accuracy of kVp settings is the kVp test cassette (Fig. 41-14, *A*). The cassette works on the principle that kVp can be determined by the amount of attenuation that occurs in a filtered beam. The specially designed cassette contains a copper filter, a series of *stepwedges,* and an optical attenuator built into the cassette. The cassette works on the principle that the effective kVp defines the step of the wedge that attenuates the radiation equal to the attenuation of the intensifying screen light by the optical attenuator. The attenuation effects are recorded as radiographic densities on film that has been exposed in the cassette at a given kVp setting (Fig. 41-14, *B*). By matching the step density produced by the stepwedge attenuator to the density produced by the optical attenuator, the effective kVp can be determined from a calibration curve supplied with the cassette. The measured effective kVp should be within ±4 kVp of the kVp setting tested.

Exposure reproducibility and linearity. Predictable radiographic exposures are essential for consistent radiographic images. The test for *exposure reproducibility* (repeatability) determines whether the same results are attained every time the same technique factors are used. *Linearity* (reciprocity) tests are done to determine that the same exposure is obtained at a given milliampere-second selection, without regard to the combination of milliampere and exposure time selections chosen to achieve the milliampere-second setting. The reproducibility/linearity test can be accomplished qualitatively by repeatedly exposing a stepwedge with the same mA/exposure time combination to determine the exposure reproducibility. To test for exposure linearity the stepwedge should be repeatedly exposed using the same total mAs but in different mA/exposure time combinations. By matching the radiographic densities of the stepwedge images, the accuracy of the parameters can be evaluated (Fig. 41-15). A dosimeter can also be used to record the output of the exposures that are compared quantitatively to determine their accuracy. An x-ray unit should produce reproducible exposures to within 5% of their average. Exposure linearity should not exceed 10%.

Focal spot size. The recorded detail in a radiographic image is partially dependent on the size of the x-ray tube's focal spot. As the size of the focal spot increases, the ability to define small structures is diminished. In addition, a change in focal spot size over time may be symptomatic of the x-ray tube's deterioration. A slit camera is used to measure the physical size of the focal spot. This device is used by physicists or other appropriately trained individuals to obtain accurate, quantitative focal spot measurements.

An easy test to determine changes in focal spot size over time is to periodically evaluate its resolving capability. A *resolution* test pattern (Fig. 41-16, *A*), which is comprised of groups of different sized bar patterns (line pairs), is radiographed using a direct exposure technique (Fig. 41-16, *B*). The radiograph of the test pattern is evaluated to determine the smallest group of line pairs that can be seen clearly (Fig. 41-16, *C* and *D*). Tables are available that equate the effective focal spot size to the smallest pattern resolved. The star test pattern is another type of resolution test pattern that is often used. This pattern provides more accurate information but is more difficult to use. Determining the resolving capability of a focal spot should be considered a qualitative test due to its inability to accurately measure the true physical size of the focal spot.

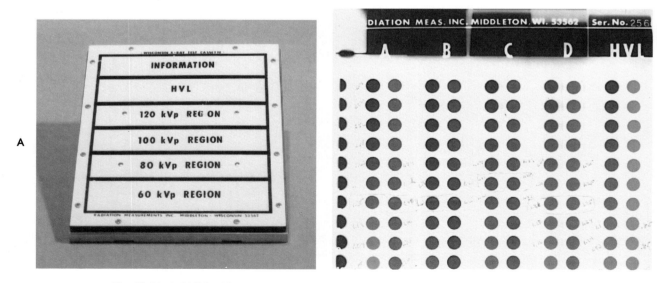

Fig. 41-14. A, RMI 8 × 10 in kVp test cassette. Can be used to measure the accuracy of 60, 80, 100, and 120 kVp settings. Cassette can also be used to measure HVL. **B,** kVp test radiograph. By measuring the densities of the adjacent dots with a densitometer, an accuracy of ±2 kVp can be achieved.

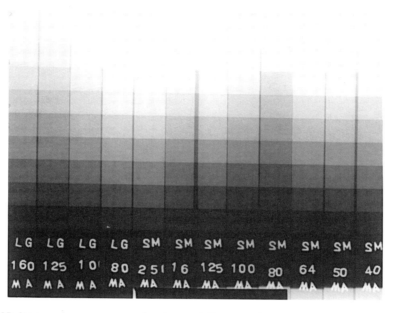

Fig. 41-15. Stepwedge exposures of various mA/time combinations can be used to check linearity. Density should not vary more than one step between exposures.

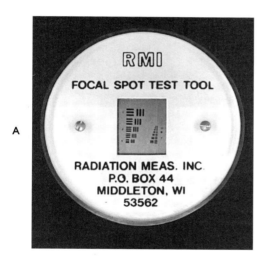

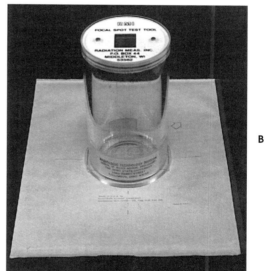

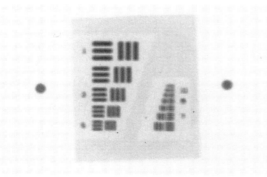

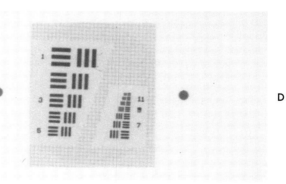

Fig. 41-16. A, RMI resolution test pattern used to measure focal spot size. **B,** Set-up of focal spot test tool. **C,** Test results on a large focal spot, showing the effective size to be 1.4 mm. **D,** Test results on a small focal spot, showing the effective size to be 0.6 mm.

Image receptors

The image receptor most commonly used in diagnostic radiology is a cassette containing intensifying screens and radiographic film. The cassette is a rigid, light-proof holder that compresses the screens and film together when closed. The care and condition of the image receptor have a direct bearing on radiographic image quality.

Cassettes. Loss of cassette integrity may produce unsharp or fogged radiographs. Cassettes should be physically inspected periodically for wearing of the latches and hinges, warping of the cassette frame, and deterioration of the foam or felt compression material. Testing for light leaks should also be a part of the inspection process. Cassettes should be repaired or replaced if they do not pass such inspections.

Intensifying screens. Dirty and worn intensifying screens can cause radiographic artifacts. It is important to visually inspect the screens for wear, abrasions, and stains and to clean them on a routine basis. Screens should be cleaned with a soft cloth and a recommended screen cleaner or a mild soap and water solution. The screens must be thoroughly dry before they are returned to service.

The speed (sensitivity) of similar intensifying screens may vary as they age or as new cassettes and screens are added to service. This lack of uniformity results in radiographic density variations. To test for screen-speed uniformity, the following steps are observed:

- Use a reliable generator and the appropriate exposure technique to produce a radiographic density of approximately 1.5.
- Identify all the similar screened cassettes in service with lead markers.
- Expose each cassette using the same technique.
- Use a densitometer to measure the density of each of the radiographs. The measured density variation between the radiographs should not exceed ± 0.2.

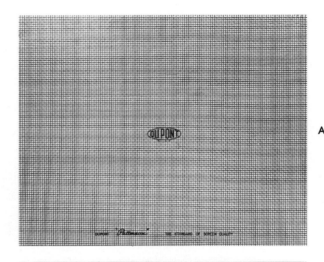

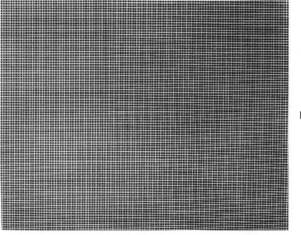

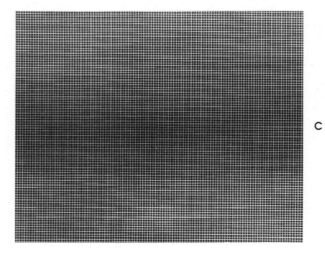

Fig. 41-17. A, Wire mesh test tool. **B,** Test radiograph exhibiting acceptable film-screen contact. **C,** Test radiograph exhibiting unacceptable film-screen contact.

Film-screen contact. Poor contact between the intensifying screens and the radiographic film reduces the contrast and recorded detail in the radiographic image. Radiographic cassettes should be periodically tested for poor film contact. A wire mesh test object is used for this purpose (Fig. 41-17, *A*). The wire mesh test object is placed on top of the cassette and radiographed. The radiographic image of the wire mesh should have a uniform radiographic density. Any areas that appear darker indicate poor contact (Fig. 41-17, *B* and *C*). Cassettes that exhibit areas of poor contact in the central portion of the cassette should be repaired or replaced.

Grids

Misaligned grids attenuate an increased portion of the primary radiation beam, resulting in increased patient radiation dose and a reduction in radiographic image quality. The loss of image quality caused by improper grid alignment can be subtle and is often attributed to other causes. A simple test to evaluate grid alignment requires radiographing a 14 × 17 inch homogeneous phantom, such as water, aluminum, or fiberboard using the following steps:

- Expose the phantom crosswise on the radiographic table.
- Place a 14 × 17 inch cassette crosswise in the Bucky tray.
- Select an exposure technique that will produce a radiographic density of approximately 1.5. A properly aligned grid will produce an even density across the radiograph. An uneven density indicates the need for corrective maintenance.

Illuminators

An important but often overlooked aspect of radiographic quality control is the evaluation of illuminator performance. Illuminator variations affect radiographic density and contrast. Illuminator output changes as the illuminator ages, and the output intensity is affected by the type of light source used. Illuminators with a reduced light intensity increase the density of the radiograph being viewed. Lack of uniformity between illuminators may cause radiographs to appear underexposed when using one illuminator and overexposed when using another, resulting in reduced contrast in both situations. A photographic or optical light meter can measure illuminator intensity and check for variation among illuminators. Gross mismatches should be corrected.

Visual inspections

Periodically, but at least annually, a thorough visual inspection of the radiographic and fluoroscopic equipment and accessory devices should be made to assess their mechanical integrity and safety. Some of the more important visual checks include the following:

1. *Overhead tube cranes:* Inspect the stability, movement, detent operation, lock function, SID and angulation indicator function, Bucky center light and light localizer brightness and accuracy, and the condition of the high tension cables.
2. *Radiographic table:* Check for the proper functioning of Bucky tray and cassette locks, power top and angulation switches, and table angulation indicator; and inspect the stability and function of foot and shoulder braces.
3. *Control panel:* Check for the proper functioning of panel lights/meters and switches, overload protection indicator, and tube heat sensors; the availability and currentness of technique charts; and an unobstructed view of the exposure room through the control panel window.
4. *Fluoroscopic systems:* Check for the proper functioning of fluoroscopic lights, meters, switches, locks, and Bucky slot cover; the presence and integrity of lead tower drapes; and the smoothness of movement of the power assist.
5. *Protective lead apparel:* Lead aprons and gloves should be either radiographed or viewed fluoroscopically to determine if any cracks are present. When not in use they should be stored on appropriate hangers to prevent cracks from forming. Lead sheets used for masking cassettes for multiple exposures should also be checked in the same manner.
6. *Miscellaneous:* Positioning aids should be examined for foreign substances that could produce artifacts on radiographs, such as barium stains on sponges. These items should be either radiographed or fluoroscoped to rule out any such possible contamination. Check the mechanical integrity of additional equipment, such as foot stools, IV stands, and upright support devices.

ADDITIONAL QUALITY CONTROL TESTS

The quality control tests previously described can be considered basic tests for monitoring the film processor and radiographic units. Similar quality control tests should be used to monitor fluoroscopic equipment, mammography equipment, and mobile radiographic units. Quality control tests are also designed for image intensifiers, tomographic equipment, automatic exposure control devices, computerized tomography systems, magnetic resonance imaging systems, and sonography units. Quality control should also be extended to include nuclear medicine and radiation therapy if such facilities exist.

Summary

Radiographic quality assurance programs can play a major role in the improvement of patient care, the reduction of unnecessary radiation to both personnel and patients, and the containment of costs of radiologic health care delivery. Although this chapter has dealt primarily with quality assurance in the context of the technical elements of the radiographic system, medical radiation personnel must remember that their responsibilities to the patient extend beyond the technical aspects of image production.

Definition of Terms

alignment Closeness of agreement of the centers and edges of the x-ray beam and collimator light fields.

attenuator Object that reduces the intensity of an x-ray beam.

base plus fog Density of unexposed processed radiographic film resulting from opacity of film base and density inherent to film emulsion.

beam hardening Increasing the mean energy of the x-ray beam spectrum by removal of the low-energy photons.

beam quality Energy of an x-ray beam.

congruence Closeness of agreement in position and size of x-ray beam and collimator light fields.

control strip Radiographic film that has been exposed by a sensitometer or radiation passing through a stepwedge.

densitometer A device used to measure the optical density of photographic film.

diagnostic radiology facility Any establishment using an x-ray system in procedures involving the radiation of the human body for the purpose of diagnosis or visualization.

exposure reproducibility The ability to obtain the same exposure output using the same mA and exposure time from one exposure to the next.

half-value layer (HVL) Thickness of an absorber that will reduce the intensity of an x-ray beam by one half.

linearity The ability to obtain the same exposure for the same mAs, regardless of mA and exposure time used.

NCDRH National Center for Devices and Radiological Health, previously called the Bureau of Radiological Health (BRH).

objective Standards of image quality that relate to aspects that can be directly measured.

quality administration procedures Management procedures that provide for the organization of the quality assurance program.

quality assurance (QA) Planned and organized efforts within a diagnostic radiology facility to ensure the production of consistent optimal quality images with minimal radiation exposure and cost to the patient consumer.

quality assurance program A distinct organized structure designed to furnish quality assurance for a diagnostic radiology facility.

quality control (QC) Methods and procedures used in the testing and maintenance of the components of an x-ray system.

reject analysis The study of repeated radiographs to determine the cause for their being discarded.

resolution Ability to record separate images of small objects that are placed very close together.

sensitometer A device designed to give precise, reproducible, and graduated light exposures to photographic film.

stepwedge A device used to put a series of increasing exposures on a radiographic film when exposed by a radiographic beam.

subjective Standards of image quality that are expressed by feelings, perceptions, and thoughts of the observer rather than by direct measurement.

x-ray system The collection of components for the production, recording, and viewing of radiographic images.

SELECTED BIBLIOGRAPHY

Barber TC et al: Radiologic quality control manual, Reston, VA, 1984, Reston Publishing Co.

Basic quality control in diagnostic radiology. Report No 4, Chicago, 1978, American Association of Physicists in Medicine.

Burkhart RL: Diagnostic radiology quality assurance catalog. HEW Publication No (FDA) 77-8028. Washington, DC, 1977, US Dept of Health, Education and Welfare.

Burkhart RL: Diagnostic radiology quality assurance catalog: supplement. HEW Publication No (FDA) 78-8028. Washington, DC, 1978, US Dept of Health, Education and Welfare.

Burkhart RL: Quality assurance programs for diagnostic radiology facilities. HEW Publication No (FDA) 80-8110. Washington, DC, 1980. US Dept of Health, Education and Welfare.

Burkhart RL: Checklist for establishing a diagnostic radiology quality assurance program, HHS Publication No (FDA) 83-8219. Washington, DC, 1983, US Dept of Health and Human Services.

Burkhart RL: A basic quality assurance program for small diagnostic radiology facilities, HHS Publication No (FDA) 83-8218, Washington, DC, 1983, US Dept of Health and Human Services.

Carlton R: Establishing a total quality assurance program in diagnostic radiology, Radiol Technol 35:23-38, 1980.

Goldman LW: Analysis of retakes: understanding, managing and using an analysis of retakes program for quality assurance. HEW Publication No (FDA) 79-8097. Washington, DC, 1979, US Dept of Health, Education and Welfare.

Gray JE: Photographic quality assurance in diagnostic radiology, nuclear medicine, and radiation therapy, vol 1, The basic principles of daily photographic quality assurance. HEW Publication No (FDA) 76-8043. Washington, DC, 1976, US Dept of Health, Education and Welfare.

Gray JE: Photographic quality assurance in diagnostic radiology, nuclear medicine and radiation therapy, vol 2, Photographic processing, quality assurance and the evaluation of photographic materials. HEW Publication No (FDA) 77-8018. Washington, DC, 1977, US Dept of Health, Education and Welfare.

Gray JE et al: Mammography quality control: Radiologic technologist's manual, 1992, American College of Radiology and the American Cancer Society.

Gray JE et al: Quality control in diagnostic imaging, Baltimore, 1983, University Park Press.

Hendee WR et al: Quality assurance for radiographic x-ray units and associated equipment. HEW Publication No (FDA) 79-8094. Washington, DC, 1979, US Dept of Health, Education and Welfare.

Hendee WR et al: Quality assurance for fluoroscopic x-ray units and associated equipment. HEW Publication No (FDA) 80-8095, Washington, DC, 1980, US Dept of Health Education and Welfare.

Hendee WR et al: Quality assurance for conventional tomographic x-ray units. HEW Publication No (FDA) 80-8096. Washington, DC, 1980, US Dept of Health, Education and Welfare.

Lawrence DJ: A simple method of processor control, Med Radiogr Photogr 49(1):2-6, 1973.

McKinney WE: Radiographic processing and quality control, Philadelphia, 1988, JB Lippincott.

McLemore JM: Quality assurance in diagnostic radiology, St Louis, 1981, Mosby.

Nelson RE et al: Economic analysis of a comprehensive quality assurance program, Radiol Technol 49:129-134, 1977.

Noyes RS: The economics of quality assurance, RNM Mag 10(6):7-9, 24, 28, Dec. 1980.

Quality assurance for diagnostic imaging equipment. NCRP Report No 99, Bethesda, MD, 1988, National Council on Radiation Protection and Measurements.

Quality assurance programs for diagnostic radiology facilities, final recommendation, Federal Register 44:71728-71740, 1979.

Quality assurance in diagnostic radiology and nuclear medicine—the obvious decision. HHS Publication No (FDA) 81-8141. Washington, DC, 1981, US Dept of Health and Human Services.

Radiologic image quality (formerly QC News), Department of Medical Physics, Univ of Wisconsin, 1983, Madison, WI.

Tortorici M: Concepts in Medical Radiographic Imaging, Philadelphia, 1992, WB Saunders.

BIBLIOGRAPHY

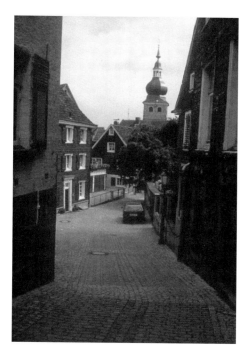

A winding and narrow street leading towards the town square in Lennep, Germany.

PEDIATRIC RADIOGRAPHY

For bibliographic citations before 1964, please see the fifth edition of this ATLAS. For citations from 1964 through 1974, see the sixth or seventh edition.

1975   Gooding CA, et al: Adverse reactions to intravenous pyelography in children, AJR 123:802-804, 1975.

Haller JO and Slovis TL: Importance of horizontal beam for lateral view of skull in pediatric radiography, Radiol Technol 47:150-152, 1975.

Holbert CL, et al: Radiographic technique, safety, and interpretation in the newborn nursery, J Pediatr 87:968-972, 1975.

Knake JE: A device to aid in positioning for the Andren von Rosen hip view, Radiology 117:735-736, 1975.

1976   Buckle CM: Immobilization of the patient in pediatric radiography, Radiography 42:195-196, 1976.

Poznanski AK: Practical approaches to pediatric radiology, Chicago, 1976, Mosby.

1977   Barry JF et al: Metrizamide in pediatric myelography, Radiology 124:409-418, 1977.

Eklof O, editor: Current concepts in pediatric radiology, New York, 1977, Springer-Verlag.

Hass EA and Solomon DJ: Telling children about diagnostic radiology procedures, Radiology 124:521, 1977.

Hirsch DJ et al: Evaluation for hip dysplasia in infancy: the significance of x-ray in diagnosis, J Med Soc NJ 74:528-532, 1977.

1978   American Academy of Pediatrics, Committee on Radiology: Water-soluble contrast material, Pediatrics 62:114-116, 1978.

Hernandez R, Gutowski D and Poznanski AK: A simple method of using a shadow gonadal shield with closed incubators, Radiology 128:821-822, 1978.

Merten DF: Comparison radiographs in extremity injuries of childhood: current application in radiological practice, Radiology 126:209-210, 1978.

1979   Cohen MD: Intravenous urography in neonates and infants: what dose of contrast media should be used? Br J Radiol 52:942-944, 1979.

Kalender W, Reither M and Schuster W: Reduction of dose in pelvic examinations of infants using modern x-ray techniques, Pediatr Radiol 8:233-235, 1979.

1980   Anderson RE et al: Impact of a "fast" scanner on image quality in pediatric computed tomography, Radiology 34:251-252, 1980.

Brodeur AE et al: The many advantages of direct microfocus roentgenographic magnification in pediatric radiology, Am J Dis Child 134:245-247, 1980.

Heller RM et al: Diagnostic imaging in pediatric emergencies, South Med J 73:844-849, 1980.

Leonidas JC: Avoiding unnecessary x-ray exposure in children, Compr Ther 6:46-54, 1980.

Lonnerholm T: Arthrography of the hip in children: technique, normal anatomy, and findings in unstable hip joints, Acta Radiol 21:279-292, 1980.

Pritchard C: Radiation protection of personnel during pediatric radiodiagnostic examination, Radiography 46:165-169, 1980.

Seibert JJ et al: Low efficacy radiography of children, AJR 134:1219-1223, 1980.

Swischuk LE: Radiology of the newborn and young infant, Baltimore, 1980, Williams & Wilkins.

Wesenberg RL et al: Low-dose radiography of children, Radiol Technol 51:641-648, 1980.

1981   Berger PE, Kuhn JP and Brusehaber J: Techniques for computed tomography in infants and children, Radiol Clin North Am 19:399-408, 1981.

Herbert R and McGrath A: Ultrasonic investigation of the brain in neonates, Radiography 47:187-193, 1981.

Hough S: Barium feeder for babies, Radiography 47:186, 1981.

Leonidas JC, McCauley RG and Faerber EN: Pediatric radiologists in the United States and Canada: involvement with newer imaging modalities, Radiology 138:235-237, 1981.

Milne EN and Gillan GG: Technique for improving neonatal chest roentgenograms, Appl Radiol 10:45-49, 1981.

1982   Brasch RC and Gould RG: Direct magnification radiography of the newborn infant, Radiology 143:649-655, 1982.

Cherian MJ, et al: Prone films of abdomen—a diagnostic tool in intestinal obstruction, Australas Radiol 26:255-260, 1982.

Coombs AR: Adapting a lateral cassette holder for paediatric radiography, Radiography 48:151-174, 1982.

Ferry PC: Skull roentgenograms in pediatric head trauma: a vanishing necessity? Pediatrics 69:237-238, 1982.

Heller RM, Partain CL and James AE: Implications of nuclear magnetic resonance imaging for the pediatrician, Am J Dis Child 136:1045-1046, 1982.

Kaiser MC and Martin DJ: Direct coronal images—a valuable addition to pediatric body CT-scanning, Pediatr Radiol 12:295-297, 1982.

Siegle RL, Davies P and Fullerton GD: Urography with metrizamide in children, AJR 139:927-930, 1982.

White SC: Radiation safety for children, Int Dent J 32:259-264, 1982.

1983   Diament MJ and Kangarloo H: Dosage schedule for pediatric urography based on body surface, AJR 140:815-816, 1983.

Gyll C: Preventing lordotic projection of the chest, Radiography 49:291-293, 1983.

Kaufman RA: Liver-spleen computed tomography: a method tailored for infants and children, J Comput Tomogr 7:45-57, 1983.

Kirks D: Practical techniques for pediatric computed tomography, Pediatr Radiol 13:148-155, 1983.

Leonidas JC et al: The one-film urogram in urinary tract infection in children, AJR 141:61-64, 1983.

Ratcliffe JF: The small bowel enema in children: a description of a technique, Clin Radiol 34:287-289, 1983.

1984   Bolz KD, Skalpe IO and Gutteberg TJ: Iohexol and metrizoate in urography in children, comparison, Acta Radiol [Diagn] (Stockh) 25:155-158, 1984.

Cohen G et al: Dose efficiency of screen-film systems used in pediatric radiography, Radiology 152:187-193, 1984.

Kuijpers D, Blickman JG and Camps JA: The five-degree rule: optimization of the paranasal sinus examination of children, Radiology 152:814, 1984.

Libson E et al: Oblique lumbar spine radiographs: importance in young patients, Radiology 151:89-90, 1984.

McAlister WH and Siegel MJ: Fatal aspirations in infancy during gastrointestinal series, Pediatr Radiol 14:81-83, 1984.

McDaniel DL et al: Relative dose efficiencies of antiscatter grids and air gaps in pediatric radiography, Med Phys 11:508-512, 1984.

Robey G et al: Pediatric urography: comparison of metrizamide and methylglucamine, Radiology 150:61-63, 1984.

Smathers RL et al: Radiation dose reduction in the neonatal intensive care unit: comparison of three gadolinium oxysulfide screen-film combinations, Invest Radiol 19:578-582, 1984.

1985   Carlsson EC et al: Pediatric angiocardiography with iohexol, Invest Radiol 20:S75-S78, 1985.

Symposium on pediatric radiology, Pediatr Clin North Am 32:1351-1622, 1985.

1986   Altman NR et al: Three-dimensional CT reformation in children, AJR 146:1261-1267, 1986.

Ball WS Jr et al: Interventional genitourinary radiology in children: a review of 61 procedures, AJR 147:791-796, 1986.

Davies J and Russell JG: Carbon fibre faced cassettes in neonatal radiography: their use and cost effectiveness, Radiography 52:113-114, 1986.

Kendall B: Iohexol in paediatric myelography: an open non-comparative trial, Neuroradiology 28:65-68, 1986.

Majid M: Radionuclide imaging in clinical pediatrics, Pediatr Ann 15:396-402, 407-8, 1986

Merten DF and Grossman H: Diagnostic imaging in pediatrics: the state of the part, Pediatr Ann 15:355-358, 1986.

Nickel O and Hahn K: New nuclear medical technologies for pediatrics, Med Prog Technol 11:65-72, 1986.

Roberts GJ, Semple J and Gibb D: Radiographic techniques in paediatric dentistry, Radiography 52:83-87, 1986.

Sprigg A et al: Compensation filtration in paediatric double-contrast barium enema, Clin Radiol 37:599-601, 1986.

Strain JD et al: Intravenously administered pentobarbital sodium for sedation in pediatric CT, Radiology 161:105-108, 1986.

Weinreb JC et al: Imaging the pediatric liver: MRI and CT, AJR 147:785-790, 1986.

1987   Boesmi B et al: Digital angiography in children, Rays 12:47-52, 1987.

Boothroyd AE, Carty HM and Robson WJ: 'Hunt the thimble': a study of the radiology of ingested foreign bodies, Arch Emerg Med 4:33-38, 1987.

Donaldson JS, Poznanski AK and Nieves A: CT of children's feet: an immibilization technique, AJR 148:169-170, 1987.

Herman MW, Mak HK and Lachman RS: Radiation exposure reduction by use of Kevlar cassettes in the neonatal nursery, AJR 148:969-972, 1987.

Sheinfeld J et al: Octoson imaging in pediatric urology, Urology 30:232-237, 1987.

Wesenberg RL et al: Ultra-low-dose routine pediatric radiography utilizing a rare-earth filter, J Can Assoc Radiol 38:158-164, 1987.

Yoshizumi TT et al: Radiation safety and protection of neonates in radiological examinations, Radiol Technol 58:405-408, 1987.

1988   Brasch RC: Ultrafast computed tomography for infants and children, Radiol Clin North Am 26:277-286, 1988.

Cole AJ, Webb L and Cole TJ: Bone age estimation: a comparison of methods, Br J Radiol 61:683-686, 1988.

Crooks LE et al: Echo-planar pediatric imager, Radiology 166:157-163, 1988.

Diament MJ, Bird CR and Stanley P: Outpatient performance of invasive radiologic procedures in pediatric patients, Radiology 166:401-403, 1988.

Duthoy MJ and Lund G: MR imaging of the spine in children, Eur J Radiol 8:188-195, 1988

Eggleston DE, Slovis TL and Watts FB: Update on pediatric chest imaging, Pediatr Pulmonol 5:158-175, 1988.

Ehara S, el-Khoury GY and Sato Y: Cervical spine injury in children: radiologic manifestations, AJR 151:1175-1178, 1988.

Gainey MA and Capitanio MA: Recent advances in pediatric nuclear medicine, Radiol Clin North Am 26:409-418, 1988.

Gyll C: Gonad protection for the paediatric patient, Radiography 54:9-11, 1988.

Hirose K et al: Antenatal ultrasound diagnosis of the femur-fibula-ulna syndrome, JCU 16:199-203, 1988.

Kane NM et al: Pediatric abdominal trauma: evaluation by computed tomography, Pediatrics 82:11-15, 1988.

Laks Y and Barzilay Z: Foreign body aspiration in childhood, Pediatr Emerg Care 4:102-106, 1988.

Magid D et al: Two-dimensional or three-dimensional computed tomography of the pediatric hip, Radiographics 8:901-933, 1988.

Markowitz RI: The anterior junction line: a radiographic sign of bilateral pneumothorax in neonates, Radiology 167:717-719, 1988.

Nahata MC: Sedation in pediatric patients undergoing diagnostic procedures, Drug Intell Clin Pharm 22:711-715, 1988.

Recent advances in practical pediatric radiology, Radiol Clin North Am 26:181-469, 1988.

Savitt DL and Wason S: Delayed diagnosis of coin ingestion in children, Am J Emerg Med 6:378-381, 1988.

Sfakianakis GN and Sfakianaki ED: Nuclear medicine in pediatric urology and nephrology, J Nucl Med 29:1287-1300, 1988.

Simmons BP and Lovallo JL: Hand and wrist injuries in children, Clin Sports Med 7:495-512, 1988.

Steiner GM: Paediatric radiology 3: genitourinary tract, Br J Hosp Med 39:518-521, 1988.

Vanderwilde R et al: Measurements on radiographs of the foot in normal infants and children, J Bone Joint Surg [Am] 70:407-415, 1988.

1989   Ben Ami T, Rozin M and Hertz M: Imaging of children with urinary tract infection: a tailored approach, Clin Radiol 40:64-67, 1989.

Bisset GS: Pediatric thoracic applications of magnetic resonance imaging, J Thorac Imaging 4:51-57, 1989.

Calandrino C: Barium enema procedure for the pediatric patient, Radiol Technol 60:209-213, 1989.

Evans DL and Bethem D: Cervical spine injuries in children, J Pediatr Orthop 9:563-568, 1989.

Fesmire FM and Luten RC: The pediatric cervical spine: developmental anatomy and clinical aspects, J Emerg Med 7:133-142, 1989.

Fredericks BJ et al: Diseases of the spinal canal in children: diagnosis with noncontrast CT scans, AJNR 10:1233-1238, 1989.

Glasier CM et al: Extracardiac chest ultrasonography in infants and children: radiographic and clinical implications, J Pediatr 114:540-544, 1989.

Horger EO and Tsai CC: Ultrasound and the prenatal diagnosis of congenital anomalies: a medicolegal perspective, Obstet Gynecol 74:617-619, 1989.

Johnson ND et al: MR imaging anatomy of the infant hip, AJR 153:127-133, 1989.

Kaufman RA: Technical aspects of abdominal CT in infants and children, AJR 153:549-554, 1989.

Keller MS: Renal Doppler sonography in infants and children, Radiology 172:603-604, 1989.

Kogutt MS, Warren FH and Kalmar JA: Low dose imaging of scoliosis: use of a computed radiographic imaging system, Pediatr Radiol 20:85-86, 1989.

Lally KP et al: Utility of the cervical spine radiograph in pediatric trauma, Am J Surg 158:540-541, 1989.

Leighton DM and de Campo M: CT invertograms, Pediatr Radiol 19:176-178, 1989.

Merten DF et al: Rational use of diagnostic imaging in paediatrics: the report of a World Health Organization Study Group, Pediatr Radiol 19:216-218, 1989.

Pennell RG and Kurtz AB: Fetal intrathoracic and gastrointestinal anomalies, Clin Diagn Ultrasound 25:111-138, 1989.

Plowman PN, Doughty D and Harnett AN: Paediatric brachytherapy. I. The role of brachytherapy in the multidisciplinary therapy of localized cancers, Br J Radiol 62:218-222, 1989.

Revonta M and Kuuliala I: The diagnosis and follow-up of pediatric sinusitis: Water's view, Laryngoscope 99:321-324, 1989.

Thomson ES, Afshar F and Plowman PN: Paediatric brachytherapy. II. Brain implantation, Br J Radiol 62:223-229, 1989.

1990   Ackerman T, Reed MH: Osteomyelitis of the tarsal bones in children, Can Assoc Radiol J 41:69-71, 1990.

Bohn D et al: Cervical spine injuries in children, J Trauma 30:463-469, 1990.

Glasier CM et al: Screening spinal ultrasound in newborns with neural tube defects, J Ultrasound Med 9:339-343, 1990.

Hedlund GL and Kirks DR: Emergency radiology of the pediatric chest, Curr Probl Diagn Radiol 19:133-164, 1990.

Odrezin GT et al: High resolution computed tomography of the temporal bone in infants and children: a review, Int J Pediatr Otorhinolaryngol 19:15-31, 1990.

Pediatrics, Curr Opin Radiol 2:955-965, 1990.

Pinsky WW and Arciniegas E: Tetralogy of Fallot, Pediatr Clin North Am 37:179-192, 1990.

Riebel T and Wartner R: Use of non-ionic contrast media for tracheobronchography in neonates and young infants, Eur J Radiol 11:120-124, 1990.

Sartoris DJ and Resnick D: Magnetic resonance imaging of pediatric foot and ankle disorders, J Foot Surg 29:489-494, 1990.

Siegel MJ: Chest applications of magnetic resonance imaging in children, Top Magn Reson Imaging 3:1-23, 1990.

1991   Altman DI and Volpe JJ: Positron emission tomography in newborn infants, Clin Perinatol 18:549-562, 1991.

Bisset GS and Ball WS Jr: Preparation, sedation, and monitoring of the pediatric patient in the magnetic resonance suite, Semin Ultrasound CT MR 12:376-378, 1991.

Bresnahan PJ and Fung J: Magnetic resonance imaging of the foot and ankle in the pediatric patient, J Am Podiatr Med Assoc 81:112-118, 1991.

Caron KH: Magnetic resonance imaging of the pediatric abdomen, Semin Ultrasound CT MR 12:448-474, 1991.

Cobby M, Clarke N and Duncan A: Ultrasound of the infant hip, West Engl Med J 106:74-76, 1991.

Coventry DM, Martin CS and Burke AM: Sedation for paediatric computerized tomography—a double-blind assessment of rectal midazolam, Eur J Anaesthesiol 8:29-32, 1991.

Herman TE and Siegel MJ: CT of the pancreas in children, AJR 157:375-379, 1991.

Johnson KJ, Bhatia P and Bell EF: Infrared thermometry of newborn infants, Pediatrics 87:34-38, 1991.

Krasny R et al: MR anatomy of infants hip: comparison to anatomical preparations, Pediatr Radiol 21:211-215, 1991.

Long BW, Rafert JA and Cory D: Percutaneous feeding tube method for use in children, Radiol Technol 62:274-278, 1991.

Pediatrics, Curr Opin Radiol 3:967-975, 1991.

Piepsz A, Gordon I and Hahn K: Paediatric nuclear medicine, Eur J Nucl Med 18:41-66, 1991.

Towbin RB: Pediatric interventional radiology, Curr Opin Radiol 3:931-935, 1991.

1992   Ablin DS, Greenspan A and Reinhart MA: Pelvic injuries in child abuse, Pediatr Radiol 22:454-457, 1992.

Beaty JH: Fractures and dislocations about the elbow in children, Instr Course Lect 41:373-384, 1992.

Bisset GS: Magnetic resonance imaging in the pediatric patient, Pediatr Ann 21:121-6, 129-31, 1992.

Blevins SJ and Benson S: A better way to get kids through scans, RN 55:40-44, 1992.

Boyer RS: Sedation in pediatric neuroimaging: the science and the art, AJNR 13:777-783, 1992.

Brody AS: Pediatric body CT, Pediatr Ann 21:111, 114-111, 120, 1992.

Bucholtz JD: Issues concerning the sedation of children for radiation therapy, Oncol Nurs Forum 19:649-655, 1992.

Cardinal E and White SJ: Imaging pediatric hip disorders and residual dysplasia of adult hips, Curr Opin Radiol 4:83-89, 1992.

Chuang S: Contrast agents in pediatric neuroimaging, AJNR 13:785-791, 1992.

Eich GF, Babyn P and Giedion A: Pediatric pelvis: radiographic appearance in various congenital disorders, Radiographics 12:467-484, 1992.

Fernbach SK and Feinstein KA: Selected topics in pediatric ultrasonography—1992, Radiol Clin North Am 30:1011-1031, 1992.

Gennuso R et al: Lumbar intervertebral disc disease in the pediatric population, Pediatr Neurosurg 18:282-286, 1992.

Grogan DP and Ogden JA: Knee and ankle injuries in children, Pediatr Rev 13:429-434, 1992.

Gross GW: Pediatric chest imaging, Curr Opin Radiol 4:36-43, 1992.

Grossglauser L: Assessment of the quality of the neonatal chest x-ray film, Neonatal Netw 11:69-72, 1992.

Haller JO and Cohen HL: Pediatric ultrasound in the 1990s, Pediatr Ann 21:79, 82-79, 86, 1992.

Harcke HT et al: Growth plate of the normal knee: evaluation with MR imaging, Radiology 183:119-123, 1992.

Harrison LA, Pretorius DH and Budorick NE: Abnormal spinal curvature in the fetus, J Ultrasound Med 11:473-479, 1992.

Harwood-Nash DC: Pediatric neuroradiology: a perspective, AJNR 13:421-422, 1992.

Hopper KD et al: CT and MR imaging of the pediatric orbit, Radiographics 12:485-503, 1992.

Kane TJ, Henry G and Furry D: A simple roentgenographic measurement of femoral anteversion: a short note, J Bone Joint Surg Am 74:1540-1542, 1992.

Kenny N and Hill J: Gonad protection in young orthopaedic patients, BMJ 304:1411-1413, 1992.

Lee DY, Lee CK and Cho TJ: A new method for measurement of femoral anteversion: a comparative study with other radiographic methods, Int Orthop 16:277-281, 1992.

Merten DF: Perspectives on pediatric imaging: 1992, Pediatr Ann 21:76-78, 1992.

Oestreich AE: Imaging of the skeleton and soft tissues in children, Curr Opin Radiol 4:55-61, 1992.

Rothrock SG, Green SM and Hummel CB: Plain abdominal radiography in the detection of major disease in children: a prospective analysis, Ann Emerg Med 21:1423-1429, 1992.

Schlesinger AE and Hernandez RJ: Diseases of the musculoskeletal system in children: imaging with CT sonography, and MR, AJR 158:729-741, 1992.

Stanley P: Advances in pediatric interventional radiology, Curr Opin Radiol 4:73-78, 1992.

Starshak RJ and Sty JR: Trends in physiologic and pharmacologic interventions in pediatric nuclear medicine, Pediatr Ann 21:101-109, 1992.

Umezawa T et al: A computerized automatic exposure device for chest radiography in infants, Clin Pediatr (Phila) 31:751-752, 1992.

Wirth T, LeQuesne GW and Paterson DC: Ultrasonography in Legg-Calve-Perthes disease, Pediatr Radiol 22:498-504, 1992.

Zimmerman RA, Gusnard DA and Bilaniuk LT: Pediatric craniocervical spiral CT, Neuroradiology 34:112-116, 1992.

1993   Bramson RT, Sherman JM and Blickman JG: Pediatric bronchography performed through the flexible bronchoscope, Eur J Radiol 16:158-161, 1993.

Ditchfield MR and De Campo JF: Is the preliminary film necessary prior to the micturating cystourethrogram in children? Abdom Imaging 18:191-192, 1993.

Faro SH, Mahboubi S and Ortega W: CT diagnosis of rib anomalies, tumors, and infection in children, Clin Imaging 17:1-7, 1993.

Feinstein KA and Poznandki AK: Evaluation of joint disease in the pediatric hand, Hand Clin 7:167-182, 1993.

Garcia FF et al: Diagnostic imaging of childhood spinal infection, Orthop Rev 22:321-327, 1993.

Harwood-Nash DC: Edward B. D. Neuhauser Lecture: pediatric neuroradiology: its evolution as a subspecialty, AJR 160:5-14, 1993.

Kaye RD, Grifka RG and Towbin R: Intervention in the thorax in children, Radiol Clin North Am 31:693-712, 1993.

Leventhal JM et al: Fractures in young children: distinguishing child abuse from unintentional injuries, Am J Dis Child 147:87-92, 1993.

Manson D et al: CT of blunt chest trauma in children, Pediatr Radiol 23:1-5, 1993.

Patel K and Chapman S: Normal symphysis pubis width in children, Clin Radiol 47:56-57, 1993.

Slifer KJ et al: Behavior analysis of motion control for pediatric neuroimaging, J App Behav Anal 26:469-470, 1993.

Sutherland GR: Has echo/Doppler influenced the practice of paediatric cardiology? Int J Card Imaging 9(Suppl 2) :17-26, 1993.

Terjesen T, Anda S and Ronningen H: Ultrasound examination for measurement of femoral anteversion in children, Skeletal Radiol 22:33-36, 1993.

Thometz JG and Simons GW: Deformity of the calcaneocuboid joint in patients who have talipes equinovarus, J Bone Joint Surg Am 75:190-195, 1993.

Trotter C and Carey BE: How to evaluate lung fields on the neonatal chest X-ray film, Neonatal Netw 12:63-66, 1993.

Vargo L: Evaluation of cardiac size on the neonatal chest x-ray, Neonatal Netw 12:65-67, 1993.

AUTOTOMOGRAPHY

For bibliographic citations before 1964, please see the fifth edition of this atlas.

1977   Forman WH: Autotomography: a means of improving visualization of the upper cervical spine, Radiology 123:800-801, 1977.

1983   Doyle T and Tress B: Autotomography with metrizamide myelography: an aid to visualization of the cranio-cervical junction and cerebellar tonsils, Clin Radiol 34:401-403, 1983.

TOMOGRAPHY

For bibliographic citations before 1964, please see the fifth edition of this ATLAS. For citations from 1964 through 1974, see the sixth or seventh edition.

1975   Freedman GS, Putman CE and Potter GD: Critical review of tomography in radiology and nuclear medicine, Crit Rev Clin Radiol Nucl Med 6:253-294, 1975.

Norman A: The use of tomography in the diagnosis of skeletal disorders, Clin Orthop 107:139-145, 1975.

Welander V: Layer formation in narrow beam rotation radiography, Acta Radiol 16:529-540, 1975.

1976 Harding G and Day MJ: Blurring quality in spiral tomography, Acta Radiol (Ther) 15:465-480, 1976.

Littleton JT: Tomography physical principles and clinical application, Baltimore, 1976, Williams & Wilkins.

Polga JP and Watnick M: Whole lung tomography in metastatic disease, Clin Radiol 27:53-56, 1976.

Stanson AW and Baker HL: Routine tomography of the temporomandibular joint, Radiol Clin North Am 14:105-127, 1976.

1977 Helander CG, Reichmann S and Astrand K: Xeroradiographic tomography, Acta Radiol 18:369-382, 1977.

Wayrynen RE, Holland RS and Schwenker RP: Film-screen sharpness in complex motion tomography, Invest Radiol 12:195-198, 1977.

1978 Durizch ML: Technical aspects of tomography, Baltimore, 1978, Williams & Wilkins.

1979 Palmer A and Munro L: The principles of tomographic positioning with particular reference to skull tomography, Radiography 45:51-60, 1979.

1980 Eckerdal O and Nelvig P: Reproducible positioning of the skull at tomography, Acta Radiol 21:557-559, 1980.

Farber AL: Advantages of variant section of thickness relative to specific anatomy, Radiol Technol 51:793-796, 1980.

Littleton JT, Durizch ML and Callahan WP: Linear vs. pluridirectional tomography of the chest: correlative radiographic anatomic study, AJR 134:241-248, 1980.

Nakamura Y, Kiyota H and Hara K: Elimination of blur in linear tomography: a simple method using the x-ray processor, Radiology 135:232-233, 1980.

1981 Bein ME and Stone DN: Full lung linear and pluridirectional tomography: a preliminary evaluation of nodule direction, AJR 136:1013-1015, 1981.

Nehen AM et al: Computed tomography and hypocycloid tomography in lesions of the nose, paranasal sinuses, and nasopharynx, Acta Radiol 22:285-287, 1981.

Perilhou JR et al: Intensified tomography: enhancement of soft tissue discrimination in conventional tomography of the brain, Radiology 138:689-696, 1981.

1982 Anderson LD et al: The role of polytomography in the diagnosis and treatment of cervical spine injuries, Clin Orthop 165:64-67, 1982.

Wright JW Jr, Wright JW III and Hicks G: Polytomography and congenital anomalies of the ear, Ann Otol Rhinol Laryngol 91:480-484, 1982.

1983 Cade WJ and Haddaway MJ: Measurement of absorbed skin dose in tomography, Radiography 49:24-26, 1983.

Chasen MH and Yrizarry JM: Tomography of the pulmonary hili: anatomical reassessment of the conventional 55 degrees posterior oblique, Radiology 149:365-369, 1983.

Genereux GP: Conventional tomographic hilar anatomy emphasizing the pulmonary veins, AJR 141:1241-1257, 1983.

Glazer GM et al: Evaluation of the pulmonary hilum: comparison of conventional radiography, 55 degrees posterior oblique tomography, and dynamic computed tomography, J Comput Assist Tomogr 7:983-989, 1983.

Gusching AC: Frontal tomography of articulating temporomandibular joint surfaces, Angle Orthod 53:234-239, 1983.

Marlowe NA: The application of blurred undersubtraction in polytomography, Radiol Technol 54:455-465, 1983.

Stigsson L and Tylen U: 55 degrees posterior oblique tomography of the pulmonary hilum in the evaluation of lung tumors, Radiologe 23:224-228, 1983.

Westesson PL: Double-contrast arthrotomography of the temporomandibular joint, J Oral Maxillofac Surg 41:163-172, 1983.

1984 Bussard DA, Yune HY and Whitehead D: Comparison of corrected-axis and straight lateral TMJ tomograms, J Clin Orthod 18:894-898, 1984.

De la Cruz A: Polytomographic evaluation of the clivus and petrous apices: a new view, Laryngoscope 94:153-164, 1984.

Moilanen A: Panoramic zonography in the diagnosis of the maxillary sinus disease, Int J Oral Surg 13:432-436, 1984.

Moilanen A and Pitkanen M: Panoramic zonography in the radiographic diagnosis of facial and related structures: a clinical study, Roentgenblatter 37:95-99, 1984.

1985 Blair WF, Berger RA and el-Khoury GY: Arthrotomography of the wrist: an experimental and preliminary clinical study, J Hand Surg [Am] 10:350-359, 1985.

Chasen MH and McCarthy MJ: Pulmonary nodules: detection of calcification by linear and pluridirectional movement in tomographic study, Radiology 156:589-592, 1985.

Fileni A et al: Tomography in the preoperative evaluation of ear malformations, J Laryngol Otol 99:432-438, 1985.

Ghosh Roy DN et al: Selective plane removal in limited angle tomographic imaging, Med Phys 12:65-70, 1985.

Vezina JA and Beauregard CG: An update on the technique of double-contrast arthrotomography of the shoulder, J Can Assoc Radiol 36:176-182, 1985.

1986 Blickman JG et al: Reconsideration of conventional tomography versus computerized tomography in the evaluation of lung metastases, Eur J Radiol 6:259-261, 1986.

Rosenberg HM and Graczyk RJ: Temporomandibular articulation tomography: a corrected anteroposterior and lateral cephalometric technique, Oral Surg Oral Med Oral Pathol 62:198-204, 1986.

1987 Avill R et al: Applied potential tomography: a new noninvasive technique for measuring gastric emptying, Gastroenterology 92:1019-1026, 1987.

Fernandes RJ et al: A cephalometric tomographic technique to visualize the buccolingual and vertical dimensions of the mandible, J Prosthet Dent 58:466-470, 1987.

Heffez L et al: Accuracy of temporomandibular joint space measurement using corrected hypocycloidal tomography, J Oral Maxillofac Surg 45:137-142, 1987.

Huston J and Muhm JR: Solitary pulmonary opacities: plain tomography, Radiology 163:481-485, 1987.

Kobayashi H and Zusho H: Measurements of internal auditory meatus by polytomography, Br J Radiol 60:209-214, 1987.

Mangnall YF et al: Applied potential tomography: a new noninvasive technique for assessing gastric function, Clin Phys Physiol Meas 8:119-129, 1987.

1988 Ahovuo J, Paavolainen P and Jaaskinen J: Arthrotomography of the unstable shoulder, Acta Orthop Scand 59:681-683, 1988.

Eyuboglu BM and Brown BH: Methods of cardiac gating applied potential tomography, Clin Phys Physiol Meas 9:43-48, 1988.

Ludlow JB: Vertical tomography of the temporomandibular joint with the use of a dental chair and intraoral x-ray unit, Oral Surg Oral Med Oral Pathol 65:358-365, 1988.

Posner MA and Greenspan A: Trispiral tomography for the evaluation of wrist problems, J Hand Surg Am 13:175-181, 1988.

Ramthun SK and Bender CE: Tomography of the posterior cervical spine fusion: a new concept, Radiol Technol 60:27-31, 1988.

1989 Hendee WR: Cross sectional medical imaging: a history, Radiographics 9:1155-1180, 1989.

Ho C, Sartoris DJ and Resnick D: Conventional tomography in musculoskeletal trauma, Radiol Clin North Am 27:929-932, 1989.

Nakanishi T et al: Sagittal tomography in the supine patient, Radiology 171:574-576, 1989.

Pyhtinen J, Laitinen J and Jokinen K: Plain radiography and tomography of the internal auditory canal for the diagnosis of acoustic neuroma, Roentgenblatter 42:339-342, 1989.

Swensen SJ, Aughenbaugh GL and Brown LR: High-resolution computed tomography of the lung, Mayo Clin Proc 64:1284-1294, 1989.

1990 Carter LC, Dennison M and Carter JM: Panoramic zonography of the midface: a clinician's guide to vertical magnification, Todays FDA 2:1C-3C, 1990.

Lynn J: TMJ tomography, a standard of the future: a review of the A-P projection of the mandibular condyle, Funct Orthod 7:32-40, 1990.

Tehranzadeh J, Davenport J and Pais MJ: Scaphoid fracture: evaluation with flexion-extension tomography, radiology 176:167-170, 1990.

1991 Croft CB et al: Polytomographic radiology in the diagnosis and management of maxillary antral disease as determined by antroscopy, Clin Otolaryngol 16:62-69, 1991.

Danforth RA et al: Corrected TMJ tomography: effectiveness of alternatives to SMV tracing, Am J Orthod Dentofacial Orthop 100:547-552, 1991.

Herrmann A, Eckl M and Maier H: Parotid sialography with a new Zonarc program, Otolaryngol Head Neck Surg 104:421-424, 1991.

Knoernschild KL, Aquilino SA and Ruprecht A: Transcranial radiography and linear tomography: a comparative study, J Prosthet Dent 66:239-250, 1991.

Ludlow JB et al: Digitally subtracted linear tomograms: three techniques for measuring condylar displacement, Oral Surg Oral Med Oral Pathol 72:614-620, 1991.

1992 Ali YA, Saleh EM and Mancuso AA: Does conventional tomography still have a place in glottic cancer evaluation? Clin Radiol 45:114-119, 1992.

Coleman RE, Robbins MS and Siegel BA: The future of positron emission tomography in clinical medicine and the impact of drug regulation, Semin Nucl Med 22:193-201, 1992.

Ehara S, el-Khoury GY and Clark CR: Radiologic evaluation of dens fracture: role of plain radiography and tomography, Spine 17:475-479, 1992.

Karasick D, Huettl EA and Cotler JM: Value of polydirectional tomography in the assessment of the postoperative spine after anterior decompression and vertebral body autografting, Skeletal Radiol 21:359-363, 1992.

1993 Chen AC: Human brain measures of clinical pain: a review. II. Tomographic imagings, Pain 54:133-144, 1993.

Jones HW: Recent activity in ultrasonic tomography, Ultrasonics 31:353-360, 1993.

Posner MA and Beltran J: Trispiral tomography and magnetic resonance imaging of the wrist, Bull Hosp Jt Dis Orthop Inst 52:34-43, 1993.

THERMOGRAPHY

For bibliographic citations before 1964, please see the fifth edition of this ATLAS. For citations from 1964 through 1974, see the sixth or seventh edition.

1975 Egan RL: Mammography, xeroradiography, and thermography, Clin Obstet Gynecol 18:197-209, 1975.

Jones CH et al: Thermography of the female breast: a five-year study in relation to the detection and prognosis of cancer, Br J Radiol 48:532-538, 1975.

1976 Evans AL, James WB and Forrest H: Thermography in lower limb arterial disease, Clin Radiol 27:383-388, 1976.

1977 Bergqvist D, Efsing HO and Hallbk T: Thermography: a noninvasive method for diagnosis of deep venous thrombosis, Arch Surg 112:600-604, 1977.

Freundlich IM, O'Mara R and Pitt MJ: Thermographic, radionuclide, and radiographic detection of bone metastases, Radiology 122:665-668, 1977.

1978 Buchanan JB and Weisberg BF: Breast thermography, J Ky Med Assoc 76:544-546, 1978.

1980 Barrett AH, Myers PC and Sadowsky NL: Microwave thermography in the detection of breast cancer, AJR 134:365-368, 1980.

Cooke ED, Carter LM and Pilcher MF: Identifying scoliosis in the adolescent with thermography: a preliminary study, Clin Orthop 148:172-176, 1980.

Kopecky WJ: Using liquid dielectrics to obtain spatial thermal distributions, Med Phys 7:566-570, 1980.

Liu DT and Blackwell RJ: Placental localization by liquid crystal thermography, Int J Gynaecol Obstet 17:617-619, 1980.

Nudelman S and Patton DD, eds: Imaging for medicine, nuclear medicine, ultrasonics, and thermography, New York, 1980, Plenum Press.

1981 Cacak RK et al: Millimeter wavelength thermographic scanner, Med Phys 8:462-465, 1981.

Goldberg IM et al: Contact plate thermography: a new technique for diagnosis of breast masses, Arch Surg 116:271-273, 1981.

Rajapakse C et al: Thermography in the assessment of peripheral joint inflammation—a re-evaluation, Rheumatol Rehabil 20:81-87, 1981.

1982 Bosiger P and Scaroni F: A microprocessor-assisted thermography system for the on-line analysis of thermograms and dynamic thermogram sequences, Prog Clin Biol Res 107:329-337, 1982.

Gautherie M et al: Long-term assessment of breast cancer risk by liquid-crystal thermal imaging, Prog Clin Biol Res 107:279-301, 1982.

Greenblatt RB, Samaras C and Vasquez J: Mastopathies: hormonology and thermography, Prog Clin Biol Res 107:303-311, 1982.

Hobbins WB: Thermography and pain, Prog Clin Biol Res 107:361-375, 1982.

Isard HJ: Breast disease and correlation of images: mammography—thermography—diaphanography, Prog Clin Biol Res 107:321-328, 1982.

Miki Y, Kawatsu T and Matsuda K: Thermographic venography in inflammatory lower leg nodules, Prog Clin Biol Res 107:439-443, 1982.

Raflo GT, Chart P and Hurwitz JJ: Thermographic evaluation of the human lacrimal drainage system, Ophthalmic Surg 13:119-124, 1982.

Ring EF: Thermal imaging and therapeutic drugs, Prog Clin Biol Res 107:463-474, 1982.

Robillard M et al: Microwave thermography—characteristics of waveguide applicators and signatures of thermal structures, J Microw Power Electromagn Energy 17:97-105, 1982.

Rubal BJ, Traycoff RB and Ewing KL: Liquid crystal thermography: a new tool for evaluating low back pain, Phys Ther 62:1593-1596, 1982.

Sterns EE et al: Thermography in breast diagnosis, Cancer 50:323-325, 1982.

Wexler CE: Lumbar, thoracic, and cervical thermography, Prog Clin Biol Res 107:377-388, 1982.

1983 Salisbury RS et al: Heat distribution over normal and abnormal joints: thermal pattern and quantification, Ann Rheum Dis 42:494-499, 1983.

Soffin CB et al: Thermography and oral inflammatory conditions, Oral Surg 56:256-262, 1983.

1984 Font-Sastre V, Jr et al: Breast cancer screening of the high risk population with clinical examination and thermography: a combination of telethermography and plate thermography, Eur J Gynaecol Oncol 5:105-109, 1984.

Kopans DB: "Early" breast cancer detection using techniques other than mammography, AJR 143:465-468, 1984.

Kopans DB, Meyer JE and Sadowsky N: Breast imaging, N Engl J Med 310:960-967, 1984.

1985 Goblyos P et al: Liquid crystal thermography of the thyroid, Eur J Radiol 5:291-294, 1985.

Goldie I: Is thermography more than an adjuvant in orthopedic diagnostics? Orthopedics 8:1128-1129, 1985.

Taylor H and Warfield CA: Thermography of pain: instrumentation and uses, Hosp Pract [Off] 20:164, 168-164, 169, 1985.

Uematsu S: Thermographic imaging of cutaneous sensory segment in patients with peripheral nerve injury: skin-temperature stability between sides of the body, J Neurosurg 62:716-720, 1985.

1986 Bothmann G: Liquid crystal thermography of the breast, Eur J Gynaecol Oncol 7:88-92, 1986.

Edeiken J and Shaber G: Thermography: a reevaluation, Skeletal Radiol 15:545-548, 1986.

Frymoyer JW and Haugh LD: Thermography: a call for scientific studies to establish its diagnostic efficacy, Orthopedics 9:699-700, 1986.

Green J et al: Comparison of neurothermography and contrast myelography, Orthopedics 9:1699-1704, 1986.

Harway RA: Precision thermal imaging of the extremities, Orthopedics 9:379-382, 1986.

Luk KD, Yeung PS and Leong JC: Thermography in the determination of amputation levels in ischaemic limbs, Int Orthop 10:79-81, 1986.

Massa T, Pino G and Boccardo F: Correlation between mammographic and thermographic patterns: use of thermography as a possible pre-screening procedure in patients at risk for breast cancer, Eur J Gynaecol Oncol 7:39-44, 1986.

Rein H: Thermography: medical and legal implications, Leg Med 95-123, 1986.

Rothschild BM: Thermographic assessment of bone and joint disease, Orthop Rev 15:765-780, 1986.

Shevelev IA et al: Thermoencephaloscopy, Hum Physiol 12:1-8, 1986.

Steele RJ: Abdominal thermography in acute appendicitis, Scott Med J 31:229-230, 1986.

Theuvenet WJ, Koeyers GF and Borghouts MH: Thermographic assessment of perforating arteries: a preoperative screening method for fasciocutaneous and musculocutaneous flaps, Scand J Plast Reconstr Surg 20:25-29, 1986.

White BA et al: The use of infrared thermography in the evaluation of oral lesions, J Am Dent Assoc 113:783-786, 1986.

1987 Ciatto S et al: Diagnostic and prognostic role of infrared thermography, Radiol Med 74:312-315, 1987.

Fraser S, Land D and Sturrock RD: Microwave thermography—an index of inflammatory joint disease, Br J Rheumatol 26:37-39, 1987.

Goodlin RC and Brooks PG: Abdominal wall hot spots in pregnant women, J Reprod Med 32:177-180, 1987.

1988 Baer MS et al: Preliminary report on the use of liquid crystal thermography in podiatry, J Foot Surg 27:398-403, 1988.

Isard HJ, Sweitzer CJ and Edelstein GR: Breast thermography: a prognostic indicator for breast cancer survival, Cancer 62:484-488, 1988.

1989 Gratt BM et al: Electronic thermography of normal facial structures: a pilot study, Oral Surg Oral Med Oral Pathol 68:346-351, 1989.

Handelsman H: Thermography for indications other than breast lesions, Health Technol Assess Rep 1-32, 1989.

1990 The American Academy of Neurology, Therapeutics and Technology Assessment Subcommittee: Assessment: thermography in neurologic practice, Neurology 40:523-525, 1990.

Aminoff MJ, Olney RK and So YT: Thermography and the evaluation of neuromuscular disorders, Semin Neurol 10:150-155, 1990.

Beinder E, Huch A and Huch R: Peripheral skin temperature and microcirculatory reactivity during pregnancy: a study with thermography, J Perinat Med 18:383-390, 1990.

Bergqvist D and Bergentz SE: Diagnosis of deep vein thrombosis, World J Surg 14:679-687, 1990.

Garagiola U and Giani E: Use of telethermography in the management of sports injuries, Sports Med 10:267-272, 1990.

Stevenson AJ, Moss JG and Kirkpatrick AE: Comparison of temperature profiles (DeVeTherm) and conventional venography in suspected lower limb thrombosis, Clin Radiol 42:37-39, 1990.

Value of thermography, J Occup Med 32:478, 1990.

Williams KL et al: Thermography in screening for breast cancer, J Epidemiol Community Health 44:112-113, 1990.

1991 Awerbuch MS: Thermography—its current diagnostic status in musculoskeletal medicine, Med J Aust 154:441-444, 1991.

Brooks PM: Thermography—turning up the heat, Med J Aust 154:436-437, 1991.

Chan AW, MacFarlane IA and Bowsher DR: Contact thermography of painful diabetic neuropathic foot, Diabetes Care 14:918-922, 1991.

Comhaire F: Scrotal thermography in varicocele, Adv Exp Med Biol 286:267-270, 1991.

Feldman F: Thermography of the hand and wrist: practical applications, Hand Clin 7:99-112, 1991.

Gratt BM and Sickles EA: Future applications of electronic thermography, J Am Dent Assoc 122:28-36, 1991.

Hearn K: Choosing the right tools, Radiol Technol 62:240-242, 1991.

Johnson KJ, Bhatia P and Bell EF: Infrared thermometry of newborn infants, Pediatrics 87:34-38, 1991.

Pawl RP: Thermography in the diagnosis of low back pain, Neurosurg Clin North Am 2:839-850, 1991.

Weinstein SA et al: Facial thermography, basis, protocol, and clinical value, Cranio 9:201-211, 1991.

1992 Giordano N et al: Telethermographic assessment of carpal tunnel syndrome, Scand J Rheumatol 21:42-45, 1992.

Plaugher G: Skin temperature assessment for neuromusculoskeletal abnormalities of the spinal column, J Manipulative Physiol Ther 15:365-381, 1992.

Shevelev IA: Temperature topography of the brain cortex: thermoencephaloscopy, Brain Topogr 5:77-85, 1992.

Thomas D et al: Computerised infrared thermography and isotopic bone scanning in tennis elbow, Ann Rheum Dis 51:103-107, 1992.

Vecchio PC et al: Thermography of frozen shoulder and rotator cuff tendinitis, Clin Rheumatol 11:382-384, 1992.

Yang WJ and Yang PP: Literature survey on biomedical applications of thermography, Biomedical Mater Eng 2:7-18, 1992.

1993 Gorbach AM: Infrared imaging of brain function, Adv Exp Med Biol 333:95-123, 1993.

Jackson VP et al: Imaging of the radiographically dense breast, Radiology 188:297-301, 1993.

Lawson W et al: Infrared thermography in the detection and management of coronary artery disease, Am J Cardiol 72:894-896, 1993.

McCulloch J et al: Thermography as a diagnostic aid in sciatica, J spinal Disord 6:427-431, 1993.

Schuman AJ: The accuracy of infrared auditory canal thermometry in infants and children, Clin Pediatr 32:347-354, 1993.

Shevelev IA et al: Thermoimaging of the brain, J Neurosci Methods 46:49-57, 1993.

Tourangeau A, MacLeod f and Breakwell M: Tap in on ear thermometry, Can Nurse 89:24-28, 1993.

1994 Emery M, Jones J and Brown M: Clinical application of infrared thermography in the diagnosis of appendicitis, Am J Emerg Med 12:48-50, 1994.

DIAPHANOGRAPHY

1981 Angquist KA et al: Diaphanoscopy and diaphanography for breast cancer detection in clinical practice, Acta Chir Scand 147:231-238, 1981.

Isard HJ: A preliminary appraisal of diaphanography in diseases of the breast, Cancer Detect Prev 4:565-569, 1981.

1982 Brenner RJ: X-ray mammography and diaphanography in screening for breast cancer, J Reprod Med 27:679-684, 1982.

1983 McIntosh DM: Breast light scanning: a real-time breast-imaging modality, J Can Assoc Radiol 34:288-290, 1983.

1984 Fodor J, Malott JC and Moskowitz M: Diaphanography: transillumination of the breast, Radiol Technol 55:97-100, 1984.

Isard HJ: Other imaging techniques, Cancer 53:658-664, 1984.

Muirhead A and Seright W: Clinical experience with the diaphanograph machine, Ann R Coll Surg Engl 66:123-124, 1984.

Sickles EA: Breast cancer detection with transillumination and mammography, AJR 142:841-844, 1984.

1985 Donn SM and Faix RG: Transillumination in neonatal diagnosis, Clin Perinatol 12:3-20, 1985.

Drexler B, Davis JL and Schofield G: Diaphanography in the diagnosis of breast cancer, Radiology 157:41-44, 1985.

Wallberg H, Alveryd A and Carlsson K: Physical interpretation of diaphanograms using the computer-controlled image scanner OSIRIS, Acta Radiol [Diagn] (Stockh) 26:417-424, 1985.

1986 Gisvold JJ et al: Comparison of mammography and transillumination light scanning in the detection of breast lesions, AJR 147:191-194, 1986.

Lafreniere R, Ashkar FS and Ketcham AS: Infrared light scanning of the breast, Am Surg 52:123-128, 1986.

Linford J et al: Development of a tissue-equivalent phantom for diaphanography, Med Phys 13:869-875, 1986.

Wallberg H et al: The value of diaphanography as an adjunct to mammography in breast diagnostics, Acta Chir Scand Suppl 530:83-87, 1986.

1987 Bundred N et al: Preliminary results using computerized telediaphanography for investigating breast disease, Br J Hosp Med 37:70-71, 1987.

Jackson PC et al: The development of a system for transillumination computed tomography, Br J Radiol 60:375-380, 1987.

Kopans DB: Nonmammographic breast imaging techniques: current status and future developments, Radiol Clin North Am 25:961-971, 1987.

Monsees B, Destouet JM and Gersell D: Light scan evaluation of nonpalpable breast lesions, Radiology 163:467-470, 1987.

Monsees B, Destouet JM and Totty WG: Light scanning versus mammography in breast cancer detection, Radiology 163:463-465, 1987.

Sickles EA: Computed tomography scanning, transillumination, and magnetic resonance imaging of the breast, Recent Results Cancer Res 105:31-36, 1987.

1988 Key H, Jackson PC and Wells PN: New approaches to transillumination imaging, J Biomed Eng 10:113-118, 1988.

Navarro GA and Profio AE: Contrast in diaphanography of the breast, Med Phys 15:181-187, 1988.

Reassessment of transillumination light scanning for the diagnosis of breast cancer, Health Technol Assess Rep 1-7, 1988.

1989 Lefebvre JP et al: In vivo transillumination of the hand using near infrared laser pulses and differential spectroscopy, J Biomed Eng 11:293-299, 1989.

Otten FW and Grote JJ: The diagnostic value of transillumination for maxillary sinusitis in children, Int J Pediatr Otorhinolaryngol 18:9-11, 1989.

Profio AE, Navarro GA and Sartorius OW: Scientific basis of breast diaphanography, Med Phys 16:60-65, 1989.

1990 Alveryd A et al: Lightscanning versus mammography for the detection of breast cancer in screening and clinical practice. A Swedish multicenter study, Cancer 65:1671-1677, 1990.

Hebden JC and Kruger RA: Transillumination imaging performance: a time-of-flight imaging system, Med Phys 17:351-356, 1990.

Hebden JC and Kruger RA: Transillumination imaging performance: spatial resolution simulation studies, Med Phys 17:41-47, 1990.

Van Der Walt JH and Gassmanis K: Skin burns from a cold light source, Anaesth Intensive Care 18:113-115, 1990.

1991 Bhargava R and Millward SF: Contrast venography in patients with very edematous feet: use of transdermal illumination to aid in vein puncture, Radiology 179:583, 1991.

Gonsoulin SM and Broussard PC: Shedding light on i.v. therapy, Nursing 21:62-64, 1991.

Inappropriate use of transillumination for breast cancer screening—Wisconsin, 1990, MMWR 40:293-296, 1991.

Pandya AN, Buch HG and Shilotri PP: Umbilical transillumination: an accurate means to diagnose minimal ascites associated with umbilical hernias, J Assoc Physicians India 39:311-312, 1991.

1992 Jarlman O et al: Diagnostic accuracy of lightscanning and mammography in women with dense breasts, Acta Radiol 33:69-71, 1992.

1993 Alper J: Transillumination: looking right through you, Science 261:560, 1993.

Jackson VP et al: Imaging of the radiographically dense breast, Radiology 188:297-301, 1993.

COMPUTED TOMOGRAPHY

For bibliographic citations before 1964, please see the fifth edition of this ATLAS. For citations from 1964 through 1974, see the sixth or seventh edition.

1975 Wilson GH: Computed cerebral tomography, West J Med 122:316-317, 1975.

1976 Banna M: Basic introduction to computerized tomography, J Can Assoc Radiol 27:143-148, 1976.

Laffey P et al: Computerized tomography in clinical medicine, Philadelphia, 1976, Medical Direction.

1977 Huckman MS, Grainer LS and Clasen RC: The normal computed tomogram, Semin Roentgenol 12:27-38, 1977.

Ledley RS et al: Cross-sectional anatomy: an atlas for computerized tomography, Baltimore, 1977, Williams & Wilkins.

McCullough EC: Factors affecting the use of quantitative information from a CT scanner, Radiology 124:99-107, 1977.

Zata LM and Alvarez RE: An inaccuracy in computed tomography: the energy dependence of CT values, Radiology 124:91-97, 1977.

1978 Christensen EE et al: An introduction to the physics of diagnostic radiology, ed 2, Philadelphia, 1978, Lea & Febiger.

Maravilla KR and Pastel MS: Technical aspects of CT scanning, CT 2:137-144, 1978.

Meire HB and Kreel L: Computed tomography and ultrasound: a comparison, Practitioner 220:593-597, 1978.

Thompson T: A practical approach to modern x-ray equipment, Boston, 1978, Little, Brown & Co.

Tully RJ, McFarland WD and Lodwick GS: General purpose digital display system for computed tomography images, Radiology 127:539-541, 1978.

Wackenheim A: Neuroradiology and computed tomography, J Belge Radiol 61:281-286, 1978.

1979 Cohen G: Contrast-detail-dose analysis of six different computed tomographic scanners, J Comput Assist Tomogr 3:197-203, 1979.

Cohen G: The use of contrast-detail-dose evaluation of image quality in a computed tomographic scanner, J Comput Assist Tomogr 3:189-195, 1979.

Frank E: Computed tomography of the pancreas: a new roentgenographic examination, Radiol Technol 50:403-409, 1979.

Kowalski G and Wagner W: Patient dose rate: an ultimate limit for spatial and density resolution of scanning systems, Biomed Tech 24(3):38-42, 1979.

Rice JF and Banks TE: Normal and high accuracy computed tomography of the brain: dose and imaging considerations, J Comput Assist Tomogr 3:497-502, 1979.

Rice JF et al: Introduction to computed tomography, Milwaukee, 1979, General Electric Co.

1980 Ball WS, Wicks JD and Mettler FA Jr: Prone-supine change in organ position: CT demonstration, AJR 135:815-820, 1980.

Coin CG and Coin JT: Contact enhancement by xenon gas in computed tomography of the spinal cord and brain: preliminary observations, J Comput Assist Tomogr 4:217-221, 1980.

Computed tomography of the abdomen, Int Adv Surg Oncol 3:221-274, 1980.

Farber AL: Advantages of varient section of thickness relative to specific anatomy, Radiol Technol 51:793-796, 1980.

Fischer HW: Occurrence of seizure during cranial computed tomography, Radiology 137:563-564, 1980.

Ghoshhajra K and Rao KC: CT in spinal trauma, CT 4:309-318, 1980.

Hatfield KD, Segal SD and Tait K: Barium sulfate for abdominal computer assisted tomography, J Comput Assist Tomogr 4:570, 1980.

Hounsfield GN: Computed medical imaging: Nobel lecture, Dec 8, 1979, J Comput Assist Tomogr 4:665-674, 1980.

Joseph PM et al: Clinical and experimental investigation of a smoothed CT reconstruction algorithm, Radiology 134:507-516, 1980.

Kubota K et al: Some devices for computed tomography radiotherapy treatment planning, J Comput Assist Tomogr 4:677-679, 1980.

Margulis AR et al: The desirable properties of computed tomography scanners, Radiology 134:261, 1980.

Meany TF et al: Detection of low contrast lesions in computed body tomography: an experimental study of simulated lesions, Radiology 134:149-154, 1980.

Schindler E and Reck R: Value and limits of computer-assisted tomography, Head Neck Surg 2:287-292, 1980.

Scott WR: Seizures: a reaction to contrast media for computed tomography of the brain, Radiology 137:359-361, 1980.

Termote JL et al: Computed tomography of the normal and pathologic muscular system, Radiology 137:439-444, 1980.

van Hassel-Strijbosch M and van de Werf K: Value of reconstruction modes in CT scanning of the head, Radiography 46:209-212, 1980.

Williams AL, Haughton VM and Syvertsen A: Computed tomography in the diagnosis of herniated nucleus pulposus, Radiology 135:95-99, 1980.

Winter J: Edge enhancement of computed tomograms by digital unsharp masking, Radiology 135:234-235, 1980.

Young SW et al: Dynamic computed tomography body scanning, J Comput Assist Tomogr 4:168-173, 1980.

1981　Cohen Z et al: Iodinated starch particles: new contrast material for computed tomography of the liver, J Comput Assist Tomogr 5:843-846, 1981.

Egund N et al: CT of soft tissue tumors, AJR 137:725-729, 1981.

Haaga JR et al: The effect of mAs variation upon computed tomography image quality as evaluated by in vivo and in vitro studies, Radiology 138:449-454, 1981.

Hamlin DJ and Burgener FA: Positive and negative contrast agents in CT evaluation of the abdomen and pelvis, CT 5:82-90, 1981.

Jones ET: Use of computed axial tomography in pediatric orthopedics, J Pediatr Orthop 1:329-338, 1981.

Kuhn JP: CT in the evaluation of pediatric abdominal abnormalities, CRC Crit Rev Diagn Imaging 16:125-180, 1981.

Schoppe WD, Hessel SJ and Adams DF: Time requirements in performing body CT studies, J Comput Assist Tomogr 5:513-515, 1981.

Steele JR and Hoffman JC: Brainstem evaluation with CT cisternography, AJR 136:287-292, 1981.

Tianado J et al: Computed tomography of the perineum, AJR 136:475-481, 1981.

Turnipseed WD et al: Computerized arteriography of the cerebrovascular system: its use with intravenous administration of contrast material, Arch Surg 116:470-473, 1981.

1982　Beck TJ, Rosenbaum AE and Miller NR: Orbital computed tomography: technical aspects, Int Ophthalmol Clin 22:7-13, 1982.

Carmel PW and Mawad M: CT scanning of the posterior fossa, Clin Neurosurg 29:51-102, 1982.

Ekelund L, Herrlin K and Rydholm A: Comparison of computed tomography and angiography in the evaluation of soft tissue tumors of the extremities, Acta Radiol [Diagn] (Stockh) 23:15-27, 1982.

Friedmann G and Promper C: CT examination of the spine and the spinal canal, Eur J Radiol 2:60-65, 1982.

Hatten HP Jr, Walker ME and Covington MC: Range highlight facility within region of interest for air-CT cisternography and canalography, Radiol Technol 54:35-36, 1982.

Howard P and Sage MR: CT of the paranasal sinuses and face, Australas Radiol 26:130-136, 1982.

Hubbard LF, McDermott JH and Garrett G: Computed axial tomography in musculoskeletal trauma, J Trauma 22:388-394, 1982.

Kassel EE, Noyek AM and Cooper PW: High resolution computerized tomography in otorhinolaryngology, J Otolaryngol 11:297-306, 1982.

Kivisaari L, Makela P and Aarimaa M: Pancreatic mobility: an important factor in pancreatic computed tomography, J Comput Assist Tomogr 6:854-856, 1982.

LaMasters DL, et al: Multiplanar metrizamide-enhanced CT imaging of the foramen magnum, AJNR 3:485-494, 1982.

Larsson SG, Mancuso A and Hanafee W: Computed tomography of the tongue and floor of the mouth, Radiology 143:493-500, 1982.

Lee JK and Balfe DM: Computed tomography evaluation of lymphoma patients, CRC Crit Rev Diagn Imaging 18:1-28, 1982.

Lee JK et al: A support device for obtaining direct coronal computed tomographic scans of the pelvis and lower abdomen, Radiology 145:209-210, 1982.

Lee KR: Computed tomography of the gastrointestinal tract, CRC Crit Rev Diagn Imaging 18:121-165, 1982.

Martinez CR et al: Computed tomography of the neck, Ann Otol Rhinol Laryngol 99:1-31, 1982.

Olson JE, Dorwart RH and Brant WE: Use of high-resolution thin-section CT scanning of the petrous bone, Laryngoscope 92:1274-1278, 1982.

Peyster RG and Hoover ED: CT in head trauma, J Trauma 22:25-38, 1982.

Seeram E: Computed tomography technology, Philadelphia, 1982, WB Saunders Co.

Silverman PM et al: High-resolution multiplanar CT images of the larynx, Invest Radiol 17:634-637, 1982.

van Waes PF and Zonneveld FW: Direct coronal body computed tomography, J Comput Assist Tomogr 6:58-66, 1982.

1983　Berg BC: Complementary roles of radionuclide and computed tomographic imaging in evaluating trauma, Semin Nucl Med 13:86-103, 1983.

Burgener FA and Hamlin DJ: Contrast enhancement of hepatic tumors in CT: comparison, AJR 140:291-295, 1983.

Chakeres DW and Spiegel PK: A systematic technique for comprehensive evaluation of the temporal bone, Radiology 146:97-106, 1983.

Dickson DR and Maue Dickson W: Tomographic assessment of craniofacial structures: cleft lip/palate, Cleft Palate J 20:23-34, 1983.

duBoulay GH, Teather D and Wills K: CT: to enhance or not to enhance: a computer-aided study, AJNR 4:421-424, 1983.

Dunn EL, Berry PH and Connally JD: Computed tomography of the pelvis in patients with multiple injuries, J Trauma 23:378-383, 1983.

Foley WD et al: Contrast enhancement technique for dynamic hepatic computed tomographic scanning, Radiology 147:797-803, 1983.

Gamsu G and Webb WR: Computed tomography of the trachea and mainstem bronchi, Semin Roentgenol 18:51-60, 1983.

Glazer GM et al: Evaluation of the pulmonary hilum: comparison of conventional radiography, 55 degrees posterior oblique tomography, and dynamic computed tomography, J Comput Assist Tomogr 7:983-989, 1983.

Goldberg HI et al: Computed tomography in the evaluation of Crohn disease, AJR 140:277-282, 1983.

Graf von Keyserlingk D, DeBleser R and Poeck K: Stereographic reconstruction of human brain CT series, Acta Anat (Basel) 115:336-344, 1983.

Hian TW: Contrast enhancement of brain tumors in computed tomography, Diagn Imaging 52:113-116, 1983.

Jazrawy H et al: Computed tomography of the temporal bone, J Otolaryngol 12:37-44, 1983.

Kuhns L and Seeger J: Atlas of computed tomography variants, Chicago, 1983, Mosby.

Lamothe A et al: High resolution CT scan of the temporal bone, J Otolaryngol 12:119-124, 1983.

Leitman BS et al: The use of computed tomography in evaluating chest wall pathology, CT 7:399-405, 1983.

Lipton MJ et al: CT scanning of the heart, Cardiovasc Clin 13:385-401, 1983.

Marsh JL and Gado M: The longitudinal orbital CT projection: a versatile image for orbital assessment, Plast Reconstr Surg 71:308-317, 1983.

Marsh JL and Vannier MW: Surface imaging from computerized tomographic scans, Surgery 94:159-165, 1983.

Morgan CL: Atlas of computed body tomography, Baltimore, 1983, University Park Press.

Naidich DP et al: Computed tomography of the diaphragm: normal anatomy and variants, J Comput Assist Tomogr 7:633-640, 1983.

Osborne D et al: Assessment of craniocervical junction and atlantoaxial relation, AJNR 4:843-845, 1983.

Parvey LS, Grizzard M and Coburn TP: Use of infusion pump for intravenous enhanced computed tomography, J Comput Assist Tomogr 7:175-176, 1983.

Rajfer J et al: The use of computerized tomography scanning to localize the impalpable testis, J Urol 129:972-974, 1983.

Riddlesberger MM Jr and Kuhn JP: The role of computed tomography in diseases of the musculoskeletal system, CT 7:85-99, 1983.

Silverman PM and Korobkin M: High-resolution computed tomography of the normal larynx, AJR 140:875-879, 1983.

Swindell W et al: Computed tomography with a linear accelerator with radiotherapy applications, Med Phys 10:416-420, 1983.

Vigo M et al: Computerized axial tomography in the evaluation of gynecologic pelvic masses, Clin Exp Obstet Gynecol 10:210-212, 1983.

Yamamoto Y, Sakurai M and Asari S: Towne (half-axial) and semisagittal computed tomography in the evaluation of blow-out fractures of the orbit, J Comput Assist Tomogr 7:306-309, 1983.

Zeitler E et al: Experiences with Rayvist and iopromid in head and body CT, Fortschr Geb Rontgerstr Nuklearmed Erganzungsband 118:162-172, 1983.

1984   Axel L et al: Functional imaging of the liver: new information from dynamic CT, Invest Radiol 19:23-29, 1984.

Bramwit DN: Direct sagittal (lateral) computer tomography of the temporomandibular joints, J Bergen Cty Dent Soc 50:11-13, 1984.

Burk DL Jr et al: Pelvic and acetabular fractures: examination by angled CT scanning, Radiology 153:548, 1984.

Chakeres DW and Kapila A: Computed tomography of the temporal bone, Med Radiogr Photogr 60:1-32, 1984.

Chambers SE and Best JJ: A comparison of dilute barium and dilute water-soluble contrast in opacification of the bowel for abdominal computed tomography, Clin Radiol 35:463-464, 1984.

Curtin HD: CT of acoustic neuroma and other tumors of the ear, Radiol Clin North Am 22:77-105, 1984.

Daniels DL, Williams AL and Haughton VM: Jugular foramen: anatomic and computed tomographic study, AJR 142:153-158, 1984.

Dorwart RH: Computed tomography of the lumbar spine: techniques, normal anatomy, CRC Crit Rev Diagn Imaging 22:1-42, 1984.

Firooznia H et al: Computed tomography in localization of foreign bodies lodged in the extremities, Comput Radiol 8:237-239, 1984.

Goldberg HI et al: Device for performing direct coronal CT scanning of the abdomen and pelvis, AJR 143:900-902, 1984.

Griffin DJ et al: Observations on CT differentiation of pleural and peritoneal fluid, J Comput Assist Tomogr 8:24-28, 1984.

Halvorsen RA and Thompson WA: Computed tomography of the gastroesophageal junction, CRC Crit Rev Diagn Imaging 21:183-228, 1984.

Haney PJ and Whitley NO: CT of benign cystic abdominal masses in children, AJR 142:1279-1281, 1984.

Kanematsu T et al: Transparent box enables three-dimensional viewing of CT imaging of the liver, Jpn J Surg 14:94-96, 1984.

Kearfott KJ, Rottenberg DA and Knowles RI: A new headholder for PET, CT, and NMR imaging, J Comput Assist Tomogr 8:1217-1220, 1984.

Love L et al: Intravenous contrast bolus in computed tomography investigation of mass lesions, Diagn Imaging 53:57-66, 1984.

Mintz MC and Seltzer SE: Oral administration of contrast medium for rectal opacification in pelvic computed tomography, CT 8:73-74, 1984.

Ohishi H et al: Usefulness of direct coronal CT in the diagnosis of urinary bladder, Radiat Med 2:181-184, 1984.

Pastakia B and Herdt JR: Radiolucent "zones" in parietal bones seen on computed tomography: a normal anatomic variant, J Comput Assist Tomogr 8:108-109, 1984.

Patel RB, Barton P and Green L: CT of isolated elbow in evaluation of trauma: a modified technique, Comput Radiol 8:1-4, 1984.

Proto AV: Evaluation of the bronchi with CT, Semin Roentgenol 19:199-210, 1984.

Rabinov K, Kell T Jr and Gordon PH: CT of the salivary glands, Radiol Clin North Am 22:145-159, 1984.

Roberts D et al: Radiologic techniques used to evaluate the temporomandibular joint, Anesth Prog 31:241-256, 1984.

Roberts D et al: Three-dimensional imaging and display of the temporomandibular joint, Oral Surg Oral Med Oral Pathol 58:461-474, 1984.

Shetty AK, Deeb ZL and Hryshko FG: Computed tomography of spine trauma, J Comput Tomogr 8:105-112, 1984.

Symposium on CT of ear, nose, and throat, Radiol Clin North Am 22:1-284, 1984.

Tehranzadeh J and Gabriele OF: The prone position for CT of the lumbar spine, Radiology 152:817-818, 1984.

Thompson WM et al: Computed tomography of the gastroesophageal junction: value of the left lateral decubitus view, J Comput Assist Tomogr 8:346-349, 1984.

Totty WG and Vannier MW: Complex musculoskeletal anatomy: analysis using three-dimensional surface reconstruction, Radiology 150:173-177, 1984.

Whelan MA et al: CT of the base of the skull, Radiol Clin North Am 22:177-217, 1984.

1985   Altman N et al: Evaluation of the infant spine by direct sagittal computed tomography, AJNR 6:65-69, 1985.

Cayea PD and Seltzer SE: A new barium paste for computed tomography of the esophagus, J Comput Assist Tomogr 9:214-216, 1985.

Clark LR et al: Enhanced pancreatic CT imaging utilizing a geometric magnification, Invest Radiol 20:531-538, 1985.

Clouse ME et al: Lymphangiography, ultrasonography, and computed tomography in Hodgkin's disease and non-Hodgkin's lymphoma, J Comput Tomogr 9:1-8, 1985.

Conover GL: Direct sagittal CT scanning of the temporomandibular joint, CDS Review 78:28-31, 1985.

Deutsch AL, Resnick D and Mink JH: Computed tomography of the glenohumeral and sternoclavicular joints, Orthop Clin North Am 16:497-511, 1985.

Garrett JS, Higgins CB and Lipton MJ: Computed axial tomography of the heart, Int J Card Imaging 1:113-126, 1985.

Gould R, Rosenfield AT and Friedlaender GE: Loose body within the glenohumeral joint in recurrent anterior dislocation: CT demonstration, J Comput Assist Tomogr 9:404-406, 1985.

Johnson DW, Voorhees RL and Wong ML: Virtues and vagaries of high-resolution CT air cisternography in the diagnosis of acoustic neuromas, Otolaryngol Head Neck Surg 93:156-160, 1985.

Johnson JF et al: Tracheoesophageal fistula: diagnosis with CT, Pediatr Radiol 15:134-135, 1985.

Knapp RH, Vannier MW and Marsh JL: Generation of three-dimensional images for CT scans: technological perspective, Radiol Technol 56:391-398, 1985.

Lau LS, Simpson L and Murphy F: High resolution CT scanning of the bronchial tree: CT bronchography—technique and clinical application, Australas Radiol 29:323-331, 1985.

Lien HH and Lund G: Computed tomography of mediastinal lymph nodes. Anatomic review based on contrast enhanced nodes following foot lymphography, Acta Radiol [Diagn] (Stockh) 26:641-647, 1985.

Manzione JV, Rumbaugh CL and Katzberg RW: Direct sagittal computed tomography of the temporal bone, J Comput Assist Tomogr 9:417-419, 1985.

Munro CJ: Computed tomography of the adrenal glands, Radiography 51:281-285, 1985.

Noble PN: Computed tomography of the pancreas, Radiography 51:205-210, 1985.

Perkerson RB Jr et al: CT densities in delayed iodine hepatic scanning, Radiology 155:445-446, 1985.

Quint LE, Glazer GM and Orringer MB: Esophageal imaging by MR and CT: study of normal anatomy and neoplasms, Radiology 156:727-731, 1985.

Russell EJ et al: CT of the inferomedial orbit and the lacrimal drainage apparatus: normal and pathologic anatomy, AJR 145:1147-1154, 1985.

Samuelsson L and Tylen U: Delineation of the normal esophagus at computed tomography, Acta Radiol [Diagn] (Stockh) 26:665-669, 1985.

Sandler CM, Raval B and David CL: Computed tomography of the kidney, Urol Clin North Am 12:657-675, 1985.

Silverman PM, Dunnick NR and Ford KK: Computed tomography of the normal seminal vesicles, Comput Radiol 9:379-385, 1985.

Simon DC et al: Direct sagittal CT of the temporomandibular joint, Radiology 157:545, 1985.

Stork J: Intraperitoneal contrast agents for computed tomography, AJR 145:300, 1985.

Zonneveld FW: The technique of direct multiplanar high resolution CT of the temporal bone, Neurosurg Rev 8:5-13, 1985.

1986 Altman NR et al: Three-dimensional CT reformation in children, AJR 146:1261-1267, 1986.

Angtuaco EJ and Binet EF: High-resolution computed tomography in intracranial aneurysms, CRC Crit Rev Diagn Imaging 25:113-158, 1986.

Bagg MN and Anderson JE: An analysis of computed tomographic brain scans: a computer-based study, S Afr Med J 70:208-211, 1986.

Beltramello A et al: Iopamidol 150: a low iodine content non-ionic water-soluble contrast medium for CT myelocisternography, Acta Radiol Suppl 369:542-544, 1986.

Beltran J et al: Rotator cuff lesions of the shoulder: evaluation by direct sagittal CT arthrography, Radiology 160:161-165, 1986.

Boger DC: Traction device to improve CT imaging of lower cervical spine, AJNR 7:719-721, 1986.

Bradley WG Jr: Magnetic resonance imaging in the central nervous system: comparison with computed tomography, Magn Reson Annu 81-122, 1986.

Bresina SJ et al: Three-dimensional wrist imaging: evaluation of functional and pathologic anatomy by computer, Clin Plast Surg 13:389-405, 1986.

Brody AS et al: Artifacts seen during CT pelvimetry: implications for digital systems with scanning beams, Radiology 160:269-271, 1986.

Christiansen EL et al: Correlative thin section temporomandibular joint anatomy and computed tomography, Radiographics 6:703-723, 1986.

Citrin CM: High resolution orbital computed tomography, J Comput Assist Tomogr 10:810-816, 1986.

Crone-Munzebrock W and Heller M: Computed tomography of the scapula, Eur J Radiol 6:99-102, 1986.

Demas BE et al: Utility of ceruletide in promoting intestinal opacification for abdominal and pelvic computed tomography, Gastrointest Radiol 11:197-199, 1986.

Farmer D et al: High-speed (cine) computed tomography of the heart, Cardiovasc Clin 17:345-356, 1986.

Fukui K, Sadamoto K and Sakaki S: Development of the new cerebral angio-CT technique and magnetic resonance angio-imaging, Acta Radiol Suppl 369:67-68, 1986.

Gillespie JE and Isherwood I: Three-dimensional anatomical images from computed tomographic scans, Br J Radiol 59:289-292, 1986.

Helms CA et al: Cine-CT of the temporomandibular joint, Cranio 4:246-250, 1986.

Kopelman JN et al: Computed tomographic pelvimetry in the evaluation of breech presentation, Obstet Gynecol 68:455-458, 1986.

Kursunoglu S et al: Three-dimensional computed tomographic analysis of the normal temporomandibular joint, J Oral Maxillofac Surg 44:257-259, 1986.

Lassen MN: Dedicated CT technique for scanning neonates, Radiology 161:363-366, 1986.

Laval Jeantet AM et al: Influence of vertebral fat content on quantitative CT density, Radiology 159:463-466, 1986.

Leib ML: Computed tomography of the orbit, Int Ophthalmol Clin 26:103-121, 1986.

Lenke RR and Shuman WP: Computed tomographic pelvimetry, J Reprod Med 31:958-960, 1986.

Lipcamon JD and Chiu LC: Contiguous computed tomography angiography (CTA) of the chest, Radiol Technol 58:23-26, 1986.

Mostrom U and Ytterbergh C: Artifacts in computed tomography of the posterior fossa: a comparative phantom study, J Comput Assist Tomogr 10:560-566, 1986.

Nakano Y et al: Stomach and duodenum: radiographic magnification using computed tomography, Radiology 160:383-387, 1986.

Nyman U and Dinnetz G: Vascular enhancement during incremental body computed tomography: a simple and reliable technique, Acta Radiol [Diagn] (Stockh) 27:667-673, 1986.

Panzer RJ, Kido DK and Hindmarsh T: A methodologic assessment of studies comparing magnetic resonance imaging and computed tomography of the brain, Acta Radiol Suppl 369:269-274, 1986.

Pate D et al: Perspective: three-dimensional imaging of the musculoskeletal system, AJR 147:545-551, 1986.

Pozzi Mucelli RS, Muner G and Pozzi Mucelli F: Three-dimensional computed tomography of the acetabulum, Eur J Radiol 6:168-177, 1986.

Rees MR et al: Heart evaluation by cine CT: use of two new oblique views, Radiology 159:804-806, 1986.

Schnyder P, Mansouri B and Uske A: Direct coronal computed tomography of the lumbar spine: a new technical approach in supine position, Eur J Radiol 6:248-251, 1986.

Shuman WP et al: Use of a power injector during dynamic computed tomography, J Comput assist Tomogr 10:1000-1002, 1986.

Simonetti G et al: Method for angio-CT, Radiol Med 72:64-66, 1986.

Singson RD, Feldman F and Rosenberg ZS: Elbow joint: assessment with double-contrast CT arthrography, Radiology 160:167-173, 1986.

Solomon A et al: Computed tomographic air enema technique to demonstrate colonic neoplasms, Gastrointest Radiol 11:194-196, 1986.

Solomon MA et al: CT scanning of the foot and ankle. 1. Normal anatomy, AJR 146:1192-1203, 1986.

Spiegel SM et al: Increased density of tentorium and falx: a false positive CT sign of subarachnoid hemorrhage, Can Assoc Radiol J 37:243-247, 1986.

Stanford W: Cine CT today only 'tip of the iceberg', Iowa Med 76:162-163, 1986.

Staron RB and Ford E: Computed tomographic volumetric calculation reproducibility, Invest Radiol 21:272-274, 1986.

Steiner RM et al: The functional and anatomic evaluation of the cardiovascular system with rapid-acquisition computed tomography (cine CT), Radiol Clin North Am 24:503-520, 1986.

Strain JD et al: Intravenously administered pentobarbital sodium for sedation in pediatric CT, Radiology 161:105-108, 1986.

Strickland B, Brennan J and Denison DM: Computed tomography in diffuse lung disease: improving the image, Clin Radiol 37:335-338, 1986.

Unger JM: Computed tomography of the parapharyngeal space, CRC Crit Rev Diagn Imaging 26:265-290, 1986.

Vaid YN and Shin MS: Computed tomography evaluation of tracheoesophageal fistula, J Comput Tomogr 10:281-285, 1986.

van Waes PF et al: Direct coronal and direct sagittal CT of abdomen and pelvis: an approach to staging malignancies, Radiographics 6:213-244, 1986.

Virapongse C et al: Three-dimensional computed tomographic reformation of the spine, skull, and brain from axial images, Neurosurgery 18:53-58, 1986.

Wang AM and Zamani AA: Intradural herniation of thoracic disc: CT metrizamide myelography, Comput Radiol 10:115-118, 1986.

Wang H et al: Low dose cervical CT myelography: how acceptable are adverse effects at this juncture? Acta Radiol Suppl 369:539-541, 1986.

Zeman RK et al: Computed tomography of renal masses: pitfalls and anatomic variants, Radiographics 6:351-372, 1986.

Zonneveld FW and Koornneef L: Patient positioning for direct sagittal CT of the orbit parallel to the optic nerve, Radiology 158:547-549, 1986.

1987 Acheson MB et al: High-resolution CT scanning in the evaluation of cervical spine fractures: comparison with plain film examinations, AJR 148:1179-1185, 1987.

Baldwin JE et al: Image quality of abdominal computed tomography in the elderly, Age Ageing 16:261-264, 1987.

Ball JB Jr: Direct oblique sagittal CT of orbital wall fractures, AJR 148:601-608, 1987.

Biondetti PR et al: Wrist: coronal and transaxial CT scanning, Radiology 163:149-151, 1987.

Bush CH, Gillespy T III and Dell PC: High-resolution CT of the wrist: initial experience with scaphoid disorders and surgical fusions, AJR 149:757-760, 1987.

Carey RP, De Campo JF and Menelaus MB: Measurement of leg length by computerised tomographic scanography: brief report, J Bone Joint Surg [Br] 69:846-847, 1987.

Christiansen EL et al: Computed tomography of condylar and articular disk positions within the temporomandibular joint, Oral Surg Oral Med Oral Pathol 64:757-767, 1987.

Curnes JT, Banning BC and Robards JB: Cranial computed tomography in the morbidly obese patient, J Comput Assist Tomogr 11:920, 1987.

Donaldson JS, Poznanski AK and Nieves A: CT of children's feet: an immibilization technique, AJR 148:169-170, 1987.

Fajardo LL et al: Excretory urography using computed radiography, Radiology 162:345-351, 1987.

Faulkner K and Moores BM: Radiation dose and somatic risk from computed tomography, Acta Radiol 28:483-488, 1987.

Feuerstein IM and Margulis AR: Semierect computed tomography of the abdomen using the Imatron ultrafast CT scanner, J Comput Assist Tomogr 11:1107-1108, 1987.

Frey EE et al: Cine CT of the mediastinum in pediatric patients, Radiology 165:19-23, 1987.

Genant HK et al: Quantitative computed tomography: update, Calcif Tissue Int 41:179-186, 1987.

Goldstein S, Gumerlock MK and Neuwelt EA: Comparison of CT-guided and stereotaxic cranial diagnostic needle biopsies, J Neurosurg 67:341-348, 1987.

Gomori JM and Steiner I: Non-linear CT windows, Comput Radiol 11:21-27, 1987.

Gower DJ, Culp P and Ball M: Lateral lumbar spine roentgenograms: potential role in complications, Surg Neurol 27:316-318, 1987.

Greenberger R, Khangure MS and Chakera TM: The morbidity of CT air meatography: a follow-up of 84 patients, Clin Radiol 38:535-536, 1987.

Hadley MN et al: Three-dimensional computed tomography in the diagnosis of vertebral column pathological conditions, Neurosurgery 21:186-192, 1987.

Heffez L, Mafee MF and Langer B: Use of a new head holder for obtaining direct sagittal CT images of the TMJ, J Oral Maxillofac Surg 45:822-824, 1987.

Honda H et al: Optimal positioning for CT examinations of the skull base: experimental and clinical studies, Eur J Radiol 7:225-228, 1987.

Hopper JL et al: Analysis of dynamic computed tomography scan brain images, Invest Radiol 22:651-657, 1987.

Ilkko E, Leinonen K and Lahde S: Comparison of the radiation doses in lumbar CT and myelography, Eur J Radiol 7:119-120, 1987.

Jackson PC et al: The development of a system for transillumination computed tomography, Br J Radiol 60:375-380, 1987.

Jessurun W et al: Anatomical relations in the carpal tunnel: a computed tomographic study, J Hand Surg Br 12:64-67, 1987.

Katowitz JA et al: Three-dimensional computed tomographic imaging, Ophthalmic Plast Reconstr 3:243-248, 1987.

Kogutt MS: Computed radiographic imaging: use in low-dose leg length radiography, AJR 148:1205-1206, 1987.

Kornberg M: Computed tomography of the lumbar spine following discography: clinical application in selective cases, Spine 12:823-825, 1987.

Lagrange JL et al: CT measurement of lung density: the role of patient position and value for total body irradiation, Int J Radiat Oncol Biol Phys 13:941-944, 1987.

Larsson SG, Lufkin RB and Hoover LA: Computed tomography of the submandibular salivary glands, Acta Radiol 28:693-696, 1987.

Lipton MJ: Cine computerized tomography, Int J Card Imaging 2:209-221, 1987.

Lipton MJ: Computer tomography, positron emission tomography and nuclear magnetic resonance in cardiology, Herz 12:1-12, 1987.

Mafee MF et al: Dynamic computed tomography and its application to ophthalmology, Radiol Clin North Am 25:715-731, 1987.

Marchisello PJ: The use of computerized axial tomography for the evaluation of talocalcaneal coalition: a case study, J Bone Joint Surg [Am] 69:609-611, 1987

Mayo JR et al: High-resolution CT of the lungs: an optimal approach, Radiology 163:507-510, 1987.

McKean JD et al: CT guided functional stereotaxic surgery, Acta Neurochir 87:8-13, 1987.

Moilanen A: The role of primary head CT-scans in facial fractures, Int J Oral Maxillofac Surg 16:572-576, 1987.

Moon JB and Smith WL: Application of cine computed tomography to the assessment of velopharyngeal form and function, Cleft Palate J 24:226-232, 1987.

Moore SC and Judy PF: Cardiac computed tomography using redundant-ray prospective gating, Med Phys 14:193-196, 1987.

Muranaka T et al: CT retrograde pancreatography using an indwelling balloon catheter, Radiat Med 5:42-47, 1987.

Nakano Y et al: Direct radiographic magnification with computed radiography, AJR 148:569-573, 1987.

Neufang KF, Zanella FE and Ewen K: Radiation doses to the eye lenses in computed tomography of the orbit and the petrous bone, Eur J Radiol 7:203-205, 1987.

Noble PN: The changing face of computerised tomography, Radiography 53:115-121, 1987.

Raptopoulos V et al: Fat-density oral contrast agent for abdominal CT, Radiology 164:653-656, 1987.

Rhodes RA et al: Tomographic levels for intravenous urography: CT-determined guidelines, Radiology 163:673-675, 1987.

Roger DJ and Richli WR: A CT table attachment for parasagittal scanning of the axilla, AJR 149:555-556, 1987.

Rothfus WE et al: Head-hanging CT: an alternative method for evaluating traumatic CSF rhinorrhea, AJNR 8:155-156, 1987.

Salonen O: CT characteristics of expansions in the middle and posterior mediastinum, Comput Radiol 11:95-100, 1987.

Sartoris DJ and Resnick D: Pictorial review: cross-sectional imaging of the foot and ankle, Foot Ankle 8:59-80, 1987.

Savic D, Jasovic A and Djeric D: The value of computerized tomography (CT) in the evaluation of the anatomic structure of the attic, J Laryngol Otol 101:1118-1124, 1987.

Scott WW Jr, Fishman EK and Magid D: Acetabular fractures: optimal imaging, Radiology 165:537-539, 1987.

Sickles EA: Computed tomography scanning, transillumination, and magnetic resonance imaging of the breast, Recent Results Cancer Res 105:31-36, 1987.

Silverman PM et al: Computed tomography of mesenteric disease, Radiographics 7:309-320, 1987.

Stark P: Computed tomography of the sternum, CRC Crit Rev Diagn Imaging 27:321-349, 1987.

Steinbach LS et al: High resolution computed tomography of knee menisci, Skeletal Radiol 16:11-16, 1987.

Temme JB, Chu W-K and Anderson JC: CT scanograms compared with conventional orthorentgenograms in long bone measurement, Radiol Technol 59:65-68, 1987.

Thompson WM et al: Computed tomography of the rectum, Radiographics 7:773-807, 1987.

Vogelzang RL and Gore RM: Bolus-rapid infusion of contrast medium: simplified technique for optimal computed tomography pancreatography without use of dynamic scanning, J Comput Tomogr 11:1-3, 1987.

Zonneveld FW et al: Normal direct multiplanar CT anatomy of the orbit with correlative, Radiol Clin North Am 25:381-407, 1987.

1988 Adler SJ et al: Three-dimensional computed tomography of the foot: optimizing the image, Comput Med Imaging Graph 12:59-66, 1988.

Alexander MP and Warren RL: Localization of callosal auditory pathways: a CT case study, Neurology 38:802-804, 1988.

Angelelli G and Macarini L: CT of the bowel: use of water to enhance depiction, Radiology 169:848-849, 1988.

Batra P et al: Evaluation of intrathoracic extent of lung cancer by plain chest radiography, computed tomography, and magnetic resonance imaging, Am Rev Respir Dis 137:1456-1462, 1988.

Baumgartner RN et al: Abdominal composition quantified by computed tomography, Am J Clin Nutr 48:936-945, 1988.

Brasch RC: Ultrafast computed tomography for infants and children, Radiol Clin North Am 26:277-286, 1988.

Buirski G and Watt I: Dynamic CT discography: an evaluation of a new technique, Australas Radiol 32:197-202, 1988.

Chintapalli K, Wentworth W and Wilson CR: Simple radiation protection device for CT, AJR 150:199-200, 1988.

Chung JW et al: Computed tomography of cavernous sinus diseases, Neuroradiology 30:319-328, 1988.

Dobson J and Nelson J: CT pelvimetry: replacing conventional with digital, Radiography 54:18-19, 1988.

Dondelinger RF and Kurdziel JC: Computed tomographic arteriography (CTA) of the liver, Bull Soc Sci Med Grand Duche Luxemb 125:27-34, 1988.

Fava C and Preti G: Lateral transcranial radiography of temporomandibular joints. II. Image formation studied with computerized tomography, J Prosthet Dent 59:218-227, 1988.

Fishman EK et al: Three-dimensional imaging and display of musculoskeletal anatomy, J Comput Assist Tomogr 12:465-467, 1988.

Fishman EK et al: Three-dimensional imaging in orthopedics: state of the art 1988, Orthopedics 11:1021-1026, 1988.

Frank DA, Kern EB and Kispert DB: Measurement of large or irregular-shaped septal perforations, Radiol Technol 59:409-412, 1988.

Heffez L, Mafee MF and Langer B: Double-contrast arthrography of the temporomandibular joint: role of direct sagittal CT imaging, Oral Surg Oral Med Oral Pathol 65:511-514, 1988.

Herman GT: Three-dimensional imaging on a CT or MR scanner, J Comput Assist Tomogr 12:450-458, 1988.

Hishikawa Y et al: Esophageal fistula: demonstration by CT, Radiat Med 6:115-116, 1988.

Ishida Y, Suzuki K and Ohmori K: Dynamics of the spinal cord: an analysis of functional myelography by CT scan, Neuroradiology 30:538-544, 1988.

Jackler RK: CT and MRI of the ear and temporal bone: current state of the art and future prospects, Am J Otol 9:232-239, 1988.

Kane NM et al: Pediatric abdominal trauma: evaluation by computed tomography, Pediatrics 82:11-15, 1988.

Karnaze MG et al: Comparison of MR and CT myelography in imaging the cervical and thoracic spine, AJR 150:397-403, 1988.

Karssemeijer N, van Erning LJ and Eijkman EG: Recognition of organs in CT-image sequences: a model guided approach, Comput Biomed Res 21:434-448, 1988.

Kashiwagi T et al: Three-dimensional demonstration of liver and spleen by a computer, Acta Radiol 29:27-31, 1988.

Keyser CK et al: Soft-tissue abnormalities of the foot and ankle: CT diagnosis, AJR 150:845-850, 1988.

Kuhlman JE et al: Complex shoulder trauma: three-dimensional CT imaging, Orthopedics 11:1561-1563, 1988.

Levin DN et al: Retrospective geometric correlation of MR, CT, and PET images, Radiology 169:817-823, 1988.

Maciunas RJ and Juneau P: Limiting artifact in CT stereotaxic periventricular procedures: technical note, J Neurosurg 69:459-460, 1988.

Mafee MF et al: Direct sagittal CT in the evaluation of temporal bone disease, AJR 150:1403-1410, 1988.

Magid D et al: Two-dimensional and three-dimensional computed tomography of the pediatric hip, Radiographics 8:901-933, 1988.

Makin WP and Hunter RD: CT scanning in intracavitary therapy: unexpected findings in "straightforward" insertions, Radiother Oncol 13:253-255, 1988.

Mostrom U: Evaluation of CT scanners for use in neuroradiology: a study with regard to radiation dose and image quality, Acta Radiol Suppl 372:89-107, 1988.

Mudge B et al: Multiplanar imaging of the hip: a systematic approach, Radiol Technol 59:307-311, 1988.

Muller NL et al: "Density mask": an objective method to quantitate emphysema using computed tomography, Chest 94:782-787, 1988.

Murphy FB and Bernardino ME: Interventional computed tomography, Curr Probl Diagn Radiol 17:121-154, 1988.

Oloff-Solomon J and Solomon MA: Computed tomographic scanning of the foot and ankle, Clin Podiatr Med Surg 5:931-944, 1988.

Pappas CT and Rekate HL: Role of magnetic resonance imaging and three-dimensional computerized tomography in craniovertebral junction anomalies, Pediatr Neurosci 14:18-22, 1988.

Peruzzi W et al: Portable chest roentgenography and computed tomography in critically ill patients, Chest 93:722-726, 1988.

Platt JF and Glazer GM: IV contrast material for abdominal CT: comparison of three methods of administration, AJR 151:275-277, 1988.

Reed DH and Morgan S: The changing mediastinum, Br J Radiol 61:695-696, 1988.

Remy Jardin M and Remy J: Comparison of vertical and oblique CT in evaluation of bronchial tree, J Comput Assist Tomogr 12:956-962, 1988.

Robb WL: Future advances and directions in imaging research, AJR 150:39-42, 1988.

Sartoris DJ and Resnick D: Computed tomography of the lower extremity. II. Orthop Rev 17:20-24, 1988.

Sartoris DJ and Resnick D: Pictorial analysis—computed tomography of trauma to the ankle and hindfoot, J Foot Surg 27:80-91, 1988.

Schick RM et al: CT guided lateral C1-C2 puncture, J Comput Assist Tomogr 12:715-716, 1988.

Schonstrom N: The significance of oblique cuts on CT scans of the spinal canal in terms of anatomic measurements, Spine 13:435-436, 1988.

Silverman PM et al: Computed tomography of the ileocecal region, Comput Med Imaging Graph 12:293-303, 1988.

Sundram SR: Direct coronal imaging of the abdomen and pelvis, Radiography 54:86-92, 1988.

Tawn DJ, Snow M and Jeans WD: Computed tomography of the internal auditory canals, Bristol Med Chir J 103:13-15, 1988.

Thoeni RF and Filson RG: Abdominal and pelvic CT: use of oral metoclopramide to enhance bowel opacification, Radiology 169:391-393, 1988.

Van Hove JE et al: Ultrafast (cine) CT scanner—new frontier in CT scanning? Indiana Med 81:630-634, 1988.

Walter E et al: CT and MR imaging of the temporomandibular joint, Radiographics 8:327-348, 1988.

Zeman RK et al: CT of the liver: a survey of prevailing methods for administration of contrast material, AJR 150:107-109, 1988.

Zinreich SJ et al: 3-D CT for cranial, facial and laryngeal surgery, Laryngoscope 98:1212-1219, 1988.

1989 Albertyn LE: Rationales for the use of intravenous contrast medium in computed tomography, Australas Radiol 33:29-33, 1989.

Bar-Ziv J and Solomon A: The use of a modified direct coronal computed tomographic technique for assessing thoraco-abdominal problems, Gastrointest Radiol 14:205-208, 1989.

Bretan PN Jr and Lorig R: Adrenal imaging: computed tomographic scanning and magnetic resonance imaging, Urol Clin North Am 16:505-513, 1989.

Brogan M and Chakeres DW: Computed tomography and magnetic resonance imaging of the normal anatomy of the temporal bone, Semin Ultrasound CT MR 10:178-194, 1989.

Conticello S et al: Computed tomography in the study of the eustachian tube, Arch Otorhinolaryngol 246:259-261, 1989.

Deck MD: Computed tomography and magnetic resonance imaging of the skull and brain, Clin Imaging 13:95-113, 1989.

Esfahani F and Dolan KD: Air CT cisternography in the diagnosis of vascular loop causing vestibular nerve dysfunction, AJNR 10:1045-1049, 1989.

Fezoulidis I et al: Diagnostic imaging of the occipito-cervical junction in patients with rheumatoid arthritis: plain films, computed tomography, magnetic resonance imaging, Acta Radiol 9:5-11, 1989.

Finch IJ, Sun Y and Shatsky SA: Technique for cranial CT scanning of excessively obese patients, AJNR 10:434, 1989.

Foley WD: Dynamic hepatic CT, Radiology 170:617-622, 1989.

Fredericks BJ et al: Diseases of the spinal canal in children: diagnosis with noncontrast CT scans, AJNR 10:1233-1238, 1989.

Graves WA, Collins JD and Miller TQ: Why is high resolution computerized tomography scanning used in evaluating the lungs? J Natl Med Assoc 81:1041-1046, 1989.

Hammerman AM, Mirowitz SA and Susman N: The gastric air-fluid sign: aid in CT assessment of gastric wall thickening, Gastrointest Radiol 14:109-112, 1989.

Heare MM, Heare TC and Gillespy T: Diagnostic imaging of pelvic and chest wall trauma, Radiol Clin North Am 27:873-889, 1989.

Hederstrom E, Ahlgren M and Salminen H: Computed tomography for localization of intra-abdominally dislocated intrauterine devices, Acta Radiol 30:531-534, 1989.

Hillel AD and Schwartz AN: Trumpet maneuver for visual and CT examination of the pyriform sinus and retrocricoid area, Head Neck 11:231-236, 1989.

Hirsh BE, Udupa JK and Roberts D: Three-dimensional reconstruction of the foot from computed tomography scans, J Am Podiatr Med Assoc 79:384-394, 1989.

Holt WW, Wong E and Lipton MJ: Conventional and ultrafast cine-computed tomography in cardiac imaging, Curr Opin Radiol 1:159-165, 1989.

Hughes RJ, Hill V and Braun H: A mobile traction device for MR and CT imaging, Australas Phys Eng Sci Med 12:160-163, 1989.

Jackson RP et al: The neuroradiographic diagnosis of lumbar herniated nucleus pulposus. I. A comparison of computed tomography (CT), myelography, CT-myelography, discography, and CT-discography, Spine 14:1356-1361, 1989.

Jackson RP et al: The neuroradiographic diagnosis of lumbar herniated nucleus pulposus. II. A comparison of computed tomography (CT), myelography, CT-myelography, and magnetic resonance imaging, Spine 14:1362-1367, 1989.

Jensen PR, Owre A and Ahlgren P: Reaction to contrast media in contrast-enhanced CT of the brain: a comparative investigation of non-ionic ultravist and ionic urografin-meglumin, Eur J Radiol 9:144-146, 1989.

Johnson CD and Stephens DH: Computed tomography of the large bowel and appendix, Mayo Clin Proc 64:1276-1283, 1989.

Kanpolat Y et al: CT-guided percutaneous cordotomy, Acta Neurochir Suppl 46:67-68, 1989.

Kaplan IL and Swayne LC: Composite SPECT-CT images: technique and potential applications in chest and abdominal imaging, AJR 152:865-866, 1989.

Kaufman RA: Technical aspects of abdominal CT in infants and children, AJR 153:549-554, 1989.

King K: CT technologist to MRI technologist: making the transition, Radiol Technol 61:121-123, 1989.

Kogutt MS, Warren FH and Kalmar JA: Low dose imaging of scoliosis: use of a computed radiographic imaging system, Pediatr Radiol 20:85-86, 1989.

Lee BC et al: CT evaluation of the temporal bone ossicles by using oblique reformations: a technical note, AJNR 10:431-433, 1989.

Leighton DM and de Campo M: CT invertograms, Pediatr Radiol 19:176-178, 1989.

Leighton DM and de Campo M: Uses of direct coronal pelvic CT, Australas Radiol 33:157-159, 1989.

Lipton MJ and Holt WW: Value of ultrafast CT scanning in cardiology, Br Med Bull 45:991-1010, 1989.

Margulis AR: Cross-sectional imaging: present and future, Curr Opin Radiol 1:101-106, 1989.

Mattrey RF: Potential role of perfluorooctylbromide in the detection and characterization of liver lesions with CT, Radiology 170:18-20, 1989.

Merine D, Fishman EK and Jones B: CT of the small bowel and mesentery, Radiol Clin North Am 27:707-715, 1989.

Moore MM and Shearer DR: Fetal dose estimates for CT pelvimetry, Radiology 171:265-267, 1989.

Nakamura R et al: Three-dimensional CT imaging for wrist disorders, J Hand Surg [Br] 14:53-58, 1989.

Nelson RC et al: Contrast-enhanced CT of the liver and spleen: comparison of ionic and nonionic contrast agents, AJR 153:973-976, 1989.

Nemcek AA Jr: CT of acute gastrointestinal disorders, Radiol Clin North Am 27:773-786, 1989.

Neri M and Querin F: CT scan in a study of the normal anatomy of the hindfoot and midfoot, Ital J Orthop Traumatol 15:507-520, 1989.

Ney DR et al: Interactive real-time multiplanar CT imaging, Radiology 170:275-276, 1989.

Phillips MH et al: Heavy charged-particle stereotactic radiosurgery: cerebral angiography and CT in the treatment of intracranial vascular malformations, Int J Radiat Oncol Biol Phys 17:419-426, 1989.

Raptopoulos V: Technical principles in CT evaluation of the gut, Radiol Clin North Am 27:631-651, 1989.

Reinhardt HF and Landolt H: CT-guided "real time" stereotaxy, Acta Neurochir 46:107-108, 1989.

Rumberger JA and Lipton MJ: Ultrafast cardiac CT scanning, Cardiol Clin 7:713-734, 1989.

Scatarige JC and DiSantis DJ: CT of the stomach and duodenum, Radiol Clin North Am 27:687-706, 1989.

Smith FW et al: Low-field (0.08 T) magnetic resonance imaging of the pancreas: comparison with computed tomography and ultrasound, Br J Radiol 62:796-802, 1989.

Smith IM et al: CT air meatography: review of side effects in 60 patients, J Laryngol Otol 103:173-174, 1989.

Steiner RM et al: Clinical experience with rapid acquisition cardiovascular CT imaging (cine CT) in the adult patient, Radiographics 9:283-305, 1989.

Stutley J, Cooke J and Parsons C: Normal CT anatomy of the tongue, floor of mouth and oropharynx, Clin Radiol 40:248-253, 1989.

Sundram SR: Direct coronal CT of the neck, Radiogr Today 55:22-23, 1989.

Sundram SR: Direct coronal imaging in computed tomography of the lumbar spine, Radiogr Today 55:22-23, 1989.

Swensen SJ, Aughenbaugh GL and Brown LR: High-resolution computed tomography of the lung, Mayo Clin Proc 64:1284-1294, 1989.

Tyrrel RT, Kaufman SL and Bernardino ME: Straight line sign: appearance and significance during CT portography, Radiology 173:635-637, 1989.

van Waes PF, Feldberg MA and Barth P: Comparison of Telebrix Gastro and Gastrografin in abdominal computed tomography, Eur J Radiol 9:179-181, 1989.

Vanneste F et al: High resolution CT findings in diseases of the external auditory canal: a review of 31 cases, J Belge Radiol 72:199-205, 1989.

Vowden P et al: A comparison of three imaging techniques in the assessment of an abdominal aortic aneurysm, J Cardiovasc Surg 30:891-896, 1989.

Williamson BR et al: Computed tomography as a diagnostic aid in diabetic and other problem feet, Clin Imaging 13:159-163, 1989.

Yoshizumi TT, Suneja SK and Teal JS: Practical CT dosimetry, Radiol Technol 60:505-509, 1989.

Yueh N et al: Gantry tilt technique for CT-guided biopsy and drainage, J Comput Assist Tomogr 13:182-184, 1989.

Zieger A, Simon H and Dusterbehn G: Practical co-table for direct coronal CT scanning, Neurosurg Rev 12:51-53, 1989.

1990 Anslow P: Neuroradiology including magnetic resonance, Acta Neurochir Suppl 50:76-79, 1990.

Baldwin JE and Freer CE: Pituitary computed tomography: is contrast enhancement necessary? Clin Radiol 42:20-23, 1990.

Balthazar EJ and Chako AC: Computed tomography of pancreatic masses, Am J Gastroenterol 85:343-349, 1990.

Bar-Ziv J and Solomon A: Direct coronal CT scanning of tracheo-bronchial, pulmonary and thoraco-abdominal lesions in children, Pediatr Radiol 20:245-248, 1990.

Bhalla M et al: Counting ribs on chest CT, J Comput Assist Tomogr 14:590-594, 1990.

Caputo GR and Higgins CB: Advances in cardiac imaging modalities: fast computed tomography, magnetic resonance imaging, and positron emission tomography, Invest Radiol 25:838-854, 1990.

Crawley EO: In vivo tissue characterization using quantitative computed tomography: a review, J Med Eng Technol 14:233-242, 1990.

Englmeier KH et al: Methods and applications of three-dimensional imaging in orthopedics, Arch Orthop Trauma Surg 109:186-190, 1990.

Fitzgerald S and Foley WD: Advances in technique and technology in body computed tomography and magnetic resonance imaging, Curr Opin Radiol 2:526-533, 1990.

Friedman L and Halls SB: Coronal computed tomography, Can Assoc Radiol J 41:287-290, 1990.

Friedman L, Johnston GH and Yong-Hing K: Computed tomography of wrist trauma, Can Assoc Radiol J 41:141-145, 1990.

Hoffman EA and Gefter WB: Multimodality imaging of the upper airway: MRI, MR spectroscopy, and ultrafast X-ray CT, Prog Clin Biol Res 345:291-301, 1990.

Howard JD, Elster AD and May JS: Temporal bone: three-dimensional CT. I. Normal anatomy, techniques, and limitations, Radiology 177:421-425, 1990.

Howard JD, Elster AD and May JS: Temporal bone: three-dimensional CT. II. Pathologic alterations, Radiology 177:427-430, 1990.

Hughes K: A simplified anatomical approach to thin section, high resolution CT of the ear and facial nerve, Radiogr Today 56:18-23, 1990.

Isono M et al: High resolution computed tomography of auditory ossicles, Acta Radiol 31:27-31, 1990.

Kalender WA et al: Spiral volumetric CT with single-breath-hold technique, continuous transport, and continuous scanner rotation, Radiology 176:181-183, 1990.

Kelly TJ: Post-myelogram CT and the incidence of headache, Radiol Technol 62:32-34, 1990.

Kinnunen J et al: Improved visualization of posterior fossa with clivoaxial CT scanning plane, Roentgenblatter 43:539-542, 1990.

Kuhn MJ and Baker MR: Optimization of low-osmolality contrast media for cranial CT: a dose comparison of two contrast agents, AJNR 11:847-9, 1990.

Laine FJ, Nadel L and Braun IF: CT and MR imaging of the central skull base. I. Techniques, embryologic development, and anatomy, Radiographics 10:591-602, 1990.

Laine FJ, Nadel L and Braun IF: CT and MR imaging of the central skull base. II. Pathologic spectrum, Radiographics 10:797-821, 1990.

Liddell RM et al: Normal intrahepatic bile ducts: CT depiction, Radiology 176:633-635, 1990.

Littleton JT et al: Pulmonary masses: contrast enhancement, Radiology 177:861-871, 1990.

Magid D et al: Adult ankle fractures: comparison of plain films and interactive two- and three-dimensional CT scans, AJR 154:1017-1023, 1990.

Mano I et al: Computerized three-dimensional normal atlas, Radiat Med 8:50-54, 1990.

Naidich DP et al: Low-dose CT of the lungs: preliminary observations, Radiology 175:729-731, 1990.

Odrezin GT et al: High resolution computed tomography of the temporal bone in infants and children: a review, Int J Pediatr Otorhinolaryngol 19:15-31, 1990.

Offutt CJ et al: Volumetric three-dimensional imaging of computerized tomography scans, Radiol Technol 61:212-219, 1990.

Palestrant AM: Comprehensive approach to CT-guided procedures with a hand-held guidance device, Radiology 174:270-272, 1990.

Pandolfo I et al: Tumors of the ampulla diagnosed by CT hypotonic duodenography, J Comput Assist Tomogr 14:199-200, 1990.

Rigauts H et al: Initial experience with volume CT scanning, J Comput Assist Tomogr 14:675-682, 1990.

Ritman EL: Fast computed tomography for quantitative cardiac analysis—state of the art and future perspectives, Mayo Clin Proc 65:1336-1349, 1990.

Russell JL et al: Computed tomography in the diagnosis of maxillofacial trauma, Br J Oral Maxillofac Surg 28:287-291, 1990.

Seto H et al: Pancrease divisum: CT and ERCP findings, Radiat Med 8:20-21, 1990.

Simon JH: Technologic advances in computed tomography and magnetic resonance imaging in the central nervous system, Curr Opin Radiol 2:518-525, 1990.

Snow N, Bergin KT and Horrigan TP: Thoracic CT scanning in critically ill patients: information obtained frequently alters management, Chest 97:1467-1470, 1990.

Teefey SA et al: Differentiating pelvic veins and enlarged lymph nodes: optimal CT techniques, Radiology 175:683-685, 1990.

Trerotola SO, Kuhlman JE and Fishman EK: Bleeding complications of femoral catheterization: CT evaluation, Radiology 174:37-40, 1990.

Tress BM and Hare WS: CT of the spine: are plain spine radiographs necessary? Clin Radiol 41:317-320, 1990.

van der Kuijl B et al: Temporomandibular joint computed tomography: development of a direct sagittal technique, J Prosthet Dent 64:709-715, 1990.

van der Kuijl B et al: Temporomandibular joint direct sagittal computed tomography: evaluation of image-processing modalities, J Prosthet Dent 64:589-595, 1990.

Webb S: Non-standard CT scanners: their role in radiotherapy, Int J Radiat Oncol Biol Phys 19:1589-1607, 1990.

1991 Adler LP et al: Comparison of PET with CT, MRI, and conventional scintigraphy in a benign and in a malignant soft tissue tumor, Orthopedics 14:891-4, 1991.

Ambrosetto P et al: CT and MR of the sellar spine, Neuroradiology 33:465, 1991.

Aronson D and Kier R: CT pelvimetry: the foveae are not an accurate landmark for the level of the ischial spines, AJR 156:527-530, 1991.

Ashenhurst M et al: Combined computed tomography and dacryocystography for complex lacrimal problems, Can J Ophthalmol 26:27-31, 1991.

Babbel R et al: Optimization of techniques in screening CT of the sinuses, AJNR 12:849-854, 1991.

Bach DB: Telebrix: a better-tasting oral contrast agent for abdominal computed tomography, Can Assoc Radiol J 42:98-101, 1991.

Bayley JC, Kruger DM and Schlegel JM: Does the angle of the computed tomographic scan change spinal canal measurements? Spine 16:526-529, 1991.

Bernard MS, Hourihan MD and Adams H: Computed tomography of the brain: does contrast enhancement really help? Clin Radiol 44:161-164, 1991.

Bettinardi V et al: Head holder for PET, CT, and MR studies, J Comput Assist Tomogr 15:886-892, 1991.

Bingham B, Shankar L and Hawke M: Pitfalls in computed tomography of the paranasal sinuses, J Otolaryngol 20:414-418, 1991.

Bonnier L et al: Three-dimensional reconstruction in routine computerized tomography of the skull and spine: experience based on 161 cases, J Neuroradiol 18:250-266, 1991.

Borock EC et al: A prospective analysis of a two-year experience using computed tomography as an adjunct for cervical spine clearance, J Trauma 31:1001-1005, 1991.

Breidahl WH, Low V and Khangure MS: Imaging the cervical spine: a comparison of MR with myelography and CT myelography, Australas Radiol 35:306-314, 1991.

Burns MA et al: Motion artifact simulating aortic dissection on CT, AJR 157:465-467, 1991.

Chan WP et al: Three-dimensional imaging of the musculoskeletal system: an overview, J Formosan Med Assoc 90:713-722, 1991.

Chevallier JM et al: The thoracic esophagus: sectional anatomy and radiosurgical applications, Surg Radiol Anat 13:313-321, 1991.

Christiansen EL and Thompson JR: Computed tomography, Cranio Clin Int 1:17-34, 1991.

Conway WF et al: Cross-sectional imaging of the patellofemoral joint and surrounding structures, Radiographics 11:195-217, 1991.

Coventry DM, Martin CS and Burke AM: Sedation for paediatric computerized tomography—a double-blind assessment of rectal midazolam, Eur J Anaesthesiol 8:29-32, 1991.

Cox IH, Foley WD and Hoffmann RG: Right window for dynamic hepatic CT, Radiology 181:18-21, 1991.

Deconinck K, Bellemans M and Van-Herreweghe W: CT of the heel and midfoot, J Belge Radiol 74:1-9, 1991.

Ebraheim NA et al: Percutaneous computed tomography stabilization of moderate to severe slipped capital femoral epiphysis, Orthopedics 859-863, 1991.

Freeny PC: Angio-CT: diagnosis and detection of complications of acute pancreatitis, Hepatogastroenterology 38:109-115, 1991.

Gay SB et al: Dynamic CT of the neck, Radiology 180:284-285, 1991.

Grosskreutz S et al: CT of the normal appendix, J Comput Assist Tomogr 15:575-577, 1991.

Guy RL et al: A comparison of CT and MRI in the assessment of the pituitary and parasellar region, Clin Radiol 43:156-161, 1991.

Hadar H et al: Air in vagina: indicator of intrapelvic pathology on CT, Acta Radiol 32:170-173, 1991.

Herman TE and Siegel MJ: CT of the pancreas in children, AJR 157:375-379, 1991.

Imanishi Y et al: Measurement of thyroid iodine by CT, J Comput Assist Tomogr 15:287-290, 1991.

Kalender WA and Polacin A: Physical performance characteristics of spiral CT scanning, Med Phys 18:910-915, 1991.

Kingsley DP, Dale G and Wallis A: A simple technique for head repositioning in CT scanning, Neuroradiology 33:243-246, 1991.

Leonardi M et al: Curved CT reformatted images of head scans, J Comput Assist Tomogr 15:1074-1076, 1991.

Levy JM and Hupke R: Composite addition technique: a new method in CT scanning of the posterior fossa, AJNR 12:686-688, 1991.

Mackay S: Use of three-dimensional CT scanning in the lumbar spine, Radiogr Today 57:17-21, 1991.

Magid D, Thompson JS and Fishman EK: Computed tomography of the hand and wrist, Hand Clin 7:219-233, 1991.

Mayo JR: The high-resolution computed tomography technique, Semin Roentgenol 26:104-109, 1991.

McDonald JF, Pruzansky JD and Meltzer RM: Evaluation of recurrent macrodactyly with three-dimensional imaging, J Am Podiatr Med Assoc 81:84-87, 1991.

Merenich WM et al: The foramen ovale: MR and CT correlation, Clin Imaging 15:20-30, 1991.

Nelson DW and Duwelius PJ: CT-guided fixation of sacral fractures and sacroiliac joint disruptions, Radiology 180:527-532, 1991.

Nelson RC: Techniques for computed tomography of the liver, Radiol Clin North Am 29:1199-1212, 1991.

Ney DR et al: Three-dimensional volumetric display of CT data: effect of scan parameters upon image quality, J Comput assist Tomogr 15:875-885, 1991.

Ozdoba C, Voigt K and Nusslin F: New device for CT-targeted percutaneous punctures, Radiology 180:576-578, 1991.

Raman S, Samuel D and Suresh K: A comparative study of X-ray pelvimetry and CT pelvimetry, Austral N Z J Obstetr Gynaecol 31:217-220, 1991.

Richardson P et al: Value of CT in determining the need for angiography when findings of mediastinal hemorrhage on chest radiographs are equivocal, AJR 156:273-279, 1991.

Rozeik C et al: Cranial CT artifacts and gantry angulation, J Comput Assist Tomogr 15:381-386, 1991.

Sharma P and Sehgal AD: Water-soluble contrast CT cisternography in CSF fistulas, Australas Radiol 35:324-326, 1991.

Shirkhoda A: Diagnostic pitfalls in abdominal CT, Radiographics 11:969-1002, 1991.

Smith RC and McCarthy S: Improving the accuracy of digital CT pelvimetry, J Comput Assist Tomogr 15:787-789, 1991.

Spiegelmann R and Friedman WA: Rapid determination of thalamic CT-stereotactic coordinates: a method, Acta Neurochir 110:77-81, 1991.

Stanford W et al: Ultrafast computed tomography in cardiac imaging: a review, Semin Ultrasound CT MR 12:45-60, 1991.

Walkey MM: Dynamic hepatic CT: how many years will it take 'til we learn? Radiology 181:17-18, 1991.

Webb WR: High-resolution computed tomography of the lung: normal and abnormal anatomy, Semin Roentgenol 26:110-117, 1991.

Wiesen EJ et al: Improvement in CT pelvimetry, Radiology 178:259-262, 1991.

Wimmer B and Wenz W: CT-guided interventions: present and future aspects, Acta Radiol Suppl 377:46-49, 1991.

1992 Aaron A et al: Comparison of orthoroentgenography and computed tomography in the measurement of limb-length discrepancy, J Bone Joint Surg Am 74:897-902, 1992.

Barnes JE: Characteristics and control of contrast in CT, Radiographics 12:825-837, 1992.

Bell GR and Ross JS: Diagnosis of nerve root compression: myelography, computed tomography, and MRI, Orthop Clin North Am 23:405-419, 1992.

Bellon RJ and Horwitz SM: Three-dimensional computed tomography studies of the tendons of the foot and ankle, J Digit Imaging 5:46-49, 1992.

Berk M: Indications for computed tomographic brain scanning in psychiatric inpatients, S Afr Med J 82:338-340, 1992.

Billet FP, Schmitt WG and Gay B: Computed tomography in traumatology with special regard to the advances of three-dimensional display, Arch Orthop Trauma Surg 111:131-137, 1992.

Bleiweis MS, Georgiou D and Brundage BH: Ultrafast CT and the cardiovascular system, Int J Card Imaging 8:289-302, 1992.

Bradley SA and Davies AM: Computed tomographic assessment of soft tissue abnormalities following calcaneal fractures, Br J Radiol 65:105-111, 1992.

Brody AS: Pediatric body CT, Pediatr Ann 21:111, 114-111, 120, 1992.

Carlson JE et al: Safety considerations in the power injection of contrast media via central venous catheters during computed tomographic examinations, Invest Radiol 27:337-340, 1992.

Castellino RA: Diagnostic imaging studies in patients with newly diagnosed Hodgkin's disease, Ann Oncol 3(Suppl 4):45-47, 1992.

Costello P et al: Assessment of the thoracic aorta by spiral CT, AJR 158:1127-1130, 1992.

Costello P et al: Spiral CT of the thorax with reduced volume of contrast material: a comparative study, Radiology 183:663-666, 1992.

Davies AM and Wellings RM: Imaging of bone tumors, Curr Opin Radiol 4:32-38, 1992.

Davies AM, Cassar-Pullicino VN and Grimer RJ: The incidence and significance of fluid-fluid levels on computed tomography of osseous lesions, Br J Radiol 65:193-198, 1992.

Dietemann JL et al: CT, myelography and CT-myelography in the evaluation of common cervicobrachial neuralgia, J Neuroradiol 19:167-176, 1992.

Ditchfield MR, Gibson RN and Fairlie N: Liver CT: a practical approach to dynamic contrast enhancement, Australas Radiol 36:210-213, 1992.

Dupuy DE, Costello P and Ecker CP: Spiral CT of the pancreas, Radiology 183:815-818, 1992.

Ebeling U and Huber P: Localization of central lesions by correlation of CT findings and neurological deficits, Acta Neurochir 119:17-22, 1992.

Engel PA and Gelber J: Does computed tomographic brain imaging have a place in the diagnosis of dementia? Arch Intern Med 152:1437-1440, 1992.

Engelhard HH: A simplified method for CT-guided stereotactic brain biopsy, J Ky Med Assoc 90:24-27, 1992.

Farber JM: A helpful radiographic sign in CDH, Orthopedics 15:1072-1074, 1992.

Fishman EK et al: Spiral CT of the pancreas with multiplanar display, AJR 159:1209-1215, 1992.

Friedman WN and Rosenfield AT: Computed tomography in obstetrics and gynecology, J Reprod Med 37:3-18, 1992.

Gossios KJ et al: Water as contrast medium for computed tomography study of colonic wall lesions, Gastrointest Radiol 17:125-128, 1992.

Hacking JC and Dixon AK: Spiral versus conventional CT in soft tissue diagnosis, Eur J Radiol 15:224-229, 1992.

Hamm B: Contrast materials for cross-sectional imaging of the abdomen, Curr Opin Radiol 4:93-104, 1992.

Harbaugh RE et al: Three-dimensional computerized tomography angiography in the diagnosis of cerebrovascular disease, J Neurosurg 76:408-414, 1992.

Henschke CI: Image selection for computed tomography of the chest: a sampling approach, Invest Radiol 27:908-911, 1992.

Ho EK et al: A comparative study of computed tomographic and plain radiographic methods to measure vertebral rotation in adolescent idiopathic scoliosis, Spine 17:771-774, 1992.

Hopper KD et al: CT and MR imaging of the pediatric orbit, Radiographics 12:485-503, 1992.

Jahnke AH Jr et al: A prospective comparison of computerized arthrotomography and magnetic resonance imaging of the glenohumeral joint, Am J Sports Med 20:695-700, 1992.

James SE, Richards R and McGrouther DA: Three-dimensional CT imaging of the wrist: a practical system, J Hand Surg [Br] 17:504-506, 1992.

Janzen DL et al: Intraarticular fractures of the calcaneus: value of CT findings in determining prognosis, AJR 158:1271-1274, 1992.

Johnston GH, Friedman L and Kriegler JC: Computerized tomographic evaluation of acute distal radial fractures, J Hand Surg [Am] 17:738-744, 1992.

Judnick JW et al: Radiotherapy technique integrates MRI into CT, Radiol Technol 64:82-89, 1992.

Kawashima A, Fishman EK and Kuhlman JE: CT and MR evaluation of posterior mediastinal masses, CRC Crit Rev Diagn Imaging 33:311-367, 1992.

Keselbrener L, Shimoni Y and Akselrod S: Nonlinear filters applied on computerized axial tomography: theory and phantom images, Med Phys 19:1057-1064, 1992.

Kim SH and Han MC: Reversed contrast-urine levels in urinary bladder: CT findings, Urol Radiol 13:249-252, 1992.

King JM, Caldarelli DD and Petasnick JP: DentaScan: a new diagnostic method for evaluating mandibular and maxillary pathology, Laryngoscope 102:379-387, 1992.

Korobkin M et al: CT of the extraperitoneal space: normal anatomy and fluid collections, AJR 159:933-942, 1992.

Lang P et al: Imaging of the hip joint: computed tomography versus magnetic resonance imaging, Clin Orthop 135-153, 1992.

Lang TF et al: Description of a prototype emission-transmission computed tomography imaging system, J Nucl Med 33:1881-1887, 1992.

Lewis LM et al: Intracranial abnormalities requiring emergency treatment: identification by a single midline tomographic slice versus complete CT of the head, South Med J 85:348-350, 1992.

Marchal G and Baert AL: Dynamic CT of the liver, Radiologe 32:211-216, 1992.

Milants WP et al: CT imaging of soft tissue pathology of the ankle: a pictorial essay, J Belge Radiol 75:410-415, 1992.

Mousseaux E and Gaux JC: Ultrafast computed tomography of the heart, Curr Opin Radiol 4:34-40, 1992.

Ney DR et al: Comparison of helical and serial CT with regard to three-dimensional imaging of musculoskeletal anatomy, Radiology 185:865-869, 1992.

Padhani AR et al: Computed tomography in abdominal trauma: an audit of usage and image quality, Br J Radiol 65:397-402, 1992.

Patil A et al: The value of intraoperative scans during CT-guided stereotactic procedures, Neuroradiology 34:453-456, 1992.

Paulson EK et al: CT arterial portography: causes of technical failure and variable liver enhancement, AJR 159:745-749, 1992.

Pueschel SM, Moon AC and Scola FH: Computerized tomography in persons with Down syndrome and atlantoaxial instability, Spine 17:735-737, 1992.

Quint DJ: CT of scoliotic patients after myelography: value of lateral decubitus positioning, Radiology 182:276-277, 1992.

Richardson ML et al: CT measurement of the cancaneal varus angle in the normal and fractured hindfoot, J Comput Assist Tomogr 16:261-264, 1992.

Ritchie CJ et al: Minimum scan speeds for suppression of motion artifacts in CT, Radiology 185:37-42, 1992.

Rosenberg ZS et al: Osgood-Schlatter lesion: fracture of tendinitis? Scintigraphic, CT, and MR imaging features, Radiology 185:853-858, 1992.

Sartoris DJ: Diagnostic imaging insight: cross-sectional imaging of the foot (computed tomography-magnetic resonance), J Foot Surg 31:190-202, 1992.

Schlesinger AE and Hernandez RJ: Diseases of the musculoskeletal system in children: imaging with CT, sonography, and MR, AJR 158:729-741, 1992.

Schmidt J, Gassel F and Naughton S: Calculation of three-dimensional deformity in scoliosis by standard roentgenograms, Acta Orthop Belg 58(Suppl 1) :60-65, 1992.

Singer AA et al: Comparison of iohexol-240 versus iohexol-300 in abdominal CT, Gastrointest Radiol 17:122-124, 1992.

Stewart NR and Gilula LA: CT of the wrist: a tailored approach, Radiology 183:13-20, 1992.

Suojanen JN et al: Spiral CT in evaluation of head and neck lesions: work in progress, Radiology 183:281-283, 1992.

Torizuka T et al: High-resolution CT of the temporal bone: a modified baseline, Radiology 184:109-111, 1992.

Trulzsch DV et al: Gastrografin-induced aspiration pneumonia: a lethal complication of computed tomography, South Med J 85:1255-1256, 1992.

Wade JP: Accuracy of pelvimetry measurements on CT scanners, Br J Radiol 65:261-263, 1992.

Wechsler RJ, Karasick D and Schweitzer ME: Computed tomography of talocalcaneal coalition: imaging techniques, Skeletal Radiol 21:353-358, 1992.

Woodring JH and Lee C: The role and limitations of computed tomographic scanning in the evaluation of cervical trauma, J Trauma 33:698-708, 1992.

Yeoman LJ et al: Gantry angulation in brain CT: dosage implications, effect on posterior fossa artifacts, and current international practice, Radiology 184:113-116, 1992.

Zimmerman RA, Gusnard DA and Bilaniuk LT: Pediatric craniocervical spiral CT, Neuroradiology 34:112-116, 1992.

1993   Ali QM, Ulrich C and Becker H: Three-dimensional CT of the middle ear and adjacent structures, Neuroradiology 35:238-241, 1993.

Bach DB, Vellet AD and Levin MF: Dynamic abdominal computed tomography: "top-down" compared with "bottom-up" imaging, Can Assoc Radiol J 44:354-358, 1993.

Baker ME et al: Contrast material for combined abdominal and pelvic CT: can cost be reduced by increasing the concentration and decreasing the volume? AJR 160:637-641, 1993.

Becker H: New aspects in spinal diagnostics with three-dimensional computed tomography, Neurosurg Rev 16:179-182, 1993.

Bluemke DA and Fishman EK: Spiral CT of the abdomen: clinical applications, CRC Crit Rev Diagn Imaging 34:103-157, 1993.

Bluemke DA and Fishman EK: Spiral CT arterial portography of the liver, Radiology 186:576-579, 1993.

Bluemke DA and Fishman EK: Spiral CT of the liver, AJR 160:787-792, 1993.

Blum A et al: Direct coronal view of the shoulder with arthrographic CT, Radiology 188:677-681, 1993.

Caceres J et al: Increased density of the azygos lobe on frontal chest radiographs simulating disease: CT findings in seven patients, AJR 160:245-248, 1993.

Chambers TP et al: Hepatic CT enhancement: a method to demonstrate reproducibility, Radiology 188:627-631, 1993.

Cotello P and Gaa J: Clinical assessment of an interventional CT table, Radiology 189:284-285, 1993.

Dawson P and Peters M: Dynamic contrast bolus computed tomography for the assessment of renal function, Invest Radiol 28:1039-1042, 1993.

Dillon EH et al: Spiral CT angiography, AJR 160:1273-1278, 1993.

Dodd GD and Baron RL: Investigation of contrast enhancement in CT of the liver: the need for improved methods, AJR 160:643-645, 1993.

Earwaker J: Anatomic variants in sinonasal CT, Radiographics 13:381-415, 1993.

Faro SH, Mahboubi S and Ortega W: CT diagnosis of rib anomalies, tumors, and infection in children, Clin Imaging 17:1-7, 1993.

Fishman EK et al: Spiral CT of musculoskeletal pathology: preliminary observations, Skeletal Radiol 22:253-256, 1993.

Foley WD: Image quality in dynamic CT: a clinical discussion, Radiographics 13:225-233, 1993.

Fox LA: Images in clinical medicine: three-dimensional CT diagnosis of maxillofacial trauma, N Engl J Med 329:102, 1993.

Friedman L et al: A limited, low-dose computed tomography protocol to examine the sacroiliac joints, Can Assoc Radiol J 44:267-272, 1993.

Fultz PJ, Hampton WR and Totterman SM: Computed tomography of pyonephrosis, Abdom Imaging 18:82-87, 1993.

Garcia FF et al: Diagnostic imaging of childhood spinal infection, Orthop Rev 22:321-327, 1993.

Ghaziuddin M et al: Utility of the head computerized tomography scan in child and adolescent psychiatry, J Am Acad Child Adolesc Psychiatry 32:123-126, 1993.

Graeter T et al: Three-dimensional vascular imaging—an additional diagnostic took, Thorac Cardiovasc Surg 41:183-185, 1993.

Grenier P, Cordeau MP and Beigelman C: High-resolution computed tomography of the airways, J Thorac Imaging 8:213-229, 1993.

Hamano K et al: A comparative study of linear measurement of the brain and three-dimensional measurement of brain volume using CT scans, Pediatr Radiol 23:165-168, 1993.

Heiken JP, Brink JA and Vannier MW: Spiral (helical) CT, Radiology 189:647-656, 1993.

Herts BR, Einstein DM and Paushter DM: Spiral CT of the abdomen: artifacts and potential pitfalls, AJR 161:1185-1190, 1993.

Holtas S: Radiology of the degenerative lumbar spine, Acta Orthop Scand Suppl 251:16-18, 1993.

Jackson A et al: CT appearances of haematomas in the corpus callosum in patients with subarachnoid haemorrhage, Neuroradiology 35:420-423, 1993.

Koutrouvelis PG et al: A three-dimensional stereotactic device for computed tomography-guided invasive diagnostic and therapeutic procedures, Invest Radiol 28:845-847, 1993.

Malone AJ Jr et al: Diagnosis of acute appendicitis: value of unenhanced CT, AJR 160:763-766, 1993.

Manson D et al: CT of blunt chest trauma in children, Pediatr Radiol 23:1-5, 1993.

Mayo JR, Jackson SA and Muller NL: High-resolution CT of the chest: radiation dose, AJR 160:479-481, 1993.

Milants WP et al: Epidural and subdural contrast in myelography and CT myelography, Eur J Radiol 16:147-150, 1993.

Miles KA, Hayball MP and Dixon AK: Functional images of hepatic perfusion obtained with dynamic CT, Radiology 188:405-411, 1993.

Morris CW, Heggie JC and Acton CM: Computed tomography pelvimetry: accuracy and radiation dose compared with conventional pelvimetry, Australas Radiol 37:186-191, 1993.

Murray JG and Breatnach E: The American Thoracic Society lymph node map: a CT demonstration, Eur J Radiol 17:61-68, 1993.

Napel S et al: CT angiography with spiral CT and maximum intensity projection, Radiology 185:607-610, 1993.

Okudera H, Takemae T and Kobayashi S: Intraoperative computed tomographic scanning during transsphenoidal surgery: technical note, Neurosurgery 32:1041-1043, 1993.

Padley SP, Adler B and Muller NL: High-resolution computed tomography of the chest: current indications, J Thorac Imaging 8:189-199, 1993.

Padovani B et al: Chest wall invasion by bronchogenic carcinoma: evaluation with MR imaging, Radiology 187:33-38, 1993.

Rabassa AE et al: CT of the spine: value of reformatted images, AJR 161:1223-1227, 1993.

Ray CE et al: Applications of three-dimensional CT imaging in head and neck pathology, Radiol Clin North Am 31:181-194, 1993.

Rubin GD et al: Three-dimensional spiral CT angiography of the abdomen: initial clinical experience, Radiology 186:147-152, 1993.

Sawada S et al: Computed tomographic percutaneous transsplenic portography, Acta Radiol 34:529-531, 1993.

Sombeck MD et al: Correlation of lymphangiography, computed tomography, and laparotomy in the staging of Hodgkin's disease, Int J Radiat Oncol Biol Phys 25:425-429, 1993.

Soyer P, Lacheheb D and Levesque M: CT arterial portography of the abdomen: effect of injecting papaverine into the mesenteric artery on hepatic contrast enhancement, AJR 160:1213-1215, 1993.

Stern EJ, Webb WR and Gamsu G: CT gantry tilt: utility in transthoracic fine-needle aspiration biopsy. Work in progress, Radiology 187:873-874, 1993.

Tso EL et al: Cranial computed tomography in the emergency department evaluation of HIV-infected patients with neurologic complaints, Ann Emerg Med 22:1169-1176, 1993.

Watanabe H et al: Spiral volumetric CT as a routine technique for thoracic imaging, J Thorac Imaging 8:316-320, 1993.

Webb WR, Muller NL and Naidich DP: Standardized terms for high-resolution computed tomography of the lung: a proposed glossary, J Thorac Imaging 8:167-175, 1993.

Yankelevitz DF, Henschke CI and Davis SD: Percutaneous CT biopsy of chest lesions: an in vitro analysis of the effect of partial volume averaging on needle positioning, AJR 161:273-278, 1993.

Yune HY: Two-dimensional-three-dimensional reconstruction computed tomography techniques, Dent Clin North Am 37:613-626, 1993.

Zeman RK et al: Helical (spiral) CT of the abdomen, AJR 160:719-725, 1993.

Zeman RK et al: Routine helical CT of the abdomen: image quality considerations, Radiology 189:395-400, 1993.

DIGITAL RADIOGRAPHY

For bibliographic citations before 1964, please see the fifth edition of this ATLAS. For citations from 1964 through 1974, see the sixth or seventh edition.

1977 Brennecke R et al: Computerized video-image processing with application to cardioangiographic roentgen image series. In Nagel HH, editor: Digital image processing, New York, 1977, Springer-Verlag.

1978 Kruger RA et al: A digital video image processor for real time x-ray subtraction imaging, Opt Engl 17:652-657, 1978.

Ovitt TW et al: Development of a digital video subtraction system for intravenous angiography. In Miller HA, Schmidt EV and Harrison DC, editors: Noninvasive cardiovascular measurements, Bellingham, Wash, 1978, Society of Photo-optical Instrumentation Engineers.

1979 Amtey SR et al: Recent and future developments in medical imaging. II. Applications of digital processing in computed radiography, Proc Soc Photooptic Instrum Eng 206:190-192, 1979.

Cohen G et al: Applications of optical instrumentation in medicine. VII. Contrast-detail-dose evaluation of computed radiography: comparison with computed tomography (CT) and conventional radiography, Proc Soc Photooptic Instrum Eng 173:41-47, 1979.

Katragadda CS et al: Computed radiography: a new imaging system, New York, 1979, IEEE.

Katragadda CS et al: Digital radiography using a computed tomographic instrument, Radiology 133:83-87, 1979.

Kruger RA et al: Computerized fluoroscopy in real time for noninvasive visualization of the cardiovascular system: preliminary studies, Radiology 130:49-57, 1979.

Kruger RA et al: Computerized fluoroscopy techniques for intravenous study of cardiac chamber dynamics, Invest Radiol 14:279-287, 1979.

Ovitt TW et al: Development of a digital video subtraction system for intravenous angiography, Proc Soc Photooptic Instrum Eng 206:73, 1979.

Sashin D et al: Applications of optical instrumentation in medicine. VIII. Computer radiography for early detection of vascular disease, Proc Soc Photooptic Instrum Eng 173:88-97, 1979.

1980 Brody WR et al: Intravenous angiography using scanned projection radiography: preliminary investigation of a new method, Invest Radiol 15:220-223, 1980.

Christenson PC et al: Intravenous angiography using digital video subtraction: intravenous cervicocerebrovascular angiography, AJR 135:1145-1152, 1980.

Crummy AB et al: Computerized fluoroscopy: digital subtraction for intravenous angiocardiography and arteriography, AJR 135:1131-1140, 1980.

Lawson TL et al: Abdominal computed radiography: evaluation of low-contrast lesions, Invest Radiol 15:215-219, 1980.

Meaney TF et al: Digital subtraction angiography of the human cardiovascular system, AJR 135:1153-1160, 1980.

Ovitt TW et al: Intravenous angiography using digital video subtraction x-ray imaging system, Am J Neuroradiol 1:387-390, 1980.

Strother CM et al: Clinical applications of computerized fluoroscopy: the extracranial carotid arteries, Radiology 136:781-783, 1980.

1981 Brody WR et al: Intravenous carotid arteriography using line-scanned digital radiography, Radiology 139:297-300, 1981.

1982 Bjork L and Bjorkholm PJ: Xenon as a contrast agent for imaging of the airways and lungs using digital radiography, Radiology 144:475-478, 1982.

Brody WR et al: Intravenous arteriography using digital subtraction techniques, JAMA 248:671-674, 1982.

Carmody RF et al: Intracranial applications of digital intravenous subtraction angiography, Radiology 144:529-534, 1982.

Enzmann DR et al: Intracranial intravenous digital subtraction angiography, Neuroradiology 23:241-251, 1982.

Fodor J and Malott JC: Digital video angiography, Radiol Technol 54:83-90, 1982.

Harrington DP, Boxt LM and Murray PD: Digital subtraction angiography: overview of technical principles, AJR 139:781-786, 1982.

Hawkins IF: Carbon dioxide digital subtraction angiography, AJR 139:19-24, 1982.

Malott JC and Fodor J: Digital video angiography, Radiol Technol 54:83-89, 1982.

Myerowitz PD: Digital subtraction angiography: present and future uses in cardiovascular diagnosis, Clin Cardiol 5:623-629, 1982.

Nelson JA et al: Digital subtraction angiography using a temporal bypass filter: initial clinical results, Radiology 145:309-313, 1982.

Sashin D et al: Diode array digital radiography: initial clinical experience, AJR 139:1045-1050, 1982.

Seeger JF et al: Digital video subtraction angiography of the cervical and cerebral vasculature, J Neurosurg 56:173-179, 1982.

Tomsak RL, Modic MT and Weinstein MA: Intravenous digital subtraction angiography in neuro-ophthalmology, J Clin Neuro Ophthalmol 2:23-31, 1982.

1983 Cacayorin ED et al: Intravenous digital subtraction angiography with iohexol, AJNR 4:329-332, 1983.

DeBrusk DP: Digital x-ray imaging: the basics, Radiol Technol 54:280-286, 1983.

Enzmann DR et al: Low-dose, high-frame-rate versus regular-dose, low-frame-rate digital subtraction angiography, Radiology 146:669-676, 1983.

Foley WD et al: Digital subtraction angiography of the portal venous system, AJR 140:497-499, 1983.

Grondahl HG and Grondahl K: Subtraction radiography for the diagnosis of periodontal bone lesions, Oral Surg Oral Med Oral Pathol 55:208-213, 1983.

Grondahl K, Grondahl HG and Webber RL: Digital subtraction radiography for diagnosis of periodontal bone disease, Oral Surg Oral Med Oral Pathol 55:313-318, 1983.

Harrington DP: Renal digital subtraction angiography, Cardiovasc Intervent Radiol 6:214-223, 1983.

Johnson GA and Ravin CE: A survey of digital chest radiography, Radiol Clin North Am 21:655-664, 1983.

Kaufman SL et al: Intraarterial digital subtraction angiography: a comparative view, Cardiovasc Intervent Radiol 6:271-279, 1983.

Kollath J and Riemann H: Pulmonary digital subtraction angiography, Cardiovasc Intervent Radiol 6:233-238, 1983.

Kubal WS, Crummy AB, and Turnipseed WD: The utility of digital subtraction arteriography in peripheral vascular disease, Cardiovasc Intervent Radiol 6:241-249, 1983.

Malott JC and Fodor J: Digital vascular imaging: two years of clinical experience, Radiol Technol 55:633-638, 1983.

Mancini GB et al: Cardiac imaging with digital subtraction angiography, Cardiovasc Intervent Radiol 6:252-262, 1983.

Maravilla KR et al: Clinical application of digital tomosynthesis: a preliminary report, AJNR 4:277-280, 1983.

Modic MT et al: Intravenous digital subtraction angiography: peripheral versus central injection of contrast material, Radiology 147:711-715, 1983.

Passariello R et al: Digital subtraction angiography for examination of vessels of the leg: use of a 40-cm image intensifier, Radiology 149:669-674, 1983.

Riederer SJ et al: The application of matched filtering to contrast material dose reduction in digital subtraction angiography, Radiology 147:853-858, 1983.

Seldin DW et al: Left ventricular volume determined from scintigraphy and digital angiography by a semi-automated geometric method, Radiology 149:809-813, 1983.

Sider L et al: Control of swallowing by use of topical anesthesia during digital subtraction angiography, Radiology 148:563-564, 1983.

Turski PA et al: Limitations of intravenous digital subtraction angiography, AJNR 4:271-273, 1983.

Vizy KN: An overview of digital radiography systems, Cardiovasc Intervent Radiol 6:296-299, 1983.

1984 Anderson RE et al: Tomographic DSA using temporal filtration: initial neurovascular application, AJNR 5:277-280, 1984.

Arnold BA and Scheibe PO: Noise analysis of a digital radiography system, AJR 142:609-613, 1984.

Hillman BJ: Digital imaging of the kidney, Radiol Clin North Am 22:341-364, 1984.

Kaufman SL et al: Interaarterial digital subtraction angiography in diagnostic arteriography, Radiology 151:323-327, 1984.

Kinney SE and Modic MT: The role of digital subtraction angiography in diagnosis of skull-base lesions, Otolaryngol Head Neck Surg 92:151-155, 1984.

Lee BC et al: Digital intravenous cerebral angiography in neonates, AJNR 5:281-286, 1984.

Nelson JA and Kruger RA: Digital angiography, Radiologe 24:149-154, 1984.

Partridge JB and Dickinson DF: Digital subtraction imaging in cardiac investigations, Clin Radiol 35:301-306, 1984.

Smith CB: Physical principles of digital radiography, Radiography 50:41-44, 1984.

Templeton AW et al: Computer graphics for digitally formatted images, Radiology 151:527-528, 1984.

Tesic MM, Sones RA and Morgan DR: Single-slit digital radiography: some practical considerations, AJR 142:697-702, 1984.

1985 Adam P et al: Pelvimetry by digital radiography, Clin Radiol 36:327-330, 1985.

Aitken AG et al: Leg length determination by CT digital radiography, AJR 144:613-615, 1985.

Barnes GT: Detector for dual-energy digital radiography, Radiology 156:537-540, 1985.

Chakraborty DP et al: Digital subtraction angiography apparatus, Radiology 157:547, 1985.

Claussen C et al: Pelvimetry by digital radiography and its dosimetry, J Perinat Med 13:287-292, 1985.

Karoll MP et al: Air gap technique for digital subtraction angiography of the extracranial carotid arteries, Invest Radiol 20:742-745, 1985.

Lavelle MI et al: Demonstration of pancreatic parenchyma by digital subtraction techniques during endoscopic retrograde cholangiopancreatography, Clin Radiol 36:405-407, 1985.

Mendelson EB et al: Evaluation of the prone position in digital subtraction angiography, Cardiovasc Intervent Radiol 8:72-75, 1985.

Ovitt TW and Newell JD II: Digital subtraction angiography: technology, equipment, and techniques, Radiol Clin North Am 23:177-184, 1985.

Riederer SJ: Digital radiography, Crit Rev Biomed Eng 12:163-200, 1985.

Saddekni S et al: Contrast administration and techniques of digital subtraction, Radiol Clin North Am 23:275-291, 1985.

Schwenker RP and Eger H: Film-screen digital radiography, Radiography 51:233-235, 1985.

1986 Feldman L: Digital vascular imaging of the great vessels and heart, Cardiovasc Clin 17:357-384, 1986.

Foley KT, Cahan LD and Hieshima GB: Intraoperative angiography using a portable digital subtraction unit, J Neurosurg 64:816-818, 1986.

Fritz SL et al: a digital radiographic imaging system for mammography, Invest Radiol 21:581-583, 1986.

Fujita H et al: Investigation of basic imaging properties in digital radiography. V. Characteristic curves of II-TV digital systems, Med Phys 13:13-18, 1986.

Gersten K et al: Crossed-leg technique for digital subtraction angiography, AJR 146:843-844, 1986.

Giger ML, Ohara K and Doi K: Investigation of basic imaging properties in digital radiography. IX. Effect of displayed grey levels on signal detection, Med Phys 13:312-318, 1986.

Goodman LR et al: Digital and conventional chest images: observer performance with Film Digital Radiography System, Radiology 158:27-33, 1986.

Kimme Smith C et al: Diagnostic effects of edge-sharpening filtration and magnification, Med Phys 13:850-856, 1986.

Kume Y et al: Investigation of basic imaging properties in digital radiography. X. Structure mottle of II-TV digital imaging systems, Med Phys 13:843-849, 1986.

Kundel HL: Digital projection radiography of the chest, Radiology 158:274-276, 1986.

Kushner DC et al: Radiation dose reduction in the evaluation of scoliosis: an application of digital radiography, Radiology 161:175-181, 1986.

Nishitani H et al: Dual-energy projection radiography using condenser x-ray generator and digital radiography apparatus, Radiology 161:533-535, 1986.

Ohara K et al: Investigation of basic imaging properties in digital radiography: detection of simulated low-contrast objects in digital subtraction angiographic images, Med Phys 13:304-311, 1986.

1987 Albert SA, Richter JO and Rosenfield AT: Low-dose digital urography in the pregnant patient, Am J Obstet Gynecol 156:926-928, 1987.

Asaga T et al: Breast imaging: dual-energy projection radiography with digital radiography, Radiology 164:869-870, 1987.

Chan HP et al: Image feature analysis and computer-aided diagnosis in digital radiography. I. Automated detection of microcalcifications in mammography, Med Phys 14:538-548, 1987.

Fraser RG et al: Scanned projection digital radiography of the chest: a review of five years' experience, Alabama J Med Sci 24:258-266, 1987.

Giger ML and Doi K: Effect of pixel size on detectability of low-contrast signals in digital radiography, J Optical Soc Am [A] 4:966-975, 1987.

Jacobs JM and Manaster BJ: Digital subtraction arthrography of the temporomandibular joint, AJR 148:344-346, 1987.

Kume Y and Doi K: Investigation of basic imaging properties in digital radiography, Med Phys 14:736-743, 1987.

Lotz H et al: Low dose pelvimetry with biplane digital radiography, Acta Radiol 28:577-580, 1987.

Morgan DR, Sones RA and Barnes GT: Performance characteristics of a dual-energy detector for digital scan projection radiography, Med Phys 14:728-735, 1987.

Southard TE, Harris EF and Walter RG: Image enhancement of the mandibular condyle through digital subtraction, Oral Surg Oral Med Oral Pathol 64:645-647, 1987.

Suddarth SA et al: Performance of high-resolution monitors for digital chest imaging, Med Phys 14:253-257, 1987.

Trefler M and Yrizarry JM: Evaluation of dry silver hard copies in digital radiography, AJR 149:853-856, 1987.

Wilson AJ and Ramsby GR: Skeletal measurements using a flying spot digital-imaging device, AJR 149:339-343, 1987.

1988 Aspelin P, Pettersson H and Boijsen E: Digital radiography using laser stimulated luminescence for evaluation of urinary calcifications, Acta Radiol 29:277-284, 1988.

De Simone DN et al: Effect of a digital imaging network on physician behavior in an intensive care unit, Radiology 169:41-44, 1988.

Feczko PJ et al: Digital radiography of the gastrointestinal tract, Gastrointest Radiol 13:191-196, 1988.

Foster CJ, Butler P and Freer CE: Digital subtraction angiography of the left ventricle, Br J Radiol 61:1009-1013, 1988.

Fujita H, Giger ML and Doi K: Investigation of basic imaging properties in digital radiography. XII. Effect of matrix configuration on spatial resolution, Med Phys 15:384-390, 1988.

Giger ML, Doi K and MacMahon H: Image feature analysis and computer-aided diagnosis in digital radiography. III. Automated detection of nodules in peripheral lung fields, Med Phys 15:158-166, 1988.

Goodman LR, Wilson CR and Foley WD: Digital radiography of the chest: promises and problems, AJR 150:1241-1252, 1988.

Goodman LR et al: Pneumothorax and other lung diseases: effect of altered resolution and edge enhancement on diagnosis with digitized radiographs, Radiology 167:83-88, 1988.

Harrison RM: Digital radiography, Phys Med Biol 33:751-784, 1988.

Holmes RL: Computer-assisted quantitative of coronary artery stenosis, Radiol Technol 60:37-41, 1988.

Katsuragawa S, Doi K and MacMahon H: Image feature analysis and computer-aided diagnosis in digital radiography: detection and characterization of interstitial lung disease in digital chest radiographs, Med Phys 15:311-319, 1988.

Kelly TL et al: Quantitative digital radiography versus dual photon absorptiometry, J Clin Endocrinol Metab 67:839-844, 1988.

Kogutt MS, Jones JP and Perkins DD: Low-dose digital computed radiography in pediatric chest imaging, AJR 151:775-779, 1988.

Kool LJ et al: Advanced multiple-beam equalization radiography in chest radiology: a simulated nodule detection study, Radiology 169:35-39, 1988.

MacMahon H et al: Digital chest radiography: effect on diagnostic accuracy of hard copy, conventional video, and reversed gray scale video display formats, Radiology 168:669-673, 1988.

Oestmann JW et al: Subtle lung cancers: impact of edge enhancement and gray scale reversal on detection with digitized chest radiographs, Radiology 167:657-658, 1988.

Perri G et al: Digital subtraction radiography in voiding cystourethrography, Eur J Radiol 8:175-178, 1988.

Pettersson H et al: Digital radiography of the spine, large bones and joints using stimulable phosphor: early clinical experience, Acta Radiol 29:267-271, 1988.

Rogowska J, Preston K Jr and Sashin D: Evaluation of digital unsharp masking and local contrast stretching, IEEE Trans Biomed Eng 35:817-827, 1988.

Saito H et al: Digital radiography in an intensive care unit, Clin Radiol 39:127-130, 1988.

Sharma S, Mishra NK and Rajani M: Evaluation of the central injection technique for intravenous digital subtraction angiography—a preliminary report, Indian Heart J 40:12-16, 1988.

Shroy RE, Jr: Dependence of noise on array width and depth in digital radiography, Med Phys 15:64-66, 1988.

Stiles RG et al: Rotator cuff disruption: diagnosis with digital arthrography, Radiology 168:705-707, 1988.

Vlasbloem H and Kool LJ: AMBER: a scanning multiple-beam equalization system for chest radiography, Radiology 169:29-34, 1988.

Wandtke JC, Plewes DB and McFaul JA: Improved pulmonary nodule detection with scanning equalization radiography, Radiology 169:23-27, 1988.

1989   Bach EF: Digital radiography today—state of the art, Radiol Diagn 30:350-356, 1989.

Barnes GT, Lauro K: Image processing in digital radiography: basic concepts and applications, J Digit Imaging 2:132-146, 1989.

Cohen MD et al: Digital imaging of the newborn chest, Clin Radiol 40:365-368, 1989.

de Monts H and Beaumont F: A new photoconductor imaging system for digital radiography, Med Phys 16:105-109, 1989.

Dobbins JT and Powell AO: Variable compensation technique for digital radiography of the chest, Radiology 173:451-458, 1989.

Fink U et al: Subtracted versus non-subtracted digital imaging in peripheral angiography, Eur J Radiol 9:236-240, 1989.

Fisher PD and Brauer GW: Impact of image size on effectiveness of digital imaging system, J Digit Imaging 2:39-41, 1989.

Fraser RG et al: Digital imaging of the chest, Radiology 171:297-307, 1989.

Gluer CC et al: A fast low-noise line scan x-ray detector, Med Phys 16:98-104, 1989.

Goodman LR and Mistretta CA: Digital chest radiology, Curr Opin Radiol 1:34-39, 1989.

Kehler M et al: Assessment of digital chest radiography using stimulable phosphor, Acta Radiol 30:581-586, 1989.

Lee KR et al: Digital venography of the lower extremity, AJR 153:413-417, 1989.

Long BW: Computed radiography: photo-stimulable phosphor image plate technology, Radiol Technol 61:107-111, 1989.

Mansson LG et al: Digital chest radiography with a large image intensifier: an ROC study with an anthropomorphic phantom, Eur J Radiol 9:208-213, 1989.

Mansson LG et al: Digital chest radiography with a large image intensifier: evaluation of diagnostic performance and patient exposure, Acta Radiol 30:337-342, 1989.

McMillan JH et al: Digital radiography, Invest Radiol 24:735-741, 1989.

Newell JD Jr: Conventional and digital radiography of the hear, aorta, and pulmonary vascularity, Curr Opin Radiol 1:179-182, 1989.

Oestmann JW et al: Impact of postprocessing on the detection of simulated pulmonary nodules with digital radiography, Invest Radiol 24:467-471, 1989.

Oestmann JW et al: "Single-exposure" dual energy digital radiography in the detection of pulmonary nodules and calcifications, Invest Radiol 24:517-521, 1989.

Schaefer CM et al: Improved control of image optical density with low-dose digital and conventional radiography in bedside imaging, Radiology 173:713-716, 1989.

Schumacher M, Kutluk K and Ott D: Digital rotational radiography in neuroradiology, AJNR 10:644-649, 1989.

Sherrier RH et al: Image optimization in a computed-radiography/photostimulable-phosphor system, J Digit Imaging 2:212-219, 1989.

Stewart BK: Single exposure dual-energy digital radiography, Comput Methods Programs Biomed 30:127-135, 1989.

Wandtke JC and Plewes DB: Comparison of scanning equalization and conventional chest radiography, radiology 172:641-645, 1989.

1990   Abukhalil JM: Quantitative coronary cineangiogram analysis: a technical assessment, Radiol Technol 61:467-471, 1990.

Brauer GW et al: Digital chest imaging using a 57-cm image intensifier: a receiver-operating characteristic study of user performance, J Digit Imaging 3:95-100, 1990.

Cervi PM et al: Digital radiography versus conventional radiography during excretory urography: our experience, Ann Radiol 33:321-328, 1990.

Cohn M, Trefler M and Young TY: Enhancement and compression of digital chest radiographs, J Thorac Imaging 5:92-95, 1990.

Davies AM et al: Real-time digital contrast enhancement and magnification in the assessment of scaphoid and other wrist injuries, Br J Radiol 63:934-939, 1990.

Gross GW, Ehrlich SM and Wang Y: Diagnostic quality of portable abdominal radiographs in neonates with necrotizing enterocolitis: digitized vs nondigitized images, AJR 154:779-783, 1990.

Hansell DM: Digital chest radiography: current status, Clin Radiol 41:229-231, 1990.

Kling TF Jr et al: Digital radiography can reduce scoliosis x-ray exposure, spine 15:880-885, 1990.

Kreipke DL et al: Readability of cervical spine imaging: digital versus film/screen radiographs, Comput Med Imaging Graph 14:119-125, 1990.

Marglin SI, Rowberg AH and Godwin JD: Preliminary experience with portable digital imaging for intensive care radiography, J Thorac Imaging 5:49-54, 1990.

Montecalvo RM et al: Evaluation of the lacrimal apparatus with digital subtraction macrodacryocystography, Radiographics 10:483-490, 1990.

Plewes DB, McFaul J and Ivanovic M: Maximizing film contrast for scanning equalization radiography, Med Phys 17:357-361, 1990.

Sagel SS et al: Digital mobile radiography, J Thorac Imaging 5:36-48, 1990.

Tarver RD et al: Pediatric digital chest imaging, J Thorac Imaging 5:31-35, 1990.

Update on digital imaging, J Thorac Imaging 5:1-95, 1990.

Wandtke JC: Newer imaging methods in chest radiography, J Thorac Imaging 5:1-9, 1990.

1991   Hansell DM: Digital chest radiology, Curr Opin Radiol 3:364-371, 1991.

Kheddache S et al: Digital chest radiography: should images be presented in negative or positive mode? Eur J Radiol 13:151-155, 1991.

Lee KR et al: State-of-the-art digital radiography, Radiographics 11:1013-25, 1991.

Lissner J and Fink U: Digital imaging and picture archiving and communication systems, Curr Opin Radiol 3:267-274, 1991.

Lupi L et al: Diagnostic potential of double contrast arthrography of the knee with the digital technique, Skeletal Radiol 20:5-8, 1991.

MacMahon H and Doi K: Digital chest radiography, Clin Chest Med 12:19-32, 1991.

MacMahon H et al: The nature and subtlety of abnormal findings in chest radiographs, Med Phys 18:206-210, 1991.

Merlo L et al: Computed radiography in neonatal intensive care, Pediatr Radiol 21:94-96, 1991.

Rudin S, Bednared DR and Wong R: Computer frame freezing of fluoroscopic images, Radiol Technol 62:369-373, 1991.

Sanada S, Doi K and MacMahon H: Image feature analysis and computer-aided diagnosis in digital radiography: automated delineation of posterior ribs in chest images, Med Phys 18:964-971, 1991.

Sanada S et al: Comparison of imaging properties of a computed radiography system and screen-film systems, Med Phys 18:414-420, 1991.

Wandtke JC and Plewes DB: Improved imaging of bone with scan equalization radiography, AJR 157:359-364, 1991.

Wiener MD et al: Imaging of the intensive care unit patient, Clin Chest Med 12:169-198, 1991.

Wilson AJ et al: Photostimulable phosphor digital radiography of the extremities: diagnostic accuracy compared with conventional radiography, AJR 157:533-538, 1991.

1992 Arthur RJ and Pease JN: Problems associated with digital luminescence radiography in the neonate and young infant: problems with digital radiography, Pediatr Radiol 22:5-7, 1992.

Buckwalter KA and Braunstein EM: Digital skeletal radiography, AJR 158:1071-1080, 1992.

Chotas HG and Ravin CE: Digital radiography with photostimulable storage phosphors: control of detector latitude in chest imaging, Invest Radiol 27:822-828, 1992.

Cleveland RH et al: Voiding cystourethrography in children: value of digital fluoroscopy in reducing radiation dose, AJR 158:137-142, 1992.

Danza FM et al: Digital genitourinary radiography, Rays 17:516-524, 1992.

Falappa PG et al: Digital imaging: digital angiography, Rays 17:393-415, 1992.

Geleijns J et al: AMBER and conventional chest radiography: comparison of radiation dose and image quality, Radiology 185:719-723, 1992.

Gomez LP, Mejuto J and Vidal JJ: A low-cost system for digital image processing of moving images in real time: application to X-ray fluoroscopy, Comput Methods Programs Biomed 39:43-49, 1992.

Jennings P, Padley SP and Hansell DM: Portable chest radiography in intensive care: a comparison of computed and conventional radiography, Br J Radiol 65:852-856, 1992.

Kirkhorn T et al: Demonstration of digital radiographs by means of ink jet-printed paper copies: pilot study, J Digit Imaging 5:246-251, 1992.

Lyttkens K et al: Bedside chest radiography using digital luminescence: a comparison between digital radiographs reviewed on a personal computer and as hard-copies, Acta Radiol 33:427-430, 1992.

Moschini M et al: Digital radiography in neuroradiology, Rays 17:525-538, 1992.

Pastore G et al: Digital radiography in mammography, Rays 17:539-546, 1992.

Pirronti T et al: Digital radiography in chest imaging, Rays 17:469-481, 1992.

Richmond BJ et al: Diagnostic efficacy of digitized images vs plain films: a study of the joints of the fingers, AJR 158:437-441, 1992.

Sanada S, Doi K and MacMahon H: Image feature analysis and computer-aided diagnosis in digital radiography: automated detection of pneumothorax in chest images, Med Phys 19:1153-1160, 1992.

Souto M et al: Enhancement of chest images by automatic adaptive spatial filtering, J Digit Imaging 5:223-229, 1992.

Takahashi M et al: Development of a 2,048 x 2,048-pixel image intensifier-TV digital radiography system: basic imaging properties and clinical application, Invest Radiol 27:898-907, 1992.

Takahashi M et al: Gastrointestinal examinations with digital radiography, Radiographics 12:969-978, 1992.

van der Stelt PF: Improved diagnosis with digital radiography, Curr Opin Dent 2:1-6, 1992.

Zoeller G et al: Digital radiography in urologic imaging: radiation dose reduction on urethrocystography, Urol Radiol 14:56-58, 1992.

1993 Chotas HG et al: Digital chest radiography with photostimulable storage phosphors: signal-to-noise ratio as a function of kilovoltage with matched exposure risk, Radiology 186:395-398, 1993.

Dershaw DD et al: Use of digital mammography in needle localization procedures, AJR 161:559-562, 1993.

Doi K et al: Digital radiography: a useful clinical tool for computer-aided diagnosis by quantitative analysis of radiographic images, Acta Radiol 34:426-439, 1993.

Frank MS et al: High-resolution computer display of portable, digital, chest radiographs of adults: suitability for primary interpretation, AJR 160:473-477, 1993.

Hansell DM: Digital chest radiography, Br J Hosp Med 49:117-120, 1993.

Langen HJ et al: Comparative evaluation of digital radiography versus conventional radiography of fractured skulls, Invest Radiol 28:686-689, 1993.

Morgan RA et al: Detection of pneumothorax with lateral shoot-through digital radiography, Clin Radiol 48:249-252, 1993.

Niklason LT et al: Portable chest imaging: comparison of storage phosphor digital, asymmetric screen-film, and conventional screen-film systems, Radiology 186:387-393, 1993.

Prokop M et al: Improved parameters for unsharp mask filtering of digital chest radiographs, Radiology 187:521-526, 1993.

MAGNETIC RESONANCE IMAGING

For bibliographic citations before 1964, please see the fifth edition of this ATLAS. For citations from 1964 through 1974, see the sixth or seventh edition.

1976 Lautebur PC et al: Digest of the Fourth International Conference on Medical Physics, Phys Can 32, 1976. (Special issue) Abstract: Phys Can 33:9, 1976.

1977 Hinshaw WS, Bottomley PA and Holland GN: Radiographic thin-section image of the human wrist by nuclear magnetic resonance, Nature 270:722-723, 1977.

1978 Damadian R et al: Field-focusing nuclear magnetic resonance (FONAR) and the formation of chemical scans in man, Naturwissenschaften 65:250-252, 1978.

Goldsmith M, Koutcher JA and Damadian R: NMR in cancer. XIII. Application of NMR malignancy index to human mammary tumours, Br J Cancer 38:547-554, 1978.

Hinshaw WS et al: Display of cross-sectional anatomy by nuclear magnetic resonance imaging, Br J Radiol 51:273-280, 1978.

1979 Budinger T: Thresholds for physiological effects due to RF and magnetic fields used in NMR imaging, IEEE Trans Nucl Sci NS:2821-2825, April 1979.

Mansfield P et al: Carcinoma of the breast imaged by nuclear magnetic resonance (NMR), Br J Radiol 52:242-243, 1979.

1980 Damadian R: Field focusing NMR (FONAR) and the formation of chemical images in man, Philos Trans R Soc Lond (Biol) 289:389-500, 1980.

Goldman MR et al: Nuclear magnetic resonance imaging: potential cardiac applications, Am J Cardiol 46:1278-1283, 1980.

Hawkes RC et al: NMR tomography of the brain: a preliminary assessment with demonstration of pathology, J Comput Assist Tomogr 4:577-586, 1980.

Holland GN, Moore WS and Hawkes RC: Nuclear magnetic resonance tomography of the brain, J Comput Assist Tomogr 4:1-3, 1980.

Partain CL et al: Nuclear magnetic resonance and computed tomography: comparison of normal body images, Radiology 136:767-770, 1980.

Wolff S et al: Tests for DNA and chromosomal damage induced by nuclear magnetic resonance imaging, Radiology 136:707-710, 1980.

1981 Crooks L et al: Nuclear magnetic resonance imaging, Prog Nucl Med 7:149-163, 1981.

Gore JC et al: Medical nuclear magnetic resonance imaging. I. Physical principles, Invest Radiol 16:269-274, 1981.

Harwell, Dodcot and Oxon: Exposure to nuclear magnetic resonance clinical imaging, Radiography 47:258-260, 1981.

Smith FW et al: Clinical application of nuclear magnetic resonance, Lancet 1:78-79, 1981.

Smith FW et al: Nuclear magnetic resonance tomographic imaging in liver disease, Lancet 1:963-966, 1981.

Smith FW et al: Oesophageal carcinoma demonstrated by whole-body nuclear magnetic resonance imaging, Br Med J 282:510-512, 1981.

1982 Brady TJ et al: NMR imaging of forearms in healthy volunteers and patients with giant-cell tumor of the bone, Radiology 144:549-552, 1982.

Bydder GM and Steiner RE: NMR imaging of the brain, Neuroradiology 23:231-240, 1982.

Doyle FH et al: Nuclear magnetic resonance imaging of the liver: initial experience, AJR 138:193-200, 1982.

Katims LM: Nuclear magnetic resonance imaging: methods and current status, Med Instrum 16:213-216, 1982.

Margulis AR: Nuclear magnetic resonance imaging—present status, J Can Assoc Radiol 33:131-136, 1982.

McCullough EC and Baker HL Jr: Nuclear magnetic resonance imaging, Radiol Clin North Am 20:3-7, 1982.

Rollo FD: New imaging modalities: positron emission tomography and nuclear magnetic resonance, Med Instrum 16:53-54, 1982.

Ross RJ et al: Nuclear magnetic resonance imaging and evaluation of human breast tissue: preliminary clinical trials, Radiology 143:195-205, 1982.

1983 Brasch RC, et al: Brain nuclear magnetic resonance imaging enhanced by a paramagnetic nitroxide contrast agent: preliminary report, AJR 141:1019-1023, 1983.

Crooks LE et al: Clinical efficiency of nuclear magnetic resonance imaging, Radiology 146:123-128, 1983.

Edelstein WA et al: Signal, noise, and contrast in nuclear magnetic resonance (NMR) imaging, J Comput Assist Tomogr 7:391-401, 1983.

Ellis JH, Dallas CS and Russell RJ: Communications device for patients undergoing nuclear magnetic resonance imaging, Radiology 149:855, 1983.

Gamsu G et al: Nuclear magnetic resonance imaging of the thorax, Radiology 147:473-480, 1983.

Higgins CB et al: Clinical nuclear magnetic resonance imaging of the body, Semin Nucl Med 13:347-363, 1983.

Hricak H et al: Anatomy and pathology of the male pelvis by magnetic resonance imaging, AJR 141:1101-1110, 1983.

Karstaedt N et al: Nuclear magnetic resonance imaging, Surg Neurol 19:206-214, 1983.

Modic MT et al: Nuclear magnetic resonance imaging of the spine, Radiology 148:757-762, 1983.

New PF et al: Potential hazards and artifacts of ferromagnetic and nonferromagnetic surgical and dental materials and devices in nuclear magnetic resonance imaging, Radiology 147:139-148, 1983.

Norman D et al: Magnetic resonance imaging of the spinal cord and canal: potentials and limitations, AJR 141:1147-1152, 1983.

Pykett IL: Instrumentation for nuclear magnetic resonance imaging, Semin Nucl Med 13:319-328, 1983.

Ratner AV, Okada RD and Brady TJ: Nuclear magnetic resonance imaging of the heart, Semin Nucl Med 13:339-346, 1983.

Rosen BR and Brady TJ: Principles of nuclear magnetic resonance for medical applications, Semin Nucl Med 13:308-318, 1983.

1984 Bradley WG, Opel W and Kassabian JP: Magnetic resonance installation: sitting and economic considerations, Radiology 151:719-721, 1984.

Brasch RC et al: Magnetic resonance imaging of the thorax in childhood: work in progress, Radiology 150:463-467, 1984.

Crooks LE et al: High-resolution magnetic resonance imaging: technical concepts and their implementation, Radiology 150:163-171, 1984.

Crooks LE et al: Magnetic resonance imaging: effects of magnetic field strength, Radiology 151:127-133, 1984.

El-Yousef SJ et al: Magnetic resonance imaging of the breast: work in progress, Radiology 150:761-766, 1984.

Fodor J and Malott JC: Magnetic resonance: a new imaging modality, Radiol Technol 56:17-21, 1984.

Han JS et al: Magnetic resonance imaging in the evaluation of the brainstem, Radiology 150:705-712, 1984.

Hendee WR and Morgan C: Introduction to nuclear magnetic resonance imaging, Denver, 1984, Multi-Media Publications.

Higgins CB et al: Multiplane magnetic resonance imaging of the heart and major vessels: studies in normal volunteers, AJR 142:661-667, 1984.

Hillman BJ et al: Adoption and diffusion of a new imaging technology: a magnetic resonance imaging prospective, AJR 143:913-917, 1984.

Kearfott KJ, Rottenberg DA and Knowles RJ: A new headholder for PET, CT, and NMR imaging, J Comput Assist Tomogr 8:1217-1220, 1984.

Roberts D et al: Radiologic techniques used to evaluate the temporomandibular joint, Anesth Prog 31:241-256, 1984.

Runge VM et al: Intravascular contrast agents suitable for magnetic resonance imaging, Radiology 153:171-176, 1984.

Thickman D et al: Nuclear magnetic resonance imaging in gynecology, Am J Obstet Gynecol 149:835-840, 1984.

Webb WR et al: Nuclear magnetic resonance of pulmonary arteriovenous fistula, J Comput Assist Tomogr 8:155-157, 1984.

1985 Nelson TR et al: Magnetic resonance imaging: the basic physical and clinical concepts. I. Radiol Technol 56:410-415, 1985.

Nelson TR et al: Magnetic resonance imaging: the basic physical and clinical concepts. II. Radiol Technol 57:26-30, 1985.

Nelson TR et al: Magnetic resonance imaging: the basic physical and clinical concepts. III. Radiol Technol 57:142-150, 1985.

Quint LE, Glazer GM and Orringer MB: Esophageal imaging by MR and CT: study of normal anatomy and neoplasms, Radiology 156:727-731, 1985.

Stark DD et al: Pelvimetry by magnetic resonance imaging, AJR 144:947-950, 1985.

Wedeen VJ et al: Projective imaging of pulsatile flow with magnetic resonance, Science 230:946-948, 1985.

1986 Bradley WG Jr: Magnetic resonance imaging in the central nervous system: comparison with computed tomography, Magn Reson Annu 81-122, 1986.

Dillon WP: Magnetic resonance imaging of head and neck tumors, Cardiovasc Intervent Radiol 8:275-282, 1986.

Dumoulin CL and Hart HR Jr: Magnetic resonance angiography, Radiology 161:717-720, 1986.

Fukui K, Sadamoto K and Sakaki S: Development of the new cerebral angio-CT technique and magnetic resonance angio-imaging, Acta Radiol Suppl 369:67-68, 1986.

Gibson MJ et al: Magnetic resonance imaging and discography in the diagnosis of disc degeneration: a comparative study of 50 discs, J Bone Joint Surg Br 68:369-373, 1986.

Mezrich RS et al: Strip scan: a method for faster MR imaging, Radiographics 6:833-845, 1986.

Mitchell MR et al: Spin echo technique selection: basic principles for choosing MRI, Radiographics 6:245-260, 1986.

Newhouse JH: Image contrast and pulse sequences in urinary tract magnetic resonance imaging, Urol Radiol 8:120-126, 1986.

Niendorf HP et al: Some aspects of the use of contrast agents in magnetic resonance imaging, Diagn Imaging Clin Med 55:25-36, 1986.

Panzer RJ, Kido DK and Hindmarsh T: A methodologic assessment of studies comparing magnetic resonance imaging and computed tomography of the brain, Acta Radiol Suppl 369:269-274, 1986.

Revel D et al: Gd-DTPA contrast enhancement and tissue, Radiology 158:319-323, 1986.

Rholl KS et al: Oblique magnetic resonance imaging of the cardiovascular system, Radiographics 6:177-188, 1986.

Russell R, Dallas-Huitema C and Cohen M: Magnetic resonance imaging techniques in children, Radiol Technol 57(5):428-430, 1986.

Tadmor R et al: Magnetic resonance imaging of the thoracical spinal cord and spine with surface coils, Acta Radiol Suppl 369:475-480, 1986.

Zimmerman RA et al: Magnetic resonance imaging of the pediatric spinal cord and canal, Acta Radiol Suppl 369:649-650, 1986.

1987 Akins EW et al: Preoperative evaluation of the thoracic aorta using MRI and angiography, Ann Thorac Surg 44:499-507, 1987.

Balter S: An introduction to the physics of magnetic resonance imaging, Radiographics 7:371-383, 1987.

Brooks RA and Di Chiro G: Magnetic resonance imaging of stationary blood: a review, Med Phys 14:903-913, 1987.

Brooks WM, Brereton IM and Doddrell DM: RAPID—a new method for fast imaging using a single slice of Z-magnetization, Magn Reson Med 5:191-195, 1987.

Ceckler TL, Bryant RG and Hornak JP: Noise reduction in wide-bore magnets using a patient cage, Magn Reson Med 5:173-174, 1987.

Champetier J et al: Magnetic resonance imaging of the liver by frontal (coronal) sections, Surg Radiol Anat 9:107-121, 1987.

Dumoulin CL, Souza SP and Hart HR: Rapid scan magnetic resonance angiography, Magn Reson Med 5:238-245, 1987.

Falke TH et al: Magnetic resonance imaging of the adrenal glands, Radiographics 7:343-370, 1987.

Fraass BA et al: Integration of magnetic resonance imaging into radiation therapy, Int J Radiat Oncol Biol Phys 13:1897-1908, 1987.

Gangarosa RE et al: Operational safety issues in MRI, Magn Reson Imaging 5:287-292, 1987.

Hajek PC et al: Potential contrast agents for MR arthrography: in vitro evaluation, AJR 149:97-104, 1987.

Hamm B, Wolf KJ and Felix R: Conventional and rapid MR imaging of the liver with Gd-DTPA, Radiology 164:313-320, 1987.

Jacobs AM et al: Magnetic resonance imaging of the foot and ankle, Clin Podiatr Med Surg 4:903-924, 1987.

Lipton MJ: Computer tomography, positron emission tomography and nuclear magnetic resonance in cardiology, Herz 12:1-12, 1987.

Mathur De Vre R: Safety aspects of magnetic resonance imaging and magnetic resonance: recommendations for MR exposures in clinical practice, Arch Belg 45:425-438, 1987.

Merritt CR: Magnetic resonance imaging—a clinical perspective: image quality, Radiographics 7:1001-1016, 1987.

Naito Y et al: Magnetic resonance imaging of the eustachian tube: a correlative anatomical study, Arch Otolaryngol Head Neck 113:1281-1284, 1987.

Patton JA et al: Techniques, pitfalls and artifacts in magnetic resonance imaging, Radiographics 7:505-519, 1987.

Pavlicek W: MR instrumentation and image formation, Radiographics 7:809-814, 1987.

Resnick MI, Kursh ED and Bryan PJ: Magnetic resonance imaging of the prostate, Prog Clin Biol Res 243B:89-96, 1987.

Sartoris DJ and Resnick D: Magnetic resonance imaging of the foot: technical aspects, J Foot Surg 26:351-358, 1987.

Sartoris DJ and Resnick D: MR imaging of the musculoskeletal system: current and future status, AJR 149:457-467, 1987.

Sartoris DJ and Resnick D: Pictorial review: cross-sectional imaging of the foot and ankle, Foot Ankle 8:59-80, 1987.

Sickles EA: Computed tomography scanning, transillumination, and magnetic resonance imaging of the breast, Recent Results Cancer Res 105:31-36, 1987.

Tonami H et al: Surface coil MR imaging of orbital blowout fractures: a comparison with reformatted CT, AJNR 8:445-449, 1987.

Van Rossum AG et al: Oblique views in magnetic resonance imaging of the heart by combined axial rotations, Acta Radiol 28:497-503, 1987.

Wang HZ, Riederer SJ and Lee JN: Optimizing the precision in T1 relaxation estimation using limited flip angles, Magn Reson Med 5:399-416, 1987.

Young IR and Payne JA: Slice-shape artifact changes with precession angle in rapid MR imaging, Magn Reson Med 5:177-181, 1987.

1988   Akber SF: Influence of anesthetics on relaxation times, Anesthesiology 69:290-291, 1988.

Atlas SW: Intracranial vascular malformations and aneurysms: current imaging, Radiol Clin North Am 26:821-837, 1988.

Atlas SW et al: STIR MR imaging of the orbit, AJR 151:1025-1030, 1988.

Barnett GH, Ropper AH and Johnson KA: Physiological support and monitoring of critically ill patients, J Neurosurg 68:246-250, 1988.

Batra P et al: Evaluation of intrathoracic extent of lung cancer by plain chest radiography, computed tomography, and magnetic resonance imaging, Am Rev Respir Dis 137:1456-1462, 1988.

Batra P et al: MR imaging of the thorax: a comparison of axial, coronal, and sagittal imaging planes, J Comput Assist Tomogr 12:75-81, 1988.

Beers GJ et al: MR imaging in acute cervical spine trauma, J Comput Assist Tomogr 12:755-761, 1988.

Bellon EP et al: Chemical shift imaging, J Belge Radiol 71:21-30, 1988.

Bird CR et al: Gd-DTPA-enhanced MR imaging in pediatric patients after brain tumor, Radiology 169:123-126, 1988.

Blumenkopf B and Juneau PA: Three-dimensional: magnetic resonance imaging (MRI) of thoracolumbar fractures, J Spinal Disord 1:144-150, 1988.

Brosnan T et al: Noise reduction in magnetic resonance imaging, Magn Reson Med 8:394-409, 1988.

Burbank F, Parish D and Wexler L: Echocardiographic-like angled views of the heart by MR imaging, J Comput Assist Tomogr 12:181-195, 1988.

Chang Y and Hricak H: Magnetic resonance imaging of the prostate gland, Semin Ultrasound CT MR 9:343-351, 1988.

Crooks LE et al: Echo-planar pediatric imager, Radiology 166:157-163, 1988.

Curati WL and Greco A: Magnetic resonance imaging of the abdomen—1988, Br J Hosp Med 40:121-123, 1988.

Czervionke LF and Daniels DL: Cervical spine anatomy and pathologic processes: applications of new MR imaging techniques, Radiol Clin North Am 26:921-947, 1988.

Czervionke LF et al: Cervical neural foramina: correlative anatomic and MR imaging study, Radiology 169:753-759, 1988.

Czervionke LF et al: The MR appearance of gray and white matter in the cervical spinal cord, AJNR 9:557-562, 1988.

Daniels DL et al: The effect of patient positioning on MR imaging of the internal auditory canal, Neuroradiology 30:395-398, 1988.

Dumoulin CL et al: Time-resolved magnetic resonance angiography, Magn Reson Med 6:275-286, 1988.

Durick DA and Phillips MLW: Diffusion of an Innovation: adoption of MRI, Radiol Technol 59:239-241, 1988.

Duthoy MJ and Lund G: MR imaging of the spine in children, Eur J Radiol 8:188-195, 1988.

Egglin TK, Hahn PF and Stark DD: MRI of the adrenal glands, Semin Roentgenol 23:280-287, 1988.

Ehrhardt JC, Tian ZC and Chang W: Reduced MR acquisition time with the CROCUS technique, J Comput Assist Tomogr 12:468-473, 1988.

Elder JA et al: Nonionizing radiation protection: radiofrequency radiation, WHO Reg Publ Eur Ser 25:117-173, 1988.

Enzmann DR and Rubin JB: Cervical spine: MR imaging with a partial flip angle, gradient-refocused pulse sequence. I. General considerations, Radiology 166:467-472, 1988.

Epstein NE et al: "Dynamic" MRI scanning of the cervical spine, Spine 13:937-938, 1988.

Evancho AM et al: MR imaging diagnosis of rotator cuff tears, AJR 151:751-754, 1988.

Frahm J et al: Rapid line scan NMR angiography, Magn Reson Med 7:79-87, 1988.

Fritzsche PJ: MRI of the scrotum, Urol Radiol 10:52-57, 1988.

Gibby WA: MR contrast agents: an overview, Radiol Clin North Am 26:1047-1058, 1988.

Glazer GM: MR imaging of the liver, kidneys, and adrenal glands, Radiology 166:303-312, 1988.

Goddard P and Jackson P: The physics of magnetic resonance imaging: a simplified approach, Bristol Med Chir J 103:7, 1988.

Goldberg AL et al: The impact of magnetic resonance on the diagnostic evaluation of acute cervicothoracic spinal trauma, Skeletal Radiol 17:89-95, 1988.

Greco A et al: MR imaging of lymphomas: impact on therapy, J Comput Assist Tomogr 12:785-791, 1988.

Gyngell ML: The application of steady-state free precession in rapid 2DFT NMR, Magn Reson Imaging 6:415-419, 1988.

Hennig J and Friedburg H: Clinical applications and methodological developments of the RARE, Magn Reson Imaging 6:391-395, 1988.

Hennig J et al: Fast and exact flow measurements with the fast Fourier flow technique, Magn Reson Imaging 6:369-372, 1988.

Herman GT: Three-dimensional imaging on a CT or MR scanner, J Comput Assist Tomogr 12:450-458, 1988.

Higgins CB and Auffermann W: MR imaging of thyroid and parathyroid glands: a review of current, AJR 151:1095-1106, 1988.

Hinks RS and Quencer RM: Motion artifacts in brain and spine MR, Radiol Clin North Am 26:737-753, 1988.

Hricak H, Chang YC and Thurnher S: Vagina: evaluation with MR imaging. I. Normal anatomy and congenital anomalies, Radiology 169:169-174, 1988.

Hyman RA and Gorey MT: Imaging strategies for MR of the brain, Radiol Clin North Am 26:471-503, 1988.

Imaging strategies in MRI, Radiol Clin North Am 26:471-699, 1988.

Jackler RK: CT and MRI of the ear and temporal bone: current state of the art and future prospects, Am J Otol 9:232-239, 1988.

Karlik SJ et al: Patient anesthesia and monitoring at a 1.5-T MRI installation, Magn Reson Med 7:210-221, 1988.

Karnaze MG et al: Comparison of MR and CT myelography in imaging the cervical and thoracic spine, AJR 150:397-403, 1988.

Kingston S: Magnetic resonance imaging of the ankle and foot, Clin Sports Med 7:15-28, 1988.

Krol G, Sze G and Amster J: Table-top support plate for imaging the entire spine with surface-coil MR, AJNR 9:396-397, 1988.

Lee JK: Magnetic resonance imaging of the retroperitoneum, Urol Radiol 10:48-51, 1988.

Levin DN et al: Retrospective geometric correlation of MR, CT, and PET images, Radiology 169:817-823, 1988.

Lipcamon JD et al: MRI of the upper abdomen using motion artifact suppression technique, Radiol Technol 59:415-418, 1988.

Listinsky JJ and Bryant RG: Gastrointestinal contrast agents: a diamagnetic approach, Magn Reson Med 8:285-292, 1988.

Lufkin R and Hanafee W: MRI of the head and neck, Magn Reson Imaging 6:69-88, 1988.

Lufkin R et al: Automated MR imaging protocols for improved patient throughout, Comput Med Imaging Graph 12:85-88, 1988.

Lufkin R et al: Magnetic resonance imaging of the craniocervical junction, Comput Med Imaging Graph 12:281-292, 1988.

Lufkin R et al: MR body stereotaxis: an aid for MR-guided biopsies, J Comput Assist Tomogr 12:1088-1089, 1988.

Lufkin R et al: A technique for MR-guided needle placement, AJR 151:193-196, 1988.

MacManus D and Bartlett P: Magnetic resonance imaging (MRI) of the orbit, Radiogr Today 54:40-41, 1988.

Martin JF et al: Inflatable surface coil for MR imaging of the prostate, Radiology 167:268-270, 1988.

Mitchell DG et al: Multiple spin-echo MR imaging of the body: image contrast and motion-induced artifact, Magn Reson Imaging 6:535-546, 1988.

Muller RN et al: The importance of nuclear magnetic relaxation dispersion (NMRD), Invest Radiol 23:6229-6231, 1988.

Norris DG, Jones RA and Hutchison JM: Projective Fourier angiography, Magn Reson Med 7:1-10, 1988.

Pappas CT and Rekate HL: Role of magnetic resonance imaging and three-dimensional computerized tomography in cranioverterbral junction anomalies, Pediatr Neurosci 14:18-22, 1988.

Pusey E et al: Aliasing artifacts in MR imaging, Comput Med Imaging Graph 12:219-224, 1988.

Redpath TW and Jones RA: FADE—a new fast-imaging sequence, Magn Reson Med 6:224-234, 1988.

Runge VM and Wood ML: Fast imaging and other motion artifact reduction schemes: a pictorial overview, Magn Reson Imaging 6:595-607, 1988.

Runge VM et al: FLASH: clinical three-dimensional magnetic resonance imaging, Radiographics 8:947-965, 1988.

Runge VM et al: Gd DTPA: future applications with advanced imaging techniques, Radiographics 8:161-179, 1988.

Runge VM et al: The straight and narrow path to good head and spine MRI, Radiographics 8:507-531, 1988.

Shellock FG and Crues JV: Temperature changes caused by MR imaging of the brain with a head coil, AJNR 9:287-291, 1988.

Shetty AN: Suppression of radiofrequency interference in cardiac gated MRI, Magn Reson Med 8:84-88, 1988.

Solomon MA and Oloff-Solomon J: Magnetic resonance imaging in the foot and ankle, Clin Podiatr Med Surg 5:945-965, 1988.

Spickler E, McKenna KM and Lufkin RB: Approaches to MR angiography, Comput Med Imaging Graph 12:211-217, 1988.

Thomson JL: A simple skin marker for magnetic resonance imaging, Br J Radiol 61:638-639, 1988.

Turner DA et al: Carcinoma of the breast: detection with MR imaging versus xeromammography, Radiology 168:49-58, 1988.

Underwood SR et al: Left ventricular volume measured rapidly by oblique magnetic resonance imaging, Br Heart J 60:188-195, 1988.

Valvassori GE and Guzman M: Magnetic resonance imaging of the posterior cranial fossa, Ann Otol Rhinol Laryngol 97:594-598, 1988.

van der Meulen P et al: Fast field echo imaging: an overview and contrast calculations, Magn Reson Imaging 6:355-368, 1988.

Van Hecke PE, Marchal GJ and Baert AL: Use of shielding to prevent folding in MR imaging, Radiology 167:557-558, 1988.

Walter E et al: CT and MR imaging of the temporomandibular joint, Radiographics 8:327-348, 1988.

Weisz GM, Lamond TS and Kitchener PN: Spinal imaging: will MRI replace myelography? Spine 13:65-68, 1988.

Wendt RE III et al: Electrocardiographic gating and monitoring in NMR imaging, Magn Reson Imaging 6:89-95, 1988.

Williamson MR et al: Spine: device to facilitate surface coil MR imaging, Radiology 187:273-274, 1988.

Wood ML, Runge VM and Henkelman RM: Overcoming motion in abdominal MR imaging, AJR 150:513-522, 1988.

Wright SM and Wright RM: A multi-plane scout sequence using flash imaging, Magn Reson Imaging 6:105-112, 1988.

Young IR et al: Further technical development in magnetic resonance imaging of the brain in young children, Clin Radiol 39:651-657, 1988.

1989   Atlas SW: Magnetic resonance imaging of the orbit: current status, Magn Reson Q 5:39-96, 1989.

Bisset GS: Evaluation of potential practical oral contrast agents for pediatric magnetic resonance imaging: preliminary observations, Pediatr Radiol 20:61-66, 1989.

Bisset GS: Pediatric thoracic applications of magnetic resonance imaging, J Thorac Imaging 4:51-57, 1989.

Braun IF: MRI of the nasopharynx, Radiol Clin North Am 27:315-330, 1989.

Bretan PN Jr and Lorig R: Adrenal imaging: computed tomographic scanning and magnetic resonance imaging, Urol Clin North Am 16:505-513, 1989.

Brogan M and Chakeres DW: Computed tomography and magnetic resonance imaging of the normal anatomy of the temporal bone, Semin Ultrasound CT MR 10:178-194, 1989.

Carvlin MJ et al: High-resolution MR of the spinal cord in humans and rats, AJNR 10:13-17, 1989.

Chakeres DW, Curtin A and Ford G: Magnetic resonance imaging of pituitary and parasellar abnormalities, Radiol Clin North Am 27:265-281, 1989.

Collins JD et al: Anatomy of the abdomen, back, and pelvis as displayed by magnetic resonance imaging. I. J Natl Med Assoc 81:680-684, 1989.

Collins JD et al: Anatomy of the abdomen, back and pelvis as displayed by magnetic resonance imaging. II. J Natl Med Assoc 81:809-813, 1989.

Collins JD et al: Anatomy of the abdomen, back, and pelvis as displayed by magnetic resonance imaging. III. J Natl Med Assoc 81:857-861, 1989.

Constable RT et al: High quality zoomed MR images, J Comput Assist Tomogr 13:179-181, 1989.

Crim JR et al: Magnetic resonance imaging of the hindfoot, Foot Ankle 10:1-7, 1989.

Curtin AJ et al: MR imaging artifacts of the axial internal anatomy of the cervical spinal cord, AJR 152:835-842, 1989.

Deck MD: Computed tomography and magnetic resonance imaging of the skull and brain, Clin Imaging 13:95-113, 1989.

Deck MD et al: Computed tomography versus magnetic resonance imaging of the brain: a collaborative interinstitutional study, Clin Imaging 13:2-15, 1989.

Dortzbach RK, Kronish JW and Gentry LR: Magnetic resonance imaging of the orbit. I. Physical principles, Ophthal Plast Reconstr Surg 5:151-159, 1989.

Duckwiler G, Lufkin RB and Hanafee WN: MR-directed needle biopsies, Radiol Clin North Am 27:255-263, 1989.

Erickson SJ et al: MR imaging of the finger: correlation with normal anatomic sections, AJR 152:1013-1019, 1989.

Fezoulidis I et al: Diagnostic imaging of the occipito-cervical junction in patients with rheumatoid arthritis: plain films, computed tomography, magnetic resonance imaging, Acta Radiol 9:5-11, 1989.

Fisher MR: Magnetic resonance for evaluation of the thorax, Chest 95:166-173, 1989.

Gamsu G and Sostman D: Magnetic resonance imaging of the thorax, Am Rev Respir Dis 139:254-274, 1989.

Gift DA, Pera A and Moore JB: Introduction to magnetic resonance imaging, J Am Osteopath Assoc 89:315-321, 1989.

Hall AS et al: Use of solvent suppression technique to enhance changes due to susceptibility variations in magnetic resonance imaging, Magn Reson Med 9:411-418, 1989.

Harris TM and Cohen MD: Abdominal magnetic resonance imaging, Pediatr Radiol 20:10-19, 1989.

Hatatu H et al: Pulmonary vasculature: high-resolution MR imaging. Work in progress, Radiology 171:391-395, 1989.

Ho PS et al: MR appearance of gray and white matter at the cervicomedullary region, AJNR 10:1051-1055, 1989.

Holliday RA and Reede DL: MRI of mastoid and middle ear disease, Radiol Clin North Am 27:283-299, 1989.

Hughes RJ, Hill V and Braun H: A mobile traction device for MR and CT imaging, Australas Phys Eng Sci Med 12:160-163, 1989.

Jackson RP et al: The neuroradiographic diagnosis of lumbar herniated nucleus pulposus. II. A comparison of computed tomography (CT), myelography, CT-myelography, and magnetic resonance imaging, Spine 14:1362-1367, 1989.

Johnson DW et al: MR imaging of the pars interarticularis, AJR 152:327-332, 1989.

Johnson ND et al: MR imaging anatomy of the infant hip, AJR 153:127-133, 1989.

Kassel EE, Keller MA and Kucharczyk W: MRI of the floor of the mouth, tongue and orohypopharynx, Radiol Clin North Am 27:331-351, 1989.

Keigley BA et al: Primary tumors of the foot: MR imaging, Radiology 171:755-759, 1989.

King K: CT technologist to MRI technologist: making the transition, Radiol Technol 61:121-123, 1989.

Kornberg M: Discography and magnetic resonance imaging in the diagnosis of lumbar disc disruption, Spine 14:1368-1372, 1989.

Larsson EM et al: Coil selection for magnetic resonance imaging of the cervical and thoracic spine using a vertical magnetic field, Acta Radiol 30:141-146, 1989.

Makow LC: Magnetic resonance imaging: a brief review of image contrast, Radiol Clin North Am 27:195-218, 1989.

Margulis AR: Cross-sectional imaging: present and future, Curr Opin Radiol 1:101-106, 1989.

Meyerhoff WL et al: Magnetic resonance imaging in the diagnosis of temporal bone and skull base lesions, Am J Otol 10:131-137, 1989.

Millen SJ, Daniels DL and Meyer GA: Gadolinium-enhanced magnetic resonance imaging in the temporal bone lesions, Laryngoscope 99:257-260, 1989.

Miller GM, Forbes GS and Onofrio BM: Magnetic resonance imaging of the spine, Mayo Clin Proc 64:986-1004, 1989.

Mitchell MJ, Sartoris DJ and Resnick D: The foot and ankle, Top Magn Reson Imaging 1:57-73, 1989.

MRI in the abdomen and pelvis, Semin Ultrasound CT MR 10:1-77, 1989.

MRI of the thorax: state of the art, J Thorac Imaging 4:1-92, 1989.

Quirk ME et al: Anxiety in patients undergoing MR imaging, Radiology 170:463-466, 1989.

Raghavan N et al: MR imaging in the tethered spinal cord syndrome, AJR 152:843-852, 1989.

Ragnarsson JI et al: Low field magnetic resonance imaging of femoral neck fractures, Acta Radiol 30:247-252, 1989.

Rapp JH et al: "Angiography" by magnetic resonance imaging: detailed vascular anatomy without ionizing radiation or contrast media, Surgery 105:662-667, 1989.

Ross JS et al: Magnetic resonance angiography of the extracranial carotid arteries and intracranial vessels: a review, Neurology 39:1369-1376, 1989.

Rusinek H et al: Volumetric rendering of MR images, Radiology 171:269-272, 1989.

Sartoris DJ and Resnick D: Magnetic resonance imaging of the diabetic foot, J Foot Surg 28:485-491, 1989.

Sartoris DJ and Resnick D: Magnetic resonance imaging of tendons in the foot and ankle, J Foot Surg 28:370-377, 1989.

Satragno L, Martinoli C and Cittadini G: Magnetic resonance imaging of the penis: normal anatomy, Magn Reson Imaging 7:95-100, 1989.

Scotti G et al: New imaging techniques in endocrinology: magnetic resonance of the pituitary gland and sella turcica, Acta Pediatr Scand Suppl 356:5-14, 1989.

Shapiro MD and Som PM: MRI of the paranasal sinuses and nasal cavity, Radiol Clin North Am 27:447-475, 1989.

Shellock FG, Schaefer DJ and Crues JV: Alterations in body and skin temperatures caused by magnetic resonance imaging: is the recommended exposure for radiofrequency radiation too conservative? Br J Radiol 62:904-909, 1989.

Shellock FG, Schaefer DJ and Crues JV: Exposure to a 1.5-T static magnetic field does not alter body and skin temperatures in man, Magn Reson Med 11:371-375, 1989.

Smith FW et al: Low-field (0.08 T) magnetic resonance imaging of the pancreas: comparison with computed tomography and ultrasound, Br J Radiol 62:796-802, 1989.

Spritzer C, Gamsu G and Sostman HD: Magnetic resonance imaging of the thorax: techniques, current applications, and future directions, J Thorac Imaging 4:1-18, 1989.

Swartz JD: Current imaging approach to the temporal bone, Radiology 171:309-317, 1989.

Swensen SJ, Ehman RL and Brown LR: Magnetic resonance imaging of the thorax, J Thorac Imaging 4:19-33, 1989.

Tabor EK and Curtin HD: MR of the salivary glands, Radiol Clin North Am 27:379-392, 1989.

Teresi LM, Lufkin RB and Hanafee WN: Magnetic resonance imaging of the larynx, Radiol Clin North Am 27:393-406, 1989.

Tien R et al: A simple method for spinal localization in MR imaging, AJNR 10:1232, 1989.

Towler CR and Young SW: Magnetic resonance imaging of the larynx, Magn Reson Q 5:228-241, 1989.

Vaughan B: Magnetic resonance imaging: physics and technical aspects, Australas Radiol 33:34-39, 1989.

Weissleder R and Stark DD: Magnetic resonance imaging of the liver, Magn Reson Q 5:97-121, 1989.

Yoffie RL et al: Three-dimensional magnetic resonance imaging of the heart, Radiol Technol 60:303-309, 1989.

Yuh WT et al: Application of magnetic resonance imaging in pancreas transplant, Diabetes 38(Suppl 1):27-29, 1989.

Yuh WT et al: Pancreatic transplants: evaluation with MR imaging, Radiology 170:171-177, 1989.

1990 Anslow P: Neuroradiology including magnetic resonance, Acta Neurochir Suppl 50:76-79, 1990.

Avrahami E: Panic attacks during MR imaging: treatment with i.v. diazepam, AJNR 11:833-835, 1990.

Beltran J et al: The diabetic foot: magnetic resonance imaging evaluation, Skeletal Radiol 19:37-41, 1990.

Beltran J: Technology evaluation and clinical trials of magnetic resonance imaging, Curr Opin Rheumatol 2:379-383, 1990.

Berquist TH: Magnetic resonance imaging of the foot and ankle, Semin Ultrasound CT MR 11:327-345, 1990.

Caputo GR and Higgins CB: Advances in cardiac imaging modalities: fast computed tomography, magnetic resonance imaging, and positron emission tomography, Invest Radiol 25:838-854, 1990.

Clayman DA, Murakami ME and Vines FS: Compatibility of cervical spine braces with MR imaging: a study of nine nonferrous devices, AJNR 11:385-390, 1990.

Cole PR et al: High resolution, high field magnetic resonance imaging of joints: unexpected features in proton images of cartilage, Br J Radiol 63:907-909, 1990.

DeLuca SA and Castronovo FP Jr: Hazards of magnetic resonance imaging, Am Fam Physician 41:145-146, 1990.

DeMarco JK and Dillon WP: Orbital magnetic resonance imaging, Curr Opin Radiol 2:112-117, 1990.

Dorfman RE and Spickler EM: Current status of magnetic resonance imaging of the orbit, Top Magn Reson Imaging 2:17-26, 1990.

Fitzgerald S and Foley WD: Advances in technique and technology in body computed tomography and magnetic resonance imaging, Curr Opin Radiol 2:526-533, 1990.

Gundry CR et al: Is MR better than arthrography for evaluating the ligaments of the wrist? In vitro study, AJR 154:337-341, 1990.

Hamm B, Laniado S and Saini S: Contrast-enhanced magnetic resonance imaging of the abdomen and pelvis, Magn Reson Q 6:108-135, 1990.

Hashimoto K et al: Magnetic resonance imaging of lumbar disc herniation: comparison with myelography, Spine 15:1166-1169, 1990.

Hoffman EA and Gefter WB: Multimodality imaging of the upper airway: MRI, MR spectroscopy, and ultrafast X-ray CT, Prog Clin Biol Res 345:291-301, 1990.

Hyde JS et al: Facial surface coil for MR imaging, Radiology 174:276-279, 1990.

Jabour BA, Lufkin RB and Hanafee WN: Magnetic resonance imaging of the larynx, Top Magn Reson Imaging 2:60-68, 1990.

Kanal E and Shellock FG: Burns associated with clinical MR examinations, Radiology 175:585, 1990.

Kanal E, Shellock FG and Talagala L: Safety considerations in MR imaging, Radiology 176:593-606, 1990.

Kerr R and Forrester DM: Magnetic resonance imaging of foot and ankle trauma, Orthop Clin North Am 21:591-601, 1990.

Kimura F et al: MR imaging of the normal and abnormal clivus, AJR 155:1285-1291, 1990.

Kirsch DL et al: MRI of the skull, Magn Reson Imaging 8:217-222, 1990.

Laine FJ, Nadel L and Braun IF: CT and MR imaging of the central skull base. I. Techniques, embryologic development, and anatomy, Radiographics 10:591-602, 1990.

Laine FJ, Nadel L and Braun IF: CT and MR imaging of the central skull base. II. Pathologic spectrum, Radiographics 10:797-821, 1990.

Lanzieri CF and Bangert B: Magnetic resonance imaging of the nasopharynx, Top Magn Reson Imaging 2:39-47, 1990.

Laptook AR: Magnetic resonance: safety considerations and future directions, Semin Perinatol 14:189-192, 1990.

Linson MA and Crowe CH: Comparison of magnetic resonance imaging and lumbar discography in the diagnosis of disc degeneration, Clin Orthop 160-163, 1990.

Litt AW et al: Role of slice thickness in MR imaging of the internal auditory canal, J Comput Assist Tomogr 14:717-720, 1990.

Lubat E and Weinreb JC: Magnetic resonance imaging of the kidneys and adrenals, Top Magn Reson Imaging 2:17-36, 1990.

Mano I et al: Computerized three-dimensional normal atlas, Radiat Med 8:50-54, 1990.

McKenna KM et al: Magnetic resonance imaging of the tongue and oropharynx, Top Magn Reson Imaging 2:49-59, 1990.

Morrison DS and Ofstein R: The use of magnetic resonance imaging in the diagnosis of rotator cuff tears, Orthopedics 13:633-637, 1990.

Nagata K et al: Clinical value of magnetic resonance imaging for cervical myelopathy, Spine 15:1088-1096, 1990.

Newhouse JH: MRI of the adrenal gland, Urol Radiol 12:1-6, 1990.

Niemi P et al: Superparamagnetic particles as gastrointestinal contrast agent in magnetic resonance imaging of lower abdomen, Acta Radiol 31:409-411, 1990.

Olcott EW: Magnetic resonance angiography, angiographic contrast media, and digital angiography, Curr Opin Radiol 2:252-258, 1990.

Pollei SR and Schellhas KP: Magnetic resonance imaging of the temporomandibular joint, Semin Ultrasound CT MR 11:346-361, 1990.

Rafal RB, Kosovsky PA and Markisz JA: Magnetic resonance imaging of the adrenal glands: a subject review, Clin Imaging 14:1-10, 1990.

Rothschild PA, Crooks LE and Margulis AR: Direction of MR imaging, Invest Radiol 25:275-281, 1990.

Saab MH, Dietrich RB and Lufkin RB: MR imaging of the calvarium: pictorial essay, Surg Radiol Anat 12:215-218, 1990.

Sartoris DJ and Resnick D: Magnetic resonance imaging of pediatric foot and ankle disorders, J Foot Surg 29:489-494, 1990.

Schnall MD and Pollack HM: Magnetic resonance imaging of the prostate gland, Urol Radiol 12:109-114, 1990.

Schnall MD et al: Magnetic resonance imaging of the prostate, Magn Reson Q 6:1-16, 1990.

Shellock FG and Slimp G: Halo vest for cervical spine fixation during MR imaging, AJR 154:631-632, 1990.

Siegel MJ: Chest applications of magnetic resonance imaging in children, Top Magn Reson Imaging 3:1-23, 1990.

Simon JH: Technologic advances in computed tomography and magnetic resonance imaging in the central nervous system, Curr Opin Radiol 2:518-525, 1990.

Swartz JD and Harnsberger HR: The temporal bone: magnetic resonance imaging, Top Magn Reson Imaging 2:1-16, 1990.

Sze G: New applications of MR contrast agents in neuroradiology, Neuroradiology 32:421-438, 1990.

Vassiliades VC and Bernardino ME: Magnetic resonance imaging of the liver, Top Magn Reson Imaging 2:1-16, 1990.

Zerhouni EA: New directions in cardiac magnetic resonance imaging, Top Magn Reson Imaging 2:67-71, 1990.

1991 Adler LP et al: Comparison of PET with CT, MRI, and conventional scintigraphy in a benign and in a malignant soft tissue tumor, Orthopedics 14:891-4, 1991.

al-Ahwani S et al: Magnetic resonance imaging of the female bony pelvis: MRI pelvimetry, J Belge Radiol 74:15-18, 1991.

Ambrosetto P et al: CT and MR of the sellar spine, Neuroradiology 33:465, 1991.

Bell GR and Stearns KL: Flexion-extension MRI of the upper rheumatoid cervical spine, Orthopedics 14:969-973, 1991.

Bettinardi V et al: Head holder for PET, CT, and MR studies, J Comput Assist Tomogr 15:886-892, 1991.

Brahme SK and Resnick D: Magnetic resonance imaging of the wrist, Rheum Dis Clin North Am 17:721-739, 1991.

Breidahl WH, Low V and Khangure MS: Imaging the cervical spine: a comparison of MR with myelography and CT myelography, Australas Radiol 35:306-314, 1991.

Bresnahan PJ and Fung J: Magnetic resonance imaging of the foot and ankle in the pediatric patient, J Am Podiatr Med Assoc 81:112-118, 1991.

Bryan RN: MR of the temporal bone, AJNR 12:17-18, 1991.

Caron KH: Magnetic resonance imaging of the pediatric abdomen, Semin Ultrasound CT MR 12:448-474, 1991.

Chevallier JM et al: The thoracic esophagus: sectional anatomy and radiosurgical applications, Surg Radiol Anat 13:313-321, 1991.

Collins JD et al: Anatomy of the thorax and shoulder girdle displayed by magnetic resonance imaging, J Natl Med Assoc 83:26-32, 1991.

Conway WF et al: Cross-sectional imaging of the patellofemoral joint and surrounding structures, Radiographics 11:195-217, 1991.

Coulden RA et al: Magnetic resonance imaging: when is one sequence sufficient? Clin Radiol 44:393-396, 1991.

DeSimone D et al: Evaluation of the safety and efficacy of gadoteridol injection (a low osmolal magnetic resonance contrast agent): clinical trials report, Invest Radiol 26(Suppl 1):S212-6, 1991.

Ebraheim NA et al: The effect of matallic implants on magnetic resonance imaging: a brief note, J Bone Joint Surg [Am] 73:1397-1398, 1991.

Ellis JH et al: Magnetic resonance imaging of the normal craniovertebral junction, Spine 16:105-111, 1991.

Erickson SJ et al: Effect of tendon orientation on MR imaging signal intensity: a manifestation of the "magic angle" phenomenon, Radiology 181:389-392, 1991.

Feldman F, Staron RB and Haramati N: Magnetic resonance imaging of the foot and ankle, Rheum Dis Clin North Am 17:617-636, 1991.

Ferkel RD, Flannigan BD and Elkins BS: Magnetic resonance imaging of the foot and ankle: correlation of normal anatomy with pathologic conditions, Foot Ankle 11:289-305, 1991.

Fry ME et al: High-resolution magnetic resonance imaging of the interphalangeal joints of the hand, Skeletal Radiol 20:273-277, 1991.

Future directions in MRI of diffusion and microcirculation. Society of Magnetic Resonance in Medicine (SMRM) workshop. Bethesda, Maryland, June 7-8, 1990, Magn Reson Med 19:209-333, 1991.

Grevers G et al: Three-dimensional magnetic resonance imaging in skull base lesions, Am J Otolaryngol 12:139-145, 1991.

Guy RL et al: A comparison of CT and MRI in the assessment of the pituitary and parasellar region, Clin Radiol 43:156-161, 1991.

Hahn PF: Advances in contrast-enhanced MR imaging: gastrointestinal contrast agents, AJR 156:252-254, 1991.

Hamm B: Advances in contrast-enhanced MR imaging: nonneurologic applications, AJR 156:245-252, 1991.

Ho CP and Sartoris DJ: Magnetic resonance imaging of the elbow, Rheum Dis Clin North Am 17:705-720, 1991.

Hricak H et al: Female urethra: MR imaging, Radiology 178:527-535, 1991.

Jones AA et al: Potential hazard: traction weights and magnetic resonance imaging, Spine 16:364-365, 1991.

Kerr R and Frey C: MR imaging in tarsal tunnel syndrome, J Comput Assist Tomogr 15:280-286, 1991.

Kido DK et al: Evaluation of the carotid artery bifurcation: comparison of magnetic resonance angiography and digital subtraction arch aortography, Neuroradiology 33:48-51, 1991.

Koch M and von Schulthess GK: Magnetic resonance angiography in the abdomen and pelvis, Curr Opin Radiol 3:463-470, 1991.

Krasny R et al: MR anatomy of infants hip: comparison to anatomical preparations, Pediatr Radiol 21:211-215, 1991.

Kressel HY: Insights of an abdominal imager: what do we need for MRI enhancement? Magn Reson Med 22:314-318, 1991.

Kruyt RH et al: Normal anorectum: dynamic MR imaging anatomy, Radiology 179:159-163, 1991.

Lim KO et al: Hepatobiliary MR imaging: first human experience with MnDPDP, Radiology 178:79-82, 1991.

Link KM et al: Clinical utility of three-dimensional magnetic resonance angiographic imaging, Clin Neurosurg 37:275-288, 1991.

Lloyd GA and Barker PB: Subtraction magnetic resonance for tumours of the skull base and sinuses: a new imaging technique, J Laryngol Otol 105:628-631, 1991.

Mattrey RF: Magnetic resonance imaging of the scrotum, Semin Ultrasound CT MR 12:95-108, 1991.

McElveen JT Jr et al: Magnetic resonance angiography: technique and skull-base applications, Am J Otol 12:323-328, 1991.

Merenich WM et al: The foramen ovale: MR and CT correlation, Clin Imaging 15:20-30, 1991.

Minami M et al: MR study of normal joint function using a low field strength system, J Comput Assist Tomogr 15:1017-1023, 1991.

Mirowitz SA et al: Dynamic gadolinium-enhanced MR imaging of the spleen: normal enhancement patterns and evaluation of splenic lesions, Radiology 179:681-686, 1991.

Mitchell DG et al: Comparison of Kaopectate with barium for negative and positive enteric contrast at MR imaging, Radiology 181:475-480, 1991.

Modic MT: Advances in contrast-enhanced MR imaging: neurologic applications, AJR 156:239-245, 1991.

Murakami DM, Bassett LW and Seeger LL: Advances in imaging of rheumatoid arthritis, Clin Orthop 265:83-95, 1991.

Oksendal AN et al: Superparamagnetic particles as an oral contrast agent in abdominal magnetic resonance imaging, Invest Radiol 26 Suppl 1:S67-70, 1991.

Runge VM and Gelblum DY: Future directions in magnetic resonance contrast media, Top Magn Reson Imaging 3:85-97, 1991.

Saini S: Advances in contrast-enhanced MR imaging: principles, AJR 156:236-239, 1991.

Schultz-Lampel D et al: MRI for evaluation of scrotal pathology, Urol Res 19:289-292, 1991.

Secaf E et al: MR imaging of the seminal vesicles, AJR 156:989-994, 1991.

Shellock FG and Kanal E: Policies, guidelines, and recommendations for MR imaging safety and patient management: SMRI Safety Committee, JMRI 1:97-101, 1991.

Simmons JW et al: Awake discography: a comparison study with magnetic resonance imaging, Spine 16:S216-S221, 1991.

Spring BI and Schiebler ML: Normal anatomy of the thoracic inlet as seen on transaxial MR images, AJR 157:707-710, 1991.

Stark DD: Physiological principles for the design of hepatic contrast agents, Magn Reson Med 22:324-8, 1991.

Tan SB, Kozak JA and Mawad ME: The limitations of magnetic resonance imaging in the diagnosis of pathologic vertebral fractures, Spine 16:919-923, 1991.

Tart RP et al: Enteric MRI contrast agents: comparative study of five potential agents in humans, Magn Reson Imaging 9:559-568, 1991.

Tham RT et al: Cystic fibrosis: MR imaging of the pancreas, Radiology 179:183-186, 1991.

Tilcock C et al: Polymeric gastrointestinal MR contrast agents, J Magn Reson Imaging 1:463-467, 1991.

von Roemeling R, Lanning RM and Eames FA: MR imaging of patients with implanted drug infusion pumps, J Magn Reson Imaging 1:77-81, 1991.

Watt I: Magnetic resonance imaging in orthopaedics, J Bone Joint Surg [Br] 73:539-550, 1991.

Weinreb JC and Naidich DP: Thoracic magnetic resonance imaging, Clin Chest Med 12:33-54, 1991.

Yu S, Haughton VM and Rosenbaum AE: Magnetic resonance imaging and anatomy of the spine, Radiol Clin North Am 29:691-710, 1991.

1992 Ainsworth JR et al: Indications for and accuracy of magnetic resonance imaging and computed tomography in orbital disease, Scott Med J 37:11-17, 1992.

Athey TW: Current FDA guidance for MR patient exposure and considerations for the future, Ann N Y Acad Sci 649:242-257, 1992.

Balzarini L et al: Magnetic resonance imaging of the gastrointestinal tract: investigation of baby milk as a low cost contrast medium, Eur J Radiol 15:171-174, 1992.

Bell GR and Ross JS: Diagnosis of nerve root compression: myelography, computed tomography, and MRI, Orthop Clin North Am 23:405-419, 1992.

Birney TJ et al: Comparison of MRI and discography in the diagnosis of lumbar degenerative disc disease, J Spinal Disord 5:417-423, 1992.

Bisset GS: Magnetic resonance imaging in the pediatric patient, Pediatr Ann 21:121-6, 129-31, 1992.

Blevins SJ and Benson S: A better way to get kids through scans, RN 55:40-44, 1992.

Bondestam S et al: Tissue characterization by image processing subtraction: windowing of specific T1 values, Magn Reson Imaging 10:989-995, 1992.

Boothroyd AE et al: The magnetic resonance appearances of the normal thymus in children, Clin Radiol 45:378-381, 1992.

Bosmans H et al: MRA review, Clin Imaging 16:152-167, 1992.

Bradley WG: Recent advances in magnetic resonance angiography of the brain, Curr Opin Neurol Neurosurg 5:859-862, 1992.

Bradley WG Jr: Future applications of contrast agents for magnetic resonance imaging of the central nervous system, Invest Radiol 27 Suppl 1:S58-S60, 1992.

Brockway JP and Bream PR Jr: Does memory loss occur after MR imaging? JMRI 2:721-728, 1992.

Carpenter JP et al: Magnetic resonance angiography of peripheral runoff vessels, J Vasc Surg 16:807-813, 1992.

Carvlin MJ, De Simone DN and Meeks MJ: Phase II clinical trial of gadoteridol injection, a low-osmolal magnetic resonance imaging contrast agent, Invest Radiol 27 Suppl 1:S16-S21, 1992.

Case TC et al: Magnetic resonance imaging in human lymphedema: comparison with lymphangioscintigraphy, Magn Reson Imaging 10:549-558, 1992.

Castellino RA: Diagnostic imaging studies in patients with newly diagnosed Hodgkin's disease, Ann Oncol 3(Suppl 4):45-47, 1992.

Cooper TG and Gift DA: Prospects for the future: magnetic resonance fast scanning and flow quantitation, Semin Ultrasound CT MR 13:303-310, 1992.

Davies AM and Wellings RM: Imaging of bone tumors, Curr Opin Radiol 4:32-38, 1992.

Downey DJ, Drennan JC and Garcia JF: Magnetic resonance image findings in congenital talipes equinovarus, J Pediatr Orthop 12:224-228, 1992.

Edelman RR: Basic principles of magnetic resonance angiography, Cardiovasc Intervent Radiol 15:3-13, 1992.

Eggli KD: The newer radiographic contrast media, Clin Pediatr 31:554-8, 1992.

Finn JP, Clarke MP and Goldmann A: MR angiography of the liver, Semin Ultrasound CT MR 13:367-376, 1992.

Finn JP and Longmaid HE: Abdominal magnetic resonance venography, Cardiovasc Intervent Radiol 15:51-59, 1992.

Gudinchet F et al: Magnetic resonance imaging of nontraumatic shoulder instability in children, Skeletal Radiol 21:19-21, 1992.

Hamed MM et al: Dynamic MR imaging of the abdomen with gadopentetate dimeglumine: normal enhancement patterns of the liver, spleen, stomach, and pancreas, AJR 158:303-307, 1992.

Harcke HT et al: Growth plate of the normal knee: evaluation with MR imaging, Radiology 183:119-123, 1992.

Harms SE and Flamig DP: Magnetic resonance angiography: application to the peripheral circulation, Invest Radiol 27 Suppl 2:S80-S83, 1992.

Herzog RJ: Imaging of the knee, Orthop Rev 21:1409-1417, 1992.

Hopper KD et al: CT and MR imaging of the pediatric orbit, Radiographics 12:485-503, 1992.

Horton WC and Daftari TK: Which disc as visualized by magnetic resonance imaging is actually a source of pain? A correlation between magnetic resonance imaging and discography, spine 17:S164-S171, 1992.

Imaeda T et al: Magnetic resonance imaging in scaphoid fractures, J Hand Surg Br 17:20-27, 1992.

Jahnke AH Jr et al: A prospective comparison of computerized arthrotomography and magnetic resonance imaging of the glenohumeral joint, Am J Sports Med 20:695-700, 1992.

Judnick JW et al: Radiotherapy technique integrates MRI into CT, Radiol Technol 64:82-89, 1992.

Kanal E and Shellock FG: Policies, guidelines, and recommendations for MR imaging safety and patient management: SMRI Safety Committee, J Magn Reson Imaging 2:247-248, 1992.

Kandarpa K et al: Prospective double-blinded comparison of MR imaging and aortography in the preoperative evaluation of abdominal aortic aneurysms, J Vasc Interv Radiol 3:83-89, 1992.

Kawashima A, Fishman EK and Kuhlman JE: CT and MR evaluation of posterior mediastinal masses, CRC Crit Rev Diagn Imaging 33:311-367, 1992.

Kneeland JB and Dalinka MK: Magnetic resonance imaging of the foot and ankle, Magn Reson Q 8:97-115, 1992.

Kono M, Kusumoto M and Adachi S: Thoracic magnetic resonance imaging, Curr Opin Radiol 4:62-68, 1992.

Lang P et al: Imaging of the hip joint: computed tomography versus magnetic resonance imaging, Clin Orthop 135-153, 1992.

Larsson EM: Magnetic resonance imaging of the cervical and thoracic spine and the spinal cord: a study using a 0.3 T vertical magnetic field, Acta Radiol Suppl Stockh 378:71-92, 1992.

Levy AS et al: Magnetic resonance imaging evaluation of calcaneal fat pads in patients with os calcis fractures, Foot Ankle 13:57-62, 1992.

Mattle HP and Edelman RR: Cerebral magnetic resonance angiography, Neurological Research 14:118-121, 1992.

Mayer DP et al: Magnetic resonance arthrography of the ankle, J Foot Surg 31:584-587, 1992.

McCauley TR et al: effect of prone versus supine patient positioning on pelvic magnetic resonance image quality, Invest Radiol 27:1005-1008, 1992.

Mirowitz SA and Susman N: Use of nutritional support formula as a gastrointestinal contrast agent for MRI, J Comput Assist Tomogr 16:908-915, 1992.

Mitchell DG: Chemical shift magnetic resonance imaging: applications in the abdomen and pelvis, Top Magn Reson Imaging 4:46-63, 1992.

Mitchell DG et al: Pancreatic disease: findings on state-of-the-art MR images, AJR 159:533-538, 1992.

Muller-Schimpfle M et al: MRI and MRA in treatment planning of subdiaphragmatic radiation therapy, J Comput Assist Tomogr 16:110-119, 1992.

Munk PL et al: Current status of magnetic resonance imaging of the ankle and the hindfoot, Can Assoc Radiol J 43:19-30, 1992.

Murphy BJ: MR imaging of the elbow, Radiology 184:525-529, 1992.

Olson MC et al: MR imaging of the female pelvic region, Radiographics 12:445-465, 1992.

Otto PM et al: Screening test for detection of metallic foreign objects in the orbit before magnetic resonance imaging, Invest Radiol 27:308-311, 1992.

Patten RM et al: OMR, a positive bowel contrast agent for abdominal and pelvic MR imaging: safety and imaging characteristics, J Magn Reson Imaging 2:25-34, 1992.

Pavone P et al: Gadopentetate dimeglumine-barium paste for opacification of the esophageal lumen on MR images, AJR 159:762-764, 1992.

Pavone P et al: A new imaging modality— MRI: its clinical indication in the study of the gastrointestinal system, Eur J Cancer Prevention 1(Suppl 3):71-79, 1992.

Perneczky G et al: Diagnosis of cervical disc disease: MRI versus cervical myelography, Acta Neurochir 116:44-48, 1992.

Price RR et al: Magnetic resonance angiography techniques, Invest Radiol 27:27-32, 1992.

Principles for the protection of patients and volunteers during clinical magnetic resonance diagnostic procedures, Ann N Y Acad Sci 649:372-375, 1992.

Reijnierse M et al: The signal intensity of the normal odontoid process (dens) displayed on magnetic resonance images, Skeletal Radiol 21:519-521, 1992.

Riles TS et al: Comparison of magnetic resonance angiography, conventional angiography, and duplex scanning, Stroke 23:341-346, 1992.

Rosenberg ZS et al: Osgood-Schlatter lesion: fracture or tendinitis? Scintigraphic, CT, and MR imaging features, Radiology 185:853-858, 1992.

Ross JS: MR imaging of the cervical spine: techniques for two- and three-dimensional imaging, AJR 159:779-786, 1992.

Saini S: Future applications of magnetic resonance contrast agents in the abdomen, Invest Radiol 27(Suppl 1):S61-S63, 1992.

Saloner D and Anderson CM: Instrumentation for magnetic resonance angiography, Cardiovasc Intervent Radiol 15:14-22, 1992.

Sartoris DJ: Diagnostic imaging insight: cross-sectional imaging of the foot (computed tomography-magnetic resonance), J Foot Surg 31:190-202, 1992.

Schiebler ML and Listerud J: Common artifacts encountered in thoracic magnetic resonance imaging: recognition, derivation, and solutions, Top Magn Reson Imaging 4:1-17, 1992.

Schiebler ML et al: Magnetic resonance angiography of the pelvis and lower extremities. Works in progress, Invest Radiol 27(Suppl 2):S90-S96, 1992.

Tehranzadeh J, Kerr R and Amster J: Magnetic resonance imaging of tendon and ligament abnormalities. I. Spine and upper extremities, Skeletal Radiol 21:1-9, 1992.

Tehranzadeh J, Kerr R and Amster J: Magnetic resonance imaging of tendon and ligament abnormalities. II. Pelvis and lower extremities, Skeletal Radiol 21:79-86, 1992.

Tehranzadeh J, Wang F and Mesgarzadeh M: Magnetic resonance imaging of osteomyelitis, CRC Crit Rev Diagn Imaging 33:495-534, 1992.

Vahlensieck M, Resendes M and Genant HK: MRI of the shoulder, Bildgebung 59:123-132, 1992.

VanDyke CW et al: Three-dimensional MR myelography, J Comput Assist Tomogr 16:497-500, 1992.

Weber AL: Magnetic resonance imaging and computed tomography of the internal auditory canal and cerebellopontine angle, Israel J Med Sci 28:173-182, 1992.

Weiss J et al: Bio-effects of high magnetic fields: a study using a simple animal model, Magn Reson Imaging 10:689-694, 1992.

White RD, Ehman RL and Weinreb JC: Cardiovascular MR imaging: current level of clinical activity, J Magn Reson Imaging 2:365-370, 1992.

Whitten CG et al: The use of intravenous gadopentetate dimeglumine in magnetic resonance imaging of synovial lesions, Skeletal Radiol 21:215-218, 1992.

Wright AR, Cameron HM and Lind T: Magnetic resonance imaging pelvimetry: a useful adjunct in the management of the obese patient, Br J Obstet Gynaecol 99:852-853, 1992.

Wright AR et al: MR pelvimetry—a practical alternative, Acta Radiol 33:582-587, 1992.

Yone K et al: Preoperative and postoperative magnetic resonance image evaluations of the spinal cord in cervical myelopathy, Spine 17:388-392, 1992.

Zisch RJ, Hollenbach HP and Artmann W: Lumbar myelography with three-dimensional MR imaging, J Magn Reson Imaging 2:731-734, 1992.

Zlatkin MB and Greenan T: Magnetic resonance imaging of the wrist, Magn Reson Q 8:65-96, 1992.

1993 Atlas SW: MR imaging is highly senseitive for acute subarachnoid hemorrhage . . . not, Radiology 186:319-322, 1993.

Baldor RA, Quirk ME and Dohan D: Magnetic resonance imaging use by primary care physicians, J Fam Pract 36:281-285, 1993.

Baleriaux D, Matos C and De Greef D: Gadodiamide injection as a contrast medium for MRI of the central nervous system: a comparison with gadolinium-DOTA, Neuroradiology 35:490-494, 1993.

Barnes PD et al: Atypical idiopathic scoliosis: MR imaging evaluation, Radiology 186:247-253, 1993.

Blatter DD et al: Cervical carotid MR angiography with multiple overlapping thin-slab acquisition: comparison with conventional angiography, AJR 161:1269-1277, 1993.

Brady AP et al: A technique for magnetic resonance imaging of the temporomandibular joint, Clin Radiol 47:127-133, 1993.

Buijs PC et al: Carotid bifurcation imaging: magnetic resonance angiography compared to conventional angiography and Doppler ultrasound, Eur J Vasc Surg 7:245-251, 1993.

Bulte JW et al: Magnetite as a potent contrast-enhancing agent in magnetic resonance imaging to visualize blood-brain barrier disruption, Acta Neurochir Suppl 57:30-34, 1993.

Carpenter JP et al: Magnetic resonance venography for the detection of deep venous thrombosis: comparison with contrast venography and duplex Doppler ultrasonography, J Vasc Surg 18:734-741, 1993.

Chambon C et al: Superparamagnetic iron oxides as positive MR contrast agents: in vitro and in vivo evidence, Magn Reson Imaging 11:509-519, 1993.

Chou CK et al: Abdominal MR imaging following antegrade air introduction into the intestinal loops, Abdom Imaging 18:205-210, 1993.

Chou CK et al: Retrograde air insufflation in MRI: a technical note, Abdom Imaging 18:211-214, 1993.

Cohen MS and Fordham J: Developments in magnetic resonance imaging, Invest Radiol 28 Suppl 4:S32-S37, 1993.

Drayer BP: MR imaging advances in practice, J Comput Assist Tomogr 17(Suppl 1):S30-S35, 1993.

Dumoulin CL et al: Reduction of artifacts from breathing and peristalsis in phase-contrast MRA of the chest and abdomen, J Comput Assist Tomogr 17:328-332, 1993.

Edelman RR and Warach S: Magnetic resonance imaging. II. N Engl J Med 328:785-791, 1993.

Erickson SJ and Rosengarten JL: MR imaging of the forefoot: normal anatomic findings, AJR 160:565-571, 1993.

Fulbright R, Ross JS and Sze G: Application of contrast agents in MR imaging of the spine, J Magn Reson Imaging 3:219-232, 1993.

Garcia FF et al: Diagnostic imaging of childhood spinal infection, Orthop Rev 22:321-327, 1993.

Goldberg RA, Heinz GW and Chiu L: Gadolinium magnetic resonance imaging dacryocystography, Am J Ophthalmol 115:738-741, 1993.

Graeter T et al: Three-dimensional vascular imaging—an additional diagnostic tool, Thorac Cardiovasc Surg 41:183-185, 1993.

Hanna SL et al: MR imaging of infradiaphragmatic lymphadenopathy in children and adolescents with Hodgkin disease: comparison with lymphography and CT, J Magn Reson Imaging 3:461-470, 1993.

Holder LE, Merine DS and Yang A: Nuclear medicine, contrast angiography, and magnetic resonance imaging for evaluating vascular problems in the hand, Hand Clin 9:85-113, 1993.

Holtas S: Radiology of the degenerative lumbar spine, Acta Orthop Scand Suppl 251:16-18, 1993.

Hricak H and Kim B: Contrast-enhanced MR imaging of the female pelvis, J Magn Reson Imaging 3:297-306, 1993.

Kier R: MR imaging of foot and ankle tumors, Magn Reson Imaging 11:149-162, 1993.

Klein MA and Spreitzer AM: MR imaging of the tarsal sinus and canal: normal anatomy, pathologic findings, and features of the sinus tarsi syndrome, Radiology 186:233-240, 1993.

Lang P et al: Acute fracture of the femoral neck: assessment of femoral head perfusion with gadopentetate dimeglumine-enhanced MR imaging, AJR 160:335-341, 1993.

Lerski RA and de Certaines JD: Performance assessment and quality control in MRI by Eurospin test objects and protocols, Magn Reson Imaging 11:817-833, 1993.

Link KM et al: Magnetic resonance imaging of the mediastinum, J Thorac Imaging 8:34-53, 1993.

Lomas DJ, Mackenzie R and Dixon A: Magnetic resonance imaging of the knee: does foot restraint improve the examination? Br J Radiol 66:497-502, 1993.

MacVicar D et al: Phase III trial of oral magnetic particles in MRI of abdomen and pelvis, Clin Radiol 47:183-188, 1993.

Martin SD, Healey JH and Horowitz S: Stress fracture MRI, Orthopedics 16:75-78, 1993.

Mayo JR: Thoracic magnetic resonance imaging: physics and pulse sequences, J Thorac Imaging 8:1-11, 1993.

Melendez JC and McCrank E: Anxiety-related reactions associated with magnetic resonance imaging examinations, JAMA 270:745-747, 1993.

Mirowitz SA: Contrast enhancement of the gastrointestinal tract on MR images using intravenous gadolinium-DTPA, Abdom Imaging 18:215-219, 1993.

Mirowitz SA, Brown JJ and Heiken JP: Evaluation of the prostate and prostatic carcinoma with gadolinium-enhanced endorectal coil MR imaging, Radiology 186:153-157, 1993.

Mistretta CA: Relative characteristics of MR angiography and competing vascular imaging modalities, J Magn Reson Imaging 3:685-698, 1993.

Mitchell DG: Hepatic imaging: techniques and unique applications of magnetic resonance imaging, Magn Reson Q 9:84-112, 1993.

Neelin P et al: Validation of an MRI/PET landmark registration method using three-dimensional simulated PET images and point simulations, Comput Med Imaging Graph 17:351-356, 1993.

Padovani B et al: Chest wall invasion by bronchogenic carcinoma: evaluation with MR imaging, Radiology 187:33-38, 1993.

Patten RM et al: Positive bowel contrast agent for MR imaging of the abdomen: phase II and III clinical trials, Radiology 189:277-283, 1993.

Posner MA and Beltran J: Trispiral tomography and magnetic resonance imaging of the wrist, Bull Hosp Jt Dis Orthop Inst 52:34-43, 1993.

Ramchandani P and Schnall MD: Magnetic resonance imaging of the prostate, Semin Roentgenol 28:74-82, 1993.

Randall PA et al: MR imaging in the evaluation of the chest after uncomplicated median sternotomy, Radiographics 13:329-340, 1993.

Rizzo PF et al: Diagnosis of occult fractures about the hip: magnetic resonance imaging compared with bone-scanning, J Bone Joint Surg Am 75:395-401, 1993.

Rosen BR and Brady TJ: Future uses of MR imaging agents, J Comput assist Tomogr 17 Suppl 1:S36-S42, 1993.

Schenck RC Jr and Heckman JD: Injuries of the knee, Clin Symp 45:1-32, 1993.

Schnall M: Magnetic resonance imaging of the scrotum, Semin Roentgenol 28:19-30, 1993.

Schuhmann-Giampieri G: Liver contrast media for magnetic resonance imaging: interrelations between pharmacokinetics and imaging, Invest Radiol 28:753-761, 1993.

Slifer KJ et al: Behavior analysis of motion control for pediatric neuroimaging, J Appl Behav Anal 26:469-470, 1993.

Stark DD, Fahlvik AK and Klaveness J: Abdominal imaging, J Magn Reson Imaging 3:285-295, 1993.

Stone LG: Molecules and magnets, N Y State J Med 93:49, 1993.

Van Wagoner M and Worah D: Gadodiamide injection: first human experience with the nonionic magnetic resonance imaging enhancement agent, Invest Radiol 28(Suppl 1):S44-S48, 1993.

Winalski CS et al: Enhancement of joint fluid with intravenously administered gadopentetate dimeglumine: technique, rationale, and implications, Radiology 187:179-185, 1993.

Woodward PJ, Wagner BJ and Farley TE: MR imaging in the evaluation of female infertility, Radiographic 13:293-310, 1993.

1994 Boutin RD, Briggs JE and Williamson MR: Injuries associated with MR imaging: survey of safety records and methods used to screen patients for metallic foreign bodies before imaging, AJR 162:189-194, 1994.

Elster AD, Link KM and Carr JJ: Patient screening prior to MR imaging: a practical approach synthesized from protocols at 15 U. S. medical center, AJR 162:195-199, 1994.

DIAGNOSTIC MEDICAL SONOGRAPHY

For bibliographic citations before 1964, please see the fifth edition of this ATLAS. For citations from 1964 through 1974, see the sixth or seventh edition.

1975 David H, Weaver JB and Pearson JF: Doppler ultrasound and fetal activity activity, Br Med J 2:62-64, 1975.

Fitzgerald DE and Carr J: Doppler ultrasound diagnosis and classification as an alternative to arteriography, Angiology 26:283-288, 1975.

1976 Leopold GR et al: Gray-scale ultrasonic cholecystography: a comparison with conventional radiographic techniques, Radiology 121:445-448, 1976.

1977 Bartrum RJ Jr, Crow HC and Foote SR: Ultrasonic and radiographic cholecystography, N Engl J Med 296:538-541, 1977.

Baum G: Ultrasound mammography, Radiology 122:199-205, 1977.

Edelstone DI: Placental localization by ultrasound, Clin Obstet Gynecol 20:285-296, 1977.

Smith RP: Basic physics of ultrasound, Clin Obstet Gynecol 20:231-241, 1977.

1978 Behan M and Kazam E: Sonography of the common bile duct: value of the right anterior oblique view, AJR 130:701-709, 1978.

Crade M, Taylor KJ and Rosenfeld AT: Water distention of the gut in the evaluation of the pancreas by ultrasound, AJR 131:348-349, 1978.

Goldberg HI et al: Capability of CT body scanning and ultrasonography to demonstrate the status of the biliary ductal system in patients with jaundice, Radiology 129:731-737, 1978.

1979 Leopold GR and Felson B: Radiology: ultrasound, JAMA 241:1389-1390, 1979.

1980 Detwiler RP et al: Ultrasonography and oral cholecystography: a comparison of their use in the diagnosis of gall bladder disease, Arch Surg 115:1096-1098, 1980.

Haller JO et al: Sonographic evaluation of the chest in infants and children, AJR 134:1019-1027, 1980.

Janus C and Janus S: Ultrasound: patients' views, JCU 8:17-20, 1980.

Leslie EV et al: Computed tomography of the abdomen, Int Adv Surg Oncol 3:221-274, 1980.

Lewis E and Ritchie WG: A simple ultrasonic method for assessing renal size, JCU 8:417-420, 1980.

Meire HB et al: The influence of ultrasound on obstetric radiography, Br J Radiol 53:1087, 1980.

Morgan CL et al: Ultrasound patterns of disorders affecting the gastrointestinal tract, Radiology 135:129-135, 1980.

Nudelman S and Patton DD, eds: Imaging for medicine, nuclear medicine, ultrasonics, and thermography, New York, 1980, Plenum Press.

Seltzer SE, Finberg HJ and Weissman BN: Arthrosonography—technique, sonographic anatomy, and pathology, Invest Radiol 15:19-28, 1980.

1981 Cole-Beuglet C et al: Ultrasound mammography: a comparison with radiographic mammography, Radiology 139:693-698, 1981.

Edwards MK et al: Cribside neurosonography: real-time sonography for intracranial investigation of the neonate, AJR 136:271-275, 1981.

Engel JM and Deitch EE: Sonography of the anterior abdominal wall, AJR 137:73-77, 1981.

Fleischer AC et al: Sonographic assessment of the bowel wall, AJR 136:887-891, 1981.

Foley WD et al: Reformatted coronal display of upper abdominal computed tomography: comparison with ultrasonography, J Comput Assist Tomogr 5:496-502, 1981.

Grant EG et al: Real-time sonography of the neonatal and infant head, AJR 136:265-270, 1981.

Hessler PC et al: High accuracy sonographic recognition of gallstones, AJR 136:517-520, 1981.

Slovis TL and Kuhns LR: Real-time sonography of the brain through the anterior fontanelle, AJR 136:277-286, 1981.

Timor-Tritsch IE, Itskovitz J and Brandes JM: Estimation of fetal weight by real-time sonography, Obstet Gynecol 57:653-656, 1981.

1982 Bernardino ME, Thomas JL and Maklad N: Hepatic sonography: technical considerations, present applications, and possible future, Radiology 142:249-251, 1982.

Burt TB, Knochel JQ and Lee TG: Gas as a contrast agent and diagnostic aid in abdominal sonography, J Ultrasound Med 1:179-184, 1982.

Cole-Beuglet C et al: Clinical experience with a prototype real-time dedicated breast scanner, AJR 139:905-911, 1982.

McGahan JP, Phillips HE and Cox KL: Sonography of the normal pediatric gallbladder and biliary tract, Radiology 144:873-875, 1982.

Simeone JF et al: Sonography of the bile ducts after a fatty meal: an aid in detection of obstruction, Radiology 143:211-215, 1982.

Waldman WJ: Biological interactions of ultrasound, Radiol Technol 54:106-113, 1982.

1983 Bluth EI: Ultrasound evaluation of small bowel abnormalities, Am J Gastroenterol 78:788-793, 1983.

Carroll BA and Gross DM: High-frequency scrotal sonography, AJR 140:511-515, 1983.

Dunne MG and Cunat JS: Sonographic determination of fetal gender before 25 weeks gestation, AJR 140:741-743, 1983.

Dunne MG and Weksberg AP: Portable real-time sonography—a valuable adjunct to computed tomography, CT 7:285-294, 1983.

Hagan-Ansert SL: Textbook of diagnostic ultrasonography, St. Louis, 1983, Mosby.

Krebs CA and Carson J: Gallbladder examinations: a comparison between sonography and radiography, Radiol Technol 54:181-188, 1983.

Ralls PW: Sonography in rheumatology, Clin Rheum Dis 9:443-451, 1983.

Slasky BS, Auerbach D and Skolnick ML: Value of portable real-time ultrasound in the ICU, Crit Care Med 11:160-164, 1983.

Wicks JD and Howe KS: Fundamentals of ultrasonographic technique, Chicago, 1983, Mosby.

1984 Amis ES, Jr and Hartman DS: Renal ultrasonography 1984: a practical overview, Radiol Clin North Am 22:315-332, 1984.

Barnett E and Morley P: Clinical diagnostic ultrasound, Chicago, 1984, Mosby.

de Lacey G et al: Should cholecystography or ultrasound be the primary investigation for gallbladder disease? Lancet 1:205-207, 1984.

Egan RL and Egan KL: Detection of breast carcinoma: comparison of automated water-path whole-breast sonography, mammography, and physical examination, AJR 143:493-497, 1984.

Fukuda M et al: Endoscopic ultrasonography in the diagnosis of pancreatic carcinoma: the use of a liquid-filled stomach method, Scand J Gastroenterol 94(suppl):65-76, 1984.

Han BK, Babcock DS and Oestreich AE: Sonography of brain tumors in infants, AJR 143:31-36, 1984.

Lux G, Heyder N and Lutz H: Ultrasound tomography of the upper gastrointestinal tract: orientation and diagnostic possibilities, Scand J Gastroenterol 94:13-20, 1984.

Montalvo BM et al: Intraoperative sonography in spinal trauma, Radiology 153:125-134, 1984.

O'Brien WF, Buck DR and Nash JD: Evaluation of sonography in the initial assessment of the gynecologic patient, Am J Obstet Gynecol 149:598-602, 1984.

Rosenberg ER et al: Extracranial cribside sonography in infants, South Med J 77:968-971, 1984.

Shawker TH, Sonies BC and Stone M: Soft tissue anatomy of the tongue and floor of the mouth: an ultrasound demonstration, Brain Lang 21:335-350, 1984.

Stannard MW, Binet EF and Jimenez JF: Cranial sonography: anatomic and pathological correlation, CRC Crit Rev Diagn Imaging 22:163-268, 1984.

Strohm WD and Classen M: Anatomical aspects in ultrasonic endoscopy, Scand J Gastroenterol 94(suppl):21-33, 1984.

Valdes C, Malini S and Malinak LR: Ultrasound evaluation of female genital tract anomalies: a review of 64 cases, Am J Obstet Gynecol 149:285-292, 1984.

1985 Butch RJ, Simeone JF and Mueller PR: Thyroid and parathyroid ultrasonography, Radiol Clin North Am 23:57-71, 1985.

Cooper C et al: Ultrasound evaluation of the normal fetal upper airway and esophagus, J Ultrasound Med 4:343-346, 1985.

Holen J, Waag RC and Gramiak R: Representations of rapidly oscillating structures on the Doppler display, Ultrasound Med Biol 11:267-272, 1985.

Kimme-Smith C et al: Ultrasound mammography: effects of focal zone placement, Radiographics 5:955-969, 1985.

Krebs CA and Eisenberg RL: Ultrasound imaging of the adrenal glands, Radiol Technol 56:421-423, 1985.

Lewin A and Schenker JG: On the safety of diagnostic ultrasonography in obstetrics and gynecology, Rev Environ Health 5:129-134, 1985.

O'Leary DH: Vascular ultrasonography, Radiol Clin North Am 23:39-56, 1985.

Rubin E et al: Hand-held real-time breast sonography, AJR 144:623-627, 1985.

Trotnow S et al: A new set of instruments for sonographically controlled follicular puncture, Arch Gynecol 236:211-217, 1985.

1986 Bartrum RJ Jr: Ultrasound instrumentation, CRC Crit Rev Diagn Imaging 25:279-303, 1986.

DePietro MA, Brody BA and Teele RL: Peritrigonal echogenic "blush" on cranial sonography: pathologic correlates, AJR 146:1067-1072, 1986.

DiPietro MA, Faix RG and Donn SM: Procedural hazards of neonatal ultrasonography, ICU 14:361-366, 1986.

Fornage BD: Normal US anatomy of the prostate, Ultrasound Med Biol 12:1011-1021, 1986.

Gutman H, Golimbu M and Subramanyam BR: Diagnostic ultrasound of scrotum, Urology 27:72-75, 1986.

Jackson VP et al: Mammography and ultrasonography for breast cancer detection, Indiana Med 79:749-752, 1986.

Kremkau FW and Taylor KJ: Artifacts in ultrasound imaging, J Ultrasound Med 5:227-237, 1986.

Maron BJ: Structural features of the athlete heart as defined by echocardiography, J Am Coll Cardiol 7:190-203, 1986.

McClure RD and Hricak H: Scrotal ultrasound in the infertile man: detection of subclinical unilateral and bilateral varicoceles, J Urol 135:711-715, 1986.

Mole R: Possible hazards of imaging and Doppler ultrasound in obstetrics, Birth 13:29-38, 1986.

Needleman L and Rifkin MD: Vascular ultrasonography: abdominal applications, Radiol Clin North Am 24:461-484, 1986.

Oakley A: The history of ultrasonography in obstetrics, Birth 13:8-13, 1986.

Parulekar SG: Evaluation of the prone view for cholecystosonography, J Ultrasound Med 5:617-624, 1986.

1987 Barry R and Nel CJ: Comparison of duplex Doppler scanning with contrast angiography in carotid artery disease, S Afr Med J 72:851-852, 1987.

Bassett LW et al: Automated and hand-held breast US: effect on patient management, Radiology 165:103-108, 1987.

Buckley AR et al: Intraoperative imaging of the biliary tree: sonography vs. operative cholangiography, J Ultrasound Med 6:589-595, 1987.

Carroll R and Gombergh R: Empty-bladder (hysterographic) view on US for evaluation of intrauterine devices. Work in progress, Radiology 163:822-823, 1987.

Dudley NJ, Lamb MP and Copping C: A new method for fetal weight estimation using real-time ultrasound, Br J Obstet Gynaecol 94:110-114, 1987.

Fornage BD: The hypoechoic normal tendon: a pitfall, J Ultrasound Med 6:19-22, 1987.

Granberg S and Wikland M: Comparison between endovaginal and transabdominal transducers for measuring ovarian volume, J Ultrasound Med 6:649-653, 1987.

Kawahara H et al: Normal development of the spinal cord in neonates and infants seen on ultrasonography, Neuroradiology 29:50-52, 1987.

Lees WR and Heron CW: US-guided percutaneous pancreatography: experience in 75 patients, Radiology 165:809-813, 1987.

Levine RA: Orbital ultrasonography, Radiol Clin North Am 25:447-469, 1987.

McLeary RD: Future developments in ultrasonic imaging of the prostate, Prog Clin Biol Res 237:209-211, 1987.

Op den Orth JO: Sonography of the pancreatic head aided by water and glucagon, Radiographics 7:85-100, 1987.

Pilu G et al: Ultrasound investigation of the posterior fossa in the fetus, Am J Perinatol 4:155-159, 1987.

Porena M et al: Real-time transrectal sonographic voiding cystourethrography, 30:171-175, 1987.

Taavitsainen M et al: Ultrasonically guided fine-needle aspiration biopsy in focal pancreatic lesions, Acta Radiol 28:541-543, 1987.

Upadhyay SS, O'Neil T, Burwell RG and Moulton A: A new method using ultrasound for measuring femoral anteversion (torsion): technique and reliability, Br J Radiol 60:519-523, 1987.

1988 Beynon J, Mortensen NJ and Rigby HS: Rectal endosonography, a new technique for the preoperative staging of rectal carcinoma, Eur J Surg Oncol 14:297-309, 1988.

Birnholz J and Hrozencik D: Technical improvement for ultrasonic study of the endometrium, Int J Fertil 33:194-200, 1988.

Davison GB and Leeton J: A case of female infertility investigated by contrast-enhanced echo-gynecography, JCU 16:44-47, 1988.

Druce HM: The use of ultrasound as an imaging technique in the diagnosis of sinusitis, N Engl Reg Allergy Proc 9:109-112, 1988.

Fornage BD and Rifkin MD: Ultrasound examination of the hand and foot, Radiol Clin North Am 26:109-129, 1988.

Fornage BD and Rifkin MD: Ultrasound examination of tendons, Radiol Clin North Am 26:87-107, 1988.

Grant EB, Tessler F and Perrella R: Infant cranial sonography, Radiol Clin North Am 26:1089-1110, 1988.

Guyer PB: Direct-contact B-scan sonomammography—an aid to X-ray mammography, Ultrasound Med Biol 14 (Suppl 1): 49-52, 1988.

Hirose K et al: Antenatal ultrasound diagnosis of the femur-fibula-ulna syndrome, JCU 16:199-203, 1988.

Kimme-Smith C et al: Ultrasound artifacts affecting the diagnosis of breast masses, Ultrasound Med Biol 1(suppl):203-210, 1988.

Lyons EA et al: In utero exposure to diagnostic ultrasound: a 6-year follow-up, Radiology 166:687-690, 1988.

Pierard GE: Ultrasound imaging of the skin: how and which future in practice? Dermatologica 177:329-331, 1988.

Quinn MK et al: Transvaginal endosonography: a new method to study the anatomy of the lower urinary tract in urinary stress incontinence, Br J Urol 62:414-419, 1988.

Rifkin MD et al: Ultrasound for guidance of breast mass removal, J Ultrasound Med 7:261-263, 1988.

Rothlin M, Metzger U and Largiader F: Present indications and future expectations of ultrasound in surgery, Surg Endosc 2:176-179, 1988.

Rouse GA et al: Current concepts in sonographic diagnosis of fetal renal disease, Radiographics 8:119-132, 1988.

Schwartz GF et al: Ultrasonographic localization of nonpalpable breast masses, Ultrasound Med Biol 14:23-25, 1988.

Schwartz GF et al: Ultrasonography: an alternative to x-ray-guided needle localization of nonpalpable breast masses, Surgery 104:870-873, 1988.

Seward JB et al: Transesophageal echocardiography: technique, anatomic correlations, Implementation, and clinical applications, Mayo Clin Proc 63:649-680, 1988.

Wells PN: Ultrasound imaging, J Biomed Eng 10:548-554, 1988.

Verschakelen J et al: Ultrasound of the chest, J Belge Radiol 71:615-621, 1988.

Yeh HC: Ultrasonography of the adrenals, Semin Roentgenol 23:250-258, 1988.

Ziskin MC and Petitti DB: Epidemiology of human exposure to ultrasound: a critical review, Ultrasound Med Biol 14:91-96, 1988.

1989 Benson CB, Doubilet PM and Richie JP: Sonography of the male genital tract, AJR 153:705-713, 1989.

Bernaschek G and Deutinger J: Endosonography in obstetrics and gynecology: the importance of standardized image display, Obstet Gynecol 74:817-820, 1989.

Boscaini M: Lower gastrointestinal endoultrasound, Surg Endosc 3:29-32, 1989.

Carroll BA: US of the gastrointestinal tract, Radiology 172:605-608, 1989.

Crawford ED: The role of ultrasound in prostatic imaging: introduction and overview, Urology 33(suppl 6):2-6, 1989.

Elam EA et al: The lack of sonographic image degradation after barium upper gastrointestinal examination, AJR 153:993-994, 1989.

Glasier CM et al: Extracardiac chest ultrasonography in infants and children: radiographic and clinical implications, J Pediatr 114:540-544, 1989.

Goyal AK et al: Can sonography replace splenoportovenography in evaluation of patients with portal hypertension? Indian J Gastroenterol 8:157-159, 1989.

Grant ES, Tessler FN and Perrella RR: Clinical Doppler imaging, AJR 152:707-717, 1989.

Hall-Craggs MA: Interventional abdominal ultrasound: recent advances, Br J Hosp Med 42:176-182, 1989.

Heckmatt J et al: Quantitative sonography of muscle, J Child Neurol 4(Suppl):S101-S106, 1989.

Herment A et al: High-resolution, reflection mode tomographic imaging. I. Principles and methods, Ultrason Imaging 11:1-21, 1989.

Herment A et al: High-resolution, reflection mode tomographic imaging. II. Application to echography, Ultrason Imaging 11:22-41, 1989.

Hirooka N et al: Sono-enterocolonography by oral water administration, JCU 17:585-589, 1989.

Horger EO and Tsai CC: Ultrasound and the prenatal diagnosis of congenital anomalies: a medicolegal perspective, Obstet Gynecol 74:617-619, 1989.

Jansen CA and van Os HC: Value and limitations of vaginal ultrasonography—a review, Hum Reprod 4:858-868, 1989.

Keller MS: Renal Doppler sonography in infants and children, Radiology 172:603-604, 1989.

Kerzel W et al: Extracorporeal piezoelectric shockwave lithotripsy of multiple pancreatic duct stones under ultrasonographic control, Endoscopy 21:229-231, 1989.

Kossoff G et al: A sonographic technique to reduce beam distortion by curved interfaces, Ultrasound Med Biol 15:375-382, 1989.

Lee F et al: Transrectal ultrasound in the diagnosis and staging of prostatic carcinoma, Radiology 170:609-615, 1989.

Lewis BD and James EM: Current applications of duplex and color Doppler ultrasound imaging: abdomen, Mayo Clin Proc 64:1158-1169, 1989.

Maulik D: Biologic effects of ultrasound, Clin Obstet Gynecol 32:645-659, 1989.

Mhaskar R et al: Fetal foot length—a new parameter for assessment of gestational age, Int J Gynaecol Obstet 29:35-38, 1989.

Ophir J and Parker KJ: Contrast agents in diagnostic ultrasound, Ultrasound Med Biol 15:319-333, 1989.

Patel PJ and Pareek SS: scrotal ultrasound in male infertility, Eur Urol 16:423-425, 1989.

Pennell RG and Kurtz AB: Fetal intrathoracic and gastrointestinal anomalies, Clin Diagn Ultrasound 25:111-138, 1989.

Rifkin MD: Prostate sonography: clinical indications and implications, Urol Radiol 11:238-240, 1989.

Smith FW et al: Low-field (0.08 T) magnetic resonance imaging of the pancreas: comparison with computed tomography and ultrasound, Br J Radiol 62:796-802, 1989.

Ueda D: Sonographic measurement of the pancreas in children, JCU 17:417-423, 1989.

Verschakelen JA et al: Sonographic appearance of the diaphragm: a cadaver study, JCU 17:222-227, 1989.

Vilaro MM et al: Hand-held and automated sonomammography: clinical role relative to X-ray mammography, J Ultrasound Med 8:95-100, 1989.

Vowden P et al: A comparison of three imaging techniques in the assessment of an abdominal aortic aneurysm, J Cardiovasc Surg 30:891-896, 1989.

Worlicek H, Dunz D and Engelhard K: Ultrasonic examination of the wall of the fluid-filled stomach, JCU 17:5-14, 1989.

Yock PG, Linker DT and Angelsen BA: Two-dimensional intravascular ultrasound: technical development and initial clinical experience, J Am Soc Echocardiogr 2:296-304, 1989.

Zanette EM et al: Comparison of cerebral angiography and transcranial Doppler sonography in acute stroke, Stroke 20:899-903, 1989.

Zierler RE: Doppler techniques for lower extremity arterial diagnosis, Herz 14:126-133, 1989.

1990 Akizuki H, Yoshida H and Michi K: Ultrasonographic evaluation during reduction of zygomatic arch fractures, J Craniomaxillofac Surg 18:263-266, 1990.

Alvord LS: Uses of ultrasound in audiology, J Am Acad Audiol 1:227-235, 1990.

Annuar Z et al: Ultrasound in the diagnosis of palpable abdominal masses in children, Med J Malaysia 45:281-287, 1990.

Barker CS and Lindsell DR: Ultrasound of the palpable abdominal mass, Clin Radiol 41:98-99, 1990.

Black IW et al: The clinical role of transoesophageal echocardiography, Aust N Z J Med 20:759-764, 1990.

Blyme PJ et al: Ultrasonographic detection of foreign bodies in soft tissue: a human cadaver study, Arch Orthop Trauma Surg 110:24-25, 1990.

Bogdahn U et al: Transcranial color-coded real-time sonography in adults, Stroke 21:1680-1688, 1990.

Breart G and Ringa V: Routine or selective ultrasound scanning, Baillieres Clin Obstet Gynaecol 4:45-63, 1990.

Bronshtein M et al: Early determination of fetal sex using transvaginal sonography: technique and pitfalls, JCU 18:302-306, 1990.

Charnley RM and Hardcastle JD: Intraoperative abdominal ultrasound, Gut 31:368-369, 1990.

Cooner WH: Reducing rectal injury from sonographically-guided transrectal needle biopsy of prostate. The "rule of finger," Urology 36:191-192, 1990.

Dodson MG and Deter RL: Definition of anatomical planes for use in transvaginal sonography, JCU 18:239-242, 1990.

Eidt JF et al: Current status of duplex Doppler ultrasound in the examination of the abdominal vasculature, Am J Surg 160:604-609, 1990.

Endoscopic ultrasonography, Gastrointest Endosc 36:S1-46, 1990.

Fleischer AC et al: Transvaginal scanning of the endometrium, JCU 18:337-349, 1990.

Glasier CM et al: Screening spinal ultrasound in newborns with neural tube defects, J Ultrasound Med 9:339-343, 1990.

Harcke HT and Grissom LE: Performing dynamic sonography of the infant hip, AJR 155:837-844, 1990.

Hildebrandt U and Feifel G: Endorectal sonography, Surg Annu 22:169-183, 1990.

Itskovitz J et al: Transvaginal ultrasonography in the diagnosis and treatment of infertility, JCU 18:248-256, 1990.

Joharjy IA, Mustafa MA and Zaidi AJ: Fluid-aided sonography of the stomach and duodenum in the diagnosis of peptic ulcer disease in adult patients, J Ultrasound Med 9:77-84, 1990.

Laing FC: Technical aspects of vaginal ultrasound, Semin Ultrasound CT MR 11:4-11, 1990.

Lewit N, Thaler I and Rottem S: The uterus: a new look with transvaginal sonography, JCU 18:331-336, 1990.

Machi J et al: Operative ultrasound guidance for various surgical procedures, Ultrasound Med Biol 16:37-42, 1990.

Matalon TA and Silver B: US guidance of interventional procedures, Radiology 174:43-47, 1990.

McGeorge DD and McGeorge S: Diagnostic medical ultrasound in the management of hand injuries, J Hand Surg [Br] 15:256-261, 1990.

Medearis AL and Platt LD: Ultrasound imaging of the cranium and spine, Clin Perinatol 17:597-609, 1990.

Nakamura H et al: Esophageal varices evaluated by endoscopic ultrasonography: observation of collateral circulation during non-shunting operations, Surg Endosc 4:69-74, 1990.

Nolsoe C et al: Major complications and deaths due to interventional ultrasonography: a review of 8000 cases, JCU 18:179-184, 1990.

Pow-Sang JM, Pow-Sang JE and Benavente V: Transrectal ultrasound of the prostate, Semin Surg Oncol 6:234-235, 1990.

Reece EA et al: The safety of obstetric ultrasonography: concern for the fetus, Obstet Gynecol 76:139-146, 1990.

Rifkin MD, Dahnert W and Kurtz AB: State of the art: endorectal sonography of the prostate gland, AJR 154:691-700, 1990.

Rosch T, Lorenz R and Classen M: Endoscopic ultrasonography in the evaluation of colon and rectal disease, Gastrointest Endosc 36:S33-S39, 1990.

Rosi P et al: Diuretic ultrasound: a non-invasive technique for the assessment of upper tract obstruction, Br J Urol 65:566-569, 1990.

Sheikh KH: Interventional ultrasound: incongruity in terms or a reality? J Am Coll Cardiol 15:352-353, 1990.

Spada I, Taylor G and McWeeny K: Endoscopic ultrasonography, Gastroenterol Nurs 13:24-30, 1990.

Thaler I and Manor D: Transvaginal imaging: applied physical principles and terms, JCU 18:235-238, 1990.

van Velthoven V and Auer LM: Practical application of intraoperative ultrasound imaging, Acta Neurochir 105:5-13, 1990.

Vick CW and Bell SA: Rotator cuff tears: diagnosis with sonography, AJR 154:121-123, 1990.

Vogel HJ, Schipper J and Hermans J: Abdominal ultrasonography: improved image quality with the combined use of a diet and laxatives, JCU 18:627-630, 1990.

Wells PN: Future developments in Doppler ultrasound, Clin Diagn Ultrasound 26:165-173, 1990.

Wozniak-Petrofsky J: Transrectal ultrasonography in prostatic carcinoma, Urol Nurs 10:12-16, 1990.

1991 Banerjee B and Brett I: Ultrasound diagnosis of horseshoe kidney, Br J Radiol 64:898-900, 1991.

Banerjee B and Das RK: Sonographic detection of foreign bodies of the extremities, Br J Radiol 64:107-112, 1991.

Benson JT, Sumners JE and Pittman JS: Definition of normal female pelvic floor anatomy using ultrasonographic techniques, JCU 19:275-282, 1991.

Bruggemann A, Greie A and Lepsien G: Real-time sonography of the mediastinum in adults: a study in 100 healthy volunteers, Surg Endosc 5:150-153, 1991.

Cameron J: Using Doppler to diagnose leg ulcers, Nurs Stand 5:25-27, 1991.

Christiansen TG, et al: Diagnostic value of ultrasound in scaphoid fractures, Injury 22:397-399, 1991.

Clewes J and Swallow J: The development of protocols for trans-vaginal sonography, Radiogr Today 57:19-22, 1991.

Cobby M, Clarke N and Duncan A: Ultrasound of the infant hip, West Engl Med J 106:74-76, 1991.

Cohen SM and Kurtz AB: Biliary sonography, Radiol Clin North Am 29:1171-1198, 1991.

Coy KM, Maurer G and Siegel RJ: Intravascular ultrasound imaging: a current perspective, J AM Coll Cardiol 18:1811-1823, 1991.

Eber J and Villasenor C: Ultrasound: advantages, disadvantages, and controversies, Nurse Pract 2:239-242, 1991.

· Hadlock FP, Harrist RB and Martinez-Poyer J: How accurate is second trimester fetal dating? J Ultrasound Med 10:557-561, 1991.

Haller JO: Sonography of the biliary tract in infants and children, AJR 157:1051-1058, 1991.

Holm HH: Interventional ultrasound, Br J Radiol 64:379-385, 1991.

Lieb WE et al: Color Doppler imaging of the eye and orbit: technique and normal vascular anatomy, Arch Ophthalmol 109:527-531, 1991.

Maresca G and Colagrande C: Diversified application of Doppler US as related to the different US and radiological problems, Rays 16:141-152, 1991.

McNicholas MM, Griffin JF and Cantwell DF: Ultrasound of the pelvis and renal tract combined with a plain film of abdomen in young women with urinary tract infection: can it replace intravenous urography? A prospective study, Br J Radiol 64:221-224, 1991.

Miller DL: Update on safety of diagnostic ultrasonography, JCU 19:531-540, 1991.

Ooms HW et al: Ultrasonography in the diagnosis of acute appendicitis, Br J Surg 78:315-318, 1991.

Pamilo M et al: Ultrasonography of breast lesions detected in mammography screening, Acta Radiol 32:220-225, 1991.

Peters AJ and Coulam CB: Hysterosalpingography with color Doppler ultrasonography, Am J Obstet Gynecol 164:1530-2, 1991.

Rosenfield AT: Artifacts in urinary tract ultrasonography, Urol Radiol 12:228-232, 1991.

Safford RE, Blackshear JL and Kapples EJ: Clinical utility of transesophageal echocardiography, South Med J 84:611-618, 1991.

Schlief R and Deichert U: Hysterosalpingo-contrast sonography of the uterus and fallopian tubes: results of a clinical trial of a new contrast medium in 120 patients, Radiology 178:213-215, 1991.

Schneider K: Sonographic imaging of the thyroid in children, Prog Pediatr Surg 26:1-14, 1991.

Sheikh KH et al: Comparison of intravascular ultrasound, external ultrasound and digital angiography for evaluation of peripheral artery dimensions and morphology, Am J Cardiol 67:817-822, 1991.

Stevens JK and Miller JI: Transrectal ultrasound: an aid to diagnosing prostate cancer, AORN 53:1166-70, 1172-8, 1991.

Stott MA et al: Ultrasound of the common bile duct in patients undergoing cholecystectomy, JCU 19:73-76, 1991.

Suzuki S et al: Ultrasound diagnosis of pathology of the anterior and posterior cruciate ligaments of the knee joint, Arch Orthop Trauma Surg 110:200-203, 1991.

Venezia R and Zangara C: Echohysterosalpingography: new diagnostic possibilities with S HU 450 Echovist, Acta Eur Fertil 22:279-282, 1991.

Yamashita T and Ogawa A: Transperineal ultrasonic voiding cystourethrography using a newly devised chair, J Urol 146:819-823, 1991.

1992 Apuzzio JJ et al: Prenatal ultrasonographic fetal iliac bone measurement: correlation with gestational age, J Reprod Med 37:348-350, 1992.

Archer RJ: Intrathoracic right kidney diagnosed by ultrasound, Australas Radiol 36:271-273, 1992.

Aspelin P et al: Ultrasound examination of soft tissue injury of the lower limb in athletes, Am J Sports Med 20:601-603, 1992.

Bagley DH, Liu JB and Goldberg BB: Use of endoluminal ultrasound of the ureter, Semin Urol 10:194-198, 1992.

Bartram CI: Anal endosonography, Ann Gastroenterol Hepatol 28:185-189, 1992.

Beach KW: 1975-2000: a quarter century of ultrasound technology, Ultrasound Med Biol 18:377-388, 1992.

Bluth EI and Merritt CR: Doppler color imaging: carotid and vertebral arteries, Clin Diagn Ultrasound 27:61-96, 1992.

Brakel K et al: Accuracy of ultrasound and oral cholecystography in assessing the number and size of gallstones: implications for non-surgical therapy, Br J Radiol 65:779-783, 1992.

Buchberger W et al: Carpal tunnel syndrome: diagnosis with high-resolution sonography, AJR 159:793-798, 1992.

Chervenak FA and McCullough LB: Ethical issues in obstetric ultrasonography, Clin Obstet Gynecol 35:758-762, 1992.

Chowdhury V et al: Cranial sonography in preterm infants, Indian Pediatr 29:411-415, 1992.

Cohen HL, Haller JO and Gross BR: Diagnostic sonography of the fetus: a guide to the evaluation of the neonate, Pediatr Ann 21:87, 91-6, 98-9, 1992.

Fernbach SK and Feinstein KA: Selected topics in pediatric ultrasonography—1992, Radiol Clin North Am 30:1011-1031, 1992.

Grant EG et al: Color Doppler imaging of the hepatic vasculature, AJR 159:943-950, 1992.

Harrison LA, Pretorius DH and Budorick NE: Abnormal spinal curvature in the fetus, J Ultrasound Med 11:473-479, 1992.

Kremkau FW: Doppler principles, Semin Roentgenol 27:6-16, 1992.

Lam AH and Firman K: Value of sonography including color Doppler in the diagnosis and management of long standing intussusception, Pediatr Radiol 22:112-114, 1992.

Maffulli N, Hughes T and Fixsen JA: Ultrasonographic monitoring of limb lengthening, J Bone Joint Surg [Br] 74:130-132, 1992.

Maroulis GB, Parsons AK and Yeko TR: Hydrogynecography: a new technique enables vaginal sonography to visualize pelvic adhesions and other pelvic structures, Fertil Steril 58:1073-1075, 1992.

Merritt CR: Doppler color imaging: abdomen, Clin Diagn Ultrasound 27:141-194, 1992.

Merritt CR: Doppler color imaging: intraoperative and cranial applications, Clin Diagn Ultrasound 27:249-271, 1992.

Merritt CR: Doppler color imaging: introduction, Clin Diagn Ultrasound 27:1-6, 1992.

Merritt CR: Evaluation of peripheral venous disease, Clin Diagn Ultrasound 27:113-140, 1992.

Nasri MN: Transvaginal versus transrectal sonography in postmenopausal women, Br J Obstet Gynaecol 99:932-933, 1992.

Olive JR Jr and Marsh HO: Ultrasonography of rotator cuff tears, Clin Orthop 282:110-113, 1992.

Papachrysostomou M et al: Anal endosonography: which endoprobe? Br J Radiol 65:715-717, 1992.

Paushter DM and Borkowski GP: Doppler color imaging: scrotum, breast, thyroid, and extremities, Clin Diagn Ultrasound 27:225-248, 1992.

Pellerito JS and Taylor KJ: Doppler color imaging: peripheral arteries, Clin Diagn Ultrasound 27:97-112, 1992.

Printz H et al: Intraoperative ultrasonography in surgery for chronic pancreatitis, Int J Pancreatol 12:233-237, 1992.

Ranke C et al: Color and conventional image-directed Doppler ultrasonography: accuracy and sources of error in quantitative blood flow measurements, JCU 20:187-193, 1992.

Read JW and Raleigh J: Diagnostic ultrasound, Aust Fam Physician 21:582-587, 1992.

Reading CC: Endorectal sonography, CRC Crit Rev Diagn Imaging 33:1-28, 1992.

Riechelmann H and Mann W: Ultrasonography of paranasal sinus lesions, Rhinology 14(Suppl):136-140, 1992.

Riles TS et al: Comparison of magnetic resonance angiography, conventional angiography, and duplex scanning, Stroke 23:341-346, 1992.

Rioux M: Sonographic detection of the normal and abnormal appendix, AJR 158:773-778, 1992.

Robie BH: Noninvasive diagnosis of cardiovascular disease using ultrasound imaging, J Cardiovasc Nurs 6:36-42, 1992.

Schiller VL and Grant EG: Doppler ultrasonography of the pelvis, Radiol Clin North Am 30:735-742, 1992.

Schlesinger AE and Hernandez RJ: Diseases of the musculoskeletal system in children: imaging with CT, sonography, and MR, AJR 158:729-741, 1992.

Schmidt J, Gassel F and Naughton S: Calculation of three-dimensional deformity in scoliosis by standard roentgenograms, Acta Orthop Belg 58(Suppl 1):60-65, 1992.

Steiner GM and Sprigg A: The value of ultrasound in the assessment of bone, Br J Radiol 65:589-593, 1992.

Taylor KJ et al: Doppler color imaging: obstetric and gynecologic applications, Clin Diagn Ultrasound 27:195-223, 1992.

Thornton KL: Principles of ultrasound, J Reprod Med 37:27-32, 1992.

Tytgat GN and Fockens P: Endoscopic ultrasonography, Scand J Gastroenterol Suppl 192:80-87, 1992.

Wagner JR, Morgan AS and Lane V: Portable ultrasonography in critical care, Am Surg 58:391-394, 1992.

Wirth T, LeQuesne GW and Paterson DC: Ultrasonography in Legg-Calve-Perthes disease, Pediatr Radiol 22:498-504, 1992.

Yasuda K et al: Clinical application of ultrasonic probes in the biliary and pancreatic duct, Endoscopy 24(Suppl 1):370-375, 1992.

Yu CJ et al: Diagnostic and therapeutic use of chest sonography: value in critically ill patients, AJR 159:695-701, 1992.

1993 Balasubramaniam C, Seshardi S and Suresh I: Intraoperative sonography in neurosurgery, Ann Acad Med Singapore 22:513-515, 1993.

Balen FG et al: Three-dimensional reconstruction of ultrasound images of the uterine cavity, Br J Radiol 66:588-591, 1993.

Balen FG et al: Ultrasound contrast hysterosalpingography—evaluation as an outpatient procedure, Br J Radiol 66:592-599, 1993.

Buijs PC et al: Carotid bifurcation imaging: magnetic resonance angiography compared to conventional angiography and Doppler ultrasound, Eur J Vasc Surg 7:245-251, 1993.

Chang TS, Bohm-Velez M and Mendelson EB: Nongynecologic applications of transvaginal sonography, AJR 160:87-93, 1993.

Cronan JJ: Venous thromboembolic disease: the role of US, Radiology 186:619-630, 1993.

Cushing GL et al: Intraluminal ultrasonography during ERCP with high-frequency ultrasound catheters, Gastrointest Endosc 39:432-435, 1993.

Di Mario C et al: Intravascular ultrasound, Ann Chir Gynaecol 82:101-108, 1993.

Evans DH: Techniques for color-flow imaging, Clin Diagn Ultrasound 28:87-107, 1993.

Fan P et al: Comparison of various agents in contrast enhancement of color Doppler flow images: an in vitro study, Ultrasound Med Biol 19:45-57, 1993.

Finet G et al: Artifacts in intravascular ultrasound imaging: analyses and implications, Ultrasound Med Biol 19:533-547, 1993.

Goldberg BB et al: Sonographically guided laparoscopy and mediastinoscopy using miniature catheter-based transducers, J Ultrasound Med 12:49-54, 1993.

Gordon PB, Goldenberg SL and Chan NH: Solid breast lesions: diagnosis with US-guided fine-needle aspiration biopsy, Radiology 189:573-580, 1993.

Hamper UM and Sheth S: Prostate ultrasonography, Semin Roentgenol 28:57-73, 1993.

Harris RA and Wells PN: Ultimate limits in ultrasound image resolution, Clin Diagn Ultrasound 28:109-123, 1993.

Harris RD and Barth RA: Sonography of the gravid uterus and placenta: current concepts, AJR 160:455-465, 1993.

Hughes TH, Maffulli N and Fixsen JA: Ultrasonographic appearance of regenerate bone in limb lengthening, J R Soc Med 86:18-20, 1993.

Hutchinson DT: Color duplex imaging: applications to upper-extremity and microvascular surgery, Hand Clin 9:47-57, 1993.

Jones HW: Recent activity in ultrasonic tomography, Ultrasonics 31:353-360, 1993.

Levine WN and Leslie BM: The use of ultrasonography to detect a radiolucent foreign body in the hand: a case report, J Hand Surg [Am] 18:218-220, 1993.

Longley DG, Finlay DE and Letourneau JG: Sonography of the upper extremity and jugular veins, AJR 160:957-962, 1993.

Montefusco von Kleist CM et al: Comparison of duplex ultrasonography and ascending contrast venography in the diagnosis of venous thrombosis, Angiology 44:169-175, 1993.

Richard WD et al: A method for three-dimensional prostate imaging using transrectal ultrasound, Comput Med Imaging Graph 17:73-79, 1993.

Rittoo D et al: The comparative value of transesophageal and transthoracic echocardiography before and after percutaneous mitral balloon valvotomy: a prospective study, Am Heart J 125:1094-1105, 1993.

Stiegmann GV and McIntyre R: Principles of endoscopic and laparoscopic ultrasound, Surg Endosc 7:360-361, 1993.

Sudakoff GS, Montazemi M and Rifkin MD: The foramen magnum: the underutilized acoustic window to the posterior fossa, J Ultrasound Med 12:205-210, 1993.

Terjesen T, Anda S and Ronningen H: Ultrasound examination for measurement of femoral anteversion in children, Skeletal Radiol 22:33-36, 1993.

van der Heijden FH et al: Value of Duplex scanning in the selection of patients for percutaneous transluminal angioplasty, Eur J Vasc Surg 7:71-76, 1993.

Walter DF et al: Colonic sonography: preliminary observations, Clin Radiol 47:200-204, 1993.

Weill FS, Rohmer P and Parizet C: Work in progress CAVUS: transcaval ultrasonography of abdominal organs. Preliminary results, J Ultrasound Med 12:91-95, 1993.

Wells PN: The present status of ultrasonic imaging in medicine, Ultrasonics 31:345-352, 1993.

Wells PN: Advances in imaging techniques, Clin Diagn Ultrasound 28:47-53, 1993.

1994 Evans JL et al: Arterial imaging with a new forward-viewing intravascular ultrasound catheter. I. Initial studies, Circulation 89:712-717, 1994.

Ng KH et al: Arterial imaging with a new forward-viewing intravascular ultrasound catheter. II. Three-dimensional reconstruction and display of data, Circulation 89:718-723, 1994.

NUCLEAR MEDICINE

For bibliographic citations before 1964, please see the fifth edition of this ATLAS. For citations from 1964 through 1974, see the sixth or seventh edition.

1976 Strauss HW: Cardiovascular nuclear medicine: a new look at an old problem, Radiology 121:257-268, 1976.

1977 Freundlich IM, O'Mara R and Pitt MJ: Thermographic, radionuclide, and radiographic detection of bone metastases, Radiology 122:665-668, 1977.

1978 Groch MW et al: Radionuclide kymography for the assessment of regional myocardial wall motion, J Nucl Med 19:1131-1137, 1978.

1979 Maynard CD: The relationship of nuclear medicine to other diagnostic studies, Semin Nucl Med 9:4-7, 1979.

Nusynowitz ML: Nuclear medicine, JAMA 241:1388-1389, 1979.

1980 Ashare AB: Radiocolloid liver scintigraphy: a choice and an echo, Radiol Clin North Am 18:315-319, 1980.

Kaul A, Henrichs K and Roedler HD: Radionuclide biokinetics and internal dosimetry in nuclear medicine, Ric Clin Lab 10:629-660, 1980.

Nudelman S and Patton DD, eds: Imaging for medicine, nuclear medicine, ultrasonics, and thermography, New York, 1980, Plenum Press.

1981 Batillas J et al: Bone scanning in the detection of occult fractures, J Trauma 21:564-569, 1981.

Beierwaltes WH: New horizons for therapeutic nuclear medicine in 1981, J Nucl Med 22:549-554, 1981.

Ell PJ and Khan O: Emission computerized tomography: clinical applications, Semin Nucl Med 11:50-60, 1981.

Malmud LS and Fisher RS: Scintigraphic evaluation of disorders of the esophagus, stomach, and duodenum, Med Clin North Am 65:1291-1310, 1981.

Oldendorf WH: Nuclear medicine in clinical neurology: an update, Ann Neurol 10:207-213, 1981.

Polak JF and Holman BL: Cardiac nuclear medicine, part I: the methods, Med Instrum 15:174-177, 1981.

Pollet JE et al: Intravenous radionuclide cystography for the detection of vesicorenal reflux, J Urol 125:75-78, 1981.

Sodee DB and Early PJ: Mosby's manual of nuclear medicine, ed 3, St Louis, 1981, Mosby.

1982 Abdel-Dayem HM, Barodawala YK and Papademetriou T: Scintographic arthrography: comparison with contrast arthrography and future applications, Clin Nucl Med 7:516-522, 1982.

Aw SE et al: Nuclear medicine—an overview, Ann Acad Med Singapore 11:464-468, 1982.

Blahd WH and Rose JG: Nuclear medicine in diagnosis and treatment of diseases of the head and neck. II. Head Neck Surg 4:213-226, 1982.

Blaufox MD et al: Applications of nuclear medicine in genitourinary imaging, Urol Radiol 4:155-164, 1982.

Chandra R: Introductory physics of nuclear medicine, Philadelphia, 1982, Lea & Febiger.

Doucet TW, Hurwitz JJ and Chin-Sang H: Lacrimal scintillography: advances and functional applications, Surv Ophthalmol 27:105-113, 1982.

Greer KL, Jaszczak RJ and Coleman RE: An overview of a camera-based SPECT system, Med Phys 9:455-463, 1982.

1983 Adams FG and Shirley AW: Factors influencing bone scan quality, Eur J Nucl Med 8:436-439, 1983.

Berg BC: Complementary roles of radionuclide and computed tomographic imaging in evaluating trauma, Semin Nucl Med 13:86-103, 1983.

Croll MN, Brady LW and Dadparvar S: Implications of lymphoscintigraphy in oncologic practice: principles and differences vis-a-vis other imaging modalities, Semin Nucl Med 13:4-8, 1983.

Goetz WA, Hendee WR and Gilday DL: In vivo diagnostic nuclear medicine: pediatric experience, Clin Nucl Med 8:434-439, 1983.

Lull RJ et al: Radionuclide evaluation of lung trauma, Semin Nucl Med 13:223-237, 1983.

Rudavsky AZ and Moss CM: Radionuclide evaluation of peripheral vascular injuries, Semin Nucl Med 13:142-152, 1983.

Uthoff LB et al: A prospective study comparing nuclear scintigraphy and computerized axial tomography in the initial evaluation of the trauma patient, Ann Surg 198:611-616, 1983.

Wilson R, McKusick K and Strauss HW: Cardiovascular nuclear medicine current applications and the outlook for 1985, Eur Radiol 3:264-267, 1983.

1984 Cowan RJ and Moody DM: Radionuclide techniques for brain imaging, Neurol Clin 2:835-851, 1984.

Fink-Bennett DM and Shapiro EE: The angle of Louis: a potential pitfall ("Louie's hot spot") in bone scan interpretation, Clin Nucl Med 9:352-354, 1984.

Froelich JW and Swanson D: Imaging of inflammatory processes with labeled cells, Semin Nucl Med 14:128-140, 1984.

Gross MD et al: The scintigraphic imaging of endocrine organs, Endocr Rev 5:221-281, 1984.

Kramer EL and Sanger JJ: Radionuclide scanning—new applications in urology, Urology 23:468-477, 1984.

Packer S: Ocular anatomy for nuclear medicine, Semin Nucl Med 14:3-7, 1984.

Pauwels EK and Cleton FJ: Radiolabelled monoclonal antibodies: a new diagnostic tool in nuclear medicine, Radiother Oncol 1:333-338, 1984.

Pozen MW et al: Cardiac nuclear imaging: adoption of an evolving technology, Med Care 22:343-348, 1984.

Sundrehagen E: A new technique for formation of 99mTc-labelled blood leucocytes and platelets, Int J Appl Radiat Isot 35:365-366, 1984.

1985 Beller G: Nuclear cardiology: current indications and clinical usefulness, Curr Prob Cardiol 10:1-76, 1985.

Clarke LP et al: SPECT imaging of [131]I (364 keV): importance of collimation, Nucl Med Commun 6:41-47, 1985.

Dale S et al: Ectomography—a tomographic method for gamma camera imaging, Phys Med Biol 30:1237-1249, 1985.

English RJ, Holman BL and Tu'meh SS: Computed tomography in nuclear medicine, Radiol Technol 56:291-295, 1985.

Garver PR et al: Appearance of breast attenuation artifacts with thallium myocardial SPECT imaging, Clin Nucl Med 10:694-696, 1985.

Heyman S, Katowitz JA and Smoger B: Dacryoscintigraphy in children, Ophthal Surg 16:703-709, 1985.

Lopez-Majano V, Sansi P and Colter R: Nuclear medicine in the diagnosis of cardiac contusion, Eur J Nucl Med 11:290-294, 1985.

Moreno AJ et al: The gallium-67 citrate bone scan, Clin Nucl Med 10(8):594-595, 1985.

Nimmo MKJ, Merrick MV and Millar AM: A comparison of the economics of xenon 127, xenon 133 and krypton 81m for routine ventilation imaging of the lungs, Br J Radiol 58:635-636, 1985.

Seagrave V: Radionuclide imaging, Radiography 51:55-56, 1985.

Taaning E et al: Comparison of 99Tcm lymphoscintigraphy and lymphangiography in patients with malignant lymphomas, Acta Radiol [Diagn] (Stockh) 26:79-83, 1985.

Wackers FJ et al: Quantitative planar thallium-201 stress scintigraphy: a critical evaluation of the method, Semin Nucl Med 15:46-66, 1985.

1986 Britton KE: Searching for the ideal kidney agent, Nucl Med Commun 7:145-147, 1986.

Brunner MC et al: Prosthetic graft infection: limitations of indium white blood cell scanning, J Vasc Surg 3:42-48, 1986.

Carson RE: A maximum likelihood method for region-of-interest evaluation in emission tomography, J Comput Assist Tomogr 10:654-663, 1986.

Coleman RE, Blinder RA and Jaszczak RJ: Single photon emission computed tomography (SPECT). II. Clinical applications, Invest Radiol 21:1-11, 1986.

Fraxedas R, Franquiz JM and Meneses A: Radiation dose to personnel working with single photon emission computed tomography (SPECT), Radiol Diagn 27:615-619, 1986.

Grime JS et al: A method of radionuclide angiography and comparison with contrast aortography in the assessment of aorto-iliac disease, Nucl Med Commun 7:45-52, 1986.

Marmor AT et al: Improved radionuclide method for assessment of pulmonary artery pressure in COPD, Chest 89:64-69, 1986.

Mettler FA Jr et al: Estimation of the genetically significant dose from diagnostic nuclear medicine examinations in the United States: 1980, Health Phys 51:377-379, 1986.

Mueller SP et al: Collimator selection for SPECT brain imaging: the advantage of high resolution, J Nucl Med 27:1729-1738, 1986.

Murata K et al: Ventilation imaging with positron emission tomography and nitrogen 13, Radiology 158:303-307, 1986.

Murphy PH: Guidelines for radiation protection, Semin Nucl Med 16:131-141, 1986.

Nickel O and Hahn K: New nuclear medical technologies for pediatrics, Med Prog Tech 11:65-72, 1986.

Nuclear medicine and the environment. II. Semin Nucl Med 16:157-230, 1986.

Romney BM et al: Radionuclide administration to nursing mothers: mathematically derived guidelines, Radiology 160:549-554, 1986.

Shore RM and Hendee WR: Radiopharmaceutical dosage selection for pediatric nuclear medicine, J Nucl Med 27:287-298, 1986.

St. Germain J: Radiation protection programs in nuclear medicine, Semin Nucl Med 16:198-202, 1986.

St. Germain J: The radioactive patient, Semin Nucl Med 16:179-183, 1986.

Techner LM, Eiser CA and Laine W: Indium-111 imaging in osteomyelitis and neuroarthropathy: review and case report, J Am Podiatr Med Assoc 76:23-29, 1986.

Tsui BM et al: Design and clinical utility of a fan beam collimator for SPECT imaging of the head, J Nucl Med 27:810-819, 1986.

Webb S et al: single photon emission computed tomographic imaging and volume estimation of the thyroid using fan-beam geometry, Br J Radiol 59:951-955, 1986.

Wells RG, Ruskin JA and Sty JR: Lymphoscintigraphy: lower extremity lymphangioma, Clin Nucl Med 11:523, 1986.

Westerman BR: Licensing criteria for nuclear medicine, Semin Nucl Med 16:171-178, 1986.

Williams ED et al: Multiple-section radionuclide tomography of the kidney: a clinical evaluation, Br J Radiol 59:975-983, 1986.

1987 Adam WE: A general comparison of functional imaging in nuclear medicine with other modalities, Semin Nucl Med 17:3-17, 1987.

Collier BD Jr, Hellman RS and Krasnow AZ: bone SPECT, Semin Nucl Med 17:247-266, 1987.

Franken PR et al: Measurement of right ventricular volumes from ECG gated steadystate krypton-81m angiocardiography, Nucl Med Commun 8:365-373, 1987.

Heller SL and Goodwin PN: SPECT instrumentation: performance, lesion detection, and recent innovations, Semin Nucl Med 17:184-199, 1987.

Hutton BF et al: Artefact reduction in dual-radionuclide subtraction studies, Phys Med Biol 32:477-493, 1987.

Iskandrian AS et al: Thallium imaging with single photon emission computed tomography, Am Heart J 114:852-865, 1987.

Keller DC et al: Quantitative radionuclide scanning of the temporomandibular joint: an initial study, Cranio 5:152-156, 1987.

Kereiakes JG: The history and development of medical physics instrumentation: nuclear medicine, Med Phys 14:146-155, 1987.

Kershaw A: Radionuclide imaging. II. Renal studies in nuclear medicine, Radiography 53:244-248, 1987.

Kircos LT, Carey JE Jr and Keyes JW Jr: Quantitative organ visualization using SPECT, J Nucl Med 28:334-341, 1987.

Knesaurek K: Comparison of 360 degrees and 180 degrees data collection in SPECT imaging, Phys Med Biol 32:1445-1456, 1987.

McAfee JG: Radionuclide imaging in metabolic and systemic skeletal diseases, Semin Nucl Med 17:334-349, 1987.

Murphy PH: Acceptance testing and quality control of gamma cameras, including SPECT, J Nucl Med 28:1221-1227, 1987.

Protection of the patient in nuclear medicine, Ann ICRP 17:1-37, 1987.

Schelbert HR: Current status and prospects of new radionuclides and radiopharmaceuticals for cardiovascular nuclear medicine, Semin Nucl Med 17:145-181, 1987.

Shulkin BL et al: Iodine-131 MIBG scintigraphy of the extremities in metastatic pheochromocytoma and neuroblastoma, J Nucl Med 28:315-318, 1987.

Shulkin BL and Wahl RL: SPECT imaging of myocarditis, Clin Nucl Med 12:841-842, 1987.

Spies SM et al: Considerations for tomographic imaging of monoclonal antibodies, Semin Nucl Med 17:267-272, 1987.

van Giessen JW et al: Two devices for longitudinal emission tomography of the thyroid, J Nucl Med 28:1892-1900, 1987.

Van Heertum RL, Brunetti JC and Yudd AP: Abdominal SPECT imaging, Semin Nucl Med 17:230-246, 1987.

Yano Y: Essentials of a rubidium-82 generator for nuclear medicine, Int J Rad Appl Instrum [A] 38:205-211, 1987.

1988 Bellotti C et al: Cerebral scintigraphy with lilindium oxine-labelled leukocytes in the differential diagnosis of intracerebral cystic lesions, Acta Neurochir Suppl 42:221-224, 1988.

Buell U: Positron versus single-photon ECT or PET complementing SPECT: what can be done with PET beyond research? Make PET go bedside, Nuklearmedizin 27:2-4, 1988.

Chen JJ et al: Single photon emission computed tomography of the thyroid, J Clin Endocrinol Metab 66:1240-1246, 1988.

Dendy PP, Barber RW and Bayliss CC: An experimental study of the relationship between image quality and spatial resolution of the gamma camera, Eur J Nucl Med 14:579-585, 1988.

Gainey MA and Capitanio MA: Recent advances in pediatric nuclear medicine, Radiol Clin North Am 26:409-418, 1988.

Halama JR, Henkin RE and Friend LE: Gamma camera radionuclide images: improved contrast with energy-weighted acquisition, Radiology 169:533-538, 1988.

Israel O et al: Normal and abnormal single photon emission computed tomography of the skull: comparison with planar scintigraphy, J Nucl Med 29:1341-1346, 1988.

Jaszczak RJ and Coleman RE: Instrumentation for single-photon-emission computed tomographic studies of the brain, Am J Physiol Imaging 3:67-70, 1988.

Jaszczak RJ, Greer KL and Coleman RE: SPECT using a specially designed cone beam collimator, J Nucl Med 29:1398-1405, 1988.

Karl RD and Hammes CS: Nuclear medicine imaging in podiatric disorders, Clin Podiatr Med Surg 5:909-929, 1988.

Norton MY, Walton S and Evans NT: Gated cardiac tomography Eur J Nucl Med 14:472-276, 1988.

Sfakianakis GN and Sfakianaki ED: Nuclear medicine in pediatric urology and nephrology, J Nucl Med 29:1287-1300, 1988.

Shih WJ et al: Application of I-123 HIPDM as a lung imaging agent, Eur J Nucl Med 14:21-24, 1988.

Sodee DB: Routine single-photon-emission computed tomographic brain imaging, Am J Physiol Imaging 3:41-47, 1988.

Weber DA: Options in camera technology for the bone scan: role of SPECT, Semin Nucl Med 18:78-89, 1988.

Welch MJ: Production of positron-emitting radiopharmaceuticals, Am J Physiol Imaging 3:71, 1988.

Wong DF and Kuhar MJ: In vivo PET and SPECT receptor imaging: new technology and tactics for receptor measurement, Adv Exper Med Biol 236:181-193, 1988.

1989 Chen CC, Hoffer PB and Swett HA: Hypermedia in radiology: computer-assisted education, J Digit Imaging 2:48-55, 1989.

Cho YD, Yum HY and Park YH: Hepatocellular carcinoma with skeletal metastasis: management with intraarterial radioactive iodine, J Belge Radiol 72:267-271, 1989.

Cosgriff PS and Sharp PF: Nuclear medicine software: safety aspects, Nucl Med Commun 10:535-538, 1989.

Deland FH: A perspective of monoclonal antibodies: past, present, and future, Semin Nucl Med 19:158-165, 1989.

DeNardo GL et al: Quantitative SPECT of uptake of monoclonal antibodies, Semin Nucl Med 19:22-32, 1989.

Dymond DS: Technical introduction to nuclear imaging, Br Med Bull 45:838-847, 1989.

Franken PR et al: Clinical usefulness of ultrashort-lived iridium-191m from a carbon-based penetration system for the evaluation of the left ventricular function, J Nucl Med 30:1025-1031, 1989.

Galli G, Salvatori M and Valenza V: Hepatobiliary scintigraphy, Rays 14:57-63, 1989.

Kaplan IL and Swayne LC: Composite SPECT-CT images: technique and potential applications in chest and abdominal imaging, AJR 152:865-866, 1989.

McAfee JG: Update on radiopharmaceuticals for medical imaging, Radiology 171:593-601, 1989.

Ott RJ: Nuclear medicine in the 1990s: a quantitative physiological approach, Br J Radiol 62:421-432, 1989.

Sardi A et al: Localization by hand-held gamma probe of tumor labeled with antibody "cocktail," J Surg Res 47:227-234, 1989.

Segall GM and Davis MJ: Prone versus supine thallium myocardial SPECT: a method to decrease artifactual inferior wall defects, J Nucl Med 30:548-555, 1989.

Sikora K: Imaging with radiolabelled monoclonal antibodies, Clin Radiol 40:32-34, 1989.

Smith ML and Wraight EP: Oblique views in thyroid imaging, Clin Radiol 40:505-507, 1989.

Taylor A Jr and Halkar R: Radionuclide renal studies, Curr Opin Radiol 1:460-467, 1989.

Thrall JH and Swanson DP: Diagnostic interventions in nuclear medicine, Curr Probl Diagn Radiol 18:1-37, 1989.

van der Weiden RM and van Zijl J: Radiation exposure of the ovaries during hysterosalpingography: is radionuclide hysterosalpingography justified? Br J Obstet Gynaecol 96:471-472, 1989.

Wagner HN Jr: Nuclear medicine, JAMA 261:2860-2862, 1989.

Wiener SN, Neumann DR and Rzeszotarski MS: Comparison of magnetic resonance imaging and radionuclide bone imaging of vertebral fractures, Clin Nucl Med 14:666-670, 1989

Wirth V: Effective energy resolution and scatter rejection in nuclear medicine, Phys Med Biol 34:85-90, 1989.

1990 Abdel-Dayem HM and Turoglu HT: Radionuclide renal studies, Curr Opin Radiol 2:834-843, 1990.

Britton KE: Tracers and methods of nuclear medicine, Clin Physiol 10:281-285, 1990.

Collier BD et al: Nuclear medicine techniques, Curr Opin Rheumatol 2:365-368, 1990.

Correia JA: Registration of nuclear medicine images, J Nucl Med 31:1227-1229, 1990.

Dale S and Bone D: Tomography using a rotating slant-hole collimator and a large number of projections, J Nucl Med 31:1675-1681, 1990.

Ell PJ: Single photon emission computed tomography (SPECT) of the brain, J Neurosci Methods 34:207-217, 1990.

Freeman LM: The radionuclide renal scan: past, present and future, Contrib Nephrol 79:87-98, 1990.

Ghosh PR: Current applications of computer in nuclear medicine, J Nucl Med 31:20A-22A, 25A, 1990.

Harding LK et al: The radiation dose to accompanying nurses, relatives and other patients in a nuclear medicine department waiting room, Nucl Med Commun 11:17-22, 1990.

Henze E et al: The orthopan tomoscintigram—a new application of emission computed tomography for facial bone scanning, Eur J Nucl Med 16:97-101, 1990.

Kim EE and Podoloff DA: Radionuclide studies of the liver and hepatobiliary system, Curr Opin Radiol 2:844-850, 1990.

Kramer EL: Lymphoscintigraphy: radiopharmaceutical selection and methods, Int J Rad Appl Instrum [B], 17:57-63, 1990.

Kung HF, Ohmomo Y and Kung MP: Current and future radiopharmaceuticals for brain imaging with single photon emission computed tomography, Semin Nucl Med 20:290-302, 1990.

Lette J et al: Standing views to differentiate gall bladder or bile leak from duodenal activity on cholescintigrams, Clin Nucl Med 15:231-236, 1990.

McAfee JG, Kopecky RT and Frymoyer PA: Nuclear medicine comes of age: its present and future roles in diagnosis, Radiology 174:609-620, 1990.

McGuire EL and Dalrymple GV: Beta and electron dose calculations to skin due to contamination by common nuclear medicine radionuclides, Health Phys 58:399-403, 1990.

Palmer J and Wollmer P: Pinhole emission computed tomography: method and experimental evaluation, Phys Med Biol 35:339-350, 1990.

1991 Adler LP et al: Comparison of PET with CT, MRI, and conventional scintigraphy in a benign and in a malignant soft tissue tumor, Orthopedics 14:891-4, 1991.

Batchelor S et al: Radiation dose to the hands in nuclear medicine, Nucl Med Commun 12:439-444, 1991.

Beierwaltes WH: Endocrine imaging: parathyroid, adrenal cortex and medulla, and other endocrine tumors. II. J Nucl Med 32:1627-1639, 1991.

Clorius JH and Irngartinger G: Renal studies in nuclear medicine, Curr Opin Radiol 3:828-839, 1991.

Coleman RE: Single photon emission computed tomography and positron emission tomography in cancer imaging, Cancer 67:1261-1270, 1991.

Gurgan T et al: Radionuclide hysterosalpingography: a simple and potentially useful method of evaluating tubal patency, J Reprod Med 36:789-792, 1991.

Mountford PJ: Techniques for radioactive decontamination in nuclear medicine, Semin Nucl Med 21:82-89, 1991.

Piepsz A, Gordon I and Hahn K: Paediatric nuclear medicine, Eur J Nucl Med 18:41-66, 1991.

Stabin M and Schlafke-Stelson A: A list of nuclear medicine radionuclides and potential contaminants for operators of in-vivo counters, Health Phys 61:427-430, 1991.

Thrall JH: Nuclear medicine, JAMA 265:3137-3139, 1991.

Urman M et al: The role of bone scintigraphy in the evaluation of talar dome fractures, J Nucl Med 32:2241-2244, 1991.

Verani MS: Adenosine thallium 201 myocardial perfusion scintigraphy, Am Heart J 122:269-278, 1991.

1992 Chisin R et al: Contribution of nuclear medicine to the diagnosis and management of extracranial head and neck diseases (excluding thyroid and parathyroid), Isr J Med Sci 28:254-261, 1992.

Clarke EA et al: Radiation doses from nuclear medicine patients to an imaging technologist: relation to ICRP recommendations for pregnant workers, Nucl Med Commun 13:795-798, 1992.

Ell PJ: Challenges for nuclear medicine in the 1990s, Nucl Med Commun 13:65-75, 1992.

Iannotti F: Functional imaging of blood brain barrier permeability by single photon emission computerised tomography and positron emission tomography, Adv tech Stand Neurosurg 19:103-119, 1992.

Johansson L et al: Effective dose from radiopharmaceuticals, Eur J Nucl Med 19:933-938, 1992.

Lang TF et al: Description of a prototype emission-transmission computed tomography imaging system, J Nucl Med 33:1881-1887, 1992.

Lee JD, Kim SM and Park CH: Tc-99m MIBI uptake in the sternum, Clin Nucl Med 17:819, 1992.

Nuclear Cardiology Today: II International Symposium: Cesena, Italy, May 28-30, 1992, J Nucl Biol Med 36:1-167, 1992.

Paludetti G et al: Functional study of the eustachian tube with sequential scintigraphy, ORL 54:76-79, 1992.

Papachrysostomou M et al: A method of computerised isotope dynamic proctography, Eur J Nucl Med 19:431-435, 1992.

Rosenberg ZS et al: Osgood-Schlatter lesion: fracture or tendinitis? Scintigraphic, CT, and MR imaging features, Radiology 185:853-858, 1992.

Segall GM et al: Functional imaging of peripheral vascular disease: a comparison between exercise whole-body thallium perfusion imaging and contrast arteriography, J Nucl Med 33:1797-1800, 1992.

Starshak RJ and Sty JR: Trends in physiologic and pharmacologic interventions in pediatric nuclear medicine, Pediatr Ann 21:101-109, 1992.

Strauss HW: Controversies in cardiovascular nuclear medicine, J Nucl Biol Med 36:291-295, 1992.

Van Heertum RL et al: Hepatic SPECT imaging in the detection and clinical assessment of hepatocellular disease, Clin Nucl Med 17:948-953, 1992.

Verlooy H et al: Quantitative scintigraphy of the sacroiliac joints, Clin Imaging 16:230-233, 1992.

Yang KT et al: Radionuclide hysterosalpingography with technetium-99m-pertechnetate: application and radiation dose to the ovaries, J Nucl Med 33:282-286, 1992.

1993 Brundin J et al: Developmental steps for radionuclide hysterosalpingography, Gynecol Obstet Invest 36:34-38, 1993.

Cambria RA et al: Noninvasive evaluation of the lymphatic system with lymphoscintigraphy: a prospective, semiquantitative analysis in 386 extremities, J Vasc Surg 18:773-782, 1993.

Cox PH: Criteria for the use of monoclonal antibodies, legislation and ethical considerations, Nucl Med Commun 14:653-657, 1993.

Even Sapir E et al: Role of SPECT in differentiating malignant from benign lesions in the lower thoracic and lumbar vertebrae, Radiology 187:193-198, 1993.

Holder LE, Merine DS and Yang A: Nuclear medicine, contrast angiography, and magnetic resonance imaging for evaluating vascular problems in the hand, Hand Clin 9:85-113, 1993.

Jacobson A and Uszler JM: A simplified technique for radionuclide hysterosalpingography, J Assist Reprod Genet 10:4-10, 1993.

McKusick KA and Quaife MA: Current procedural terminology coding of nuclear medicine procedures, Semin Nucl Med 23:59-66, 1993.

Reba RC: Nuclear medicine, JAMA 270:230-232, 1993.

Rizzo PF et al: Diagnosis of occult fractures about the hip: magnetic resonance imaging compared with bone-scanning, J Bone Joint Surg Am 75:395-401, 1993.

Roman KM: Overdoses of nuclear medicine cause concern for hospitals, physicians, patients—and for the Nuclear Regulatory Commission, J Arkansas Med Soc 90:263-264, 1993.

Rossleigh MA, Leighton DM and Farnsworth RH: Diuresis renography: the need for an additional view after gravity-assisted drainage, Clin Nucl Med 18:210-213, 1993.

Wald A et al: Scintigraphic studies of rectal emptying in patients with constipation and defecatory difficulty, Dig Dis Sci 38:353-358, 1993.

West JH, Seymour JC and Drane WE: Combined transmission-emission imaging in lymphoscintigraphy, Clin Nucl Med 18:762-764, 1993.

POSITRON EMISSION TOMOGRAPHY

1980 Geltman EM, Roberts R and Sobel BE: Cardiac positron tomography: current status and future directions, Herz 5:107-119, 1980.

1981 Bergstrom M et al: Head fixation device for reproducible position alignment in transmission CT and positron emission tomography, J Comput Assist Tomogr 5:136-141, 1981.

Lenzi GL, Jones T and Frackowiak RS: Positron emission tomography: state of the art in neurology, Prog Nucl Med 7:118-137, 1981.

Ter-Pogossian MM et al: Photon time-of-flight-assisted positron emission tomography, J Comput Assist Tomogr 5:227-239, 1981.

1982 Rollo FD: New imaging modalities: positron emission tomography and nuclear magnetic resonance, Med Instrum 16:53-54, 1982.

1983 Bergstrand G et al: Cerebrospinal fluid circulation: evaluation by single-photon and positron emission tomography, AJNR 4:557-559, 1983.

Di-Chiro G et al: Metabolic imaging of the brain stem and spinal cord: studies with positron emission tomography using 18F-2-deoxyglucose in normal and pathological cases, J Comput Assist Tomogr 7:937-945, 1983.

Wong WH et al: Image improvement and design optimization of the time-of-flight PET, J Nucl Med 24:52-60, 1983.

1984 Budinger TF, Derenzo SE and Huesman RH: Instrumentation for positron emission tomography, Ann Neurol 15(Suppl):35-43, 1984.

Ginsberg MD, Howard BE and Hassel WR: Emission tomographic measurement of local cerebral blood flow in humans by an in vivo autoradiographic strategy, Ann Neurol 15(Suppl):12-18, 1984.

Hoffman EJ et al: Prospects for both precision and accuracy in positron emission tomography, Ann Neurol 15(Suppl):25-34, 1984.

Kearfott KJ, Rottenberg DA and Knowles RJ: A new headholder for PET, CT, and NMR imaging, J Comput Assist Tomogr 8:1217-1220, 1984.

Kuhl DE: Imaging local brain function with emission computed tomography, Radiology 150:625-631, 1984.

Lockwood AH: Functional evaluation of the blood-brain barrier using positron emission tomography, Ann Neurol 15(Suppl):103-106, 1984.

1985 Correia JA and Alpert NM: Positron emission tomography in cardiology, Radiol Clin North Am 23:783-793, 1985.

1986 Carson RE: A maximum likelihood method for region-of-interest evaluation in emission tomography, J Comput Assist Tomogr 10:654-663, 1986.

Mazoyer BM et al: Dynamic PET data analysis, J Comput Assist Tomogr 10:645-653, 1986.

Muehllehner G and Karp JS: Positron emission tomography imaging—technical considerations, Semin Nucl Med 16:35-50, 1986.

Ott RJ et al: Three-dimensional positron emission tomography: preliminary results, Br J Radiol 59:419-422, 1986.

1987 Chugani HT: Positron emission tomography: principles and applications in pediatrics, Mead Johnson Symp Perinat Dev Med 15-18, 1987.

Comar D, Crouzel C and Maziere B: Positron emission tomography: standardisation of labelling procedures, Int J Rad Appl Instrum [A], 38:587-596, 1987.

Daube-Witherspoon ME and Muehllehner G: Treatment of axial data in three-dimensional PET, J Nucl Med 28:1717-1724, 1987.

Ell PJ et al: Functional imaging of the brain, Semin Nucl Med 17:214-229, 1987.

Guzzardi R and Licitra G: A critical review of Compton imaging, Crit Rev Biomed Eng 15:237-268, 1987.

Lipton MJ: Computer tomography, positron emission tomography and nuclear magnetic resonance in cardiology, Herz 12:1-12, 1987.

Ott RJ et al: Measurement of radiation dose to the thyroid using positron emission tomography, Br J Radiol 60:245-251, 1987.

1988 ACNP/SNM Task Force on Clinical PET: Positron emission tomography: clinical status in the United States in 1987, J Nucl Med 29:1136-1143, 1988.

Buell U: Positron versus single-photon ECT or PET complementing SPECT: what can be done with PET beyond research? Make PET go bedside, Nuklearmedizin 27:2-4, 1988.

Chen JJ et al: Single photon emission computed tomography of the thyroid, J Clin Endocrinol Metab 66:1240-1246, 1988.

Council on Scientific Affairs: Application of positron emission tomography in the heart: report of the Positron Emission Tomography Panel, JAMA 259:2438-2445, 1988.

Council on Scientific Affairs: Instrumentation in positron emission tomography: report of the Positron Emission Tomography Panel, JAMA 259:1531-1536, 1988.

Council on Scientific Affairs: Positron emission tomography in oncology, JAMA 259:2126-2131, 1988.

Levin DN et al: Retrospective geometric correlation of MR, CT, and PET images, Radiology 169:817-823, 1988.

Spinks TJ, Guzzardi R and Bellina CR: Performance characteristics of a whole-body positron tomograph, J Nucl Med 29:1833-1841, 1988.

Volkow ND, Mullani NA and Bendriem B: Positron emission tomography instrumentation: an overview, Am J Physiol Imaging 3:142-153, 1988.

Webb S, Ott RJ and Flower MA: Three-dimensional shaded-surface images from positron tomography using MUP-PET, Br J Radiol 61:1172-1175, 1988.

Wong DF and Kuhar MJ: In vivo PET and SPECT receptor imaging: new technology and tactics for receptor measurement, Adv Exp Med Biol 236:181-193, 1988.

1989 Brunken RC and Schelbert HR: Positron emission tomography in clinical cardiology, Cardiol Clin 7:607-629, 1989.

Esser PD, Jakimcius A and Foley L: The peanut orbit: a modified elliptical orbit for single photon emission computed tomography imaging, Med Phys 16:114-118, 1989.

Frackowiak RS and Jones T: PET scanning, BMJ 298:693-694, 1989.

Hicks K et al: Automated quantitation of three-dimensional cardiac positron emission tomography for routine clinical use, J Nucl Med 30:1787-1797, 1989. SPET of the brain—patient positioning, Radiogr Today 55:39, 1989.

Mintun MA, Fox PT and Raichle ME: A highly accurate method of localizing regions of neuronal activation in the human brain with positron emission tomography, J Cereb Blood Flow Metab 9:96-103, 1989.

Strauss LG et al: Imaging positron emitting radionuclides generated during radiation therapy, Eur J Radiol 9:200-202, 1989.

Tamaki N et al: Positron emission tomography using fluorine-18 deoxyglucose in evaluation of coronary artery bypass grafting, Am J Cardiol 64:860-865, 1989.

1990 Bench CJ et al: Positron emission tomography in the study of brain metabolism in psychiatric and neuropsychiatric disorders, Br J Psychiatry Suppl 82-95, 1990.

Caputo GR and Higgins CB: Advances in cardiac imaging modalities: fast computed tomography, magnetic resonance imaging, and positron emission tomography, Invest Radiol 25:838-854, 1990.

Defrise M, Townsend D and Geissbuhler A: Implementation of three-dimensional image reconstruction for multi-ring positron tomographs, Phys Med Biol 35:1361-1372, 1990.

Herholz K, Wienhard K and Heiss WD: Validity of PET studies in brain tumors, Cerebrovasc Brain Metab Rev 2:240-265, 1990.

Jones T: Positron emission tomography, Clin Phys Physiol Meas 11(Suppl A):27-36, 1990.

Schelbert HR: Future perspectives: diagnostic possibilities with positron emission tomography, Roentgenblatter 43:384-390, 1990.

Valk PE et al: Clinical evaluation of a high-resolution (2.6-mm) positron emission tomography, Radiology 176:783-790, 1990.

1991 Adler LP et al: Comparison of PET with CT, MRI, and conventional scintigraphy in a benign and in a malignant soft tissue tumor, Orthopedics 14:891-4, 1991.

Alpert NM et al: The precision of positron emission tomography: theory and measurement, J Cereb Blood Flow Metab 11:A26-A30, 1991.

Altman DI and Volpe JJ: Positron emission tomography in newborn infants, Clin Perinatol 18:549-562, 1991.

Bettinardi V et al: Head holder for PET, CT, and MR studies, J Comput Assist Tomogr 15:886-892, 1991.

Budinger TF et al: High resolution positron emission tomography for medical science studies, Acta Radiol Suppl 376:15-23, 1991.

Carson RE: Precision and accuracy considerations of physiological quantitation in PET, J Cereb Blood Flow Metab 11:A45-A50, 1991.

Cherry SR, Dahlbom M and Hoffman EJ: Three-dimensional PET using a conventional multislice tomograph without septa, J Comput Assist Tomogr 15:655-668, 1991.

Chin HW et al: Application of positron emission tomography to neurological oncology, Nebr Med J 76:70-73, 1991.

Coleman RE: Single photon emission computed tomography and positron emission tomography in cancer imaging, Cancer 67:1261-1270, 1991.

Fischman AJ and Strauss HW: Clinical PET—a modest proposal, J Nucl Med 32:2351-2355, 1991.

Gewirtz H: PET scanning in evaluation of ischemic heart disease, R I Med J 74:527-531, 1991.

Gould KL: PET perfusion imaging and nuclear cardiology, J Nucl Med 32:579-606, 1991.

Guzzardi R et al: Methodologies for performance evaluation of positron emission tomographs, J Nucl Biol Med 35:141-157, 1991.

Instrumentation for positron emission tomography, Med Prog Tech 17:131-268, 1991.

Karp JS et al: Performance standards in positron emission tomography, J Nucl Med 32:2342-2350, 1991.

Kubo S et al: Assessment of pancreatic blood flow with positron emission tomography and oxygen-15 water, Ann Nucl Med 5:133-138, 1991.

Maziere B and Maziere M: Positron emission tomography studies of brain receptors, Fundam Clin Pharmacol 5:61-91, 1991.

McGivney WT: Hurdles to technology diffusion: what are expectations for PET? J Nucl Med 32:660-664, 1991.

Mountz JM and Wilson MW: Brain structure localization in positron emission tomography: comparison of magnetic resonance imaging and a stereotactic method, Comput Med Imaging Graph 15:17-22, 1991.

Pisani P et al: User-friendly image processing software tools: general purpose features and application to the correlation of PET-CT brain images, Med Prog Tech 17:205-209, 1991.

Powers WJ et al: Technology assessment revisited: does positron emission tomography have proven clinical efficacy? Neurology 41:1339-1340, 1991.

Schultz SJ, Foley CR and Gordon DG: Preparing your patient for a cardiac P.E.T. scan, Nursing 21:63-64, 1991.

Teras M, Parviainen S and Raunio A: Processing of blood samples in positron emission tomography, Acta Radiol Suppl 376:87-88, 1991.

Watson JD: The current state of positron emission tomography, Br J Hosp Med 46:163-166, 1991.

Welch MJ, Mathias CJ and McGuire A: Positron emission tomography: present status and future prospectives, Acta Radiol Suppl 376:24-30, 1991.

1992   Bailey DL: Three-dimensional acquisition and reconstruction in positron emission tomography, Ann Nucl Med 6:123-130, 1992.

Batchelor S, Blake GM and Saunders JE: A comparison of three commercially available PET imaging systems, Nucl Med Commun 13:20-27, 1992.

Coleman RE, Robbins MS and Siegel BA: The future of positron emission tomography in clinical medicine and the impact of drug regulation, Semin Nucl Med 22:193-201, 1992.

Dahlbom M et al: Whole-body positron emission tomography. I. Methods and performance characteristics, J Nucl Med 33:1191-1199, 1992.

Frick MP et al: Considerations in setting up a positron emission tomography center, Semin Nucl Med 22:182-188, 1992.

Hoffman JM and Coleman RE: Perfusion quantitation using positron emission tomography, Invest Radiol 27(Suppl 2):S22-S26, 1992.

Iannotti F: Functional imaging of blood brain barrier permeability by single photon emission computerised tomography and positron emission tomography, Adv Tech Stand Neurosurg 19:103-119, 1992.

Koeppe RA and Hutchins GD: Instrumentation for positron emission tomography: tomographs and data processing and display systems, Semin Nucl Med 22:162-181, 1992.

Maciunas RJ et al: Positron emission tomography imaging-directed stereotactic neurosurgery, Stereotact Funct Neurosurg 58:134-140, 1992.

Mullani NA and Volkow ND: Positron emission tomography instrumentation: a review and update, Am J Physiol Imaging 7:121-135, 1992.

Ponto LL and Ponto JA: Uses and limitations of positron emission tomography in clinical pharmacokinetics/dynamics. I. Clin Pharmacokinet 22:211-222, 1992.

1993   Adler LP and Bloom AD: Positron emission tomography of thyroid masses, Thyroid 3:195-200, 1993.

Bench CJ et al: Regional cerebral blood flow in depression measured by positron emission tomography: the relationship with clinical dimensions, Psychol Med 23:579-590, 1993.

Corbetta M et al: A PET study of visuospatial attention, J Neurosci 13:1202-1226, 1993.

Neelin P et al: Validation of an MRI/PET landmark registration method using three-dimensional simulated PET images and point simulations, Comput Med Imaging Graph 17:351-356, 1993.

Position statement: clinical use of cardiac positron emission tomography. Position paper of the Cardiovascular Council of the Society of Nuclear Medicine, J Nucl Med 34:1385-1388, 1993.

Rege SD et al: Imaging of pulmonary mass lesions with whole-body positron emission tomography and fluorodeoxyglucose, Cancer 72:82-90, 1993.

Wang GJ et al: Comparison of two PET radioligands for imaging extrastriatal dopamine receptors in the human brain, Synapse 15:246-249, 1993.

1994   Wienhard K et al: The ECAT EXACT HR: performance of a new high resolution positron scanner, J Comput Assist Tomogr 18:110-118, 1994.

RADIATION THERAPY

For bibliographic citations before 1964, please see the fifth edition of this ATLAS. For citations from 1964 through 1974, see the sixth or seventh edition.

1975   Pizzarello DJ and Witcofski RL: Basic radiation biology, Philadelphia, 1975, Lea & Febiger.

1976   Kramer S: Definitive radiation therapy, CA 26:269-273, 1976.

Selman J: The basic physics of radiation therapy, ed 2, Springfield, Ill, 1976, Charles C Thomas, Publisher.

1977   del Regato JA and Spjut MJ: Ackerman and del Regato's cancer: diagnosis, treatment, and prognosis, ed 5, St Louis, 1977, Mosby.

Sachs MC: Introduction to pion radiotherapy, Radiol Technol 49:11-14, 1977.

Walter J: Cancer and radiotherapy, ed 2, Edinburgh, 1977, Churchill Livingstone.

1978   Kogelnik HD and Withers HR: Radiobiological considerations in multifraction irradiation, Radiol Clin 47:362-369, 1978.

Levene MB et al: Computer controlled radiation therapy, Radiology 129:769-775, 1978.

Rubin P et al: Clinical oncology for medical students and physicians, ed 5, Rochester, NY, 1978, American Cancer Society, Inc.

1979   Moore JL et al: Treatment time and sublethal repair in radiotherapy, Br J Radiol 52:978-983, 1979.

Moss WT, Brand WN and Battifora H: Radiation oncology: rationale, technique, results, ed 5, St. Louis, 1979, Mosby.

1980   Cooper JS and Pizzarello DJ: Concepts in cancer care, Philadelphia, 1980, Lea & Febiger.

Essentials and guidelines of an accredited educational program for the radiation therapy technologist, Radiol Technol 51:651-662, 1980.

Smith LL: Cancer patients' evaluations of radiation therapy services, Radiol Technol 51:603-609, 1980.

VanDyk J et al: A technique for the treatment of large irregular fields, Radiology 134:543-544, 1980.

Wang CC: Primer on radiation therapy technology, Boston, 1980, (pamphlet) Department of Radiation Sciences, Massachusetts General Hospital.

1981   Edwards M et al: A computed tomography-radiation therapy treatment planning system utilizing a whole body CT scanner, Med Phys 8:242-248, 1981.

1982   Taylor HF: Intraoperative radiotherapy, Radiol Technol 54:23-25, 1982.

1983 Badcock PC: The role of computed tomography in the planning of radiotherapy fields, Radiology 147:241-244, 1983.

Bova FJ and Hill LW: Surface doses for acrylic versus lead acrylic blocking trays for Co-60, 8-MV, and 17-MV photons, Med Phys 10:254-256, 1983.

Brady LW: The changing role of radiation oncology in cancer management, Cancer 51:2506-2514, 1983.

Goitein M and Abrams M: Multi-dimensional treatment planning. I. Delineation of anatomy, Int J Radiat Oncol Biol Phys 9:777-787, 1983.

1984 Dewit L and van der Schueren E: Radiation treatment planning for the localized prostatic carcinoma: methods and rationale, Strahlentherapie 160:474-484, 1984.

Gerber RL: Quality assurance in radiation therapy: clinical and physical aspects: manpower requirements in training and certification of technologists and dosimetrists, Int J Radiat Oncol Biol Phys 10 (Suppl 1):127-130, 1984.

McLees E, Thompson P and Faulwell M: Radiation therapy technology: profile of a profession, Radiol Technol 55:25-33, 1984.

Pizzarello DJ et al: The carcinogenicity of radiation therapy, Surg Gynecol Obstet 159:189-200, 1984.

Suntharalingam N: Quality assurance in radiation therapy: future plans in physics, Int J Radiat Oncol Biol Phys 10:43-44, 1984.

1985 Hassey KM: Radiation therapy for breast cancer: a historic review, Semin Oncol Nurs 1:181-188, 1985.

Shuman WP et al: The impact of CT CORRELATE ScoutView images on radiation therapy planning, AJR 145:633-638, 1985.

Starkschall G: Analytic evaluation of depths of dose calculation points for external beam radiation therapy treatment planning, Med Phys 12:477-479, 1985.

Vick NA and Wilson CB: Total care of the patient with a brain tumor with consideration of some ethical issues, Neurol Clin 3:705-710, 1985.

1986 Ashayer E et al: Anesthesia in intraoperative radiotherapy patients, J Natl Med Assoc 78:193-199, 1986.

Biggs PJ, Wang CC and Gitterman MM: An afterloading vaginal applicator, Int J Radiat Oncol Biol Phys 12:247-249, 1986.

Brady LW, Markoe AM and Fisher S: Cancer cure with organ preservation using radiation therapy, Radiology 160:1-8, 1986.

Brett CM, Wara WM and Hamilton WK: Anesthesia for infants during radiotherapy: an insufflation technique, Anesthesiology 64:402-405, 1986.

Bulski W and Dade M: Treatment planning software for afterloading brachytherapy, Radiother Oncol 5:59-64, 1986.

Griffiths SE: Reproducibility in radiotherapy, Radiography 52:167-169, 1986.

Lee DJ et al: A new design of microwave interstitial applicators for hyperthermia with improved treatment volume, Int J Radiat Oncol Biol Phys 12:2003-2008, 1986.

Mantell BS, Klevenhagen SC and Afshar F: An afterloaded applicator for the interstitial irradiation of brain tumours, Clin Radiol 37:35-38, 1986.

McEwan AC and Smyth VG: The effect of scattered radiation in ^{60}Co beams on wall correction factors for ionization chambers, Med Phys 13:117-118, 1986.

Reed CE, Marks RD Jr and Crawford FA Jr: Use of brachytherapy in lung cancer, J S C Med Assoc 82:589-591, 1986.

Sause WT: Technical advances in radiation therapy, Urol Clin North Am 13:501-523, 1986.

Scrimger JW and Connors SG: Performance characteristics of a widely used orthovoltage x-ray therapy machine, Med Phys 13:267-269, 1986.

1987 Apuzzo ML et al: Interstitial radiobrachytherapy of malignant cerebral neoplasms: rationale, Methodology, prospects, Neurolog Res 9:91-100, 1987.

Bagne F and Dobelbower RR: Modified mesh panel for radiation therapy treatment table, Radiology 163:579-580, 1987.

Berry RJ: Therapeutic uses of X-rays, Int J Radiat Biol Related Studies Phys Chem Med 51:873-895, 1987.

Blanco S, Lopex-Bote MA and Desco M: Quality assurance in radiation therapy: systematic evaluation of errors during the treatment execution, Radiother Oncol 8:253-256, 1987.

Brahme A: Design principles and clinical possibilities with a new generation of radiation therapy equipment: a review, Acta Oncol 26:403-412, 1987.

Buck BA: Radiation therapy technologists: a profile, Radiol Technol 59:151-158, 1987.

Croft MJ: Film dosimetry for shaped electron fields, Radiol Technol 58:333-337, 1987.

Digel CA, Lastner GMF and Zinreich ES: The use of transmission block in the radiation therapy protal for treatment of the inguinal nodes in late stage pelvic malignancies, Radiol Technol 58:227-231, 1987.

Dyck P, Bouzaglou A and Gruskin P: Stereotactic biopsy and brachytherapy of brain tumours, Neurol Res 9:69-90, 1987.

Engelmeier RL: Patient alignment device for cobalt-60 radiation therapy, J Prosthet Dent 58:620-622, 1987.

Granville-White M: Quality assurance errors in radiotherapy: an overview, Radiography 53:135-139, 1987.

Griffiths SE, Pearcey RG and Thorogood J: Quality control in radiotherapy: the reduction of field placement errors, Int J Radiat Oncol Biol Phys 13:1583-1588, 1987.

Harrison LB and Weissberg JB: a technique for interstitial nasopharyngeal brachytherapy, Int J Radiat Oncol Biol Phys 13:451-453, 1987.

Hilaris BS, Nori D and Anderson LL: New approaches to brachytherapy, Imp Adv Oncol 237-261, 1987.

Jakobsen A et al: A new system for patient fixation in radiotherapy, Radiother Oncol 8:145-151, 1987.

Maddock PG: Brachytherapy sources and applicators, Semin Oncol Nurs 3:15-22, 1987.

McCarthy CP: The role of interstitial implantation in the treatment of primary breast cancer, Semin Oncol Nurs 3:47-53, 1987.

Niroomand-Rad A et al: Performance characteristics of an orthovoltage x-ray therapy machine, Med Phys 14:874-878, 1987.

Niwa K and Fujikawa K: New equipment for a radiation therapy simulator: a device for simplifying irregular field shaping and integrating simulator and therapy machine, Radiat Med 5:27-29, 1987.

Pla C, Evans MD and Podgorsak EB: Dose distributions around selectron applicators, Int J Radiat Oncol Biol Phys 13:1761-1766, 1987.

Poulsen MG and Fitchew RS: A simple device for calculating removal times for brachytherapy sources, Australas Radiol 31:428-430, 1987.

Rosenow UF, Findlay PA and Wright DC: The NCI-atlas of dose distributions for regular 125I brain implants, Radiother Oncol 10:127-139, 1987.

Rothwell BR: Prevention and treatment of the orofacial complications of radiotherapy, J Am Dent Assoc 114:316-322, 1987.

Strohl RA: Head and neck implants, Semin Oncol Nurs 3:30-46, 1987.

Tanaka S et al: Sonographic positioning of endouterine applicator, Radiat Med 5:92-93, 1987.

Trott NG: Radionuclides in brachytherapy: radium and after, Br J Radiol Suppl 21:1-54, 1987.

Uyeda LM: Permanent dots in radiation therapy, Radiol Technol 58:409-411, 1987.

Vojnovic B, Sehmi DS and Newman RG: A simple radiation beam position monitor, Phys Med Biol 32:1179-1185, 1987.

1988 Balducci M et al: Dosage-clinical problems related to a method of patient immobilization by mask during external beam radiotherapy, Rays 13:129-136, 1988.

Barish RJ and Barish SV: A new stereotactic X-ray knife, Int J Radiat Oncol Biol Phys 14:1295-1298, 1988.

Bedford J: Iridium Implants, Radiography 54:100-103, 1988.

Brahme A: Optimal setting of multileaf collimators in stationary beam radiation therapy, Strahlenther Onkol 164:343-350, 1988.

Carabetta RJ: Island custom blocking technique, Med Dosim 13:13-14, 1988.

Conte S et al: Three-field isocentric technique for breast irradiation using individualized shielding blocks, Int J Radiat Oncol Biol Phys 14:1299-1305, 1988.

Cox JD: Time, dose, and fractionation in radiation therapy: an historical perspective, Front Radiat Ther Oncol 22:14-18, 1988.

Glicksman AS and Leith JT: Radiobiological considerations of brachytherapy, Oncology (Williston Park) 2:25-32, 1988.

Hilaris BS and Martini N: The current state of intraoperative interstitial brachytherapy in lung cancer, Int J Radiat Oncol Biol Phys 15:1347-1354, 1988.

Makin WP and Hunter RD: CT scanning in intracavitary therapy: unexpected findings in "straightforward" insertions, Radiother Oncol 13:253-255, 1988.

Maruyama Y: Neutron brachytherapy for the treatment of malignant neoplasia, Int J Radiat Oncol Biol Phys 15:1415-1429, 1988.

Mood DW, Cook CA and Chadwell DK: Increasing patients' knowledge of radiation therapy, Int J Radiat Oncol Biol Phys 15:989-993, 1988.

Rassow J: Quality control of radiation therapy equipment, Radiother Oncol 12:45-55, 1988.

Rozenfeld M: Treatment planning with external beams: introduction and historical overview, Radiographics 8:557, 1988.

Saw CB and Suntharalingam N: Reference dose rates for single- and double-plane 192Ir implants, Med Phys 15:391-396, 1988.

Suit HD et al: Potential for improvement in radiation therapy, Int J Radiat Oncol Biol Phys 14:777-786, 1988.

VanAken ML et al: Incorporation of patient immobilization, tissue compensation and matchline junction technique for three-field breast treatment, Med Dosim 13:131-135, 1988.

Withers HR: Some changes in concepts of dose fractionation over 20 years, Front Radiat Ther Oncol 22:1-13, 1988.

1989 Aird EG: Radiotherapy today and tomorrow—an introduction to optimisation of conformal radiotherapy, Phys Med Biol 34:1345-1348, 1989.

Bomford CK et al: Treatment simulators, Br J Radiol Suppl 23:1-49, 1989.

Brandt BB and Harney J: An overview of interstitial brachytherapy and hyperthermia, Oncol Nurs Forum 16:833-841, 1989.

Brenner DJ: Precision and accuracy in radiotherapy, Radiother Oncol 14:159-167, 1989.

Carter SS, Torp-Pedersen ST and Holm HH: Ultrasound-guided implantation techniques in treatment of prostate cancer, Urol Clin North Am 16:751-762, 1989.

Cho YD, Yum HY and Park YH: Hepatocellular carcinoma with skeletal metastasis: management with intraarterial radioactive iodine, J Belge Radiol 72:267-271, 1989.

Chu JC et al: Patterns of change in the physics and technical support of radiation therapy in the USA 1975-1986, Int J Radiat Oncol Biol Phys 17:437-442, 1989.

Clarke DH et al: The clinical advantages of I-125 seeds as a substitute for Ir-192 seeds in temporary plastic tube implants, Int J Radiat Oncol Biol Phys 17:859-863, 1989.

Daniel TM et al: A new, rapid safe method for local radiation of intrathoracic sites, Am Surg 55:560-562, 1989.

Heifetz MD: Stereotactic radiosurgery for fractionated radiation: a proposal applicable to linear accelerator and proton beam programs, Stereotact Funct Neurosurg 53:167-177, 1989.

Joffe SN et al: Laserthermia. A new method of interstitial local hyperthermia using the contact Nd:YAG laser, Radiol Clin North Am 27:611-620, 1989.

Jones D, Armstrong J and Hafermann MD: A port film marker, Int J Radiat Oncol Biol Phys 17:225-226, 1989.

Kennedy DK et al: Design and dose distribution for rectal applicators for the high dose rate remote afterloading iridium-192 brachytherapy system, Med Dosim 14:209-218, 1989.

Kim TH et al: An afterloading brachytherapy device utilizing thermoplastic material, Radiother Oncol 15:341-344, 1989.

Laughlin JS: Development of the technology of radiation therapy, Radiographics 9:1245-1266, 1989.

Marsh BR: Bronchoscopic brachytherapy, Laryngoscope 99:1-13, 1989.

McCunniff AJ and Liang MJ: Radiation tolerance of the cervical spinal cord, Int J Radiat Oncol Biol Phys 16:675-678, 1989.

McGowan KL: Radiation therapy: saving your patient's skin, RN 52:24-27, 1989.

Mountford PJ and Coakley AJ: Radioactive patients, BMJ 298:1538-1539, 1989.

Ohara K et al: Irradiation synchronized with respiration gate, Int J Radiat Oncol Biol Phys 17:853-857, 1989.

Ostertag CB: Stereotactic interstitial radiotherapy for brain tumors, J Neurosurg Sci 33:83-89, 1989.

Plowman PN, Doughty D and Harnett AN: Paediatric brachytherapy. I. The role of brachytherapy in the multidisciplinary therapy of localized cancers, Br J Radiol 62:218-222, 1989.

Sardi A et al: Localization by hand-held gamma probe of tumor labeled with antibody "cocktail," J Surg Res 47:227-234, 1989.

Shapiro SJ and Perez CA: Management of sequelae of chest irradiation, Mo Med 86:746-750, 1989.

Thomson ES, Afshar F and Plowman PN: Paediatric brachytherapy. II. Brain implantation, Br J Radiol 62:223-229, 1989.

Tiver K: Treatment of CNS tumours with conventional radiotherapy: the importance of dose & volume factors in tumour control & CNS radiation tolerance, Australas Radiol 33:15-22, 1989.

Visser AG: An intercomparison of the accuracy of computer planning systems for brachytherapy, Radiother Oncol 15:245-258, 1989.

1990 Bentel GC: Positioning and immobilization device for patients receiving radiation therapy for carcinoma of the breast, Med Dosim 15:3-6, 1990.

Buscher M: The building of free-form customized immobilizers, Med Dosim 15:17-18, 1990.

Cotter GW: Adjustable field shaping for external-beam radiation therapy, Radiology 174:892-893, 1990.

Croft MJ: Stereotactic radiosurgery of arteriovenous malformations, Radiol Technol 61:375-379, 1990.

del Regato JA: Fractionation: a panoramic view, Int J Radiat Oncol Biol Phys 19:1329-1331, 1990.

Edwards EK Jr and Edwards EK: Grenz ray therapy, Int J Dermatol 29:17-18, 1990.

Griffiths S: Radiotherapy quality control—portal and verification films, Radiogr Today 56:17, 1990.

Lowdermilk DL: Nursing care update: internal radiation therapy, NAACOGS Clin Issu Perinat Womens Health Nurs 1:532-540, 1990.

Merkle K, Lessel A and Huttner J: Quality assurance in radiotherapy—a clinical view-point, Radiobiologia, Radiotherapia 31:19-23, 1990.

Morrison R: Interrelationship of the mind, body and emotions in the cancer fight, Radiol Technol 62:28-31, 1990.

Munro P, Rawlinson JA and Fenster A: Therapy imaging: a signal-to-noise analysis of a fluoroscopic imaging system for radiotherapy localization, Med Phys 17:763-772, 1990.

Ortin TT, Shostak CA and Donaldson SS: Gonadal status and reproductive function following treatment for Hodgkin's disease in childhood: the Stanford experience, Int J Radiat Oncol Biol Phys 19:873-880, 1990.

Schlom J et al: Innovations that influence the pharmacology of monoclonal antibody guided tumor targeting, Cancer Res 50:820-827, 1990.

Shanahan TG et al: Minimization of small bowel volume within treatment fields utilizing customized "belly boards," Int J Radiat Oncol Biol Phys 19:469-476, 1990.

Silber JH, Littman PS and Meadows AT: Stature loss following skeletal irradiation for childhood cancer, J Clin Oncol 8:304-312, 1990.

Smithson P: Radiotherapy QA—a systematic approach, Radiogr Today 56:12-13, 1990.

Swann-D'Emilia B, Chu JC and Daywalt J: Misadministration of prescribed radiation dose, Med Dosim 15:185-191, 1990.

Walls C: Portal films and their use in quality assurance—cranial irradiation, Radiogr Today 56:15-18, 1990.

Webb S: Non-standard CT scanners: their role in radiotherapy, Int J Radiat Oncol Biol Phys 19:1589-1607, 1990.

1991 Bertelrud K et al: Bellyboard device reduces small bowel displacement, Radiol Technol 6:284-287, 1991.

Biggs PJ: Analysis of field and custom block sizes used in radiation therapy—implications for multileaf collimator design, Med Dosim 16:169-172, 1991.

Chin HW et al: Application of positron emission tomography to neurological oncology, Nebr Med J 76:70-73, 1991.

del Regato JA: Milestones in therapeutic radiology, Front Radiat Ther Oncol 25:4-9, 1991.

Frith B: Giving information to radiotherapy patients, Nurs Stand 5:33-35, 1991.

Hellmann K and Rhomberg W: Radiotherapeutic enhancement by razoxane, Cancer Treat Rev 18:225-240, 1991.

Jaeger SS, Chin HW and Frank AR: Standardization of dosimetry chart checks, Med Dosim 16:143-146, 1991.

Jones LW: Port film dosage in radiation therapy, Radiol Technol 62:362-368, 1991.

Kun LE: Radiation therapy: trends in treatment, Neurologic Clinics 9:337-350, 1991.

Leach VE: Elbow and knee pads provide comfort to patients, Oncol Nurs Forum 18:785, 1991.

Lilley P: The educational needs of radiotherapy patients, Radiogr Today 57:13-14, 1991.

Sullivan DM: Quality assurance in radiation therapy, Oncol Nurs Forum 18:787, 1991.

Tatsuzaki H and Urie MM: Importance of precise positioning for proton beam therapy in the base of skull and cervical spine, Int J Radiat Oncol Biol Phys 21:757-765, 1991.

Vijayakumar S et al: Estimation of doses to heart, coronary arteries, and spinal cord in mediastinal irradiation for Hodgkin's disease, Med Dosim 16:237-241, 1991.

Yankelevitz DF et al: Effect of radiation therapy on thoracic and lumbar bone marrow: evaluation with MR imaging, AJR 157:87-92, 1991.

1992 Barlow A: Radiolabeled antibodies in cancer treatment, Radiol Technol 63:324-329, 1992.

Boyer AL et al: A review of electronic portal imaging devices (EPIDs), Med Phys 19:1-16, 1992.

Boyer AL et al: Clinical dosimetry for implementation of a multileaf collimator, Med Phys 19:1255-1261, 1992.

Bucholtz JD: Issues concerning the sedation of children for radiation therapy, Oncol Nurs Forum 19:649-655, 1992.

Fallone BG, Evans MDC and Parmar D: Technique to improve lateral cervicothoracic radiographs, Radiol Technol 64:104-107, 1992.

Fiorino C et al: Skin dose measurements for head and neck radiotherapy, Med Phys 19:1263-1266, 1992.

Horiuchi K and Miyamoto T: Radioreductive effect of bestatin (Ubenimex) in BALB/c mice, Int J Radiat Biol 62:73-80, 1992.

Judnick JW et al: Radiotherapy technique integrates MRI into CT, Radiol Technol 64:82-89, 1992.

Kaanders JH et al: Devices valuable in head and neck radiotherapy, Int J Radiat Oncol Biol Phys 23:639-645, 1992.

Kihlen B: Regular processor control improves portal film quality, Radiol Technol 63:244-247, 1992.

Lagendik JJ and Hofman P: A standardized multifield irradiation technique for breast tumours using asymmetrical collimators and beam angulation, Br J Radiol 65:56-62, 1992.

Loeffler JS and Larson DA: Subspecialization in radiation oncology: impact of stereotactic radiosurgery, Int J Radiat Oncol Biol Phys 24:885-887, 1992.

Meli JA and Vatali PE: A simple eye-lens shielding technique compatible with independent jaws of a linear accelerator, Med Dosim 17:221-223, 1992.

Mijnheer BJ: Quality assurance in radiotherapy: physical and technical aspects, Qual Assur Health Care 4:9-18, 1992.

Mughnaw SB: An overview of methods in stereotactic radiosurgery, Radiol Technol 63:402-405, 1992.

Muller-Schimpfle M et al: MRI and MRA in treatment planning of subdiaphragmatic radiation therapy, J Comput Assist Tomogr 16:110-119, 1992.

Schot LJ et al: Late effects of radiotherapy on hearing, Eur Arch Otorhinolaryngol 249:305-308, 1992.

1993 Baughan CA et al: A randomized trial to assess the efficacy of 5-aminosalicylic acid for the prevention of radiation enteritis, Clin Oncol R Coll Radiol 5:19-24, 1993.

Hazuka MB et al: Prostatic thermoluminescent dosimeter analysis in a patient treated with 18 MV X rays through a prosthetic hip, Int J Radiat Oncol Biol Phys 25:339-343, 1993.

Herbert SH et al: Volumetric analysis of small bowel displacement from radiation portals with the use of a pelvic tissue expander, Int J Radiat Oncol Biol Phys 25:885-893, 1993.

Hindley A and Cole H: Use of peritoneal insufflation to displace the small bowel during pelvic and abdominal radiotherapy in carcinoma of the cervix, Br J Radiol 66:67-73, 1993.

Kao GD, Whittington R and Coia L: Anatomy of the celiac axis and superior mesenteric artery and its significance in radiation therapy, Int J Radiat Oncol Biol Phys 25:131-134, 1993.

Kostich MV: An arms-up positioning device for treatment of malignancies of the intrathoracic region, Med Dosim 18:81-84, 1993.

Mackie TR et al: Tomotherapy: a new concept for the delivery of dynamic conformal radiotherapy, Med Phys 20:1709-1719, 1993.

Mattsson O: Optical radiation-field indication in X-ray tubes with more than one focus, Acta Radiol 34:197-199, 1993.

1994 Schain WS et al: Mastectomy versus conservative surgery and radiation therapy: psychosocial consequences, Cancer 73:1221-1228, 1994.

STEREOTACTIC SURGERY

For bibliographic citations before 1964, please see the fifth edition of this ATLAS. For citations from 1964 through 1974, see the sixth or seventh edition.

1975 Yoshida T et al: Stereotactic operations with the help of a skull x-ray apparatus, Confin Neurol 37:291-295, 1975.

1979 Brown RA: A computerized tomography—computer graphics approach to stereotaxic localization, J Neurosurg 50:715-720, 1979.

1980 Bergstrom M, Greitz T and Steiner L: An approach to stereotaxic radiography, Acta Neurochir 54:157-165, 1980.

Boethius J et al: CT localization of stereotactic surgery, Appl Neurophysiol 43:164-169, 1980.

Perry JH et al: Computed tomography/guided stereotactic surgery: conception and development of a new stereotactic methodology, Neurosurgery 7:376-381, 1980.

1981 Colombo F et al: A new method for utilizing CT data in stereotactic surgery: measurement and transformation technique, Acta Neurochir 57:195-203, 1981.

1982 Lunsford LD, Rosenbaum AE and Perry J: Stereotactic surgery using the "therapeutic" CT scanner, Surg Neurol 18:116-122, 1982.

Rhodes ML et al: Stereotactic neurosurgery using 3-D image data from computed tomography, J Med Syst 6:105-119, 1982.

1983 Gildenberg PL: Stereotactic neurosurgery and computerized tomographic scanning, Appl Neurophysiol 46:170-179, 1983.

Giorgi C et al: Neuroanatomical digital image processing in CT-guided stereotactic operations, Appl Neurophysiol 46:236-239, 1983.

Hardy TL, Koch J and Lassiter A: Computer graphics with computerized tomography for functional neurosurgery, Appl Neurophysiol 46:217-226, 1983.

Levy WJ: Simple plastic stereotactic unit for use in the computed tomographic scanner, Neurosurgery 13:182-185, 1983.

Lunsford LD, Leksell L and Jernberg B: Probe holder for stereotactic surgery in the CT scanner: a technical note, Acta Neurochir 69:297-304, 1983.

Olivier A and Bertrand G: A new head clamp for stereotactic and intracranial procedures, Appl Neurophysiol 46:272-275, 1983.

1984 Alker G and Kelly PJ: An overview of CT based stereotactic systems for the localization of intracranial lesions, Comput Radiol 8:193-196, 1984.

Lunsford LD and Martinez AJ: Stereotactic exploration of the brain in the era of computed tomography, Surg Neurol 22:222-230, 1984.

1985   Fox PT, Perlmutter JS and Raichle ME: A stereotactic method of anatomical localization for positron emission tomography, J Comput Assist Tomogr 9(1):141-153, 1985.

Iseki H et al: A new apparatus for CT-guided stereotactic surgery, Appl Neurophysiol 48(1-6):50-60, 1985.

1986   Bergstrom M, Greitz T and Ribbe T: A method of stereotaxic localization adopted for conventional and digital radiography, Neuroradiology 28:100-104, 1986.

Engle DJ, Lunsford LD and Panichelli T: Rigid head fixation for intraoperative computed tomography, Neurosurgery 19:258-262, 1986.

Lunsford LD, Martinez AJ and Latchaw RE: Stereotaxic surgery with a magnetic resonance and computerized tomography compatible system, J Neurosurg 64:872-878, 1986.

Patil AA and Woosley RE: Scalp marking of intracranial lesions using computed tomography (CT) images: a technical note, Acta Neurochir 80:62-64, 1986.

Peters TM et al: Integrated stereotaxic imaging with CT, MR imaging, and digital subtraction angiography, Radiology 161:821-826, 1986.

1987   Banks G, Vries JK and McLinden S: Radiologic automated diagnosis (RAD), Comput Methods Programs Biomed 25:157-167, 1987.

Bergstrom M, Greitz T and Ribbe T: An adaptor to the Leksell stereotaxic instrument for digital coordinate determination in radiography, Neuroradiology 29:585-587, 1987.

Giorgi C et al: Three-dimensional reconstruction of cerebral angiography in stereotactic neurosurgery, Acta Neurochir Suppl 39:13-14, 1987.

Kall BA: The impact of computer and imaging technology on stereotactic surgery, Appl Neurophysiol 50:9-22, 1987.

McKean JD et al: CT guided functional stereotaxic surgery, Acta Neurochir 87:8-13, 1987.

Mechanic A and Markowitz R: CT-guided stereotaxic biopsy of brain tumors: new technology for an old problem, Am J Clin Oncol 10:285-288, 1987.

Peters TM et al: Stereotactic surgical planning with magnetic resonance imaging, digital subtraction angiography and computed tomography, Appl Neurophysiol 50:33-38, 1987.

Watanabe E et al: Three dimensional digitizer (neuronavigator): new equipment for computed tomography—guided stereotaxic surgery, Surg Neurol 27:543-547, 1987.

1988   Chuang KS, Liou NH and Liu JC: New stereotactic technique for percutaneous thermocoagulation upper thoracic ganglionectomy in cases of palmar hyperhidrosis, Neurosurgery 22:600-604, 1988.

Griffin BR et al: Stereotactic neutron radiosurgery for arteriovenous malformations of the brain, Med Dosim 13:179-182, 1988.

Jenny AB et al: The computer and stereotactic surgery in neurological surgery, Comput Med Imaging Graph 12:75-83, 1988.

Lufkin R et al: MR body stereotaxis: an aid for MR-guided biopsies, J Comput Assist Tomogr 12:1088-1089, 1988.

Moringlane JR, Lippitz B and Ostertag CB: Cerebral angiography under stereotactic conditions: technical note, Acta Neurochir 91:147-150, 1988.

Redmond MJ, Saines NS and Coroneos M: The use of computed tomographic directed stereotaxis in the diagnosis of intracerebral lesions, Med J Aust 149:468-472, 1988.

Rossitch E Jr et al: The use of computed tomography guided stereotactic techniques in the treatment of brainstem abscesses, Clin Neurol Neurosurg 90:365-368, 1988.

1989   Gower DJ: Image guided stereotaxic surgery, J Okla State Med Assoc 82:265-268, 1989.

Hardy TL: A method for MRI and CT mapping of diencephalic somatotopography, Stereotact Funct Neurosurg 52:242-249, 1989.

Heifetz MD et al: Rapid method for determination of isocenter of radiation gantry and alignment of laser beams for stereotactic radiosurgery, Stereotact Funct Neurosurg 53:46-48, 1989.

Kanpolat Y et al: CT-guided percutaneous cordotomy, Acta Neurochir Suppl 46:67-68, 1989.

Loeffler JS et al: Stereotactic radiosurgery for intracranial arteriovenous malformations using a standard linear accelerator, Int J Radiat Oncol Biol Phys 17:673-677, 1989.

Phillips MH et al: Heavy charged-particle stereotactic radiosurgery: cerebral angiography and CT in the treatment of intracranial vascular malformation, Int J Radiat Oncol Biol Phys 17:419-426, 1989.

Podgorsak EB et al: Radiosurgery with high energy photon beams: a comparison among techniques, Int J Radiat Oncol Biol Phys 16:857-865, 1989.

Reinhardt HF and Landolt H: CT-guided "real time" stereotaxy, Acta Neurochir 46:107-108, 1989.

1990   Hariz MI and Bergenheim AT: A comparative study on ventriculographic and computerized tomography-guided determinations of brain targets in functional stereotaxis, J Neurosurg 73:565-571, 1990.

Lofgren M, Andersson I and Lindholm K: Stereotactic, x-ray guided, fine needle aspiration biopsy of nonpalpable breast lesions: comparison with the coordinate grid localization technique, Recent Results Cancer Res 119:100-104, 1990.

Menhinick S: Computed tomography aided, stereotactic localisation of intracranial lesions, Radiogr Today 55:13-15, 1990.

Peters TM et al: Integration of stereoscopic DSA with three-dimensional image reconstruction for stereotactic planning, Stereotact Funct Neurosurg 55:471-476, 1990.

van Velthoven V and Auer LM: Practical application of intraoperative ultrasound imaging, Acta Neurochir 105:5-13, 1990.

1991   Giunta F and Gilardoni C: Digital x-ray apparatus especially designed for precise biometry in stereotactic surgical procedures, Acta Neurochir 52:61-63, 1991.

Goncalves-Ferreira A: Stereotactic anatomy of the posterior cranial fossa: a study of the transcerebellar approach to the brainstem, Acta Neurochir 113:149-165, 1991.

Henri CJ, Collins DL and Peters TM: Multimodality image integration for stereotactic surgical planning, Med Phys 18:167-177, 1991.

Mountz JM and Wilson MW: Brain structure localization in positron emission tomography: comparison of magnetic resonance imaging and a stereotactic method, Comput Med imaging Graph 15:17-22, 1991.

Spiegelmann R and Friedman WA: Rapid determination of thalamic CT-stereotactic coordinates: a method, Acta Neurochir 110:77-81, 1991.

Tal H and Moses O: A comparison of panoramic radiography with computed tomography in the planning of implant surgery, Dentomaxillofac Radiol 20:40-42, 1991.

1992   Barnett GH, Kormos DW and Steiner CP: Stereotactic magnetic resonance angiography, Stereotact Funct Neurosurg 58:118-120, 1992.

Black KL, Mazziotta JC and Toga AW: Imaging and functional localization for brain tumors, Clin Neurosurg 39:475-481, 1992.

Ehricke HH et al: Use of MR angiography for stereotactic planning, J Comput Assist Tomogr 16:35-40, 1992.

Guo WY et al: Stereotaxic angiography in gamma knife radiosurgery of intracranial arteriovenous malformations, AJNR 13: 1107-1114, 1992.

Jolesz FA and Shtern F: The operating room of the future: report of the national Cancer Institute Workshop, "Imaging-guided stereotactic tumor diagnosis and treatment," Invest Radiol 27:326-328, 1992.

Kondziolka D et al: A comparison between magnetic resonance imaging and computed tomography for stereotactic coordinate determination, Neurosurgery 30:402-406, 1992.

Loeffler JS and Larson DA: Subspecialization in radiation oncology: impact of stereotactic radiosurgery, Int J Radiat Oncol Biol Phys 24:885-887, 1992.

Maciunas RJ et al: Positron emission tomography imaging-directed stereotactic neurosurgery, Stereotact Funct Neurosurg 58:134-140, 1992.

Mughnaw SB: An overview of methods in stereotactic radiosurgery, Radiol Technol 63:402-405, 1992.

Patil A et al: The value of intraoperative scans during CT-guided stereotactic procedures, Neuroradiology 34:453-456, 1992.

Tian ZM et al: CT -guided stereotactic injection of radionuclide for treatment of brain tumors, Stereotact Funct Neurosurg 59: 169-173, 1992.

1993 Black PM et al: Sterotactic techniques in managing pediatric brain tumors, Childs Nerv Syst 9:343-346, 1993.

Coste E et al: Frameless method of stereotaxic localization with DSA, Radiology 189:829-834, 1993.

De la Porte C: Technical possibilities and limitations of stereotaxy, Acta Neurochir 124:3-6, 1993.

Gildenberg PL: Stereotactic versus stereotaxic, Neurosurgery 32:965-966, 1993.

Hussman K et al: MR mammographic localization. Work in progress, Radiology 189:915-917, 1993.

Jones AP: Diagnostic imaging as a measureing device for stereotactic neurosurgery, Physiol Meas 14:91-112, 1993.

Koutrouvelis PG et al: A three-dimensional stereotactic device for computed tomography-guided invasive diagnostic and therapeutic procedures, Invest Radiol 28:845-847, 1993.

Koutrouvelis PG et al: Stereotactic percutaneous lumbar discectomy, Neurosurgery 32:582-586, 1993.

Prasad SC et al: A simple approach to the technical aspects of radiosurgery treatments, Med Dosim 18:113-117, 1993.

Thomas DG and Kitchen ND: Stereotactic techniques for brain biopsies, Arch Dis Child 69:621-622, 1993.

INDEX

Index

Index

Index

Index

Research applications of ionizing radiation, **1:**22-23
Resistive magnet
 defined, **3:**203
 in magnetic resonance imaging, **3:**185
Resnick method for lungs, **1:**467
Resolution, **3:**247
 in computed tomography, **3:**130, **3:**143, **3:**144
 defined, **3:**207, **3:**320
 focal spot size and, **3:**316
 positron emission tomography and, **3:**277, **3:**290
 spatial, **3:**130, **3:**143
  defined, **3:**152
Resonance, **3:**183
 defined, **3:**203
Resonant frequency, **3:**210, **3:**247
Respirations; *see also* Breathing
 gravid patient and, **2:**204
Respiratory excursion, **1:**404
Respiratory system, **1:**436-439; *see also* Lung
 nuclear medicine and, **3:**267
Response time, defined, **3:**126
Rete testis, **2:**197
Retention catheters, **2:**122
Retention tips, rectal, **2:**122
Retina, **2:**288
Retinoblastoma, **3:**300
Retrieval, defined, **3:**152
Retrograde cystography, **2:**157, **2:**183
 contrast injection method for, **2:**183
 contrast media for, **2:**182
Retrograde urography, **2:**158, **2:**179-182
 contrast media for, **2:**160-161
Retroperitoneum, ultrasound of, **3:**227-231
Reverberation, **3:**247
Reverberation artifact, **3:**212
Reverse Caldwell position for skull tomography, **3:**68
Reverse Waters method for facial bones, **2:**308, **2:**309
Rhese method
 for ethmoidal, frontal, and sphenoidal sinuses, **2:**392, **2:**393
 for optic foramen, **2:**272-275
Rheumatoid arthritis, thermography in, **3:**82
RIA; *see* Radioimmunoassay
Rib, **1:**420-431
 anatomy of, **1:**402
 axillary portion of, **1:**428-429
 false, **1:**403
 floating, **1:**403
 posterior, **1:**426-427
 projection for
  AP, **1:**426-427
  AP oblique, **1:**428-429
  PA, **1:**424-425
  PA oblique, **1:**430-431
  in RAO or LAO positions, **1:**460-461
  in RPO or LPO positions, **1:**428-429
 respiration in radiography of, **1:**422, **1:**423
 true, **1:**403
 upper anterior, **1:**424-425
Rib tubercle articular facet; *see* Costal facet
Richards method for localization of eye foreign body, **2:**293
Right anterior oblique position, **1:**53
Right colic flexure, **2:**61; *see also* Intestine, large
Right lateral decubitus position, **1:**55

Right posterior oblique position, **1:**54
Rigler method for pneumothorax, **1:**476
Rima glottidis, **2:**14; *see also* Neck
Rima vestibuli, **2:**14
Ring biliary drainage catheter, **2:**568
Risk versus benefit
 defined, **2:**492
 in mammography, **2:**458-459
RMI; *see* Radiation Measurements Incorporated
Road mapping in digital subtraction angiography, **3:**177
Robinson, Meares, and Goree method for sphenoidal sinus effusion, **2:**240
Roentgen, **1:**24
 defined, **3:**304
ROI; *see* Region of interest
Rolleston and Reay technique for hydronephrosis, **2:**174
ROM; *see* Read only memory
Roseno and Jepkins introduction of intravenous pyelography, **2:**160
Rotation, **1:**57
Rotational tomography, **2:**368-369
Rotator cuff, sectional anatomy of, **2:**602
Round window; *see* Fenestra cochlea
Rowntree first use of contrast media in urinary tract, **2:**160
Rubin, Gray, and Green method for shoulder, **1:**142, **1:**143
Rugae; *see* Gastric folds
Runström method for otitis media, **2:**406

S
Saccule; *see* Sacculus
Sacculus, **2:**229; *see also* Ear
Sacral cornu; *see* Sacral horns
Sacral horns, **1:**323; *see also* Sacrum and coccyx
Sacral promontory, **1:**275
Sacral vertebral canal
 axial projection for, **1:**390-391
 Nölke method for, **1:**390-391
Sacroiliac joint, **1:**274, **1:**323, **1:**378-383
 Brower and Kransdorf method for, **1:**378-379
 Chamberlain method for, **1:**384-385
 Meese method for, **1:**378-379
 Nölke method for, **1:**390-391
 projection for
  AP axial, **1:**378-379
  AP oblique, **1:**380-381
  axial, **1:**390-391
  PA oblique, **1:**382-383
  in RAO or LAO positions, **1:**382-383
  in RPO or LPO positions, **1:**380-381
 sectional anatomy of, **2:**614
Sacroiliac motion, Chamberlain method for, **1:**384-385
Sacrum, sectional anatomy of, **2:**618
Sacrum and coccyx, **1:**275, **1:**386-389
 anatomy of, **1:**312, **1:**322-323
 female, **1:**322
 male, **1:**322
 projection for
  AP and PA axial, **1:**386-387
  lateral, **1:**388-389
Saddle joint, **1:**47
Sagittal image plane, **3:**213
 of neonatal skull, **3:**238
Sagittal sinuses, sectional anatomy of, **2:**599
Sagittal suture, **2:**216

Salivary glands, **2:**1-10
 anatomy of, **2:**3
 calculi of, **2:**4
 diverticulae of, **2:**4
 fistulae of, **2:**4
 function of, nuclear medicine studies of, **3:**268
 Iglauer method for, **2:**8
 parotid, **2:**5-9
 sectional anatomy of, **2:**596, **2:**599, **2:**600
 sialography and, **2:**4
 strictures of, **2:**4
 sublingual, **2:**10
 submandibular, **2:**8-9
Salter-Harris fracture, **3:**33
Sampling in positron emission tomography, **3:**286
Sandbags in pediatric immobilization, **3:**14
Sansregret modification of Chaussé method for temporal bone, **2:**418-419
Santorini's duct, **2:**35
Scan
 defined, **3:**152, **3:**247
 myocardial perfusion, **3:**258
Scan converter, **3:**211, **3:**247
Scan diameters, **3:**144
 defined, **3:**152
Scanner
 components of, **3:**135-139
 generations of, **3:**131-132
 positron emission, **3:**284-285; *see also* Positron emission tomography
 rectilinear, **3:**255, **3:**273
Scanning
 dynamic, in computed tomography, **3:**145, **3:**152
 whole-body, **3:**284, **3:**288
Scaphoid, **1:**180, **1:**181; *see also* Wrist
 anatomy of, **1:**60
 PA axial projection for, **1:**91-92
 Stecher method for, **1:**91-92
Scapula, **1:**164-173
 anatomy of, **1:**122-123
 Lilienfeld method of, **1:**168-169
 Lorenz and Lilienfeld methods for, **1:**168-169
 Marzujian method for, **1:**166, **1:**167
 McLaughlin method for, **1:**166
 projection for
  AP, **1:**164, **1:**165
  AP axial, **1:**172, **1:**173
  AP oblique, **1:**170, **1:**171
  lateral, **1:**166, **1:**167
  PA oblique, **1:**166-169
Scapular notch, **1:**123; *see also* Scapula
Scapular spine, **1:**174-177
 Laquerrière-Pierquin method for, **1:**174-175
Scapular Y projection, **1:**142, **1:**143
Scapulohumeral articulation, **1:**125; *see also* Shoulder
Scatter, **3:**247
 defined, **3:**304
 of ultrasound wave, **3:**209
Scatter radiation, **1:**24
Schencker infusion nephrotomography and nephrourography, **2:**175
Schilling's test, nuclear medicine and, **3:**269
School-age child
 approach to, **3:**6
 limb radiography in, **3:**31
 upright chest radiography of, **3:**16, **3:**17
Schüller method
 for cranial base, **2:**253-254, **2:**255